D1611861

PLUM AND POSNER'S DIAGNOSIS OF STUPOR AND COMA

Fourth Edition

SERIES EDITOR

Sid Gilman, MD, FRCP
William J. Herdman Distinguished University Professor of Neurology
University of Michigan

Contemporary Neurology Series

PLUM AND POSNER'S DIAGNOSIS OF STUPOR AND COMA

Fourth Edition

Jerome B. Posner, MD
George C. Cotzias Chair of Neuro-oncology
Evelyn Frew American Cancer Society Clinical Research Professor
Memorial Sloan-Kettering Cancer Center
New York, NY

Clifford B. Saper, MD, PhD
James Jackson Putnam Professor of Neurology and Neuroscience,
Harvard Medical School
Chairman, Department of Neurology
Beth Israel Deaconess Medical Center
Boston, MA

Nicholas D. Schiff, MD
Associate Professor of Neurology and Neuroscience
Department of Neurology and Neuroscience
Weill Cornell Medical College
New York, NY

Fred Plum, MD
University Professor Emeritus
Department of Neurology and Neuroscience
Weill Cornell Medical College
New York, NY

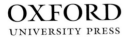
OXFORD
UNIVERSITY PRESS

2007

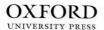

Oxford University Press, Inc., publishes works that further
Oxford University's objective of excellence
in research, scholarship, and education.

Oxford   New York
Auckland   Cape Town   Dar es Salaam   Hong Kong   Karachi
Kuala Lumpur   Madrid   Melbourne   Mexico City   Nairobi
New Delhi   Shanghai   Taipei   Toronto

With offices in
Argentina   Austria   Brazil   Chile   Czech Republic   France   Greece
Guatemala   Hungary   Italy   Japan   Poland   Portugal   Singapore
South Korea   Switzerland   Thailand   Turkey   Ukraine   Vietnam

Published by Oxford University Press, Inc.
198 Madison Avenue, New York, New York 10016

www.oup.com

Oxford is a registered trademark of Oxford University Press

Library of Congress Cataloging-in-Publication Data
Plum and Posner's diagnosis of stupor and coma / Jerome B. Posner . . . [et al.]. — 4th ed.
   p. ; cm.—(Contemporary neurology series ; 71)
Rev. ed. of: The diagnosis of stupor and coma / Fred Plum, Jerome B. Posner. 3rd ed. c1980.
Includes bibliographical references and index.
ISBN 978-0-19-532131-9
1. Coma—Diagnosis.   2. Stupor—Diagnosis.   I. Posner, Jerome B., 1932–   II. Plum, Fred, 1924–
Diagnosis of stupor and coma.   III. Title: Diagnosis of stupor and coma.   IV. Series.
[DNLM: 1. Coma—diagnosis.   2. Stupor—diagnosis.   3. Brain Diseases—diagnosis.
4. Brain Injuries—diagnosis.
W1 CO769N v.71 2007 / WB 182 P7335 2007]
RB150.C6P55 2007
616.8'49—dc22   2006103219

9 8 7 6 5 4 3 2 1

Printed in the United States of America
on acid-free paper

Jerome Posner, Clifford Saper and Nicholas Schiff dedicate this book to Fred Plum, our mentor. His pioneering studies into coma and its pathophysiology made the first edition of this book possible and have contributed to all of the subsequent editions, including this one. His insistence on excellence, although often hard to attain, has been an inspiration and a guide for our careers.

The authors also dedicate this book to our wives, whose encouragement and support make our work not only possible but also pleasant.

Preface to the Fourth Edition

Fred Plum came to the University of Washington in 1952 to head up the Division of Neurology (in the Department of Medicine) that consisted of one person, Fred. The University had no hospital but instead used the county hospital (King County Hospital), now called Harborview. The only emergency room in the entire county was at that hospital, and thus it received all of the comatose patients in the area. The only noninvasive imaging available was primitive ultrasound that could identify, sometimes, whether the pineal gland was in the midline. Thus, Fred and his residents (August Swanson, Jerome Posner, and Donald McNealy, in that order) searched for clinical ways to differentiate those lesions that required neurosurgical intervention from those that required medical treatment. The result was the first edition of *The Diagnosis of Stupor and Coma*.

Times have changed. Computed tomography (CT) and magnetic resonance imaging (MRI) have revolutionized the approach to the patient with an altered level of consciousness. The physician confronted with such a patient usually first images the brain and then if the image does not show a mass or destructive lesion, pursues a careful metabolic workup. Even the laboratory evaluation has changed. In the 1950s the only pH meter in the hospital was in our experimental laboratory and many of the metabolic tests that we now consider routine were time consuming and not available in a timely fashion. Yet the clinical approach taught in *The Diagnosis of Stupor and Coma* remains the cornerstone of medical care for comatose patients in virtually every hospital, and the need for a modern updating of the text has been clear for some time.

The appearance of a fourth edition now called *Plum and Posner's Diagnosis of Stupor and Coma* more than 25 years after the third edition is deserving of comment. There were several reasons for this delay. First, the introduction and rapid development of MRI scanning almost immediately after the publication of the last edition both stimulated the authors to prepare a new edition and also delayed the efforts, as new information using the new MRI methods accumulated at a rapid pace and dramatically changed the field over the next decade. At the same time, there was substantial progress in theory on the neural basis of consciousness, and the senior author wanted to incorporate as much of that new material as possible into the new edition. A second obstacle to the early completion of a fourth edition was the retirement of the senior author, who also developed some difficulty with expressive language. It became apparent that the senior author was not going to be able to complete the new edition with the eloquence for which he had been known. Ultimately, the two original authors asked two of their proteges, CBS and NDS, to help with the preparation of the new edition. Fred participated in the initial drafts of this edition, but not fully in the final product. Thus, the mistakes and wrongheaded opinions you might find in this edition are ours and not his. We as his students feel privileged to be able to continue and update his classic work.

One of our most important goals was to retain the clear and authoritative voice of the senior author in the current revision. Even though much of the text has been rewritten, we worked from the original organizational and conceptual context of the third edition. Fred Plum's description of how one examines an unconscious patient was, and is, classic. Accordingly, we've tried whenever possible to use his words from the first three editions. Because the clinical examination remains largely unchanged, we could use some of the case reports and many of the figures describing the clinical examination from previous editions. Fred was present at each of the critical editorial meetings, and he continued to contribute to the overall structure and scientific and clinical content of the book. Most important, he instilled his ideas and views into each of the other authors, whom he taught and mentored over many years. The primary writing tasks for the first four chapters fell to CBS, Chapters 5 to 7 to JBP, and Chapters 8 and 9 to NDS. However, each of the chapters was passed back and forth and revised and edited by each of the authors, so that the responsibility for the content of the fourth edition remains joint and several.

Most important, although the technologic evaluation of patients in coma has changed in ways that were unimaginable at the time of publication of the earlier editions, the underlying principles of evaluation and management have not. The examination of the comatose patient remains the cornerstone to clinical judgment. It is much faster and more accurate than any imaging study, and accurate clinical assessment is necessary to determine what steps are required for further evaluation, to determine the tempo of the workup, and most important, to identify those patients in critical condition who need emergency intervention. Coma remains a classic problem in neurology, in which intervention within minutes can often make the difference between life and death for the patient. In this sense, the fourth edition of *Plum and Posner's Diagnosis of Stupor and Coma* does not differ from its predecessors in offering a straightforward approach to diagnosis and management of these critically ill patients.

The authors owe a debt of gratitude to many colleagues who have helped us prepare this edition of the book. Dr. Joe Fins generously contributed a section on ethics to Chapter 8 that the other authors would not have otherwise been able to provide. Chapters were reviewed at various stages of preparation by Drs. George Richerson, Michael Ronthal, Jonathan Edlow, Richard Wolfe, Josef Parvizi, Matt Fink, Richard Lappin, Steven Laureys, Marcus Yountz, Veronique van der Horst, Amy Amick, Nicholas Silvestri, and John Whyte. These colleagues have helped us avoid innumerable missteps. The remaining errors, however, are our own. Drs. Jonathan Kleefield and Linda Heier have provided us with radiologic images and Dr. Jeffrey Joseph with pathological images. The clarity of their vision has contributed to our own, and illuminates many of the ideas in this book. We also thank Judy Lampron, who read the entire book correcting typos, spelling errors (better than spellcheck), and awkward sentences. We owe our gratitude to a series of patient editors at Oxford University Press who have worked with the authors as we have prepared this edition. Included among these are Fiona Stevens, who worked with us on restarting the project, and Craig Panner, who edited the final manuscript. Sid Gilman, the series editor, has provided continuous support and encouragement.

Finally, we want to thank the members of our families, who have put up with our intellectual reveries and physical absences as we have prepared the material in this book. It has taken much more time than any of us had expected, but it has been a labor of love.

Fred Plum, MD
Jerome B. Posner, MD
Clifford B. Saper, MD, PhD
Nicholas D. Schiff, MD

Contents

PLUM AND POSNER'S DIAGNOSIS OF STUPOR AND COMA

Fourth Edition

Chapter 1

Pathophysiology of Signs and Symptoms of Coma

ALTERED STATES OF CONSCIOUSNESS

*And men should know that from nothing else but
from the brain came joys, delights, laughter and
jests, and sorrows, griefs, despondency and lamen-
tations. And by this, in an especial manner, we acquire wisdom and knowledge, and see and hear and
know what are foul, and what are fair, what sweet
and what unsavory . . .*
— The Hippocratic Writings

Impaired consciousness is among the most difficult and dramatic of clinical problems. The an-
cient Greeks knew that normal consciousness
depends on an intact brain, and that impaired
consciousness signifies brain failure. The brain
tolerates only limited physical or metabolic injury, so that impaired consciousness is often a
sign of impending irreparable damage to the
brain. Stupor and coma imply advanced brain
failure, just as, for example, uremia means renal
failure, and the longer such brain failure lasts,

3

the narrower the margin between recovery and the development of permanent neurologic injury. The limited time for action and the multiplicity of potential causes of brain failure challenge the physician and frighten both the physician and the family; only the patient escapes anxiety.

Many conditions cause coma. Table 1–1 lists some of the common and often perplexing causes of unconsciousness that the physician may encounter in the emergency department of a general hospital. The purpose of this monograph is to describe a systematic approach to the diagnosis of the patient with reduced consciousness, stupor, or coma based on anatomic and physiologic principles. Accordingly, this book divides the causes of unconsciousness into two major categories: structural and metabolic. Chapter 1 provides background information on the pathophysiology of impaired consciousness, as well as the signs and symptoms that accompany it. In Chapter 2 this information is used to define a brief but informative neurologic examination that is necessary to

Table 1–1 Cause of Stupor or Coma in 500 Patients Initially Diagnosed as "Coma of Unknown Etiology"*

	Subtotals		Subtotals
I. Supratentorial lesions	101	B. Destructive or ischemic lesions	53
A. Rhinencephalic and subcortical destructive lesions	2	1. Pontine hemorrhage	11
		2. Brainstem infarct	40
1. Thalamic infarcts	2	3. Basilar migraine	1
B. Supratentorial mass lesions	99	4. Brainstem demyelination	1
1. Hemorrhage	76	III. Diffuse and/or metabolic brain dysfunction	326
a. Intracerebral	44	
(1) Hypertensive	36	A. Diffuse intrinsic disorders of brain	38
(2) Vascular anomaly	5	1. "Encephalitis" or encephalomyelitis	14
(3) Other	3	
b. Epidural	4	2. Subarachnoid hemorrhage	13
c. Subdural	26	3. Concussion, nonconvulsive seizures, and postictal states	9
d. Pituitary apoplexy	2	
2. Infarction	9	4. Primary neuronal disorders	2
a. Arterial occlusions	7	B. Extrinsic and metabolic disorders	288
(1) Thrombotic	5	
(2) Embolic	2	1. Anoxia or ischemia	10
b. Venous occlusions	2	2. Hypoglycemia	16
3. Tumors	7	3. Nutritional	1
a. Primary	2	4. Hepatic encephalopathy	17
b. Metastatic	5	5. Uremia and dialysis	8
4. Abscess	6	6. Pulmonary disease	3
a. Intracerebral	5	7. Endocrine disorders (including diabetes)	12
b. Subdural	1	
5. Closed head injury	1	8. Remote effects of cancer	0
II. Subtentorial lesions	65	9. Drug poisons	149
A. Compressive lesions	12	10. Ionic and acid-base disorders	12
1. Cerebellar hemorrhage	5	11. Temperature regulation	9
2. Posterior fossa subdural or extradural hemorrhage	1	12. Mixed or nonspecific metabolic coma	1
3. Cerebellar infarct	2	IV. Psychiatric "coma"	8
4. Cerebellar tumor	3	A. Conversion reactions	4
5. Cerebellar abscess	1	B. Depression	2
6. Basilar aneurysm	0	C. Catatonic stupor	2

*Represents only patients for whom a neurologist was consulted because the initial diagnosis was uncertain and in whom a final diagnosis was established. Thus, obvious diagnoses such as known poisonings, meningitis, and closed head injuries, and cases of mixed metabolic encephalopathies in which a specific etiologic diagnosis was never established are underrepresented.

determine if the reduced consciousness has a structural cause (and therefore may require immediate imaging and perhaps surgical treatment) or a metabolic cause (in which case the diagnostic approach can be more lengthy and extensive). Chapters 3 and 4 discuss pathophysiology and specific causes of structural injury to the brain that result in defects of consciousness. Chapter 5 examines the broad range of metabolic causes of unconsciousness, and the specific treatments they require. Chapter 6 explores psychiatric causes of unresponsiveness, which must be differentiated from organic causes of stupor and coma. Chapter 7 provides a systematic discussion of the treatment of both structural and metabolic coma. Chapter 8 explores the outcomes of coma of different causes, including the prognosis for useful recovery and the states of long-term impairment of consciousness. Chapter 9 reviews some ethical problems encountered in treating unconscious individuals.

DEFINITIONS

Consciousness

Consciousness is the state of full awareness of the self and one's relationship to the environment. Clinically, the level of consciousness of a patient is defined operationally at the bedside by the responses of the patient to the examiner. It is clear from this definition that it is possible for a patient to be conscious yet not responsive to the examiner, for example, if the patient lacks sensory inputs, is paralyzed (see *locked-in syndrome*, page 7), or for psychologic reasons decides not to respond. Thus, the determination of the state of consciousness can be a technically challenging exercise. In the definitions that follow, we assume that the patient is not unresponsive due to sensory or motor impairment or psychiatric disease.

Consciousness has two major components: content and arousal. The *content* of consciousness represents the sum of all functions mediated at a cerebral cortical level, including both cognitive and affective responses. These functions are subserved by unique networks of cortical neurons, and it is possible for a lesion that is strategically placed to disrupt one of the networks, causing a *fractional loss of consciousness.*[1] Such patients may have preserved awareness of most stimuli, but having suffered the loss of a critical population of neurons (e.g., for recognizing language symbol content, differences between colors or faces, or the presence of the left side of space), the patient literally becomes unconscious of that class of stimuli. Patients with these deficits are often characterized as "confused" by inexperienced examiners, because they do not respond as expected to behavioral stimuli. More experienced clinicians recognize the focal cognitive deficits and that the alteration of consciousness is confined to one class of stimuli. Occasionally, patients with right parietotemporal lesions may be sufficiently inattentive as to appear to be globally confused, but they are not sleepy and are, in fact, usually agitated.[2]

Thus, unless the damage to cortical networks is diffuse or very widespread, the level of consciousness is not reduced. For example, patients with advanced Alzheimer's disease may lose memory and other cognitive functions, but remain awake and alert until the damage is so extensive and severe that response to stimuli is reduced as well (see *vegetative state*, page 8). Hence, a reduced *level of consciousness* is not due to focal impairments of cognitive function, but rather to a global reduction in the level of behavioral responsiveness. In addition to being caused by widespread cortical impairment, a reduced level of consciousness can result from injury to a specific set of brainstem and diencephalic pathways that regulate the overall *level* of cortical function, and hence consciousness (Figure 1–1). The normal activity of this arousal system is linked behaviorally to the appearance of wakefulness. It should be apparent that cognition is not possible without a reasonable degree of arousal.

Sleep is a recurrent, physiologic, but not pathologic, form of reduced consciousness in which the responsiveness of brain systems responsible for cognitive function is globally reduced, so that the brain does not respond readily to environmental stimuli. Pathologic alteration of the relationships between the brain systems that are responsible for wakefulness and sleep can impair consciousness. The systems subserving normal sleep and wakefulness are reviewed later in this chapter. A key difference between sleep and coma is that sleep is intrinsically reversible: sufficient stimulation will return the individual to a normal waking state. In contrast, if patients with pathologic alterations of consciousness can be awakened at all, they rapidly fall back into a sleep-like state when stimulation ceases.

Patients who have a sleep-like appearance and remain behaviorally unresponsive to all external stimuli are unconscious by any definition. However, continuous sleep-like coma as a result of brain injury rarely lasts more than 2 to 4 weeks.

Acutely Altered States of Consciousness

Clouding of consciousness is a term applied to minimally reduced wakefulness or awareness, which may include hyperexcitability and irritability alternating with drowsiness. A key distinction must be made in such patients between those who are confused (i.e., do not respond appropriately to their environment) because of a focal deficit of cognitive function versus those who have more global impairment. The beclouded patient is usually incompletely oriented to time and sometimes to place. Such patients are inattentive and perform poorly on repeating numbers backward (the normal range is at least four or five) and remembering details or even the meaning of stories. Drowsiness is often prominent during the day, but agitation may predominate at night.

The pathophysiology of brain function in such patients has rarely been studied, but Posner and Plum[3] found that cerebral oxygen consumption had declined by 20% below normal levels in patients with hepatic encephalopathy with lethargy and global confusion, and Shimojyo and colleagues noted similar reductions in patients with lethargy and global confusion due to Wernicke's encephalopathy.[4] More recently, Trzepacz and colleagues have identified decreased regional cerebral blood flow (CBF) bilaterally in the frontotemporal cortex and right basal ganglia of patients with subclinical hepatic encephalopathy.[5] Increases in CBF during treatment of cobalamin deficiency correlate with clinical improvement.[6] Other studies have implicated reduced cholinergic function; excess release of dopamine, norepinephrine, and glutamate; and both decreased and increased serotonergic and gamma-aminobutyric acid (GABA) activity.[7] The pathogenesis of clouding of consciousness and delirium is discussed in more detail in Chapter 5.

Delirium, from the Latin "to go out of the furrow," is a more floridly abnormal mental state characterized by misperception of sensory stimuli and, often, vivid hallucinations. Delirium is defined by the *Diagnostic and Statistical Manual of Mental Disorders*, 4th edition (*DSM-IV*),[8] as follows: "A. Disturbance of consciousness (i.e., reduced clarity of awareness of the environment) with reduced ability to focus, sustain or shift attention. B. A change in cognition (such as memory deficit, disorientation, language disturbance) or the development of a perceptual disturbance that is not better accounted for by a pre-existing, established or evolving dementia. C. The disturbance develops over a short period of time (usually hours to days) and tends to fluctuate during the course of the day."

Delirious patients are disoriented, first to time, next to place, and then to persons in their environment. Rarely are patients unaware of who they are, although sometimes married women will revert to their maiden name. Patients are often fearful or irritable and may overreact or misinterpret normal activities of physicians and nurses. Delusions or hallucinations may place the patient completely out of contact with the environment and the examiner. Full-blown delirious states tend to come on rapidly and rarely last more than 4 to 7 days. However, fragments of misperceptions may persist for several weeks, especially among alcoholics and patients with cerebral involvement from collagen vascular diseases.

Delirium with agitation occasionally may be seen as a consequence of focal lesions of the right parieto-occipitotemporal cortex,[2,9] but generally is indicative of bilateral impairment of cortical function in toxic-metabolic states, such as atropine poisoning, alcohol or sedative drug (e.g., benzodiazepine) withdrawal, acute porphyria, or hepatic or renal failure. It also occurs with systemic infectious processes or as a component of encephalitis, during which immune mediators such as cytokines and eicosanoid derivatives may cloud mental function.

Obtundation, from the Latin "to beat against or blunt," literally means mental blunting or torpidity. In a medical setting, such patients have a mild to moderate reduction in alertness, accompanied by a lesser interest in the environment. Such patients have slower psychologic responses to stimulation. They may have an increased number of hours of sleep and may be drowsy between sleep bouts.

Stupor, from the Latin "to be stunned," is a condition of deep sleep or similar behavioral unresponsiveness from which the subject can be aroused only with vigorous and continuous stimulation. Even when maximally aroused, the level of cognitive function may be impaired. Such patients can be differentiated from those with psychiatric impairment, such as catatonia or severe depression, because they can be aroused by vigorous stimulation to respond to simple stimuli.

Coma, from the Greek "deep sleep or trance," is a state of unresponsiveness in which the patient lies with eyes closed and cannot be aroused to respond appropriately to stimuli even with vigorous stimulation. The patient may grimace in response to painful stimuli and limbs may demonstrate stereotyped withdrawal responses, but the patient does not make localizing responses or discrete defensive movements. As coma deepens, the responsiveness of the patient, even to painful stimuli, may diminish or disappear. However, it is difficult to equate the lack of motor responses to the depth of the coma, as the neural structures that regulate motor responses differ from those that regulate consciousness, and they may be differentially impaired by specific brain disorders.

The locked-in syndrome describes a state in which the patient is de-efferented, resulting in paralysis of all four limbs and the lower cranial nerves. This condition has been recognized at least as far back as the 19th century, but its distinctive name was applied in the first edition of this monograph (1966), reflecting the implications of this condition for the diagnosis of coma and for the specialized care such patients require. Although not unconscious, locked-in patients are unable to respond to most stimuli. A high level of clinical suspicion is required on the part of the examiner to distinguish a locked-in patient from one who is comatose. The most common cause is a lesion of the base and tegmentum of the midpons that interrupts descending cortical control of motor functions. Such patients usually retain control of vertical eye movements and eyelid opening, which can be used to verify their responsiveness. They may be taught to respond to the examiner by using eye blinks as a code. Rare patients with subacute motor neuropathy, such as Guillain-Barré syndrome, also may become completely de-efferented, but there is a history of subacute paralysis. In both instances, electroencephalographic (EEG) examination discloses a reactive posterior alpha rhythm[10] (see *EEG* section, page 82).

It is important to identify locked-in patients so that they may be treated appropriately by the medical and nursing staff. At the bedside, discussion should be *with* the patient, not, as with an unconscious individual, *about* the patient. Patients with large midpontine lesions often are awake most of the time, with greatly diminished sleep on physiologic recordings.[11] They may suffer greatly if they are treated by hospital staff as if they are nonresponsive.

As the above definitions imply, each of these conditions includes a fairly wide range of behavioral responsiveness, and there may be some overlap among them. Therefore, it is generally best to describe a patient by indicating what stimuli do or do not result in responses and the kinds of responses that are seen, rather than using less precise terms.

Subacute or Chronic Alterations of Consciousness

Dementia defines an enduring and often progressive decline in mental processes owing to an organic process not usually accompanied by a reduction in arousal. Conventionally, the term implies a diffuse or disseminated reduction in cognitive functions rather than the impairment of a single psychologic activity such as language. *DSM-IV* defines dementia as follows: "A. The development of multiple cognitive defects manifested by both: (1) Memory impairment (impaired ability to learn new information or to recall previously learned information); (2) One (or more) of the following cognitive disturbances: aphasia (language disturbance), apraxia (impaired ability to carry out motor activities despite intact motor function), agnosia (failure to recognize or identify objects despite intact sensory function), disturbance in executive function (i.e., planning, organization, sequencing, abstracting)."

The reader will recognize this definition as an arbitrary restriction. Usually, the term *dementia* is applied to the effects of primary disorders of the cerebral hemispheres, such as degenerative conditions, traumatic injuries, and neoplasms. Occasionally, dementia can be at least partially reversible, such as when it accompanies thyroid or vitamin B_{12} deficiency or results from a reversible communicating hydrocephalus; more often, however, the term applies to chronic conditions carrying limited hopes for improvement.

Patients with dementia are usually awake and alert, but as the dementia worsens, may become less responsive and eventually evolve into a vegetative state (see below). Patients with dementia are at significantly increased risk of developing delirium when they become medically ill or develop comorbid brain disease.

Hypersomnia refers to a state characterized by excessive but normal-appearing sleep from which the subject readily, even if briefly, awakens when stimulated. Many patients with either acute or chronic alterations of consciousness sleep excessively. However, when awakened, consciousness is clearly clouded. In the truly hypersomniac patient, sleep appears normal and cognitive functions are normal when patients are awakened. Hypersomnia results from hypothalamic dysfunction, as indicated later in this chapter.[12]

Abulia (from the Greek for "lack of will") is an apathetic state in which the patient responds slowly if at all to verbal stimuli and generally does not initiate conversation or activity. When sufficiently stimulated, however, cognitive functions may be normal. Unlike hypersomnia, the patient usually appears fully awake. Abulia is usually associated with bilateral frontal lobe disease and, when severe, may evolve into akinetic mutism.

Akinetic mutism describes a condition of silent, alert-appearing immobility that characterizes certain subacute or chronic states of altered consciousness in which sleep-wake cycles have returned, but externally obtainable evidence for mental activity remains almost entirely absent and spontaneous motor activity is lacking. Such patients generally have lesions including the hypothalamus and adjacent basal forebrain.

The *minimally conscious state* (MCS) is a concept that was recently developed by the Aspen Workgroup, a consortium of neurologists, neurosurgeons, neuropsychologists, and rehabilitation specialists.[13] MCS identifies a condition of severely impaired consciousness in which minimal but definite behavioral evidence of self (this can only be assessed verbally, of course) or environmental awareness is demonstrated.

Like the vegetative state, MCS often exists as a transitional state arising during recovery from coma or worsening of progressive neurologic disease. In some patients, however, it may be an essentially permanent condition. For a detailed discussion of the clinical criteria for the diagnosis of the minimally conscious state, see Chapter 9.

The *vegetative state* (VS) denotes the recovery of crude cycling of arousal states heralded by the appearance of "eyes-open" periods in an unresponsive patient. Very few surviving patients with severe forebrain damage remain in eyes-closed coma for more than 10 to 30 days. In most patients, vegetative behavior usually replaces coma by that time. Patients in the vegetative state, like comatose patients, show no evidence of awareness of self or their environment. Unlike brain death, in which the cerebral hemispheres and the brainstem both undergo overwhelming functional impairment, patients in vegetative states retain brainstem regulation of cardiopulmonary function and visceral autonomic regulation. Although the original term *persistent vegetative state* (PVS) was not associated with a specific time, the use of PVS is now commonly reserved for patients remaining in a vegetative state for at least 30 days. The American Neurological Association advises that PVS be applied only to patients in the state for 1 month. Some patients recover from PVS (see Chapter 9). Other terms in the literature designating the vegetative state include *coma vigil* and the *apallic state*.

Brain death is defined as the irreversible loss of all functions of the entire brain,[14] such that the body is unable to maintain respiratory and cardiovascular homeostasis. Although vigorous supportive care may keep the body processes going for some time, particularly in an

Table 1–2 **Terms Used to Describe Disorders of Consciousness**

Acute	Subacute or Chronic
Clouding	Dementia
Delirium	Hypersomnia
Obtundation	Abulic
Stupor	Akinetic mutism
Coma	Minimal consciousness
Locked in (not coma; see text)	Vegetative
	Brain death

otherwise healthy young person, the loss of brain function eventually results in failure of the systemic circulation within a few days or, rarely, after several weeks. That the brain has been dead for some time prior to the cessation of the heartbeat is attested to by the fact that the organ in such cases is usually autolyzed (respirator brain) when examined postmortem.[15] Because function of the cerebral hemispheres depends on the brainstem (see *ascending arousal system* section below), and because cerebral hemisphere function is extremely difficult to assess when the brainstem is nonfunctioning, physicians in the United Kingdom have developed the concept of *brainstem death*,[16] defined as "irreversible loss of the capacity for consciousness, combined with irreversible loss of the capacity to breathe." The criteria for the diagnosis of brain death and brainstem death are almost identical. They are detailed in Chapter 8.

Acute alterations of consciousness are discussed in Chapters 2 through 5. Subacute and chronic alterations of consciousness are discussed in Chapter 9.

APPROACH TO THE DIAGNOSIS OF THE COMATOSE PATIENT

Determining the cause of an acutely depressed level of consciousness is a difficult clinical challenge. The clinician must determine rapidly whether the cause of the impairment is structural or metabolic, and what treatments must be instituted to save the life of the patient. Since the last edition of this monograph in 1980, there has been a revolution in brain imaging. Computed tomography (CT) scans and sometimes magnetic resonance imaging (MRI) are immediately available in the emergency room to evaluate acutely ill patients. In appropriate clinical circumstances, if the initial examination suggests structural brain damage, a scan may identify the cause of the alteration of consciousness and dictate the therapy. However, when the scan does not give the cause, there is no simple solution; usually no single laboratory test or screening procedure will sift out the critical initial diagnostic categories as effectively as a careful clinical evaluation.

If the cause of coma is structural, it generally is due to a focal injury along the course of the neural pathways that generate and maintain a normal waking brain. *Therefore, the clinical diagnosis of structural coma depends on the recognition of the signs of injury to structures that accompany the arousal pathways through the brain.* Structural processes that impair the function of the arousal system fall into two categories: (1) supratentorial mass lesions, which may compress deep diencephalic structures and hence impair the function of both hemispheres, and (2) infratentorial mass or destructive lesions, which directly damage the arousal system at its source in the upper brainstem. The remainder of Chapter 1 will systematically examine the major arousal systems in the brain and the physiology and pathophysiology of consciousness. Chapter 2 addresses examination of the patient with a disturbance of consciousness, particularly those components of the examination that assay the function of the arousal systems and the major sensory, motor, and autonomic systems that accompany them. Once the examination is completed, the examiner should be able to determine whether the source of the impairment of consciousness is caused by a structural lesion (Chapters 3 and 4) or a diffuse and therefore presumably metabolic process (Chapter 5).

Although it is important to question family members or attendants who may have details of the history, including emergency medical personnel who bring the patient into the emergency department, the history for comatose patients is often scant or absent. The neurologic examination of a patient with impaired consciousness, fortunately, is brief, because the patient cannot detect sensory stimuli or provide voluntary motor responses. The key components of the examination, which can be completed by a skillful physician in just a few minutes, include (1) the level of consciousness of the patient, (2) the pattern of breathing, (3) the size and reactivity of the pupils, (4) the eye movements and oculovestibular responses, and (5) the skeletal motor responses. From this information, the examiner must be able to reconstruct the type of the lesion and move swiftly to lifesaving measures. Before reviewing the components of the coma examination in detail, however, it is necessary to understand the basic pathways in the brain that sustain wakeful, conscious behavior. Only from this perspective is it possible to understand how the components of the coma examination test pathways that are intertwined with those that maintain consciousness.

Box 1–1 Constantin von Economo and the Discovery of Intrinsic Wake and Sleep Systems in the Brain

Baron Constantin von Economo von San Serff was born in 1876, the son of Greek parentage. He was brought up in Austrian Trieste, studied medicine in Vienna, and in 1906 took a post in the Psychiatric Clinic under Professor Julius von Wagner-Jauregg. In 1916 during World War I, he began seeing cases of a new and previously unrecorded type of encephalitis and published his first report of this illness in 1917. Although subsequent accounts have often confused this illness with the epidemic of influenza that swept through Europe and then the rest of the world during World War I, von Economo was quite clear that encephalitis lethargica was not associated with respiratory symptoms, and that its appearance preceded the onset of the latter epidemic. Von Economo continued to write and lecture about this experience for the remainder of his life, until his premature death in 1931 from heart disease.

Based on his clinical observations, von Economo proposed a dual center theory for regulation of sleep and wakefulness: a waking influence arising from the upper brainstem and passing through the gray matter surrounding the cerebral aqueduct and the posterior third ventricle; and a rostral hypothalamic sleep-promoting area. These observations became the basis for lesion studies done by Ranson in 1939,[20] by Nauta in 1946,[21] and by Swett and Hobson in 1968,[22] in which they showed that the posterior lateral hypothalamic lesions in monkeys, rats, and cats could reproduce the prolonged sleepiness that von Economo had observed. The rostral hypothalamic sleep-promoting area was confirmed experimentally in rats by Nauta in 1946[21] and in cats by Sterman and Clemente in the 1960s.[23]

Interestingly, von Economo also identified a third clinical syndrome, which appeared some months after the acute encephalitis in some patients who had

Sleep as a Problem of Localization*

Baron
Constantin von Economo

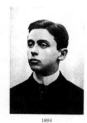

1894

* Read before the College of Physicians and Surgeons, Columbia University, December 3, 1929. Reprinted, by permission, from *The Journal of Nervous and Mental Disease*, Vol. 71, No. 3, March, 1930.

Figure B1–1A. A photograph of Baron Constantin von Economo, and excerpts from the title page of his lecture on the localization of sleep and wake promoting systems in the brain. (From von Economo,[19] with permission.)

(continued)

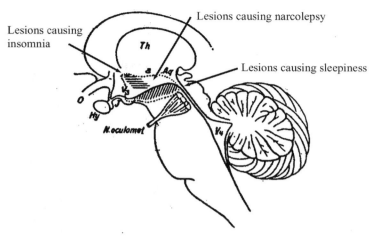

Lesions causing narcolepsy

Lesions causing insomnia

Lesions causing sleepiness

Schema of the median section of the interbrain; the dotted line is the boundary of the field, in which the center for sleep regulation is lying.

Figure B1–1B. Von Economo's original drawing of the localization of the lesions in the brain that caused excessive sleepiness and insomnia. (Modified from von Economo,[19] with permission.)

posterior hypothalamic lesions, as they were beginning to recover. These individuals would develop episodes of sleep attacks during which they had an overwhelming need to sleep. He noted that they also had attacks of cataplexy in which they lost all muscle tone, often when excited emotionally. Von Economo noted accurately that these symptoms were similar to the rare condition previously identified by Gelinaux as narcolepsy. S.A. Kinnier Wilson described a cohort of similar patients in London in 1928.[24] He also noted that they had developed symptoms of narcolepsy after recovering from encephalitis lethargica with posterior hypothalamic lesions. Wilson even described examining a patient in his office, with the young house officer McDonald Critchley, and that the patient indeed had atonic paralysis, with loss of tendon reflexes and an extensor plantar response during the attack.

Von Economo's theory was highly influential during this period, and a great deal of what was subsequently learned about the organization of brain systems controlling sleep and wakefulness owes its origins to his careful clinicopathologic observations and his imaginative and far-reaching vision about brain organization.

PHYSIOLOGY AND PATHOPHYSIOLOGY OF CONSCIOUSNESS AND COMA

The Ascending Arousal System

In the late 19th century, the great British neurologist John Hughlings-Jackson[17] proposed that consciousness was the sum total of the activity in human cerebral hemispheres. A corollary was that consciousness could only be eliminated by lesions that simultaneously damaged both cerebral hemispheres. However, several clinical observations challenged this view. As early as 1890, Mauthner[18] reported that stupor in patients with Wernicke's encephalopathy was associated with lesions involving the gray matter surrounding the cerebral aqueduct and the caudal part of the third ventricle. The nascent field of neuro-surgery also began to contribute cases in which loss of consciousness was associated with lesions confined to the upper brainstem or caudal di-encephalon. However, the most convincing body of evidence was assembled by Baron Constantin von Economo,[19] a Viennese neurologist who recorded his observations during an epidemic of a unique disorder, encephalitis lethargica, that occurred in the years surrounding World War I. Most victims of encephalitis lethargica were very sleepy, spending 20 or more hours per day asleep, and awakening only briefly to eat. When awakened, they could interact in a relatively unimpaired fashion with the examiner, but soon fell asleep if not continuously stimulated. Many of these patients suffered from oculomotor abnormalities, and when they died, they were found to have lesions involving the paramedian reticular formation of the midbrain at the junction with the diencephalon. Other patients during the same epidemic developed prolonged wakefulness, sleeping at most a few hours per day. Movement disorders were also common. Von Economo identified the causative lesion in the gray matter surrounding the anterior part of the third ventricle in the hypothalamus and extending laterally into the basal ganglia at that level.

Von Economo suggested that there was specific brainstem circuitry that causes arousal or wakefulness of the forebrain, and that the hypothalamus contains circuitry for inhibiting this system to induce sleep. However, it was difficult to test these deductions because naturally occurring lesions in patients, or experimental lesions in animals that damaged the brainstem, almost invariably destroyed important sensory and motor pathways that complicated the interpretation of the results. As long as the only tool for assessing activity of the cerebral hemispheres remained the clinical examination, this problem could not be resolved.

In 1929, Hans Berger, a Swiss psychiatrist, reported a technologic innovation, the electro-encephalogram (EEG), which he developed to assess the cortical function of his psychiatric patients with various types of functional impairment of responsiveness.[25] He noted that the waveform pattern that he recorded from the scalps of his patients was generally sinusoidal, and that the amplitude and frequency of the waves in the EEG correlated closely with the level of consciousness of the patient.

Shortly afterward, in 1935, the Belgian neurophysiologist Frederic Bremer[28] (see also[29]) examined the EEG waveforms in cats into which he had placed lesions of the brainstem. He found that after a transection between the medulla and the spinal cord, a preparation that he called the *encephale isole*, or isolated brain, animals showed a desynchronized (low voltage, fast, i.e., waking) EEG pattern and appeared to be fully awake. However, when he transected the neuraxis at the level between the superior and inferior colliculus, a preparation he called the *cerveau isole*, or isolated cerebrum, the EEG showed a synchronized, or high-voltage, slow-wave pattern indicative of deep sleep and the animals were behaviorally unresponsive. Bremer concluded that the forebrain fell asleep due to the lack of somatosensory and auditory sensory inputs. He did not address why the animals failed to respond to visual inputs either with EEG desynchronization or by making vertical eye movements (as do patients who are locked in).

This issue was addressed after World War II by Moruzzi and Magoun,[30] who placed more selective lesions in the lateral part of the midbrain tegmentum in cats, interrupting the ascending somatosensory and auditory lemniscal pathways, but leaving the paramedian reticular core of the midbrain intact. Such animals were deaf and did not appear to appreciate somatosensory stimuli, but were fully awake, as indicated both by EEG desynchronization and motor responses to visual stimuli. Conversely, when they placed lesions in the paramedian reticular formation of the midbrain, the animals still showed cortical-evoked responses to somatosensory or auditory stimuli, but the background EEG was synchronized and the animals were behaviorally unresponsive. Later studies showed that electrical stimulation of the midbrain reticular core could excite forebrain desynchronization.[31] These observations emphasized the midbrain reticular core as relaying important arousing influences to the cerebral cortex, and this pathway was labeled the ascending reticular activating system. The origin of the pathway was not established in this early work.

Subsequent studies, in which transecting lesions were placed sequentially at different levels of the brainstem in cats, demonstrated that transections at the midpontine level or caudally down to the lower medulla resulted in animals that acutely spent most of their time in

Box 1–2 The Thalamus, Basal Forebrain, and Generation of EEG Waves

The origin of the sinusoidal appearance of the waveforms in the EEG remained a mystery until the 1980s. Although it was understood that the EEG voltages are due to the summated excitatory postsynaptic potentials in dendrites of cortical neurons, the reason for the synchronous waves of dendritic potentials remained elusive. The waves of postsynaptic potentials in the cerebral cortex are now understood to be due to the intrinsic burst firing of neurons in the thalamus, basal forebrain, and the cortex itself, which produce waves of postsynaptic potentials in cortical neurons.

When the membrane potential of burst neurons is close to their firing threshold, they fire single action potentials that transmit sensory and other information. However, when burst neurons have been hyperpolarized to membrane potentials far below their usual threshold for firing sodium action potentials, a low-threshold calcium channel is deinactivated. When the low-threshold calcium channel is triggered, calcium entry brings the membrane potential to a plateau that is above the threshold for firing sodium action potentials. As a result, a series of sodium spikes are fired, until sufficient calcium has entered the cell to activate a calcium-activated potassium current. This potassium current then brings the cell back to a hyperpolarized state, terminating the burst of action potentials. The more deeply the resting

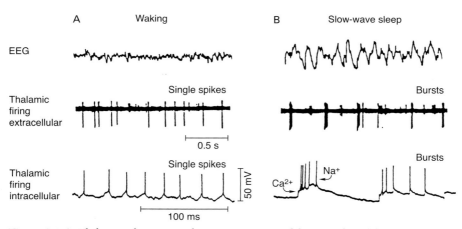

Figure B1–2. Thalamic relay neurons have transmission and burst modes of firing. (A) During transmission mode, which operates mainly during wakefulness, individual neurons in the thalamus fire single spikes in patterns that reflect their incoming afferent inputs. This correlates with a desynchronized electroencephalogram. (B) During burst mode, the thalamic neurons are hyperpolarized by gamma-aminobutyric acid (GABA)-ergic afferents, deinactivating a low-threshold calcium current with a long plateau. This brings the cell above the threshold for firing sodium action potentials, which are fired in a burst, until this is terminated by a calcium-activated potassium current that hyperpolarizes and silences the cell. These bursts tend to fire rhythmically, in correspondence with high-voltage slow waves in the EEG, which reflect large volleys of synchronized excitatory inputs reaching cortical dendrites. (From Saper, C. Brain stem modulation of sensation, movement, and consciousness. Chapter 45 in: Kandel, ER, Schwartz, JH, Jessel, TM. *Principles of Neural Science.* 4th ed. McGraw-Hill, New York, 2000, pp. 871–909. By permission of McGraw-Hill.)

(continued)

Box 1–2 The Thalamus, Basal Forebrain, and Generation of EEG Waves (cont.)

membrane potential of the cells is hyperpolarized, the less frequent but longer the bursts become.

The bursting behavior of neurons in the thalamic relay nuclei, which are a major source of cortical inputs, is often thought to be a major source of cortical EEG. The synchrony is credited to the thalamic reticular nucleus, which is a thin sheet of GABAergic neurons that covers the thalamus like a shroud. Thalamic axons on their way to the cerebral cortex, and cortical projections to the thalamus, give off collaterals to the reticular nucleus as they pass through it. Neurons in the reticular nucleus provide GABAergic inputs to the thalamic relay nuclei, which hyperpolarizes them and sets them into bursting mode.

However, there is evidence that the synchrony of EEG rhythms across the cerebral cortex is due in large part to corticocortical connections, and that even isolated slabs of cortex can set up rhythmic slow-wave potentials.[26] Recent evidence suggests that the basal forebrain may play a critical role in entraining cortical rhythmic activity. Basal forebrain neurons also fire in bursts that are time-locked to cortical rhythms. In addition, cell-specific lesions of the basal forebrain can eliminate fast cortical rhythms, including those associated with wakefulness and rapid eye movement (REM) sleep, whereas large cell-specific thalamic lesions have surprisingly little effect on the cortical EEG.[27]

Thus, the waveforms of the cortical EEG appear to be due to complex interactions among the burst neurons in the thalamus, cortex, and basal forebrain, all of which receive substantial inputs from the ascending arousal system.

---

a wakeful state.[32] Thus, the lower brainstem was thought to play a synchronizing, or sleep-promoting, role.[33] Transections from the rostral pons forward produced EEG slowing and behavioral unresponsiveness. Periods of forebrain arousal returned after several days if the animals were kept alive. However, it is clear that the slab of tissue from the rostral pons through the caudal midbrain (the mesopontine tegmentum) contains neural structures that are critically important to forebrain arousal, at least in the acute setting.

At the time, little was known about the origins of ascending projections from the mesopontine tegmentum to the forebrain, and the arousal effect was attributed to neurons in the reticular formation. However, more recent studies have shown that projections from the mesopontine tegmentum to the forebrain arise from several well-defined populations of neurons. The major source of mesopontine afferents that span the entire thalamus is a collection of cholinergic neurons that form two large clusters, the pedunculopontine and laterodorsal tegmen-

tal nuclei.[34] These neurons project through the paramedian midbrain reticular formation to the relay nuclei of the thalamus (which innervate specific cortical regions), as well as the midline and intralaminar nuclei (which innervate the entire cortex more diffusely), and the reticular nucleus. As noted in Box 1–2, the reticular nucleus plays a critical role in regulating thalamocortical transmission by profoundly hyperpolarizing thalamic relay neurons via $GABA_B$ receptors.[35] Cholinergic inputs in turn hyperpolarize the reticular nucleus. Other neurons in the cholinergic pedunculopontine and laterodorsal tegmental nuclei send axons into the lateral hypothalamus, where they may contact populations of neurons with diffuse cortical projections (see below). Neurons in the pedunculopontine and laterodorsal tegmental nuclei fire fastest during REM sleep (see Box 1–3) and wakefulness,[36] two conditions that are characterized by a low-voltage, fast (desynchronized) EEG. They slow down during non-REM (NREM) sleep, when the EEG is dominated by high-voltage slow waves (Figure B1–3A).

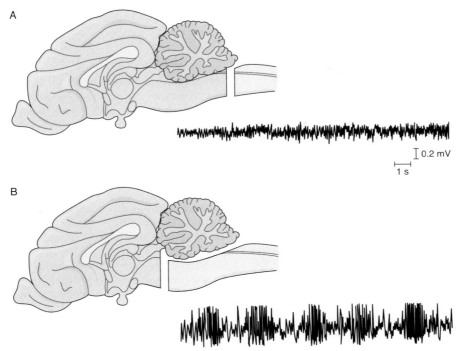

Figure 1–1. Electroencephalogram (EEG) from a cat in which Frederic Bremer transected the cervicomedullary junction (A), showing a normal, desynchronized waking activity. However, after a transection at the midcollicular level (B), the EEG consisted of higher voltage slow waves, more typical of sleep or coma. (From Saper, C. Brain stem modulation of sensation, movement, and consciousness. Chapter 45 in: Kandel, ER, Schwartz, JH, Jessel, TM. *Principles of Neural Science*. 4th ed. McGraw-Hill, New York, 2000, pp. 871–909. By permission of McGraw-Hill.)

In addition, at the mesopontine level the brainstem contains at least three different monoamine groups whose axons project through the hypothalamus to the cerebral cortex.[42] The noradrenergic locus coeruleus projects through the paramedian midbrain reticular formation and the lateral hypothalamus, innervating the entire cerebral cortex diffusely.[43] Serotoninergic neurons in the dorsal and median raphe nuclei project through a similar course.[44] Mixed in with the serotoninergic neurons are a smaller number of dopaminergic cells, which are an extension of the ventral tegmental dopamine group along the midline of the midbrain, into the area under the cerebral aqueduct.[45] These dopaminergic neurons also project through the paramedian midbrain reticular formation. Some of them innervate the midline and intralaminar nuclei of the thalamus, and others pass through the lateral hypothalamus to the basal forebrain and prefrontal cortex. Evidence from single-unit recording studies in behaving animals

indicates that neurons in these monoaminergic nuclei are most active during wakefulness, slow down during slow-wave sleep, and stop almost completely during REM sleep.[46–49]

Application of monoaminergic neurotransmitters to cortical neurons produces complex responses.[35,50–52] In most cases, there is inhibition resulting in a decrease in background firing, although firing induced by the specific stimulus to which the neuron is best tuned may not be reduced to as great a degree as background firing. In an awake and aroused individual, this alteration in firing may result in an improvement in signal-to-noise ratio, which may be critical in sharpening cortical information processing to avoid misperception of stimuli, such as occurs during a delirious state.

Although the cholinergic and monoaminergic neurons in the mesopontine tegmentum have traditionally been thought to play a major role in regulating wake-sleep states, lesions of these cell groups have relatively little effect on wake-sleep states or cortical EEG.[53] Recent studies

Box 1–3 Wake-Sleep States

In the early days of EEG recording, it was widely assumed that sleep, like coma, represented a period of brain inactivity. Hence, it was not surprising when the EEG appearance of sleep was found to resemble the high-voltage, slow waves that appear during coma. However, in 1953, Aserinsky and Kleitman[37] reported the curious observation that, when they recorded the EEG as well as the electromyogram (EMG) and the electro-oculogram (EOG) overnight, their subjects would periodically enter a state of sleep in which their eyes would move and their EEG would appear to be similar to waking states, yet their eyes were closed and they were deeply unresponsive to external stimuli.[37,38]

This condition of REM sleep has also been called desynchronized sleep (from the appearance of the EEG) as well as paradoxical sleep. More detailed study of the course of a night of sleep revealed that the REM and NREM periods tend to alternate in a rhythmic pattern through the night.[39–41]

During active wakefulness, the EEG gives the appearance of small, desynchronized waves and the EMG is active, indicating muscle activity associated with waking behavior. In quiet wakefulness, the EEG often begins to synchronize, with 8- to 12-Hz alpha waves predominating, particularly posteriorly over the hemisphere. Muscle tone may diminish as well. As sleep begins, the EEG rhythm drops to the 4- to 7-Hz theta range, muscle tone is further diminished, and slowly roving eye movements emerge (stage I NREM). The appearance of sleep spindles (waxing and waning runs of alpha frequency waves) and large waves in the 1- to 3-Hz delta range, called K complexes, denotes the onset of stage II NREM. The subject may then pass into the deeper stages of NREM, sometimes called slow-wave sleep, in which delta waves become a progressively more prominent (stage III) and then dominant (stage IV) feature. During these periods, eye movements are few and muscle tone drops to very low levels. This usually takes about 45 to 60 minutes, and then the subject often will gradually emerge from the first bout of slow-wave sleep to stage I again.

At this point, the first bout of REM sleep of the night often occurs. The subject abruptly transitions into a desynchronized, low-voltage EEG, with rapid and

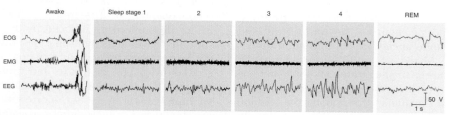

Figure B1–3A. The main features of a polysomnogram showing the eye movements (electro-oculogram [EOG]), muscle tone (electromyogram [EMG]), and electroencephalogram (EEG) across the different stages of sleep and wakefulness. During wakefulness, the EEG is desynchronized, the EMG is active, and there are spontaneous eye movements. During non-rapid eye movement (NREM) sleep, the EEG becomes progressively slower, the EMG less active, and eye movements slow down or become slowly roving. During REM sleep, there is a rapid transition to a desynchronized EEG, and irregular, rapid eye movements, but the EMG becomes minimal, consistent with atonia. (From Rechtschaffen, A, and Siegel, J. Sleep and dreaming. Chapter 47 in: Kandel, ER, Schwartz, JH, Jessel, TM. *Principles of Neural Science.* 4th ed. McGraw-Hill, New York, 2000, pp. 936–947. By permission of McGraw-Hill.)

(continued)

vigorous eye movements and virtually complete loss of muscle tone, except in the muscles of respiration. The first bout of REM sleep during the night typically lasts only 5 to 10 minutes, and then the subject will transition into stage I NREM, and again begin to descend gradually into deeper stages of NREM sleep.

As the night progresses, the subject typically will spend progressively less time in the deeper stages of NREM sleep, and more time in REM sleep, so that most of the REM sleep for the night comes in the last few bouts. Spontaneous awakenings during the night typically occur from the lighter stages of NREM sleep. Active dreams

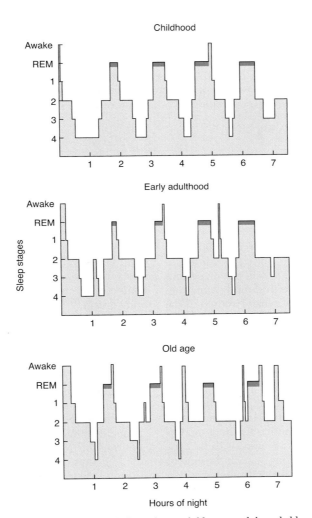

Figure B1–3B. The stages of sleep through the night in a child, young adult, and older person. There is usually regular progression from wakefulness through the stages of non-rapid eye movement (NREM) sleep into its deepest stages, then progression back to light NREM sleep before the first REM episode of the night. With successive cycles through the night, the amount of deeper NREM sleep becomes less, and the amount of REM becomes greater. With aging, the amount of deep NREM sleep diminishes, and sleep fragmentation with more frequent awakenings is seen. (From Rechtschaffen, A, and Siegel, J. Sleep and dreaming. Chapter 47 in: Kandel, ER, Schwartz, JH, Jessel, TM. *Principles of Neural Science*. 4th ed. McGraw-Hill, New York, 2000, pp. 936–947. By permission of McGraw-Hill.)

(*continued*)

Box 1–3 Wake-Sleep States (cont.)

occur predominantly during REM sleep, although many subjects report passive dreams and ideation during NREM sleep as well.

This pattern, which is typical of young adults, changes dramatically across a lifetime. Infants spend much more time asleep, and much more time in the deeper stages of NREM sleep, than adults. The amount of stages III and IV NREM sleep diminishes as children enter puberty, and it may not occur at all in some older adults. Thus, phenomena such as night terrors, bed wetting, and sleep walking tend to occur mainly during slow-wave sleep in children but disappear as the children become older and spend less time in those sleep stages. Most sedative drugs are $GABA_A$ receptor agonists that acutely increase the amount of time spent in the lighter stages of NREM sleep, but there may be little time spent in stages III or IV of NREM or in REM sleep. These drugs are thought to act directly on the arousal system, inhibiting the firing of its neurons. Newer drugs such as gaboxadol, which acts on a specific class of $GABA_A$ receptors containing delta subunits, may allow activation of the endogenous sleep system of the brain, and produce a pattern of sleep including more deep slow waves and more REM sleep.

by Lu and Saper (unpublished) have focused on neurons in the mesopontine tegmentum that provide inputs to the basal forebrain, which is critical for maintaining a wakeful state. Populations of neurons in the pre-locus coeruleus area and medial parabrachial nucleus have intense inputs to the basal forebrain. Cell-specific lesions of these neurons produce profound coma, suggesting that they may be a major source of the ascending arousal influence.

In addition, along the course of the ascending cholinergic and monoaminergic axons through the rostral midbrain reticular formation, there are many additional neurons that project to the thalamic relay, midline, and intralaminar nuclei.[34] Most of these neurons appear to be glutamatergic, and they may amplify the arousal signal that arises in the mesopontine tegmentum. On the other hand, they do not appear to be capable of maintaining a waking state in the case of acute loss of the influence from the mesopontine neurons.

Along the course of the ascending arousal systems, as they pass through the hypothalamus, are several hypothalamic cell groups that augment the ascending projection to the basal forebrain and cerebral cortex. These include histaminergic neurons in the tuberomammillary nucleus as well as several populations of neurons in the lateral hypothalamic area, all of which project diffusely to the cerebral cortex and

innervate the intralaminar and midline thalamus.[54] There is considerable evidence that the histaminergic input in particular is important for maintaining a wakeful state. Histamine H_1 blockers impair wakefulness in both animals and humans,[55] and transgenic mice lacking H_1 receptors have impairment of arousal responses induced by intraventricular injection of the peptide orexin.[56] Transgenic mice lacking histidine decarboxylase show a deficit in wakefulness induced by a novel environment, and mice injected with an inhibitor of this key enzyme for histamine synthesis similarly show less wakefulness.[57]

Some of the lateral hypothalamic neurons contain orexin,[58] a peptide that is associated with arousal, and others contain melanin-concentrating hormone[59,60] or GABA.[61] Many neurons in the lateral hypothalamic area, including those that contain orexin, fire fastest during wakefulness and slow down during both slow-wave and REM sleep.[62,63] Alternatively, the firing of some lateral hypothalamic neurons, which are likely to contain melanin-concentrating hormone, increases during REM sleep.[38,64,65]

In addition, the ascending monoaminergic and hypothalamic projections pass through the basal forebrain, and along their pathway to the cerebral cortex, they encounter and are augmented further by additional populations of

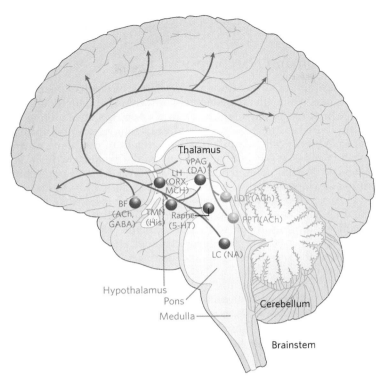

Figure 1–2. A summary diagram of the ascending arousal system. The cholinergic system, shown in yellow, provides the main input to the relay and reticular nuclei of the thalamus from the upper brainstem. This inhibits the reticular nucleus and activates the thalamic relay nuclei, putting them into transmission mode for relaying sensory information to the cerebral cortex. The cortex is activated simultaneously by a series of direct inputs, shown in red. These include monoaminergic inputs from the upper brainstem and posterior hypothalamus, such as noradrenaline (NA) from the locus coeruleus (LC), serotonin (5-HT) from the dorsal and median raphe nuclei, dopamine (DA) from the ventral periaqueductal gray matter (vPAG), and histamine (His) from the tuberomammillary nucleus (TMN); peptidergic inputs from the hypothalamus such as orexin (ORX) and melanin-concentrating hormone (MCH) both from the lateral hypothalamus (LH); and both cholinergic (ACh) and gamma-aminobutyric acid (GABA)-ergic inputs from the basal forebrain (BF). Activation of the brainstem yellow pathway in the absence of the red pathways occurs during rapid eye movement (REM) sleep, resulting in the cortex entering a dreaming state. LDT, laterodorsal tegmental nuclei; PPT, pedunculopontine. (From Saper, CB, Scammell, TE, Lu J. Hypothalamic regulation of sleep and circadian rhythms. *Nature* 437:1257–1263, 2005. By permission of Nature Publishing Group.)

cholinergic and noncholinergic neurons in the magnocellular basal forebrain nuclei.[76] These large cholinergic neurons receive afferents from virtually all of the hypothalamic and monoaminergic brainstem ascending systems and accompany them to diffusely innervate the cerebral cortex.[77,78] However, the pattern of termination of the cholinergic neurons is more specific than the monoamine inputs to the cortex. Whereas axons from individual monoaminergic neurons typically ramify widely in the cerebral cortex, axons from basal forebrain cholinergic neurons each innervate a patch of cortex of only a few millimeters in diameter.[42,54] Recordings from basal forebrain neurons in rats across the wake-sleep cycle indicate that they have a wide range

of activity patterns. Many are most active during wakefulness or during slow-wave sleep, and they fire in bursts that correlate with EEG wave patterns.[79] Interestingly, in behaving monkeys, basal forebrain neuron firing correlates best with the reward phase of complex behaviors, suggesting that these neurons may be involved in some highly specific aspect of arousal, such as focusing attention on rewarding tasks, rather than in the general level of cortical activity.[80,81]

Thus, the ascending arousal system consists of multiple ascending pathways originating in the mesopontine tegmentum, but augmented by additional inputs at virtually every level through which it passes on its way to the basal forebrain, thalamus, and cerebral cortex. These

Box 1–4 Orexin and Narcolepsy

From its first description by Gelineau in 1880,[66] narcolepsy had puzzled clinicians and scientists alike. Although Gelineau included within his definition a wide range of disorders with excessive daytime sleepiness, Gowers has been credited with limiting the term to cases with brief periods of sleep that interrupt a normal waking state. Kinnier Wilson firmly identified it with attacks of cataplexy, during which "the patient's knees give way and he may sink to the ground, without any loss of consciousness."[24] Wilson pointed out that narcolepsy had been considered a very rare condition of which he had seen only a few cases during the first 20 years of his practice, but that in the mid-1920s there was a sudden increase in the number of cases, so that he had seen six within a year in 1927; Spiller reported seeing three within a year in 1926. Wilson opined that the epidemic of new cases of narcolepsy in those years was due to the worldwide epidemic of encephalitis from about 1918 to 1925. However, the prevalence of narcolepsy has remained relatively high, with a current rate of one per 2,000 population, and it has its peak incidence during the second and third decades of life.[38]

Over the years, additional features of narcolepsy were described. About half of patients reported sleep paralysis, a curious state of inability to move during the transition from sleep to wakefulness or from wakefulness to sleep.[38] However, up to 20% of normal individuals may also experience this condition occasionally. More characteristic of narcolepsy, but occurring in only about 20% of cases, are episodes of hypnagogic hallucinations, during which the patient experiences a vivid, cartoon-like hallucination, with movement and action, against a background of wakefulness. The patient can distinguish that the hallucination is not real. EEG and EMG recordings during sleep and wakefulness show that narcoleptic patients fall asleep more frequently during the day, but they also awaken more frequently at night, so that they get about the same amount of sleep as normal individuals. However, they often enter into REM sleep very soon after sleep onset (short-onset REM periods [SOREMPs]), and during cataplexy attacks they show muscle atonia consistent with intrusion of a REM-like state into consciousness. On a multiple sleep latency test (MSLT), where the patient lies down in a quiet room five times during the course of the day at 2-hour intervals, narcoleptics typically fall asleep much faster than normal individuals (often in less than 5 minutes on repeated occasions) and show SOREMPs, which normal individuals rarely, if ever, experience.

There is a clear genetic predisposition to narcolepsy, as individuals with a first-degree relative with the disorder are 40 times more likely to develop it themselves.[38] However, there are clearly environmental factors involved, even among monozygotic twins; if one twin develops narcolepsy, the other will develop it only about 25% of the time. HLA allele DQB1*0602 is found in 88% to 98% of individuals with narcolepsy with cataplexy, but only in about 12% of white Americans and 38% of African Americans in the general population.

Scientists worked fruitlessly for decades to unravel the pathophysiology of this mysterious illness, until in 1999 two dramatic and simultaneous findings suddenly brought the problem into focus. The previous year, two groups of scientists, Masashi Yanagisawa and colleagues at the University of Texas Southwestern Medical School, and Greg Sutcliffe and coworkers at the Scripps Institute, had simultaneously identified a new pair of peptide neurotransmitters made by neurons in the lateral hypothalamus, which Yanagisawa called "orexins" (based on the pre-

(continued)

sumption of a role in feeding)[67] and Sutcliffe called "hypocretins" (because it was a hypothalamic peptide with a sequence similar to secretin).[68] Yanagisawa further showed that the type 1 orexin receptor had 10-fold specificity for orexin A, whereas the type 2 receptor was activated equally well by both orexins.[69] The orexin neurons in the lateral hypothalamus were found to have wide-ranging projections from the cerebral cortex to the spinal cord, much like the monoaminergic neurons in the brainstem.[58,70]

When Yanagisawa's group prepared mice in which the orexin gene had been deleted, they initially found that the animals had normal sleep behavior during the day.[70] However, when the mice were observed under infrared video monitoring during the night, they showed intermittent attacks of behavioral arrest during which they would suddenly fall over onto their side, twitch a bit, and lie still for a minute or two, before just as suddenly getting up and resuming their normal behaviors. EEG and EMG recordings demonstrated that these attacks have the appearance of cataplexy (sudden loss of muscle tone, EEG showing either an awake pattern or large amounts of theta activity typical of rodents during REM sleep). The animals also had short-onset REM periods when asleep, another hallmark of narcolepsy.

At the same time, Emmanuel Mignot had been working at Stanford for nearly a decade to determine the cause of genetically inherited canine narcolepsy. He finally determined that the dogs had a genetic defect in the type 2 orexin receptor.[71]

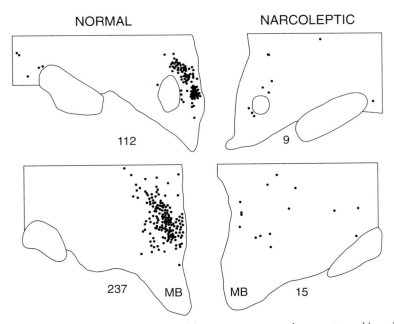

Figure B1–4A. Narcolepsy is caused by loss of the orexin neurons in the posterior and lateral hypothalamus of the human brain. The panels plot the location of orexin neurons in the posterior hypothalamus in two subjects with normal brains on the left and two patients with narcolepsy on the right. There is typically about 90% loss of orexin neurons in patients who have narcolepsy with cataplexy. (From Thannickal, TC, Moore, RY, Nienhuis, R, et al. Reduced number of hypocretin neurons in human narcolepsy. *Neuron* 27, 469–474, 2000. By permission of Elsevier B.V.)

(continued)

Box 1–4 Orexin and Narcolepsy (cont.)

The nearly simultaneous publication of the two results established firmly that narcolepsy could be produced in animals by impairment of orexin signaling.

Over the following year, it became clear that most humans with narcolepsy do not have a genetic defect either of the orexin gene or of its receptors, although a few cases with onset during infancy and particularly severe narcolepsy were found to be due to this cause.[72] Instead, postmortem studies showed that narcoleptics with cataplexy lose about 90% of their orexin neurons, and that the spinal fluid levels of orexin often are very low.[72–74] However, the nearby melanin-concentrating hormone neurons were not affected. This specificity suggested either an autoimmune or neurodegenerative cause of the orexin cell loss.

The presence of type 2 orexin receptors on histaminergic neurons, type 1 receptors in the locus coeruleus, and both types of orexin receptors on serotoninergic and other neurons in the pontine reticular formation[75] suggests that one or more of these targets may be critical for regulating the transitions to REM sleep that are disrupted in patients with narcolepsy.

different pathways may fire independently under a variety of different conditions, modulating the functional capacities of cortical neurons during a wide range of behavioral states.

Behavioral State Switching

An important feature of the ascending arousal system is its interconnectivity: the cell groups that contribute to the system also maintain substantial connections with other components of the system. Another important property of the system is that nearly all of these components receive inputs from the ventrolateral preoptic nucleus.[82–84] Ventrolateral preoptic neurons contain the inhibitory transmitters GABA and galanin; they fire fastest during sleep.[40,83,85] Lesions of the ventrolateral preoptic nucleus cause a state of profound insomnia in animals,[86,87] and such lesions undoubtedly accounted for the insomniac patients described by von Economo[19] (see Box 1–1).

The ventrolateral preoptic neurons also receive extensive inhibitory inputs from many components of the ascending arousal system. This mutual inhibition between the ventrolateral preoptic nucleus and the ascending arousal system has interesting implications for the mechanisms of the natural switching from wakefulness to sleep over the course of the day, and from slow-wave to REM sleep over the course

of the night. Electrical engineers call a circuit in which the two sides inhibit each other a "flip-flop" switch.[84] Each side of a flip-flop circuit is self-reinforcing (i.e., when the neurons are firing, they inhibit neurons that would otherwise turn them off, and hence they are disinhibited by their own activity). As a result, firing by each side of the circuit tends to be self-perpetuating, and the circuit tends to spend nearly all of its time with either one side or the other in ascendancy, and very little time in transition. These sharp boundaries between wakefulness and sleep are a key feature of normal physiology, as it would be maladaptive for animals to walk around half-asleep or to spend long portions of their normal sleep cycle half-awake.

REM sleep is a stage of sleep in which the brain enters a very different state from the high-voltage slow waves that characterize NREM sleep. As indicated in Box 1–3, during REM sleep, the forebrain shows low-voltage, fast EEG activity similar to wakefulness, and the ascending cholinergic system is even more active than during a wakeful state. However, the ascending monoaminergic systems cease firing virtually completely during REM sleep,[46–49] so that the increased thalamocortical transmission seen during REM sleep falls upon a cerebral cortex that lacks the priming to maintain a wakeful state. As a result, REM sleep is sometimes called paradoxical sleep because the cortex gives an EEG appearance of wakefulness, and yet the

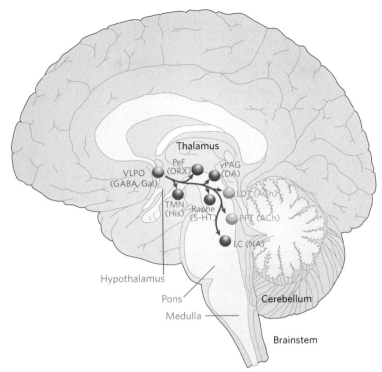

Figure 1–3. The ventrolateral preoptic nucleus (VLPO), shown in purple, inhibits the components of the ascending arousal system during sleep. VLPO neurons contain both gamma-aminobutyric acid (GABA) and an inhibitory peptide, galanin, and send axons to most of the cell groups that compose the ascending arousal system. This unique relationship allows the VLPO neurons effectively to turn off the arousal systems during sleep. Loss of VLPO neurons results in profound insomnia. 5-HT, serotonin; ACh, acetylcholine; DA, dopamine; Gal, ; His, histamine; LC, locus coeruleus; LDT, laterodorsal tegmental nuclei; NA, noradrenaline; ORX, orexin; PeF, ; PPT, pedunculopontine; TMN, tuberomammillary nucleus; vPAG, ventral periaqueductal gray matter. (From Saper, CB, Scammell, TE, Lu J. Hypothalamic regulation of sleep and circadian rhythms. *Nature* 437:1257–1263, 2005. By permission of Nature Publishing Group.)

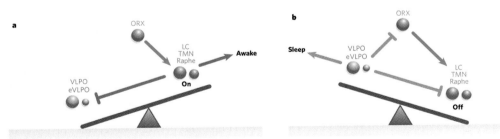

Figure 1–4. A diagram of the flip-flop relationship between the ventrolateral preoptic nucleus (VLPO), which promotes sleep, and several monoaminergic cell groups that contribute to the arousal system, including the locus coeruleus (LC), the tuberomammillary nucleus (TMN), and raphe nuclei. During wakefulness (a), the orexin neurons (ORX) are active, stimulating the monoamine nuclei, which both cause arousal and inhibit the VLPO to prevent sleep. During sleep (b), the VLPO and extended VLPO (eVLPO) inhibit the monoamine groups and the orexin neurons, thus preventing arousal. This mutually inhibitory relationship ensures that transitions between wake and sleep are rapid and complete. (From Saper, CB, Scammell, TE, Lu J. Hypothalamic regulation of sleep and circadian rhythms. *Nature* 437:1257–1263, 2005. By permission of Nature Publishing Group.)

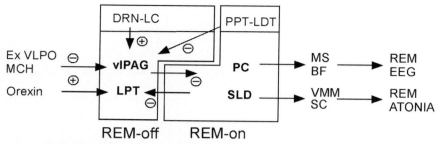

Figure 1–5. The control elements for rapid eye movement (REM) sleep also form a flip-flop switch. Gamma-aminobutyric acid (GABA)-ergic REM-off neurons in the ventrolateral periaqueductal gray matter (vlPAG) and the lateral pontine tegmentum (LPT) inhibit the REM-on neurons in the sublaterodorsal (SLD) and the precoeruleus (PC) areas, whereas GABA-ergic SLD neurons inhibit the vlPAG and the LPT. This mutual inhibition forms a second flip-flop switch that regulates transitions into and out of REM sleep, which also are generally rapid and complete. Other modulatory systems, such as the extended ventrolateral preoptic nucleus (Ex VLPO) and the melanin-concentrating hormone (MCH) and orexin neurons in the hypothalamus, regulate REM sleep by their inputs to this switch. Similarly, the monoaminergic dorsal raphe nucleus (DRN) and locus coeruleus (LC) inhibit REM sleep by activating the REM-off neurons, and cholinergic neurons in the pedunculopontine (PPT) and laterodorsal tegmental nuclei (LDT) activate REM sleep by inhibiting neurons in the REM-off region. Neurons in the SLD cause motor atonia during REM sleep by excitatory inputs to inhibitory interneurons in the ventromedial medulla (VMM) and the spinal cord (SC), which inhibit alpha motor neurons. Neurons in the PC contact the medial septum (MS) and basal forebrain (BF), which drive the electroencephalogram (EEG) phenomena associated with REM sleep. (Modified from Lu, Sherman, Devor, et al.,[53] by permission.)

individual is profoundly unresponsive to external stimuli.

A second flip-flop switch in the pons for switching from NREM to REM sleep (and back again) has recently been identified in the rostral pons. Many GABAergic neurons in the extended part of the ventrolateral preoptic nucleus are specifically active during REM sleep, suggesting that they inhibit a population of REM-off neurons.[88] In addition, the orexin neurons in the lateral hypothalamus are excitatory, but their firing inhibits REM sleep, suggesting that they may activate REM-off neurons, as patients or animals with narcolepsy who lack orexin neurons transition into REM sleep exceptionally quickly.[70,89] By searching for the intersection of these two pathways, a population of neurons was defined in the rostral pons, including the ventrolateral periaqueductal gray matter and the lateral pontine tegmentum at the level where they are adjacent to the dorsal raphe nucleus. These sites contain many GABAergic neurons, and lesions of this region increase REM sleep, confirming a REM-off influence.[53] GABAergic neurons in the REM-off area innervate an adjacent region including the sublaterodorsal nucleus and pre-coeruleus region that contain REM-active neurons. This REM-on region contains two types of neurons. GABAergic neurons, mainly in the sublaterodorsal nucleus, project back to the REM-off area. This produces a flip-

flop switch relationship accounting for the tendency for transitions into and out of REM sleep to be relatively abrupt. A second population of neurons is glutamatergic. Glutamatergic REM-on neurons in the sublaterodorsal nucleus project to the brainstem and spinal cord, where they are thought to be responsible for the motor manifestations of REM sleep, including atonia and perhaps the rapid eye movements that are the hallmarks of the state. Glutamatergic REM-on neurons in the coeruleus region target the basal forebrain where they appear to be critical for maintaining EEG phenomena associated with REM sleep.

Cholinergic and monoaminergic influences may have a modulatory effect on REM sleep by playing upon this flip-flop switch mechanism. Although lesions of these systems do not have a major effect on REM sleep, overactivity may have quite dramatic effects. For example, injections of cholinomimetic agents into the region containing the REM switch can trigger prolonged bouts of a REM-like state in animals.[90] Whether this is due to activating REM-on neurons or inhibiting REM-off neurons (or both) is not known. On the other hand, patients who take antidepressants that are either serotonin or norepinephrine reuptake inhibitors (or both) have very little REM sleep. This effect may be due to the excess monoamines activating the REM-off neurons or inhibiting the REM-on neurons (or both) and thereby locking the individual out of REM sleep.[70,89]

Relationship of Coma to Sleep

Because the brain enters a state of quiescence during sleep on a daily basis, it is natural to wonder whether coma may not be a pathologic entrance into the sleep state. In fact, both impaired states of consciousness and NREM sleep are characterized by EEG patterns that include increased amounts of high-voltage slow waves. Both conditions are due, ultimately, to lack of activity by the ascending arousal system. However, in sleep, the lack of activity is due to an intrinsically regulated inhibition of the arousal system, whereas in coma the impairment of the arousal system is due either to damage to the arousal system or to diffuse dysfunction of its diencephalic or forebrain targets.

Because sleep is a regulated state, it has several characteristics that distinguish it from coma. A key feature of sleep is that the subject can be aroused from it to wakefulness. Patients who are obtunded may be aroused briefly, but they require continuous stimulation to maintain a wakeful state, and comatose patients may not be arousable at all. In addition, sleeping subjects undergo a variety of postural adjustments, including yawning, stretching, and turning, which are not seen in patients with pathologic impairment of level of consciousness.

The most important difference, however, is the lack of cycling between NREM and REM sleep in patients in coma. Sleeping subjects undergo a characteristic pattern of waxing and waning depth of NREM sleep during the night, punctuated by bouts of REM sleep, usually beginning when the NREM sleep reaches its lightest phase. The monotonic high-voltage slow waves in the EEG of the comatose patient indicate that although coma may share with NREM sleep the property of a low level of activity in the ascending arousal systems, it is a fundamentally different and pathologic state.

The Cerebral Hemispheres and Conscious Behavior

The cerebral cortex acts like a massively parallel processor that breaks down the components of sensory experience into a wide array of abstractions that are analyzed independently and in parallel during normal conscious experience.[42] This organizational scheme predicts many of the properties of consciousness, and it sheds light on how these many parallel streams of cortical activity are reassimilated into a single conscious state.

The cerebral neocortex of mammals, from rodents to humans, consists of a sheet of neurons divided into six layers. Inputs from the thalamic relay nuclei arrive mainly in layer IV, which consists of small granule cells. Inputs from other cortical areas arrive into layers II, III, and V. Layers II and III consist of small- to medium-sized pyramidal cells, arrayed with their apical dendrites pointing toward the cortical surface. Layer V contains much larger pyramidal cells, also in the same orientation. The apical dendrites of the pyramidal cells in layers II, III, and V receive afferents from thalamic and cortical axons that course through layer I parallel to the cortical surface. Layer VI comprises a varied collection of neurons of different shapes and sizes (the polymorph layer). Layer III provides most projections to other cortical areas, whereas layer V provides long-range projections to the brainstem and spinal cord. The deep part of layer V projects to the striatum. Layer VI provides the reciprocal output from the cortex back to the thalamus.[91]

It has been known since the 1960s that the neurons in successive layers along a line drawn through the cerebral cortex perpendicular to the pial surface all tend to be concerned with similar sensory or motor processes.[92,93] These neurons form columns, of about 0.3 to 0.5 mm in width, in which the nerve cells share incoming signals in a vertically integrated manner. Recordings of neurons in each successive layer of a column of visual cortex, for example, all respond to bars of light in a particular orientation in a particular part of the visual field. Columns of neurons send information to one another and to higher order association areas via projection cells in layer III and, to a lesser extent, layer V.[94] In this way, columns of neurons are able to extract progressively more complex and abstract information from an incoming sensory stimulus. For example, neurons in a primary visual cortical area may be primarily concerned with simple lines, edges, and corners, but by integrating their inputs, a neuron in a higher order visual association area may

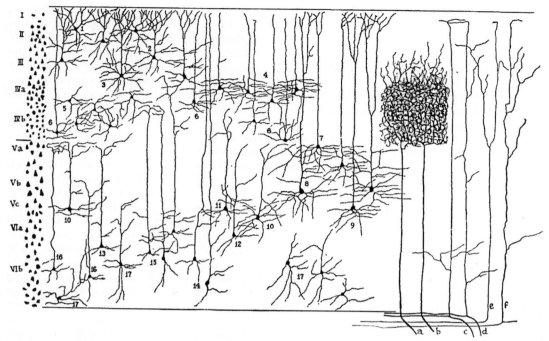

Figure 1–6. A summary drawing of the laminar organization of the neurons and inputs to the cerebral cortex. The neuronal layers of the cerebral cortex are shown at the left, as seen in a Nissl stain, and in the middle of the drawing as seen in Golgi stains. Layer I has few if any neurons. Layers II and III are composed of small pyramidal cells, and layer V of larger pyramidal cells. Layer IV contains very small granular cells, and layer VI, the polymorph layer, cells of multiple types. Axons from the thalamic relay nuclei (a, b) provide intense ramifications mainly in layer IV. Inputs from the "nonspecific system," which includes the ascending arousal system, ramify more diffusely, predominantly in layers II, III, and V (c, d). Axons from other cortical areas ramify mainly in layers II, III, and V (e, f). (From Lorente de No R. Cerebral cortex: architecture, intracortical connections, motor projections. In Fulton, JF. *Physiology of the Nervous System.* Oxford University Press, New York, 1938, pp. 291–340. By permission of Oxford University Press.)

respond only to a complex shape, such as a hand or a brush.

The organization of the cortical column does not vary much from mammals with the most simple cortex, such as rodents, to primates with much larger and more complex cortical development. The depth or width of a column, for example, is only marginally larger in a primate brain than in a rat brain. What has changed most across evolution has been the number of columns. The hugely enlarged sheet of cortical columns in a human brain provides the massively parallel processing power needed to perform a sonata on the piano, solve a differential equation, or send a rocket to another planet.

An important principle of cortical organization is that neurons in different areas of the cerebral cortex specialize in certain types of operations. In a young brain, before school age, it is possible for cortical functions to reorga-

nize themselves to an astonishing degree if one area of cortex is damaged. However, the organization of cortical information processing goes through a series of critical stages during development, in which the maturing cortex gives up a degree of plasticity but demonstrates improved efficiency of processing.[95,96] In adults, the ability to perform a specific cognitive process may be irretrievably assigned to a region of cortex, and when that area is damaged, the individual not only loses the ability to perform that operation, but also loses the very concept that the information of that type exists. Hence, the individual with a large right parietal infarct not only loses the ability to appreciate stimuli from the left side of space, but also loses the concept that there is a left side of space. We have witnessed a patient with a large right parietal lobe tumor who ate only the food on the right side of her plate; when done, she would get up and turn around to the right, until the remaining food appeared on her right side, as she was entirely unable to conceive that the plate or space itself had a left side. Similarly, a patient with aphasia due to damage to Wernicke's area in the dominant temporal lobe not only cannot appreciate the language symbol content of speech, but also can no longer comprehend that language symbols are an operative component of speech. Such a patient continues to speak meaningless babble and is surprised that others no longer understand his speech because the very concept that language symbols are embedded in speech eludes him.

This concept of fractional loss of consciousness is critical because it explains confusional states caused by focal cortical lesions. It is also a common observation by clinicians that, if the cerebral cortex is damaged in multiple locations by a multifocal disorder, it can eventually cease to function as a whole, producing a state of such severe cognitive impairment as to give the appearance of a global loss of consciousness. During a Wada test, a patient receives an injection of a short-acting barbiturate into the carotid artery to anesthetize one hemisphere so that its role in language can be assessed prior to cortical surgery. When the left hemisphere is acutely anesthetized, the patient gives the appearance of confusion and is typically placid but difficult to test due to the absence of language skills. When the patient recovers, he or she typically is amnestic for the event, as much of memory is encoded verbally. Following a right hemisphere injection, the patient also typically appears to be confused and is unable to orient to his or her surroundings, but can answer simple questions and perform simple commands. The experience also may not be remembered clearly, perhaps because of the sudden inability to encode visuospatial memory.

However, the patient does not appear to be unconscious when either hemisphere is acutely anesthetized. An important principle of examining patients with impaired consciousness is that the condition is not caused by a lesion whose acute effects are confined to a single hemisphere. A very large space-occupying lesion may simultaneously damage both hemispheres or may compress the diencephalon, causing impairment of consciousness, but an acute infarct of one hemisphere does not. Hence, loss of consciousness is not a typical feature of unilateral carotid disease unless both hemispheres

are supplied by a single carotid artery or the patient has had a subsequent seizure.

The concept of the cerebral cortex as a massively parallel processor introduces the question of how all of these parallel streams of information are eventually integrated into a single consciousness, a conundrum that has been called the binding problem.[97,98] Embedded in this question, however, is a supposition: that it is necessary to reassemble all aspects of our experience into a single whole so that they can be monitored by an internal being, like a small person or homunculus watching a television screen. Although most people believe that they experience consciousness in this way, there is no a priori reason why such a self-experience cannot be the neurophysiologic outcome of the massively parallel processing (i.e., the illusion of reassembly, without the brain actually requiring that to occur in physical space). For example, people experience the visual world as an unbroken scene. However, each of us has a pair of holes in the visual fields where the optic nerves penetrate the retina. This blind spot can be demonstrated by passing a small object along the visual horizon until it disappears. However, the visual field is "seen" by the conscious self as a single unbroken expanse, and this hole is papered over with whatever visual material borders it. If the brain can produce this type of conscious impression in the absence of reality, there is no reason to think that it requires a physiologic reassembly of other stimuli for presentation to a central homunculus. Rather, consciousness may be conceived as a property of the integrated activity of the two cerebral hemispheres and not in need of a separate physical manifestation.

Despite this view of consciousness as an "emergent" property of hemispheric information processing, the hemispheres do require a mechanism for arriving at a singularity of thought and action. If each of the independent information streams in the cortical parallel processor could separately command motor responses, human movement would be a hopeless confusion of mixed activities. A good example is seen in patients in whom the corpus callosum has been transected to prevent spread of epileptic seizures.[99] In such "split-brain" patients, the left hand may button a shirt and the right hand follow along right behind it unbuttoning. If independent action of the two hemispheres can be so disconcerting, one could only imagine the effect of each stream of cortical processing commanding its own plan of action.

The brain requires a funnel to narrow down the choices from all of the possible modes of action to the single plan of motor behavior that will be pursued. The physical substrate of this process is the basal ganglia. All cortical regions provide input to the striatum (caudate, putamen, nucleus accumbens, and olfactory tubercle). The output from the striatum is predominantly to the globus pallidus, which it inhibits by using the neurotransmitter GABA.[100,101] The pallidal output pathways, in turn, also are GABAergic and constitutively inhibit the motor thalamus, so that when the striatal inhibitory input to the pallidum is activated, movement is disinhibited. By constricting all motor responses that are not specifically activated by this system, the basal ganglia ensure a smooth and steady, unitary stream of action. Basal ganglia disorders that permit too much striatal disinhibition of movement (hyperkinetic movement disorders) result in the emergence of disconnected movements that are outside this unitary stream (e.g., tics, chorea, athetosis).

Similarly, the brain is capable of following only one line of thought at a time. The conscious self is prohibited even from seeing two equally likely versions of an optical illusion simultaneously (e.g., the classic case of the ugly woman vs. the beautiful woman illusion) (Figure 1–7). Rather, the self is aware of the two alternative visual interpretations alternately. Similarly, if it is necessary to pursue two different tasks at the same time, they are pursued alternately rather than simultaneously, until they become so automatic that they can be performed with little conscious thought. The striatal control of thought processes is implemented by the outflow from the ventral striatum to the ventral pallidum, which in turn inhibits the mediodorsal thalamic nucleus, the relay nucleus for the prefrontal cortex.[100,101] By disinhibiting prefrontal thought processes, the striatum ensures that a single line of thought and a unitary view of self will be expressed from the multipath network of the cerebral cortex.

An interesting philosophic question is raised by the hyperkinetic movement disorders, in which the tics, chorea, and athetosis are thought to represent "involuntary movements." But the use of the term "involuntary" again presupposes

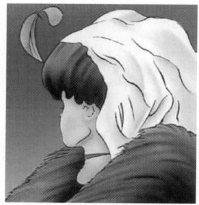

Figure 1–7. A classic optical illusion, illustrating the inability of the brain to view the same scene simultaneously in two different ways. The image of the ugly, older woman or the pretty younger woman may be seen alternately, but not at the same time, as the same visual elements are used in two different percepts. (From W.E. Hill, "My Wife and My Mother-in-Law," 1915, for *Puck* magazine. Used by permission. All rights reserved.)

a homunculus that is in control and making decisions. Instead, the interrelationship of involuntary movements, which the self feels "compelled" to make, with self-willed movements is complex. Patients with movement disorders often can inhibit the unwanted movements for a while, but feel uncomfortable doing so, and often report pleasurable release when they can carry out the action. Again, the conscious state is best considered as an emergent property of brain function, rather than directing it.

Similarly, hyperkinetic movement disorders may be associated with disinhibition of larger scale behaviors and even thought processes. In this view, thought disorders can be conceived as chorea (derailing) and dystonia (fixed delusions) of thought. Release of prefrontal cortex inhibition may even permit it to drive mental imagery, producing hallucinations. Under such conditions, we have a tendency to believe that somehow the conscious self is a homunculus that is being tricked by hallucinatory sensory experiences or is unable to command thought processes. In fact, it may be more accurate to view the sensory experience and the behavior as manifestations of an altered consciousness due to malfunction of the brain's machinery for maintaining a unitary flow of thought and action.

Neurologists tend to take the mechanistic perspective that all that we observe is due to ac-

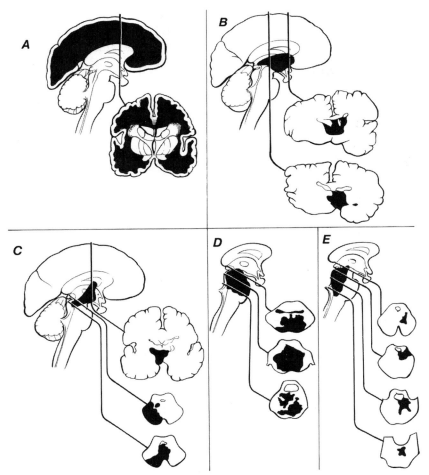

Figure 1–8. Brain lesions that cause coma. (A) Diffuse hemispheric damage, for example, due to hypoxic-ischemic encephalopathy (see Patient 1–1). (B) Diencephalic injury, as in a patient with a tumor destroying the hypothalamus. (C) Damage to the paramedian portion of the upper midbrain and caudal diencephalon, as in a patient with a tip of the basilar embolus. (D) High pontine and lower midbrain paramedian tegmental injury (e.g., in a case of basilar artery occlusion). (E) Pontine hemorrhage, because it produces compression of the surrounding brainstem, can cause dysfunction that extends beyond the area of the tissue loss. This case shows the residual area of injury at autopsy 7 months after a pontine hemorrhage. The patient was comatose during the first 2 months.

tion of the nervous system behaving according to fundamental principles. Hence, the evaluation of the comatose patient becomes an exercise in applying those principles to the evaluation of a human with brain failure.

Structural Lesions That Cause Altered Consciousness in Humans

To produce stupor or coma in humans, a disorder must damage or depress the function of either extensive areas of both cerebral hemispheres or the ascending arousal system, including the paramedian region of the upper brainstem or the diencephalon on both sides of the brain. Figure 1–8 illustrates examples of such lesions that may cause coma. Conversely, unilateral hemispheric lesions, or lesions of the brainstem at the level of the midpons or below, do not cause coma. Figure 1–9 illustrates several such cases that may cause profound sensory and motor deficits but do not impair consciousness.

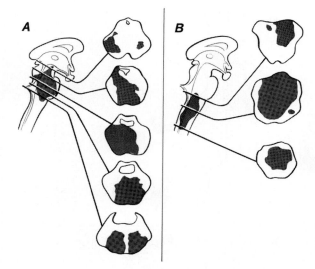

Figure 1–9. Lesions of the brainstem may be very large without causing coma if they do not involve the ascending arousal system bilaterally. (A) Even an extensive infarction at the mesopontine level that does not include the dorsolateral pons on one side and leaves intact the paramedian midbrain can result in preservation of consciousness. (B) Lesions at a low pontine and medullary level, even if they involve a hemorrhage, do not impair consciousness. (Patient 1–2, p. 33)

BILATERAL HEMISPHERIC DAMAGE

Bilateral and extensive damage to the cerebral cortex occurs most often in the context of hypoxic-ischemic insult. The initial response to loss of cerebral blood flow (CBF) or insufficient oxygenation of the blood includes loss of consciousness. Even if blood flow or oxygenation is restored after 5 or more minutes, there may be widespread cortical injury and neuronal loss even in the absence of frank infarction.[102,103] The typical appearance pathologically is that neurons in layers III and V (which receive the most glutamatergic input from other cortical areas) and in the CA1 region of the hippocampus (which receives extensive glutamatergic input from both the CA3 fields and the entorhinal cortex) demonstrate eosinophilia in the first few days after the injury. Later, the neurons undergo pyknosis and apoptotic cell death (Figure 1–10). The net result is pseudolaminar necrosis, in which the cerebral cortex and the CA1 region both are depopulated of pyramidal cells.

Alternatively, in some patients with less extreme cortical hypoxia, there may be a lucid interval in which the patient appears to recover, followed by a subsequent deterioration. Such a patient is described in the historical vignette on this and the following page. (Throughout this book we will use historical vignettes to describe cases that occurred before the modern era of neurologic diagnosis and treatment, in which

the natural history of a disorder unfolded in a way in which it would seldom do today. Fortunately, most such cases included pathologic assessment, which is also all too infrequent in modern cases.)

HISTORICAL VIGNETTE

Patient 1–1

A 59-year-old man was found unconscious in a room filled with natural gas. A companion already had died, apparently the result of an attempted double suicide. On admission the man was unresponsive. His blood pressure was 120/80 mm Hg, pulse 120, and respirations 18 and regular. His rectal temperature was 102°F. His stretch reflexes were hypoactive, and plantar responses were absent. Coarse rhonchi were heard throughout both lung fields.

He was treated with nasal oxygen and began to awaken in 30 hours. On the second hospital day he was alert and oriented. On the fourth day he was afebrile, his chest was clear, and he ambulated. The neurologic examination was normal, and an evaluation by a psychiatrist revealed a clear sensorium with "no evidence of organic brain damage." He was discharged to his relatives' care 9 days after the anoxic event.

At home he remained well for 2 days but then became quiet, speaking only when spoken to. The following day he merely shuffled about and res-

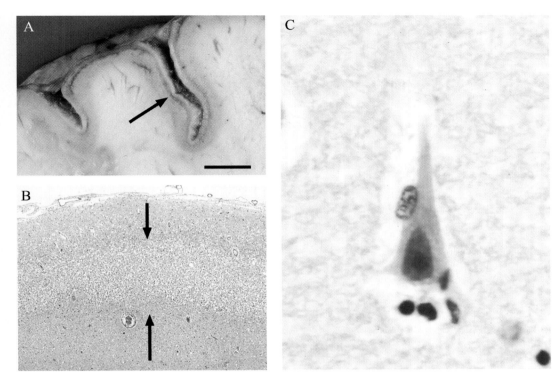

Figure 1–10. Hypoxia typically causes more severe damage to large pyramidal cells in the cerebral cortex and hippocampus compared to surrounding structures. (A) shows a low magnification view of the cerebral cortex illustrating pseudolaminar necrosis (arrow), which parallels the pial surface. At higher magnification (B), the area of necrosis involves layers II to V of the cerebral cortex, which contains the large pyramidal cells (region between the two arrows). (C) At high magnification, surviving neurons are pyknotic and eosinophilic, indicating hypoxic injury. Scale in A = 8 mm, B = 0.6 mm, and C = 15 micrometers.

ponded in monosyllables. The next day (13 days after the anoxia) he became incontinent and unable to walk, swallow, or chew. He neither spoke to nor recognized his family. He was admitted to a private psychiatric hospital with the diagnosis of depression. Deterioration continued, and 28 days after the initial anoxia he was readmitted to the hospital. His blood pressure was 170/100 mm Hg, pulse 100, respirations 24, and temperature 101°F. There were coarse rales at both lung bases. He perspired profusely and constantly. He did not respond to pain, but would open his eyes momentarily to loud sounds. His extremities were flexed and rigid, his deep tendon reflexes were hyperactive, and his plantar responses extensor. Laboratory studies, including examination of the spinal fluid, were normal. He died 3 days later.

An autopsy examination showed diffuse bronchopneumonia. The brain was grossly normal. There was no cerebral swelling. Coronal sections appeared normal with no evidence of pallidal necrosis. Histologically, neurons in the motor cortex,

hippocampus, cerebellum, and occipital lobes appeared generally well preserved, although a few sections showed minimal cytodegenerative changes and reduction of neurons. There was occasional perivascular lymphocytic infiltration. Pathologic changes were not present in blood vessels, nor was there any interstitial edema. The striking alteration was diffuse demyelination involving all lobes of the cerebral hemispheres and sparing only the arcuate fibers (the immediately subcortical portion of the cerebral white matter). Axons were also reduced in number but were better preserved than was the myelin. Oligodendroglia were preserved in demyelinated areas. Reactive astrocytes were considerably increased. The brainstem and cerebellum were histologically intact. The condition of delayed postanoxic cerebral demyelination observed in this patient is discussed at greater length in Chapter 5.

Another major class of patients with bilateral hemispheric damage causing coma is of those

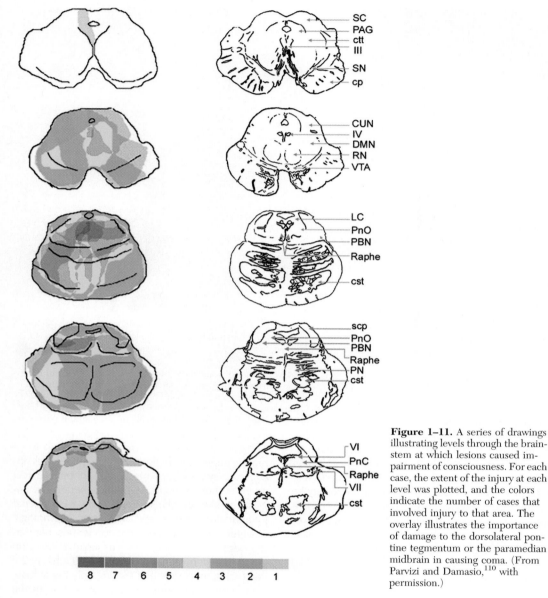

Figure 1–11. A series of drawings illustrating levels through the brainstem at which lesions caused impairment of consciousness. For each case, the extent of the injury at each level was plotted, and the colors indicate the number of cases that involved injury to that area. The overlay illustrates the importance of damage to the dorsolateral pontine tegmentum or the paramedian midbrain in causing coma. (From Parvizi and Damasio,[110] with permission.)

who suffer from brain trauma.[104] These cases usually do not present a diagnostic dilemma, as there is usually history or external evidence of trauma to suggest the cause of the impaired consciousness.

DIENCEPHALIC INJURY

The relay nuclei of the thalamus provide the largest ascending source of input to the cerebral cortex. As a result, it is no exaggeration to

say that virtually any deficit due to injury of a discrete cortical area can be mimicked by injury to its thalamic relay nucleus. Hence, thalamic lesions that are sufficiently extensive can produce the same result as bilateral cortical injury. The most common cause of such lesions is the "tip of the basilar" syndrome, in which vascular occlusion of the perforating arteries that arise from the basilar apex or the first segment of the posterior cerebral arteries can produce bilateral thalamic infarction.[105]

However, careful examination of the MRI scans of such patients, or their brains postmortem, usually shows some damage as well to the paramedian midbrain reticular formation and often in the posterior hypothalamus. Other causes of primarily thalamic damage include thalamic hemorrhage, local infiltrating tumors, and rare cases of diencephalic inflammatory lesions (e.g., Behçet's syndrome).[106,107]

Another example of severe thalamic injury causing coma was reported by Kinney and colleagues[108] in the brain of Karen Anne Quinlan, a famous medicolegal case of a woman who remained in a persistent vegetative state (Chapter 9) for many years after a hypoxic brain injury. Examination of her brain at the time of death disclosed unexpectedly widespread thalamic neuronal loss. However, there was also extensive damage to other brain areas, including the cerebral cortex, so that the thalamic damage alone may not have caused the clinical loss of consciousness. On the other hand, thalamic injury is frequently found in patients with brain injuries who eventually enter a persistent vegetative state (Chapter 9).[104]

Ischemic lesions of the hypothalamus are rare, because the hypothalamus is literally encircled by the main vessels of the circle of Willis and is fed by local penetrating vessels from all the major arteries. However, the location of the hypothalamus above the pituitary gland results in localized hypothalamic damage in cases of pituitary tumors.[109] The hypothalamus also may harbor primary lymphomas of brain, gliomas, or sarcoid granulomas. Patients with hypothalamic lesions often appear to be hypersomnolent rather than comatose. They may yawn, stretch, or sigh, features that are usually lacking in patients with coma due to brainstem lesions.

UPPER BRAINSTEM INJURY

Evidence from clinicopathologic analyses firmly establishes that the midbrain and pontine area critical to consciousness in humans includes the paramedian tegmental zone immediately ventral to the periaqueductal gray matter, from the caudal diencephalon through the rostral pons.[110] Numerous cases are on record of small lesions involving this territory bilaterally in which there was profound loss of consciousness (see Figure 1–11). On the other hand, we have not seen loss of consciousness with lesions confined to the medulla or the caudal pons. This principle is illustrated by the historical vignettes on pages 30 and below.

HISTORICAL VIGNETTES

Patient 1–2

A 62-year-old woman was examined through the courtesy of Dr. Walter Camp. Twenty-five years earlier she had developed weakness and severely impaired position and vibration sense of the right arm and leg. Two years before we saw her, she developed paralysis of the right vocal cord and wasting of the right side of the tongue, followed by insidiously progressing disability with an unsteady gait and more weakness of the right limbs. Four days before coming to the hospital, she became much weaker on the right side, and 2 days later she lost the ability to swallow.

When she entered the hospital she was alert and in full possession of her faculties. She had no difficulty breathing and her blood pressure was 162/110 mm Hg. She had upbeat nystagmus on upward gaze and decreased appreciation of pinprick on the left side of the face. The right sides of the pharynx, palate, and tongue were paralyzed. The right arm and leg were weak and atrophic, consistent with disuse. Stretch reflexes below the neck were bilaterally brisk, and the right plantar response was extensor. Position and vibratory sensations were reduced on the right side of the body and the appreciation of pinprick was reduced on the left.

The next day she was still alert and responsive, but she developed difficulty in coughing and speaking and finally she ceased breathing. An endotracheal tube was placed and mechanical ventilation was begun. Later, on that third hospital day, she was still bright and alert and quickly and accurately answered questions by nodding or shaking her head. The opening pressure of cerebrospinal fluid (CSF) at lumbar puncture was 180 mm of water, and the xanthochromic fluid contained 8,500 red blood cells/mm^3 and 14 white blood cells/mm^3.

She lived for 23 more days. During that time she developed complete somatic motor paralysis below the face. Several hypotensive crises were treated promptly with infusions of pressor agents, but no pressor drugs were needed during the last 2 weeks of life. Intermittently during those final days, she had brief periods of unresponsiveness, but then awakened and signaled quickly and appropriately to questions demanding a yes or no answer and opened or closed her eyes and moved them laterally when commanded to do so. There was no other voluntary movement. Four days before she died, she developed ocular bobbing when commanded to look laterally, but although she consistently responded to commands by moving her eyes, it was difficult to know whether or not her responses were appropriate. During the ensuing 3 days, evidence of wakefulness decreased. She died of gastrointestinal hemorrhage 26 days after entering the hospital.

The brain at autopsy contained a moderate amount of dark, old blood overlying the right lateral medulla adjacent to the fourth ventricle. A raspberry-appearing arteriovenous malformation, 1.4 cm in greatest diameter, protruded from the right lateral medulla, beginning with its lower border 2.5 cm caudal to the obex. On section, the vascular malformation was seen to originate in the central medulla and to extend rostrally to approximately 2 mm above the obex. From this point, a large hemorrhage extended forward to destroy the central medulla all the way to the pontine junction (Figure 1–9B). Microscopic study demonstrated that, at its most cranial end, the hemorrhage destroyed the caudal part of the right vestibular nuclei and most of the adjacent lower pontine tegmentum on the right. Caudal to this, the hemorrhage widened and destroyed the entire dorsal center of the medulla from approximately the plane of the nucleus of the glossopharyngeal nerve down to just below the plane of the nucleus ambiguus. From this latter point caudally, the hemorrhage was more restricted to the reticular formation of the medulla. The margins of this lesion contained an organizing clot with phagocytosis and reticulum formation indicating a process at least 2 weeks old. The center of the hemorrhage contained a degenerating clot estimated to be at least 72 hours old; at several places along the lateral margin of the lesion were small fresh hemorrhages estimated to have occurred within a few hours of death. It was considered unlikely that the lesion had changed substantially in size or extent of destruction in the few days before death.

Patient 1–3

A 65-year-old woman was admitted to the neurology service for "coma" after an anesthetic procedure. She had rheumatoid arthritis with subluxa-

tion of C1 on C2, and compression of the C2 root causing occipital neuralgia. An anesthesiologist attempted to inject the root with ethanol to eliminate the pain. Almost immediately after the injection, the patient became flaccid and experienced a respiratory arrest. On arrival in the neurology intensive care unit she was hypotensive and apneic. Mechanical ventilation was instituted and blood pressure was supported with pressors.

On examination she had spontaneous eye movements in the vertical direction only and her eyelids fluttered open and closed. There was complete flaccid paralysis of the hypoglossal, vagal, and accessory nerves, as well as all spinal motor function. Twitches of facial and jaw movement persisted. There was no response to pinprick over the face or body. CT scan showed hypodensity of the medulla and lower pons.

The patient responded to commands to open and close her eyes and learned to communicate in this way. She lived another 12 weeks in this setting, without regaining function, and rarely was observed to sleep. No postmortem examination was permitted. However, the injection of ethanol had apparently entered the C2 root sleeve and fixed the lower brainstem up through the facial and abducens nuclei without clouding the state of consciousness of the patient.

Comment: Both of these cases demonstrated the preservation of consciousness in patients with a locked-in state due to destruction of motor pathways below the critical level of the rostral pons. Chapter 2 will explore the ways in which the neurologic examination of a comatose patient can be used to differentiate these different causes of loss of consciousness.

REFERENCES

1. Scheid R, Voltz R, Guthke T, et al. Neuropsychiatric findings in anti-Ma2-positive paraneoplastic limbic encephalitis. Neurology 61, 1159–1160, 2003.
2. Mesulam MM, Waxman SG, Geschwind N, et al. Acute confusional states with right middle cerebral artery infarctions. J Neurol Neurosurg Psychiatry 39, 84–89, 1976.
3. Posner JB, Plum F. The toxic effects of carbon dioxide and acetazolamide in hepatic encephalopathy. J Clin Invest 39, 1246–1258, 1960.
4. Shimojyo S, Scheinberg P, Reinmuth O. Cerebral blood flow and metabolism in the Wernicke-Korsakoff syndrome. J Clin Invest 46, 849–854, 1967.
5. Trzepacz PT, Tarter RE, Shah A, et al. SPECT scan and cognitive findings in subclinical hepatic

encephalopathy. J Neuropsychiatry Clin Neurosci 6, 170–175, 1994.

6. Nilsson K, Warkentin S, Hultberg B, et al. Treatment of cobalamin deficiency in dementia, evaluated clinically and with cerebral blood flow measurements. Aging (Milano) 12, 199–207, 2000.

7. Van der Mast RC. Pathophysiology of delirium. J Geriatr Psychiatry Neurol 11, 138–145, 1998.

8. Frances A, Pincus HA, First MB. Diagnostic and Statistical Manuel of Mental Disorders: DSM-IV. 4th ed., 1994.

9. Peroutka SJ, Sohmer BH, Kumar AJ, et al. Hallucinations and delusions following a right temporoparieto-occipital infarction. Johns Hopkins Med J 151, 181–185, 1982.

10. Markand ON. Eectroencephalogram in "locked-in" syndrome. Electroencephalogr Clin Neurophysiol 40, 529–534, 1976.

11. Markand ON, Dyken ML. Sleep abnormalities in patients with brain stem lesions. Neurology 26, 769–776, 1976.

12. Billiard M, Dauvilliers Y. Idiopathic hypersomnia. Sleep Med Rev 5, 349–358, 2001.

13. Giacino JT. The vegetative and minimally conscious states: consensus-based criteria for establishing diagnosis and prognosis. NeuroRehabilitation 19, 293–298, 2004.

14. Schlotzhauer AV, Liang BA. Definitions and implications of death. Hematol Oncol Clin North Am 16, 1397–1413, 2002.

15. Towbin A. The respirator brain death syndrome. Hum Pathol 4, 583–594, 1973.

16. Criteria for the diagnosis of brain stem death. Review by a working group convened by the Royal College of Physicians and endorsed by the Conference of Medical Royal Colleges and their Faculties in the United Kingdom. J R Coll Physicians Lond 29, 381–382, 1995.

17. Jackson JH. Selected writings of John Hughlings Jackson. London: Hode and Stoughton, 1931.

18. Mauthner L. Zur Pathologie und Physiologie des Schlafes nebst Bermerkungen ueber die "Nona." Wien Klin Wochenschr 40, 961–1185, 1890.

19. Von Economo C. Sleep as a problem of localization. J Nerv Ment Dis 71, 249–259, 1930.

20. Ranson SW. Somnolence caused by hypothalamic lesions in monkeys. Arch Neurol Psychiat 41, 1–23, 1939.

21. Nauta WJH. Hypothalamic regulation of sleep in rats. An experimental study. J Neurophysiol 9, 285–314, 1946.

22. Swett CP, Hobson JA. The effects of posterior hypothalamic lesions on behavioral and electrographic manifestations of sleep and waking in cat. Arch Ital Biol 106, 270–282, 1968.

23. Sterman, MB, Clemente, CD. Forebrain inhibitory mechanisms: sleep patterns induced by basal forebrain stimulation in the behaving cat. Exp Neurol 6, 103–117, 1962.

24. Wilson SAK. The Narcolepsies. In: Problems in Neurology. London: Edward Arnold, pp 76–119, 1928.

25. Berger H. Ueber das electroenkephalogramm des menschen. Arch Psychiatr Nervenkr 87, 527–570, 1929.

26. Steriade M. The corticothalamic system in sleep. Front Biosci 8, d878–d899, 2003.

27. Buzsaki G, Bickford RG, Ponomareff G, et al. Nucleus basalis and thalamic control of neocortical activity in the freely moving rat. J Neurosci 8, 4007–4026, 1988.

28. Bremer F. CR. Soc Biol 118, 1235–1241, 1935.

29. Bremer F. Cerebral hypnogenic centers. Ann Neurol 2, 1–6, 1977.

30. Moruzzi G, Magoun HW. Brain stem reticular formation and activation of the EEG. 1949. J Neuropsychiatry Clin Neurosci 7, 251–267, 1995.

31. Starzl TE, Taylor CW, Magoun HW. Ascending conduction in reticular activating system, with special reference to the diencephalon. J Neurophysiol 14, 461–477, 1951.

32. Zernicki B, Gandolfo G, Glin L, et al. Cerveau isole and pretrigeminal rat preparations. Physiol Bohemoslov 34 Suppl, 183–185, 1985.

33. Magni F, Moruzzi G, Rossi GF, et al. EEG arousal following inactivation of the lower brainstem by selective injection of barbiturate into the vertebral circulation. Arch Ital Biol 97, 33–46, 1959.

34. Hallanger AE, Levey AI, Lee HJ, et al. The origins of cholinergic and other subcortical afferents to the thalamus in the rat. J Comp Neurol 262, 105–124, 1987.

35. McCormick DA, Bal T. Sleep and arousal: thalamocortical mechanisms. Annu Rev Neurosci 20, 185–215, 1997.

36. Strecker RE, Morairty S, Thakkar MM, et al. Adenosinergic modulation of basal forebrain and preoptic/anterior hypothalamic neuronal activity in the control of behavioral state. Behav Brain Res 115, 183–204, 2000.

37. Aserinsky E, Kleitman N. Regularly occurring periods of eye motility, and concomitant phenomena, during sleep. Science 118, 273–274, 1953.

38. Scammell TE. The neurobiology, diagnosis, and treatment of narcolepsy. Ann Neurol 53, 154–166, 2003.

39. Kales A, Vela-Bueno A, Kales JD. Sleep disorders: sleep apnea and narcolepsy. Ann Intern Med 106, 434–443, 1987.

40. Szymusiak R, Alam N, Steininger TL, et al. Sleep-waking discharge patterns of ventrolateral preoptic/anterior hypothalamic neurons in rats. Brain Res 803, 178–188, 1998.

41. Vgontzas AN, Kales A. Sleep and its disorders. Annu Rev Med 50, 387–400, 1999.

42. Saper CB. Diffuse cortical projection systems: anatomical organization and role in cortical function. In: F. Plum, ed. Handbook of Physiology. The Nervous System. V. Bethesda, Md.: American Physiological Society, pp 169–210, 1987.

43. Loughlin SE, Foote SL, Fallon JH. Locus coeruleus projections to cortex: topography, morphology and collateralization. Brain Res Bull 19, 287–294, 1982.

44. Bobillier P, Seguin S, Petitjean F, et al. The raphe nuclei of the cat brain stem: a topographical atlas of their efferent projections as revealed by autoradiography. Brain Res 113, 449–486, 1976.

45. Lu J, Jhou TC, Saper CB. Identification of wake-active dopaminergic neurons in the ventral periaqueductal gray matter. J Neurosci 26, 193–202, 2006.

46. Heym J, Steinfels GF, Jacobs BL. Activity of serotonin-containing neurons in the nucleus raphe pallidus of freely moving cats. Brain Res 251, 259–276, 1982.

47. Rasmussen K, Jacobs BL. Single unit activity of locus coeruleus neurons in the freely moving cat. II. Conditioning and pharmacologic studies. Brain Res 371, 335–344, 1986.

48. Steininger TL, Alam MN, Gong H, et al. Sleep-waking discharge of neurons in the posterior lateral hypothalamus of the albino rat. Brain Res 840, 138–147, 1999.

49. Wu MF, John J, Boehmer LN, et al. Activity of dorsal raphe cells across the sleep-waking cycle and during cataplexy in narcoleptic dogs. J Physiol 554, 202–215, 2004.

50. Kolta A, Reader TA. Modulatory effects of catecholamines on neurons of the rat visual cortex: single-cell iontophoretic studies. Can J Physiol Pharmacol 67, 615–623, 1989.

51. Sato H, Fox K, Daw NW. Effect of electrical stimulation of locus coeruleus on the activity of neurons in the cat visual cortex. J Neurophysiol 62, 946–958, 1989.

52. Bassant MH, Ennouri K, Lamour Y. Effects of iontophoretically applied monoamines on somatosensory cortical neurons of unanesthetized rats. Neuroscience 39, 431–439, 1990.

53. Lu J, Sherman D, Devor M, et al. A putative flip-flop switch for control of REM sleep. Nature 441, 589–594, 2006.

54. Saper CB. Diffuse cortical projection systems: anatomical organization and role in cortical function. In: F. Plum, ed. Handbook of Physiology. The Nervous System. V. Bethesda, Md.: American Physiological Society, pp 168–210, 1987.

55. Welch MJ, Meltzer EO, Simons FE. H1-antihistamines and the central nervous system. Clin Allergy Immunol 17, 337–388, 2002.

56. Huang ZL, Qu WM, Li WD, et al. Arousal effect of orexin A depends on activation of the histaminergic system. Proc Natl Acad Sci 98, 9965–9970, 2001.

57. Parmentier R, Ohtsu H, Djebbara-Hannas Z, et al. Anatomical, physiological, and pharmacological characteristics of histidine decarboxylase knock-out mice: evidence for the role of brain histamine in behavioral and sleep-wake control. J Neurosci 22, 7695–7711, 2002.

58. Peyron C, Tighe DK, van den Pol AN, et al. Neurons containing hypocretin (orexin) project to multiple neuronal systems. J Neurosci 18, 9996–10015, 1998.

59. Bittencourt JC, Frigo L, Rissman RA, et al. The distribution of melanin-concentrating hormone in the monkey brain (Cebus apella). Brain Res 804, 140–143, 1998.

60. Bittencourt JC, Presse F, Arias C, et al. The melanin-concentrating hormone system of the rat brain: an immuno- and hybridization histochemical characterization. J Comp Neurol 319, 218–245, 1992.

61. Lin CS, Nicolelis MA, Schneider JS, et al. A major direct GABAergic pathway from zona incerta to neocortex. Science 248, 1553–1556, 1990.

62. Lee MG, Hassani OK, Jones BE. Discharge of identified orexin/hypocretin neurons across the sleep-waking cycle. J Neurosci 25, 6716–6720, 2005.

63. Mileykovskiy BY, Kiyashchenko LI, Siegel JM. Behavioral correlates of activity in identified hypocretin/orexin neurons. Neuron 46, 787–798, 2005.

64. Verret L, Goutagny R, Fort P, et al. A role of melanin-concentrating hormone producing neurons in the central regulation of paradoxical sleep. BMC Neurosci 4, 19, 2003.

65. Alam MN, Gong H, Alam T, et al. Sleep-waking discharge patterns of neurons recorded in the rat perifornical lateral hypothalamic area. J Physiol 538, 619–631, 2002.

66. Gelineau JBE. De la narcolepsie. Gaz Hop (Paris) 53, 626–637, 1880.

67. Sakurai T, Amemiya A, Ishii M, et al. Orexins and orexin receptors: a family of hypothalamic neuropeptides and G protein-coupled receptors that regulate feeding behavior. Cell 92, 573–585, 1998.

68. de Lecea L, Kilduff TS, Peyron C, et al. The hypocretins: hypothalamus-specific peptides with neuroexcitatory activity. Proc Natl Acad Sci 95, 322–327, 1998.

69. Willie JT, Chemelli RM, Sinton CMYM. To eat or to sleep? Orexin in the regulation of feeding and wakefulness. Annu Rev Neurosci 24, 429–458, 2001.

70. Chimelli RM, Willie JT, Sinton CM, et al. Narcolepsy in orexin knockout mice: molecular genetics of sleep regulation. Cell 98, 437–451, 1999.

71. Lin L, Faraco J, Li R, et al. The sleep disorder canine narcolepsy is caused by a mutation in the hypocretin (orexin) receptor 2 gene. Cell 98, 365–376, 1999.

72. Peyron C, Faraco J, Rogers W, et al. A mutation in a case of early onset narcolepsy and a generalized absence of hypocretin peptides in human narcoleptic brains. Nat Med 6, 991–997, 2000.

73. Ripley B, Overeem S, Fujiki N, et al. CSF hypocretin/orexin levels in narcolepsy and other neurological conditions. Neurology 57, 2253–2258, 2001.

74. Thannickal TC, Moore RY, Nienhuis R, et al. Reduced number of hypocretin neurons in human narcolepsy. Neuron 27, 469–474, 2000.

75. Marcus JN, Aschkenasi CJ, Lee CE, et al. Differential expression of orexin receptors 1 and 2 in the rat brain. J Comp Neurol 435, 6–25, 2001.

76. Saper CB. Organization of cerebral cortical afferent systems in the rat. II. Magnocellular basal nucleus. J Comp Neurol 222, 313–342, 1984.

77. Zaborsky L, Brownstein MJ, Palkovits M. Ascending projections to the hypothalamus and limbic nuclei from the dorsolateral pontine tegmentum: a biochemical and electron microscopic study. Acta Morphol Acad Sci Hung 25, 175–188, 1977.

78. Zaborsky L, Cullinan WE, Luine VN. Catecholaminergic-cholinergic interaction in the basal forebrain. Prog Brain Res 98, 31–49, 1993.

79. Lee MG, Hassani OK, Alonso A, et al. Cholinergic basal forebrain neurons burst with theta during waking and paradoxical sleep. J Neurosci 25, 4365–4369, 2005.

80. Richardson RT, DeLong MR. Nucleus basalis of Meynert neuronal activity during a delayed response task in monkey. Brain Res 399, 364–368, 1986.

81. Richardson RT, DeLong MR. Context-dependent responses of primate nucleus basalis neuron in a go/no-go-go task. J Neurol Sci 10, 2528–2540, 1990.

82. Sherin JE, Shiromani PJ, McCarley RW, et al. Activation of ventrolateral preoptic neurons during sleep. Science 271, 216–219, 1996.

83. Sherin JE, Elmquist JK, Torrealba F, et al. Innervation of histaminergic tuberomammilary neurons by GABAergic and alaninergic neurons in the ven-

trolateral preoptic nucleus of the rat. J Neurosci 18, 4705–4721, 1998.

84. Saper CB, Chou TC, Scammell TE. The sleep switch: hypothalamic control of sleep and wakefulness. Trends Neurosci 24, 726–731, 2001.

85. Gaus SE, Strecker RE, Tate BA, et al. Ventrolateral preoptic nucleus contains sleep-active, galaninergic neurons in multiple mammalian species. Neuroscience 115, 285–294, 2002.

86. Sallanon M, Denoyer M, Kitahama K, et al. Long-lasting insomnia induced by preoptic neuron lesions and its transient reversal by muscimol injection into the posterior hypothalamus in the cat. Neuroscience 32, 669–683, 1989.

87. Lu J, Greco MA, Shiromani P, et al. Effect of lesions of the ventrolateral preoptic nucleus on NREM and REM sleep. J Neurosci 20, 3820–3842, 2000.

88. Lu J, Bjorkum AA, Xu M, et al. Selective activation of the extended ventrolateral preoptic nucleus during rapid eye movement sleep. J Neurosci 22, 4568–4576, 2002.

89. Hara J, Beuckmann CT, Nambu T, et al. Genetic ablation of orexin neurons in mice results in narcolepsy, hypophagia, and obesity. Neuron 30, 345–354, 2001.

90. Lydic R, Douglas CL, Baghdoyan HA. Microinjection of neostigmine into the pontine reticular formation of C57BL/6J mouse enhances rapid eye movement sleep and depresses breathing. Sleep 25, 835–841, 2002.

91. Lorente de No R. Cerebral cortex: architecture, intracortical connections, motor projections. In: JF Fulton, ed. Physiology of the Nervous System. New York: Oxford University Press, pp 291–340, 1938.

92. Hubel DH, Wiesel TN. Shape and arrangement of columns in cat's striate cortex. J Physiol 165, 559–568, 1963.

93. McCasland JS, Woolsey TA. High-resolution 2-deoxyglucose mapping of functional cortical columns in mouse barrel cortex. J Comp Neurol 278, 555–569, 1988.

94. Gilbert CD, Wiesel TN. Columnar specificity of intrinsic horizontal and corticocortical connections in cat visual cortex. J Neurosci 9, 2432–2442, 1989.

95. Hubel DH, Wiesel TN. The period of susceptibility to the physiological effects of unilateral eye closure in kittens. J Physiol 206, 419–436, 1970.

96. Frank MG, Issa NP, Stryker MP. Sleep enhances plasticity in the developing visual cortex. Neuron 30, 275–287, 2001.

97. Hardcastle VG. Consciousness and the neurobiology of perceptual binding. Semin Neurol 17, 163–170, 1997.

98. Revonsuo A. Binding and the phenomenal unity of consciousness. Conscious Cogn 8, 173–185, 1999.

99. Nishikawa T, Okuda J, Mizuta I, et al. Conflict of intentions due to callosal disconnection. J Neurol Neurosurg Psychiatry 71, 462–471, 2001.

100. Alexander GE, DeLong MR, Strick PL. Parallel organization of functionally segregated circuits linking basal ganglia and cortex. Annu Rev Neurosci 9, 357–381, 1986.

101. Alexander GE, Crutcher MD, DeLong MR. Basal ganglia-thalamocortical circuits: parallel substrates for motor, oculomotor, "prefrontal" and "limbic" functions. Prog Brain Res 119–146, 1990.

102. Wyrtzes LM, Chatrian GE, Shaw CM, et al. Acute failure of forebrain with sparing of brain-stem function. Electroencephalographic, multimodality evoked-potential, and pathologic findings. Arch Neurol 46, 93–97, 1989.

103. van der Knaap MS, Smit LS, Nauta JJ, et al. Cortical laminar abnormalities—occurrence and clinical significance. Neuropediatrics 24, 143–148, 1993.

104. Adams JH, Graham DI, Jennett B. The neuropathology of the vegetative state after an acute brain insult. Brain 123, 1327–1338, 2000.

105. Caplan LR. "Top of the basilar" syndrome. Neurology 30, 72–79, 1980.

106. Wechler B, Dell'Isola B, Vidailhet M, et al. MRI in 31 patients with Behcet's disease and neurological involvement: prospective study with clinical correlation. J Neurol Neurosurg Psychiatry 56, 793–798, 1993.

107. Park-Matsumoto YC, Ogawa K, Tazawa T, et al. Mutism developing after bilateral thalamo-capsular lesions by neuro-Behcet disease. Acta Neurol Scand 91, 297–301, 1995.

108. Kinney HC, Korein J, Panigrahy A, et al. Neuropathological findings in the brain of Karen Ann Quinlan. The role of the thalamus in the persistent vegetative state. N Engl J Med 330 (21), 1469–1475, 1994.

109. Reeves AG, Plum F. Hyperphagia, rage, and demential accompanying a ventromedial hypothalamic neoplasm. Arch Neurol 20, 616–624, 1969.

110. Parvizi J, Damasio AR. Neuroanatomical correlates of brainstem coma. Brain 126, 1524–1536, 2003.

Chapter 2

Examination of the Comatose Patient

OVERVIEW

Coma, indeed any alteration of consciousness, is a medical emergency. The physician encountering such a patient must begin examination and treatment simultaneously. The examination must be thorough, but brief. The examination begins by informally assessing the patient's level of consciousness. First, the physician addresses the patient verbally. If the patient does not respond to the physician's voice, the physician may speak more loudly or shake the patient. When this fails to produce a response, the physician begins a more formal coma evaluation.

The examiner must systematically assess the arousal pathways. To determine if there is a structural lesion involving those pathways, it is necessary also to examine the function of brainstem sensory and motor pathways that are adjacent to the arousal system. In particular, because the oculomotor circuitry enfolds and surrounds most of the arousal system, this part of the examination is particularly informative. Fortunately, the examination of the comatose patient can usually be accomplished very quickly because the patient has such a limited range of responses. However, the examiner must become conversant with the meaning of the signs elicited in that examination, so that decisions that may save the patient's life can then be made quickly and accurately.

The evaluation of the patient with a reduced level of consciousness, like that of any patient, requires a history (to the extent possible), physical examination, and laboratory evaluation. These are considered, in turn, in this chapter. However, *as soon as it is determined that a patient has a depressed level of consciousness, the next step is to ensure that the patient's brain is receiving adequate blood and oxygen.* The emergency treatment of the comatose patient is detailed in Chapter 7. The physiology and pathophysiology of the cerebral circulation and of respiration are considered in the paragraphs below.

HISTORY

In patients with nervous system dysfunction, the history is the most important part of the examination (Table 2–1). Of course, patients with coma or diminished states of consciousness by definition are not able to give a history. Thus, the history must be obtained if possible from relatives, friends, or the individuals, usually the emergency medical personnel, who brought the patient to the hospital.

The onset of coma is often important. In a previously healthy, young patient, the sudden onset of coma may be due to drug poisoning, subarachnoid hemorrhage, or head trauma; in the elderly, sudden coma is more likely caused

Table 2–1 **Examination of the Comatose Patient**

History (from Relatives, Friends, or Attendants)
Onset of coma (abrupt, gradual)
Recent complaints (e.g., headache, depression, focal weakness, vertigo)
Recent injury
Previous medical illnesses (e.g., diabetes, renal failure, heart disease)
Previous psychiatric history
Access to drugs (sedatives, psychotropic drugs)

General Physical Examination
Vital signs
Evidence of trauma
Evidence of acute or chronic systemic illness
Evidence of drug ingestion (needle marks, alcohol on breath)
Nuchal rigidity (assuming that cervical trauma has been excluded)

Neurologic Examination
Verbal responses
Eye opening
Optic fundi
Pupillary reactions
Spontaneous eye movements
Oculocephalic responses (assuming cervical trauma has been excluded)
Oculovestibular responses
Corneal responses
Respiratory pattern
Motor responses
Deep tendon reflexes
Skeletal muscle tone

by cerebral hemorrhage or infarction. Most patients with lesions compressing the brain either have a clear history of trauma (e.g., epidural hematoma; see Chapter 4) or a more gradual rather than abrupt impairment of consciousness. Gradual onset is also true of most patients with metabolic disorders (see Chapter 5).

The examiner should inquire about previous medical symptoms or illnesses or any recent trauma. A history of headache of recent onset points to a compressive lesion, whereas the history of depression or psychiatric disease may suggest drug intoxication. Patients with known diabetes, renal failure, heart disease, or other chronic medical illness are more likely to be suffering from metabolic disorders or perhaps brainstem infarction. A history of premonitory signs, including focal weakness such as dragging of the leg or complaints of unilateral sensory symptoms or diplopia, suggests a cerebral or brainstem mass lesion.

GENERAL PHYSICAL EXAMINATION

The general physical examination is an important source of clues as to the cause of unconsciousness. After stabilizing the patient (Chapter 7), one should search for signs of head trauma. Bilateral symmetric black eyes suggest basal skull fracture, as does blood behind the tympanic membrane or under the skin overlying the mastoid bone (Battle's sign). Examine the neck with care; if there is a possibility of trauma, the neck should be immobilized until cervical spine instability has been excluded by imaging. Resistance to neck flexion in the presence of easy lateral movement suggests meningeal inflammation such as meningitis or subarachnoid hemorrhage. Flexion of the legs upon flexing the neck (Brudzinski's sign) confirms meningismus. Examination of the skin is also useful. Needle marks suggest drug ingestion. Petechiae may suggest meningitis or intravascular coagulation. Pressure sores or bullae indicate that the patient has been unconscious and lying in a single position for an extended period of time, and are especially frequent in patients with barbiturate overdosage.[1]

LEVEL OF CONSCIOUSNESS

After conducting the brief history and examination as outlined above and stabilizing the patients' vital functions, the examiner should conduct a formal coma evaluation. In assessing the level of consciousness of the patient, it is necessary to determine the intensity of stimulation necessary to arouse a response and the quality of the response that is achieved. When the patient does not respond to voice or vigorous shaking, the examiner next provides a source of pain to arouse the patient. Several methods for providing a sufficiently painful stimulus to arouse the patient without causing tissue damage are illustrated in Figure 2–1. It is best to begin with a modest, lateralized stimulus, such as compression of the nail beds, the supraorbital ridge, or the temporomandibular joint. These give information about the lateralization of motor response (see below), but must be repeated on each side in case there is a focal lesion of the pain pathways on one side of the brain or spinal cord. If there is no response to the stimulus, a more vigorous midline stimulus may be given by the sternal rub. By vigorously pressing the examiner's knuckles into the patient's sternum and rubbing up and down the chest, it is possible to create a sufficiently painful stimulus to arouse any subject who is not deeply comatose.

The response of the patient is noted and graded. The types of motor responses seen are considered in the section on *motor responses* (page 73). However, the level of response is important to the initial consideration of the depth of impairment of consciousness. In descending order of arousability, a sleepy patient who responds to being addressed verbally or light shaking, or one who responds verbally to more intense mechanical stimulation, is said to be lethargic or obtunded. A patient whose best response to deep pain is to attempt to push the examiner's arm away is considered to be stuporous, with localizing responses. Patients who

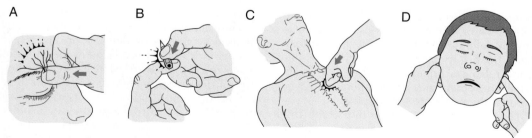

Figure 2–1. Methods for attempting to elicit responses from unconscious patients. Noxious stimuli can be delivered with minimal trauma to the supraorbital ridge (A), the nail beds or the fingers or toes (B), the sternum (C) or the temporomandibular joints (D).

Box 2–1 Coma Scales

A number of different scales have been devised for scoring patients with coma. The value of these is in providing a simple estimate of the prognosis for different groups of patients. Obviously, this is related as much to the cause of the coma (when known) as to the current status of the examination. Teasdale and Jennett's Glasgow Coma Scale (GCS),[2] devised to categorize patients with head trauma, is reproduced below. Unfortunately, when used by emergency room physicians, interrater agreement is only moderate.[3] Two simple scales, ACDU (alert, confused, drowsy, unresponsive) and AVPU (alert, response to voice, response to pain, unresponsive)[4] are about as accurate as the GCS and much easier to use.[4] The ACDU scale appears better at identifying early deterioration in level of consciousness. A recently validated coma scale, the FOUR scale (full outline of unresponsiveness), provides more neurologic detail than the GCS. However, no scale is adequate for all patients; hence, the best policy in recording the results of the coma examination is simply to describe the findings.

Nevertheless, the GCS is widely used, and still is probably the best for most trauma patients.[5] It is useful to obtain GCS scores, which can be compared against large databases to evaluate prognosis for specific etiologies of coma (see Chapter 9).

FOUR Score (Full Outline of Unresponsiveness)[109]

Eye Response

    4 = eyelids open or opened, tracking, or blinking to command
    3 = eyelids open but not tracking
    2 = eyelids closed but open to loud voice
    1 = eyelids closed but open to pain
    0 = eyelids remain closed with pain

Motor Response

    4 = thumbs-up, fist, or peace sign
    3 = localizing to pain
    2 = flexion response to pain
    1 = extension response to pain
    0 = no response to pain or generalized myoclonus status

Brainstem Reflexes

    4 = pupil and corneal reflexes present
    3 = one pupil wide and fixed
    2 = pupil or corneal reflexes absent
    1 = pupil and corneal reflexes absent
    0 = absent pupil, corneal, and cough reflex

Respiration

    4 = not intubated, regular breathing pattern
    3 = not intubated, Cheyne-Stokes breathing pattern
    2 = not intubated, irregular breathing
    1 = breathes above ventilator rate
    0 = breathes at ventilator rate or apnea

(continued)

Box 2–1 Coma Scales (cont.)

Glasgow Coma Scale

Eye Response

    4 = eyes open spontaneously
    3 = eye opening to verbal command
    2 = eye opening to pain
    1 = no eye opening

Motor Response

    6 = obeys commands
    5 = localizing pain
    4 = withdrawal from pain
    3 = flexion response to pain
    2 = extension response to pain
    1 = no motor response

Verbal Response

    5 = oriented
    4 = confused
    3 = inappropriate words
    2 = incomprehensible sounds
    1 = no verbal response

A GCS score of 13 or higher indicates mild brain injury, 9 to 12 moderate brain injury, and 8 or less severe brain injury.

AVPU

Is the patient
    Alert and oriented?
    Responding to voice?
    Responding to pain?
    Unresponsive?

ACDU

Is the patient
    Alert and oriented?
    Confused?
    Drowsy?
    Unresponsive?

make only nonspecific motor responses (wincing, restlessness, withdrawal reflexes) without a directed attempt to defend against the stimulus are considered to have a nonlocalizing response and are comatose. Patients who fail to respond at all are in the deepest stage of coma.

This rough grading system, from verbal responsiveness, to localizing responses, to nonlocalizing responses, to no response, is all that is needed for an initial assessment of the depth of unresponsiveness that can be used to follow the progress of the patient. If the initial evaluation of the level of consciousness demonstrates impairment, it is essential to progress through the next steps of the coma examination as rapidly as possible to safeguard that patient's life. More elaborate coma scales are described in Box 2–1, but many of these depend upon the results of later stages in the examination, and it is never justified to delay attending to the basics of airway, breathing, and circulation while performing a more elaborate scoring evaluation.

ABC: AIRWAY, BREATHING, CIRCULATION

It is critical to ensure that the patient's airway is maintained, that he or she is breathing adequately, and that there is sufficient arterial perfusion pressure. The first goal must be to correct any of these conditions if they are found inadequate (Chapter 7). In addition, blood pressure, heart rate, and respiration may provide valuable clues to the cause of coma.

Circulation

It is critical first to ensure that the brain is receiving adequate blood flow. Cerebral perfusion pressure is the systemic blood pressure minus the intracranial pressure. The physician can measure blood pressure but in the initial examination can only estimate intracranial pressure. Over a wide range of blood pressures, cerebral perfusion remains stable because the brain autoregulates its blood flow by mechanisms described in the paragraphs below and illustrated in Figure 2–2. If the blood pressure falls too low or becomes too high, autoregulation fails and cerebral perfusion follows perfusion pressure passively; that is, it falls as the blood pressure falls and rises as the blood pressure rises. In this situation, both too low (ischemia) and too high (hypertensive encephalopathy; see Chapter 5) a blood pressure can damage the brain. To ensure adequate

brain perfusion, the physician should attempt to maintain the blood pressure at a level normal for the individual patient. For example, a patient with chronic hypertension autoregulates at a higher level than a normotensive patient. Lowering the blood pressure to a "normal level" may deprive the brain of an adequate blood supply (see Figure 2–2). Conversely, the cerebral blood flow (CBF) in children and pregnant women, who normally run low blood pressures, is regulated at lower levels and may develop excessive perfusion if the blood pressure is raised (e.g., pre-eclampsia).

The perfusion pressure of the brain may be influenced by the position of the head. In a normal individual, as the head is raised, the systemic arterial pressure is maintained by blood pressure reflexes. At the same time, the arterial perfusion pressure to the head is reduced by the distance the head is raised above the heart, but the intracranial pressure is also reduced because of the improved venous and cerebrospinal fluid (CSF) drainage. The net effect is that there is very little change in brain perfusion pressure or CBF. On the other hand, in a patient with stenosis of a carotid or vertebral artery, the perfusion pressure for that vessel may be much lower than systemic arterial pressure. If the head of the bed is raised,

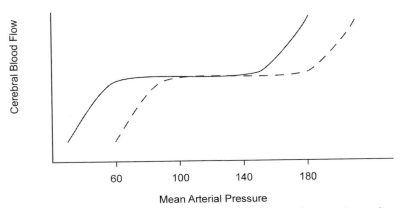

Figure 2–2. Cerebral autoregulation in hypertension. Schematic representation of autoregulation of cerebral blood flow (CBF) in normotensive (solid line) and hypertensive (dashed line) subjects. In both groups, within a range of about 100 mm Hg, increases or decreases in mean arterial pressure are associated with maintenance of CBF due to appropriate changes in arteriolar resistance. Changes in pressure outside this range are eventually associated with loss of autoregulation, leading to a reduction (with hypotension) or an elevation (with marked hypertension) in CBF. Note that hypertensive encephalopathy (increased blood flow with pressures exceeding the autoregulatory range) may occur with a mean arterial pressure below 200 mm Hg in the normotensive individual, but may require a much higher mean arterial pressure in patients who have sustained hypertension. Conversely, lowering blood pressure to the "normal range" of a mean arterial pressure of 80 mm Hg (equivalent to 120/60) may produce a clinically significant fall in CBF, particularly if there is a preexisting cerebrovascular stenosis.

perfusion pressure may fall below the threshold for autoregulation, and blood flow may be diminished below the level needed to support neurologic function. Such patients may show improvement in neurologic function when the head of the bed is flat. Conversely, in cases of head trauma where there is increased intracranial pressure, it may be important to raise the head of the bed 15 to 30 degrees to improve venous drainage to maximize cerebral perfusion pressure.[6] Similarly, it is necessary to remove tight neckwear and ensure that a cervical spine collar is not applied too tightly to a victim of head injury to avoid diminishing venous outflow from the brain.

In a patient with impaired consciousness, the blood pressure can give important clues to the level of the nervous system that has been damaged. *Damage to the descending sympathetic pathways that support blood pressure may result in a fall to levels seen after spinal transaction (mean arterial pressure about 60 to 70 mm Hg).* Blood pressure is supported by a descending sympathoexcitatory pathway from the rostral ventrolateral medulla to the spinal cord, and so damage along the course of this pathway can result in spinal levels of blood pressure. The hypothalamus in turn provides a descending sympathoexcitatory input to the medulla and the spinal cord.[7,8] As a consequence, bilateral diencephalic lesions result in a fall in sympathetic tone, including meiotic pupils (see below), decreased sweating responses, and a generally low level of arterial pressure.[9]

However, persistent hypotension below these levels in a comatose patient is almost never caused by an acute neurologic injury. One of the most common mistakes seen in evaluation of a comatose patient with a mean arterial pressure below 60 mm Hg is the assumption that a neurologic event may have caused the hypotension. This is almost never the case. A mean arterial pressure at or above 60 mm Hg is generally sufficient in a supine patient to support cerebral and systemic function. On the other hand, acute hypotension, due to cardiogenic or vasomotor shock, is a common cause of loss of consciousness and a threat to the patient's life. Thus, the initial evaluation of a comatose patient with low blood pressure should focus on identifying the cause of and correcting the hypotension.

On the other hand, *lesions that result in stimulation of the sympathoexcitatory system may cause an increase in blood pressure.* For example, pain is a major ascending sympathoexcitatory stimulus, which acts via direct collaterals from the ascending spinothalamic tract into the rostral ventrolateral medulla. The elevation of blood pressure in response to a painful stimulus applied to the body (pinch of skin, sternal rub) is evidence of intact medullospinal connections.[10,11] In a patient who is still semiwakeful after subarachnoid hemorrhage, blood pressure may be elevated as a response to headache pain. Each of these conditions is associated with a rise in heart rate as well.

Direct pressure to the floor of the medulla can activate the Cushing reflex, an increase in blood pressure and a decrease in heart rate.[12] In children, the Cushing reflex may be seen when there is a generalized increased intracranial pressure, even above the tentorium. However, the more rigid compartmentalization of intracranial contents in adults usually prevents this phenomenon unless the expansile mass is in the posterior fossa.

Activation of descending sympathoexcitatory pathways from the forebrain may also elevate blood pressure. Irritative lesions of the hypothalamus, such as occur with subarachnoid hemorrhage, may result in an excess hypothalamic input to the sympathetic and parasympathetic control systems.[13] This condition can trigger virtually any type of cardiac arrhythmia, from sinus pause to supraventricular tachycardia to ventricular fibrillation.[14] However, the most common finding in subarachnoid hemorrhage is a pattern of subendocardial ischemia. Such patients may in fact have enzyme evidence of myocardial infarction, and at autopsy demonstrate contraction band necrosis of the myocardium.[15]

Sympathoexcitation is also seen in patients who are delirious. The infralimbic and insular cortex and the central nucleus of the amygdala provide important inputs to sympathoexcitatory areas of the hypothalamus and the medulla.[8] Activation of these areas due to misperception of stimuli in the environment causing emotional responses such as fear or anger may result in hypertension, tachycardia, and enlarged pupils.

Stokes-Adams attacks are periods of brief loss of consciousness due to lack of adequate cerebral perfusion. These almost always occur in an upright position. In recumbent positions, when the head is at the same height as the heart, it takes a much steeper fall in blood pressure (below 60 to 70 mm Hg mean pressure) to cause loss of consciousness. The fall in blood pressure during a Stokes-Adams attack may reflect a failure of the baroreceptor reflex arc on assuming an upright posture (in which case it can be reproduced by testing orthostatic responses). Alternatively, hyperactivity of the baroreceptor reflex nerves may occasionally cause hypotension (e.g., in patients with carotid sinus hypersensitivity or glossopharyngeal neuralgia, where brief bursts of activity in baroreceptor nerves trigger a rapid fall in heart rate and blood pressure).[16,17] In other patients, the fall in blood pressure may be caused by an intermittent failure of the pump (i.e., cardiac arrhythmia). Thus, careful cardiologic evaluation is required if a neurologic cause is not identified.

PATHOPHYSIOLOGY

The brain ordinarily tightly controls the circulation to provide an adequate level of cerebral perfusion. It does this in two ways. First, across a wide range of arterial blood pressures, it autoregulates its own blood flow.[18–21] The mechanism for this remarkable stability of blood flow is not entirely understood, although it appears to be due to intrinsic innervation of the cerebral blood vessels and may also be regulated by local metabolism.[20,22] In general, local increases in CBF correspond to increases in local metabolic rate, allowing the use of blood flow (in positron emission tomography [PET] imaging) or local blood volume (in functional magnetic resonance imaging [MRI]) to approximate neuronal activity. However, there are also neuronal networks that regulate cerebral perfusion distinct from metabolic need. The two systems normally act in concert to ensure sufficient blood supply to allow normal cerebral function over a wide range of blood pressures but are dysregulated following some brain injuries.

Second, the brain acts through the autonomic nervous system to acutely adjust systemic arterial pressure in order to maintain a pressure head that is within the range that allows cerebral autoregulation. Blood pressure is the product of the cardiac output times the total vascular peripheral resistance. Cardiac output in turn is the product of heart rate and stroke volume. Both heart rate and stroke volume are increased by beta-1 adrenergic stimulation from sympathetic nerves (or adrenal catechols), which play a key role in regulating cardiac output. Heart rate is slowed by muscarinic cholinergic action of the vagus nerve, and hence, increased vagal tone decreases cardiac output. Peripheral resistance is regulated mainly by the level of alpha-1 adrenergic tone in small arterioles, the most important resistance vessels. Therefore, the blood pressure is regulated by the balance of sympathetic tone, which increases both cardiac output and vasoconstrictor tone, versus parasympathetic tone, which slows heart rate and therefore decreases cardiac output. The cardiac vagal tone is maintained by the nucleus ambiguus in the medulla, which contains most of the cardiac parasympathetic preganglionic neurons.[23] Sympathetic vascular and cardiac sympathetic tone is set by neurons in the rostral ventrolateral medulla that provide a tonic activating input to the sympathetic preganglionic neurons in the thoracic spinal cord.[24]

When in a lying position, the brain is at the same level as the heart, but as one rises, the brain elevates to a position 20 to 30 cm above the heart. This drop in perfusion pressure (arterial pressure minus intracranial pressure) is equivalent to 15 to 23 mm Hg, and it may be sufficient to cause a drop in cerebral perfusion pressure that would make it difficult to maintain CBF necessary to allow conscious brain function.

To defend against such a precipitous fall in perfusion pressure, the brain maintains reflex mechanisms to compensate for the hydrodynamic consequences of gravity. The level of arterial pressure is measured at two sites, the aortic arch (by the aortic depressor nerve, a branch of the vagus nerve) and the carotid bifurcation (by the carotid sinus nerve, a branch of the glossopharyngeal nerve). These two nerves terminate in the brain in the nucleus of the solitary tract, which is the main relay for all visceral sensory information in the brain.[25,26] The nucleus of the solitary tract then provides an excitatory input to the caudal ventrolateral medulla.[27]

The caudal ventrolateral medulla in turn provides an ascending inhibitory input to the tonic vasomotor neurons in the rostral ventrolateral medulla.[28] In addition, the nucleus of the solitary tract provides both direct and relayed excitatory inputs to the cardiac decelerator neurons in the nucleus ambiguus.[27] Thus, a rise in blood pressure results in a reflex fall in heart rate and vasomotor tone, re-establishing a normal arterial pressure. Conversely, a fall in blood pressure causes a reflex tachycardia and vasoconstriction, re-establishing the necessary arterial perfusion pressure. As a result, on assuming an upright posture, there is normally a small increase in both heart rate and blood pressure.

On occasion, loss of consciousness may result from failure of this baroreceptor reflex arc. In such patients, measurement of standing and supine blood pressure and heart rate discloses a fall in blood pressure on assuming an upright posture that is clinically associated with symptoms of insufficient CBF. Rigid criteria for diagnosing orthostatic hypotension (e.g., a fall in blood pressure of 10 or 15 mm Hg) are not useful, as systemic arterial pressure is usually measured in the arm but the symptoms are produced by decreased blood flow to the brain. A pressure head that is adequate to perfuse the arm (which is at the same elevation as the heart) will be reduced by 15 to 23 mm Hg at the brain in an upright posture, and if perfusion pressure to the brain falls even a few mm Hg below the level needed to maintain autoregulation, the drop in cerebral perfusion may be precipitous.

The most common nonneurologic causes of orthostatic hypotension, including low intravascular volume (often a consequence of diuretic administration or inadequate fluid intake), cardiac pump failure, and medications that impair arterial constriction (e.g., alpha blockers or direct vasodilators), do not impair the tachycardic response. Most neurologic cases of orthostatic hypotension, including peripheral autonomic neuropathy or central or peripheral autonomic degeneration, impair both the heart rate and the blood pressure responses. Put in other words, the hallmark of baroreceptor reflex failure is absence of the elevation of heart rate when arterial pressure falls in response to an orthostatic challenge.

Respiration

The brain cannot long survive without an adequate supply of oxygen. Within seconds of being deprived of oxygen, brain function begins to fail, and within minutes neurons begin to die. The physician must ensure that respiration is supplying adequate oxygenation. To do this requires examination of both respiratory exchange and respiratory pattern. Listening to the chest will ensure that there is adequate movement of air. A normal patient at rest will regularly breathe at about 14 breaths per minute and the exchange of air can be heard at both lung bases. The physician should estimate from the rate and depth of respiration whether the patient is hypo- or hyperventilating or whether respiration is normal. The patient's color is a gross indicator of oxygenation: cyanosis indicates deficient oxygenation; a cherry red color may also indicate deficient oxygenation because of CO intoxication. A better estimate of oxygenation can be achieved by placing an oximeter on the finger; many intensive care units and some emergency departments also measure expired CO_2, which correlates well with PCO_2.

This section considers the neuroanatomic basis of respiratory abnormalities that accom-

Table 2–2 **Neuropathologic Correlates of Breathing Abnormalities**

Forebrain damage
  Epileptic respiratory inhibition
  Apraxia for deep breathing or breath holding
  "Pseudobulbar" laughing or crying
  Posthyperventilation apnea
  Cheyne-Stokes respiration
Hypothalamic-midbrain damage
  Central reflex hyperpnea (neurogenic pulmonary edema)
Basis pontis damage
  Pseudobulbar paralysis of voluntary control
Lower pontine tegmentum damage or dysfunction
  Apneustic breathing
  Cluster breathing
  Short-cycle anoxic-hypercapnic periodic respiration
  Ataxic breathing (Biot)
Medullary dysfunction
  Ataxic breathing
  Slow regular breathing
  Loss of autonomic breathing with preserved voluntary control
  Gasping

pany coma (Table 2–2, Figure 2–3). Chapter 5 discusses respiratory responses to metabolic disturbances. Because neurogenic and metabolic influences on breathing interact extensively, respiratory changes must be interpreted cautiously if there is evidence of pulmonary disease.

The pattern of respiration can give important clues concerning the level of brain damage. Once assured that there is adequate exchange of oxygen, the physician should watch the patient spontaneously breathe. Irregularities of the respiratory pattern that provide clues to the level of brain damage are described in the paragraphs below.

PATHOPHYSIOLOGY

Breathing is a sensorimotor act that integrates nervous influences arising from nearly every level of the brain and upper spinal cord. In humans, respiration subserves two major func-

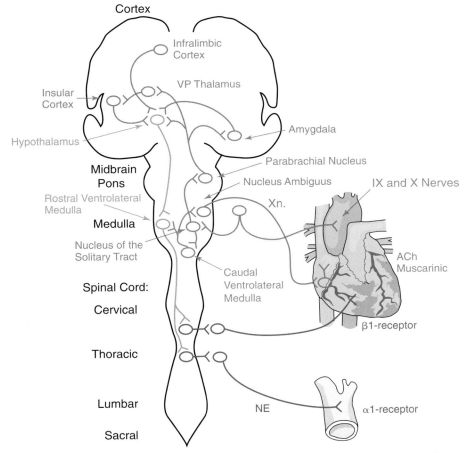

Figure 2–3. A diagram summarizing the cardiovascular control pathways in the brain. Visceral afferent information (gray) arrives from nerves IX and X into the nucleus of the solitary tract. This information is then distributed to the parabrachial nucleus, which relays it to the forebrain, and to the ventrolateral medulla, where it controls cardiovascular reflexes. These include both vagal control of heart rate (red) and medullary control (purple) of the sympathetic vasomotor control area of the rostral ventrolateral medulla (orange), which regulates sympathetic outflow to both the heart and the blood vessels (dark green). Forebrain areas that influence the cardiovascular system (brown) include the insular cortex (a visceral sensory area), the infralimbic cortex (a visceral motor area), and the amygdala, which produces autonomic emotional responses. All of these act on the hypothalamic sympathetic activating neurons (light green) in the paraventricular and lateral hypothalamic areas to provide behavioral and emotional influence over the blood pressure and heart rate. ACh, acetylcholine; NE, norepinephrine; VP, ventroposterior.

tions: one of metabolism and the other behavioral. Metabolically, respiratory control is directed principally at maintaining tissue oxygenation and normal acid-base balance. It is regulated mainly by reflex neural mechanisms located in the posterior-dorsal region of the pons and in the medulla. Behavioral control of breathing allows it to be integrated with swallowing, and in humans, with verbal and emotional communication as well as other behaviors.

Respiratory rhythm is an intrinsic property of the brainstem that is generated by a network of neurons that lie in the ventrolateral medulla, including the pre-Bötzinger complex[29,30] (see Figure 2–3). This rhythm is regulated in the intact brain by a number of influences that enter via the vagus and glossopharyngeal nerves.

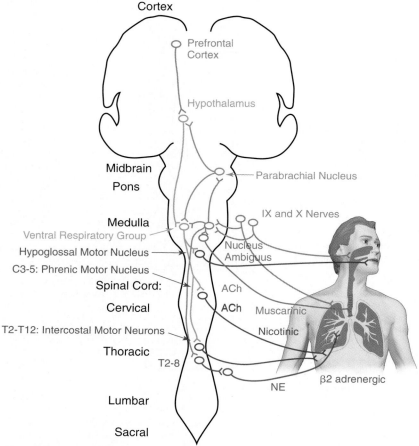

Figure 2–4. A diagram summarizing the respiratory control pathways in the brain. Afferents from the lung (pulmonary stretch), upper airway (cough reflexes), and carotid body arrive via cranial nerves IX and X in the nucleus of the solitary tract (gray), also called the dorsal respiratory group. These control airway and respiratory reflexes, analogous to the cardiovascular system, by inputs to the ventrolateral medulla. These include outputs to the airways via the vagus nerve (red) and outputs from the ventral respiratory group (orange) to the spinal cord, controlling sympathetic airway responses (green) and respiratory motor (phrenic motor nucleus, blue) and accessory motor (hypoglossal and intercostal, blue) outputs. The ventral respiratory group is responsible for generating respiratory rhythm. However, it is assisted in this process by the parabrachial nucleus (or pontine respiratory group, purple), which receives ascending respiratory afferents and integrates them with other brainstem reflexes (e.g., swallowing). The prefrontal cortex (brown) provides behavioral regulation of breathing, producing a continual breathing rhythm even in the absence of metabolic need. This influences the hypothalamus (light green), which may vary respiratory pattern in coordination with behavior or emotion. ACh, acetylcholine; NE, norepinephrine.

The carotid sinus branch of the glossopharyngeal nerve brings afferents that carry information about blood oxygen and carbon dioxide content, whereas the vagus nerve conveys pulmonary stretch afferents. These terminate in the commissural, ventrolateral, intermediate, and interstitial components of the nucleus of the solitary tract.[31–33] Chemoreceptor afferents can increase respiratory rate and depth, whereas pulmonary stretch receptors tend to inhibit lung inflation (the Herring-Breuer reflex). These influences are relayed to reticular areas in the ventrolateral medulla that regulate the onset of inspiration and expiration.[34] In addition, serotoninergic neurons in the ventral medulla may also serve as chemoreceptors and directly influence the nearby circuitry that generates the respiratory rhythm.[35,36]

The medullary circuitry that controls respiration is under the control of pontine cell groups that integrate breathing with ongoing orofacial stimuli and behaviors.[37] Neurons in the parabrachial nucleus primarily increase the rate and depth of respiration, presumably in relation to emotional responses or in anticipation of metabolic demand during various behaviors. On the other hand, neurons located more ventrally in the intertrigeminal zone, between the principal sensory and motor trigeminal nuclei, produce apneas, which are necessary during swallowing and in response to noxious chemical irritation of the airway (e.g., smoke or water in the nasal passages).[38]

Superimposed upon these metabolic demands and basic reflexes, the forebrain can command a wide range of respiratory responses. Respiration can be altered by emotional response, and it increases in anticipation of metabolic demand during voluntary exercise, even if the muscle that is to be contracted has been paralyzed (i.e., as a consequence of central command rather than metabolic reflex). The pathways that control vocalization in humans appear to originate in the frontal opercular cortex, which provides premotor and motor integration of orofacial motor actions. However, there is also a prefrontal contribution to the maintenance of respiratory rhythm, even in the absence of metabolic demand (the basis for posthyperventilation apnea, described below).

These considerations make the recognition of respiratory changes useful in the diagnosis of coma (Figure 2–5).

POSTHYPERVENTILATION APNEA

If the arterial carbon dioxide tension is lowered by a brief period of hyperventilation, a healthy awake subject will nevertheless continue to breathe with a normal rhythm, at least initially,[39] albeit at reduced volume, until the PCO_2 returns to its original level. By contrast, subjects with diffuse metabolic impairment of the forebrain, or bilateral structural damage to the frontal lobes, commonly demonstrate posthyperventilation apnea.[40] Their respirations stop after deep breathing has lowered the carbon dioxide content of the blood below its usual resting level. Rhythmic breathing returns when endogenous carbon dioxide production raises the arterial level back to normal.

The demonstration of posthyperventilation apnea requires that the patient voluntarily take several deep breaths, so that it is useful in differential diagnosis of lethargic or confused patients, but not in cases of stupor or coma. One instructs the subject to take five deep breaths. No other instructions are given. It is useful for the examiner to place a hand on the patient's chest, to make it easier later to detect when breathing has restarted, and to count the breaths. If the lungs function well, the maneuver usually lowers the arterial carbon dioxide by 8 to 14 torr. At the end of the deep breathing, wakeful patients without brain damage show little or no apnea (less than 10 seconds). However, in patients with forebrain impairment, the period of apnea may last from 12 to 30 seconds. The neural substrate that produces a continuous breathing pattern even in the absence of metabolic need is believed to include the same frontal pathways that regulate behavioral alterations of breathing patterns, as the continuous breathing pattern disappears with sleep, bilateral frontal lobe damage, or diffuse metabolic impairment of the hemispheres.

CHEYNE-STOKES RESPIRATION

Cheyne-Stokes respiration[41] is a pattern of periodic breathing with phases of hyperpnea alternating regularly with apnea. The depth of respiration waxes from breath to breath in a smooth crescendo during onset of the hyperpneic phase and then, once a peak is reached, wanes in an equally smooth decrescendo until a period of apnea, usually from 10 to 20 seconds,

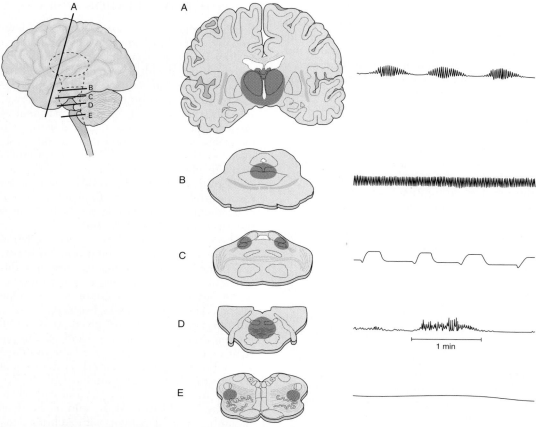

Figure 2–5. Different abnormal respiratory patterns are associated with pathologic lesions (shaded areas) at various levels of the brain. Tracings by chest-abdomen pneumography, inspiration reads up. (A) Cheyne-Stokes respiration is seen with metabolic encephalopathies and with lesions that impair forebrain or diencephalic function. (B) Central neurogenic hyperventilation is most commonly seen in metabolic encephalopathies, but may rarely be seen in cases of high brainstem tumors. (C) Apneusis, consisting of inspiratory pauses, may be seen in patients with bilateral pontine lesions. (D) Cluster breathing and ataxic breathing are seen with lesions at the pontomedullary junction. (E) Apnea occurs when lesions encroach on the ventral respiratory group in the ventrolateral medulla bilaterally. (From Saper, C. Brain stem modulation of sensation, movement, and consciousness. Chapter 45 in: Kandel, ER, Schwartz, JH, Jessel, TM. *Principles of Neural Science*. 4th ed. McGraw-Hill, New York, 2000, pp. 871–909. By permission of McGraw-Hill.)

is reached. The hyperpneic phase usually lasts longer than the apneic phase (Figure 2–5).

This rhythmic alternation in Cheyne-Stokes respiration results from the interplay of normal brainstem respiratory reflexes.[42–45] When the medullary chemosensory circuits sense adequate oxygen and carbon dioxide tension, they reduce the rate and depth of respiration, causing a gradual rise in arterial carbon dioxide tension. There is normally a short delay of a few seconds, representing the transit time for fresh blood from the lungs to reach the left heart and then the chemoreceptors in the carotid artery and the brain. By the time the brain begins increasing the rate and depth of respiration, the alveolar carbon dioxide has reached even higher levels, and so there is a gradual ramping up of respiration as the brain sees a rising level of carbon dioxide, despite its additional efforts. By the time the brain begins to see a fall in carbon dioxide tension, the levels in the alveoli may be quite low. When blood containing this low level of carbon dioxide reaches the brain, respiration slows or may even cease, thus setting off another cycle. Hence, the periodic cycling is due to the delay (*hys-*

teresis) in the feedback loop between alveolar ventilation and brain chemoreceptor sensory responses.

The Cheyne-Stokes respiratory cycle is not usually seen in normal individuals because the circulatory delay between a change in alveolar blood gases and carbon dioxide tension in the brain is only a few seconds. Even as circulatory delay rises with cardiovascular or pulmonary disease, during waking the descending pathways that prevent posthyperventilation apnea also ensure the persistence of respiration even during periods of low metabolic need, thus damping the oscillations that produce Cheyne-Stokes respiration. However, during sleep or with bilateral forebrain impairment, due either to a diffuse metabolic process such as uremia, hepatic failure, or bilateral damage such as cerebral infarcts or a forebrain mass lesion with diencephalic displacement, periodic breathing may emerge.[43–45] In patients with heart failure, the transit time for blood from the lungs to reach the carotid and cerebral chemoreceptors can become so prolonged as to produce a Cheyne-Stokes pattern of respiration, even in the absence of forebrain impairment. Thus, Cheyne-Stokes respiration is mainly useful as a sign of intact brainstem respiratory reflexes in the patients with forebrain impairment, but cannot be interpreted in the presence of significant congestive heart failure.

HYPERVENTILATION IN COMATOSE PATIENTS

Sustained hyperventilation is often seen in patients with impaired consciousness, but is usually a result of either hepatic coma or sepsis, conditions in which circulating chemical stimuli cause hyperpnea, or a metabolic acidosis, such as diabetic ketoacidosis (see Chapter 5). Other patients have meningitis caused either by infection or subarachnoid hemorrhage, which stimulates chemoreceptors in the brainstem,[46] probably by altering CSF pH.

Some patients hyperventilate when intrinsic brainstem injury or subarachnoid hemorrhage or seizures cause neurogenic pulmonary edema.[47] The ventilatory response is driven by pulmonary mechanosensory and chemosensory receptors. The pulmonary congestion lowers both the arterial carbon dioxide and the oxygen tension. Stimulation of pulmonary stretch re-

ceptors is apparently sufficient to cause reflex hyperpnea, as oxygen therapy sufficient to raise the arterial oxygen level does not always correct the overbreathing.

Another small group of patients has been identified who have hyperventilation associated with brainstem gliomas or lymphomas.[48,49] These patients have spinal fluid that is acellular, but generally acidotic compared to arterial pH. In others, the lumbar CSF may have a normal pH, but it is believed that the tumor causes local lactic acidosis, which may trigger brain chemoreceptors to cause hyperventilation (Figure 2–5).

It is theoretically possible for an irritative lesion in the region of the parabrachial nucleus or other respiratory centers to produce hyperpnea.[37] The diagnosis of such true "central neurogenic hyperventilation" requires that with the subject breathing room air, the blood gases show elevated arterial oxygen tension, decreased carbon dioxide tension, and an elevated pH. The cerebrospinal fluid likewise must show an elevated pH and be acellular. The respiratory changes must persist during sleep to eliminate psychogenic hyperventilation, and one must exclude the presence of stimulating drugs, such as salicylates, or disorders that stimulate respiration, such as hepatic failure or underlying systemic infection. Cases fulfilling all of these criteria have rarely been observed,[50,51] and none that we are aware of has come to postmortem examination of the brain.

APNEUSTIC BREATHING

Apneusis is a respiratory pause at full inspiration. Fully developed apneustic breathing, with each cycle including an inspiratory pause, is rare in humans, but of considerable localizing value. Experiments in animals indicate that apneusis develops with injury to the pontine respiratory nuclei described above, and experience with rare human cases would support this view[52,53] (see Figure 2–5).

Clinically, end-inspiratory pauses of 2 to 3 seconds usually alternate with end-expiratory pauses, and both are most frequently encountered in the setting of pontine infarction due to basilar artery occlusion. However, apneustic breathing may rarely be observed in metabolic encephalopathies, including hypoglycemia, anoxia, or meningitis. It is sometimes observed in cases of transtentorial herniation, as the brainstem dysfunction advances. At least one patient with apneusis due to a brainstem infarct responded to buspirone, a serotonin 1A receptor agonist.[53]

ATAXIC BREATHING

Irregular, gasping respiration implies damage to the respiratory rhythm generator at the pre-Bötzinger level of the upper medulla.[30] This cell group can be specifically eliminated in experimental animals by the use of a toxin that binds to neurons that express NK-1 receptors. The resulting irregular, gasping breathing is eerily similar to humans with bilateral rostral medullary lesions, and it indicates that sufficient neurons survive in the medullary reticular formation to drive primitive ventilatory efforts, despite the loss of the neurons that cause smooth to-and-fro respiration.[54] More complete bilateral lesions of the ventrolateral medullary reticular formation cause apnea, which is not compatible with life unless the patient is artificially ventilated (Figure 2–5).

A variety of intermediate types of breathing patterns are also seen with high medullary lesions. Some patients may breathe in irregular clusters or ratchet-like breaths separated by pauses. In other cases, particularly during intoxication with opiates or sedative drugs, the breathing may slow and decline in depth gradually until it fades into complete arrest.

There is a tendency in modern hospitals to intubate and ventilate patients with structural coma to protect the airway and permit treatment of respiratory failure. If the patient fights intubation or ventilation, paralytic drugs are often administered. This compromises the ability of the neurologist to assess brainstem reflexes, and in some cases may delay diagnosis and compromise care. Thus, it is important, whenever possible, to delay intubation until after the brief coma examination described here has been completed.

SLEEP APNEA AND ONDINE'S CURSE

Obstructive sleep apnea is a common disorder in which the cross-section of the upper airway is anatomically narrow.[55,56] During sleep, the muscles that keep the upper airway open, including the genioglossus muscle that pulls the tongue forward, undergo a gradual loss of tone. This results in critical narrowing of the airway and the increased rate of movement of air tends to further reduce airway pressure, resulting in sudden closure. Liable to the disorder are obese patients, because deposition of fat in neck tissue reduces airway diameter; men, because the increased ratio of the length of the airway to its diameter predisposes to collapse; and middle aged or older patients, because muscle tone is more reduced during sleep with age. However, cases may occur in thin young adults, or even in children. Sleep apnea typically occurs in cycles lasting a few minutes each when the patient falls asleep, airway tone fails and an obstructive apnea occurs, blood oxygen levels fall, carbon dioxide rises, and the patient is aroused sufficiently to resume breathing. This cycle may be repeated many times over the course of a night. The fragmentation of sleep and intermittent hypoxia result in chronic daytime sleepiness and impairment of cognitive function, particularly vigilance.

Excessive drowsiness during the day and loud snoring at night may be the only clues. Lethargy or drowsiness due to neurologic injury may induce apneic cycles in a patient with obstructive sleep apnea. However, as the level of consciousness becomes more impaired, it may be difficult to achieve the periodic arousals necessary to resume breathing.

Other patients with pauses in ventilation have central sleep apnea. Most such patients have congestive heart failure, and the pauses are thought to be analogous to the periodic breathing that is seen in patients who develop Cheyne-Stokes respiration when they fall asleep.

Failure of automatic breathing is a rare condition, sometimes called Ondine's curse, named after the mythologic wood nymph whose mortal lover lost autonomic functions whenever he went to sleep. In adults, Ondine's curse is seen after lesions of the ventrolateral medullary chemosensory areas or bilateral damage to the descending pathways that control automatic respiration in the lateral columns of the spinal cord (e.g., as a complication of cordotomy to relieve cancer pain).[57–62] In children, it is most frequently seen as a congenital condition in infants, sometimes in association with Hirschsprung's disease, and either a neuroblastoma or pheochromocytoma, often associated with a mutation in the PHOX2B gene.[63] A variety of interventions have been successful, ranging from a rocking bed, which provides continuous somatic sensory and vestibular stimulation, to negative pressure ventilation, or even diaphragmatic pacing.[64]

YAWNING, HICCUPPING, VOMITING

The neuronal pattern generators responsible for coordinating respiratory-related behaviors also are located in the ventrolateral medulla, in close proximity to the nucleus ambiguus.[65] Yawning is a motor pattern that involves deep inspiration associated with wide opening of the jaw and generalized muscle stretching.[66,67] It is seen even in patients who are locked in, and hence is apparently organized at a medullary level. Yawning may improve the compliance of the lungs and chest wall, but its function is not understood. It may be seen in lethargic patients, but yawning is also seen in complex partial seizures emanating from the medial temporal lobe, and is not of great localizing value.

Hiccups occur in patients with abdominal or subphrenic pathology (e.g., pancreatic cancer) that impinges upon the vagus nerve.[68,69] Dexamethasone may induce hiccups; the mechanism is unknown.[70] Hiccups occasionally occur with lesions in the medullary tegmentum, including neoplasms, infarction, hematomas, infections, or syringobulbia. Because stuporous patients with intracranial mass lesions are often treated with corticosteroids to reduce brain edema, it may be difficult to determine whether pressure on the floor of the fourth ventricle from the mass lesion or the treatment with corticosteroids is causing the hiccups.[71] Pathologic hiccupping is peculiarly more common in men; in a study of 220 patients at the Mayo Clinic with pathologic hiccupping, all but 39 were men.[72]

The hiccup reflex consists of a spasmodic burst of inspiratory activity, followed 35 milliseconds later by abrupt glottic closure, so that the ventilatory effect is negligible. On the other hand, if the airway is kept open artificially (e.g., by tracheostomy), the inrush of air can be sufficient to hyperventilate the patient. As an example, one patient in New York Hospital with a low brainstem infarct and tracheostomy maintained his total ventilation for several days by hiccup alone.

Pathologic hiccups are difficult to treat.[73] A number of drugs and physical approaches have been tried, most of which do not work well. Agents used to treat hiccups include phenothiazines, calcium channel blockers, baclofen, and anticonvulsants, gabapentin being the most recent.[74] In steroid-induced hiccups, decreasing the dose usually reduces the hiccups.[73]

Vomiting is a reflex response involving coordinated somatomotor (posture, abdominal muscle contraction), gastrointestinal (reversal of peristalsis), and respiratory (retching, breath holding) components that are coordinated by neurons in the ventrolateral medullary tegmentum near the compact portion of the nucleus ambiguus. The vomiting reflex may be triggered by vagal afferents[75,76] or by chemosensory neurons in the area postrema, a small group of nerve cells that sits atop the nucleus of the solitary tract in the floor of the fourth ventricle, just at the level of the obex.[77]

In patients with impaired consciousness, vomiting is frequently due to lesions involving the lateral pons or medulla, causing vestibular imbalance. It occasionally occurs in patients with irritative lesions limited to the region of the nucleus of the solitary tract.[77] Such vomiting is typically preceded by intense nausea. More commonly, however, vomiting is due to a sudden increase in intracranial pressure, such as occurs in subarachnoid hemorrhage. The pressure wave may stimulate the emetic response directly by pressure on the floor of the fourth ventricle, resulting in sudden, "projectile" vomiting, without warning. This type of vomiting is particularly common in children with posterior fossa tumors. It is also seen in adults with brain tumor, who hypoventilate during sleep, resulting in cerebral vasodilation. The small increase in intravascular blood volume, in a patient whose intracranial pressure is already elevated, may cause a sharp increase in intracranial pressure (see Chapter 3), resulting in onset of an intense headache that may waken the patient, followed shortly thereafter by sudden projectile vomiting. Children with posterior fossa tumors may simply vomit without headache.

Vomiting is also commonly seen in patients with brain tumors during chemotherapy or even radiation therapy. Tissue injury, particularly in the gut, may release emetic hormones, such as glucagon-like peptide-1 (GLP-1). GLP-1 is detected by neurons in the area postrema, and it can induce a vomiting reflex.[78] The area postrema contains both dopaminergic and serotoninergic neurons, and the latter produce emesis primarily by means of contacting $5HT_3$ receptors.[77] Hence, drugs that block dopamine D_2 receptors (e.g., chlorpromazine, metoclopramide) or serotonin $5HT_3$ receptors (ondansetron) are effective antiemetics.

PUPILLARY RESPONSES

The pupillary light reflex is one of the most basic and easily tested nervous system responses. It is controlled by a complex balance of sympathetic (pupillodilator) and parasympathetic (pupilloconstrictor) pathways (see Figure 2–6). The anatomy of these pathways is closely intertwined with the components of the ascending arousal system. In addition, the pupillary pathways are among the most resistant to metabolic insult. *Hence, abnormalities of pupillary responses are of great localizing value in diagnosing the cause of stupor and coma, and the pupillary light reflex is the single most important physical sign in differentiating metabolic from structural coma.*

Examine the Pupils and Their Responses

If possible, inquire if the patient has suffered eye disease or uses eyedrops. Observe the pupils in ambient light; if room lights are bright and pupils are small, dimming the light may make it easier to see the pupillary responses. They should be equal in size and about the same size as those of normal individuals in the same light (8% to 18% of normal individuals have anisocoria greater than 0.4 mm). Unequal pupils can result from sympathetic paralysis making the pupil smaller or parasympathetic paralysis making the pupil larger. If one suspects sympathetic paralysis (see *Horner's syndrome*, page 58), dim the lights in the room, allowing the normal pupil to dilate and thus bringing out the pupillary inequality. Unless there is specific damage to the pupillary system, pupils of stuporous or comatose patients are usually smaller than normal pupils in awake subjects. Pupillary responses must be examined with a bright light. The eyelids can be held

open while the light from a bright flashlight illuminates each pupil. Shining the light into one pupil should cause both pupils to react briskly and equally. Because the pupils are often small in stuporous or comatose patients and the light reflex may be through a small range, one may want to view the pupil through the bright light of an ophthalmoscope using a plus 20 lens or through the lens of an otoscope. Most pupillary responses are brisk, but a tonic pupil may react slowly, so the light should illuminate the eye for at least 10 seconds. Moving the light from one eye to the other may result in constriction of both pupils when the light is shined into the first eye, but paradoxically pupillary dilation when the light is shined in the other eye. This aberrant pupillary response results from damage to the retina or optic nerve on the side on which the pupil dilates (relative afferent pupillary defect [RAPD]).[79]

One of the most ominous signs in neurology is a unilateral dilated and unreactive pupil. In a comatose patient, this usually indicates oculomotor nerve compromise either by a posterior communicating artery aneurysm or by temporal lobe herniation (see *oculomotor responses*, page 60). However, the same finding can be mimicked by unilateral instillation of atropine-like eye drops. Occasionally this happens by accident, as when a patient who is using a scopolamine patch to avert motion sickness inadvertently gets some scopolamine onto a finger when handling the patch, and then rubs the eye; however, it is also seen in cases of factitious presentation. Still other times, unilateral pupillary dilation may occur in the setting of ciliary ganglion dysfunction from head or facial trauma. In most of these cases there is a fracture in the posterior floor of the orbit that interrupts the fibers of the inferior division of the oculomotor nerve.[80] Injury to the third nerve can be distinguished from atropinic blockade at the bedside by instilling a dilute solution of pilocarpine into the eye (see *pharmacology*, page 56). The denervated pupil will respond briskly, whereas the one that is blocked by atropine will not.[81]

Once both the ipsilateral and consensual pupillary light reflexes have been noted, the next step is to induce a ciliospinal reflex.[10] This can be done by pinching the skin of the neck or the face. The pupils should dilate 1 to 2 mm bilaterally. This reflex is an example of a spinobulbospinal response (i.e., the pain stimulus arises from the trigeminal or spinal dorsal horn, must ascend to brainstem autonomic control areas, and then descend again to the C8-T2 sympathetic preganglionic neurons). A normal ciliospinal response ensures integrity of these circuits from the lower brainstem to the spinal cord, thus usually placing the lesion in the rostral pons or higher.

Pathophysiology of Pupillary Responses: Peripheral Anatomy of the Pupillomotor System

The pupil is a hole in the iris; thus, change in pupillary diameter occurs when the iris contracts or expands. The pupillodilator muscle is a set of radially oriented muscle fibers, running from the edge of the pupil to the limbus (outer edge) of the iris. When these muscles contract, they open the pupil in much the way a drawstring pulls up a curtain. The pupillodilator muscles are innervated by sympathetic ganglion cells in the superior cervical ganglion. These

axons pass along the internal carotid artery, joining the ophthalmic division of the trigeminal nerve in the cavernous sinus and accompanying it through the superior orbital fissure, into the orbit. Sympathetic input to the lid retractor muscle takes a similar course, but sympathetic fibers from the superior cervical ganglion that control facial sweating travel along the external carotid artery. Hence, lesions of the ascending cervical sympathetic chain up to the superior cervical ganglion typically give rise to Horner's syndrome (ptosis, miosis, and facial anhydrosis). However, lesions along the course of the internal carotid artery may give only the first two components of this syndrome (Raeder's paratrigeminal syndrome). The sympathetic preganglionic neurons for pupillary control are found in the intermediolateral column of the first three thoracic segments. Hence, lesions of those roots, or of the ascending sympathetic trunk between T1 and the superior cervical ganglion, may also cause a Horner's syndrome with, depending on the exact site of the lesion, anhydrosis of the ipsilateral face or the face and arm.

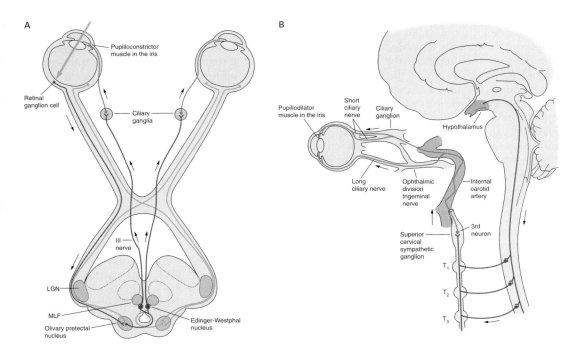

Figure 2–6. Two summary drawings indicating the (**A**) parasympathetic pupilloconstrictor pathways and (**B**) sympathetic pupillodilator pathways. LGN, lateral geniculate nucleus; MLF, medial longitudinal fasciculus. (From Saper, C. Brain stem modulation of sensation, movement, and consciousness. Chapter 45 in: Kandel, ER, Schwartz, JH, Jessel, TM. *Principles of Neural Science.* 4th ed. McGraw-Hill, New York, 2000, pp. 871–909. By permission of McGraw-Hill.)

The pupilloconstrictor muscle consists of circumferentially oriented muscle fibers that narrow the pupil when they contract, in the same manner as the drawstring of a purse. The parasympathetic neurons that supply the pupilloconstrictor muscle are located in the ciliary ganglion and in episcleral ganglion cells within the orbit. The preganglionic neurons for pupilloconstriction are located in the oculomotor complex in the brainstem (Edinger-Westphal nucleus) and they arrive in the orbit via the oculomotor or third cranial nerve. The pupilloconstrictor fibers travel in the dorsomedial quadrant of the third nerve, where they are vulnerable to compression by a number of causes (Chapter 3), often before there is clear impairment of the third nerve extraocular muscles. As a result, unilateral loss of pupilloconstrictor tone is of great diagnostic importance in patients with stupor or coma caused by supratentorial mass lesions.

Pharmacology of the Peripheral Pupillomotor System

Because the state of the pupils is of such importance in the diagnosis of patients with coma, it is sometimes necessary to explore the origin of aberrant responses. Knowledge of the pharmacology of the pupillomotor system is essential to properly interpret the findings.[82] The sympathetic preganglionic neurons in the thoracic spinal cord are cholinergic, and they act upon a nicotinic type II receptor on the sympathetic ganglion cells. The sympathetic terminals onto the pupillodilator muscle in the iris are noradrenergic, and they dilate the pupil via a beta-1 adrenergic receptor.

In the presence of a unilateral small pupil, it is possible to determine whether the cause is due to failure of the sympathetic ganglion cells or is preganglionic. In the latter case, the ganglion cells are intact, but not active. The pupil can then be dilated by instilling a few drops of 1% hydroxyamphetamine into the eye, which releases norepinephrine from surviving sympathetic terminals. Because the postsynaptic receptors have become hypersensitive due to the paucity of neurotransmitter being released, there is brisk pupillodilation after instilling the eye drops. Conversely, if the pupil is small due to loss of postganglionic neurons or receptor blockade, hydroxyamphetamine will have little if any effect. Postganglionic failure can be differentiated from receptor blockade (e.g., instillation of eyedrops containing a beta blocker such as are used to treat glaucoma) by introduction of 0.1% adrenaline drops, which have direct beta agonist effects. Denervated receptors are hypersensitive and there is brisk pupillary dilation, but a pupil that is small due to a beta blocker does not respond.

The pupilloconstrictor neurons in the oculomotor complex use acetylcholine, and they act on the ciliary and episcleral ganglion cells via a nicotinic II receptor. The parasympathetic ganglion cells, by contrast, activate the pupilloconstrictor muscle via a muscarinic cholinergic synapse. In the presence of a dilated pupil due to an injury to the third nerve or the postganglionic neurons, the hypersensitive receptors will constrict the pupil rapidly in response to a dilute solution of the muscarinic agonist pilocarpine (0.125%). However, if the enlarged pupil is due to atropine, even much stronger solutions of pilocarpine (up to 1.0%) will be unable to constrict the pupil.

CENTRAL PATHWAYS CONTROLLING PUPILLARY RESPONSES

It is important to understand the central pathways that regulate pupillary light responses, because dysfunction in these pathways causes the abnormal pupillary signs seen in patients with coma due to brainstem injury.

Preganglionic *sympathetic* neurons in the C8-T2 levels of the spinal cord, which regulate pupillodilation, receive inputs from several levels of the brain. The main input driving sympathetic pupillary tone derives from the ipsilateral hypothalamus. Neurons in the paraventricular and arcuate nuclei and in the lateral hypothalamus all innervate the upper thoracic sympathetic preganglionic neurons.[83] The orexin/hypocretin neurons in the lateral hypothalamus provide a particularly intense input to this area.[84] This input may be important, as the activity of the orexin neurons is greatest during wakefulness, when pupillodilation is maximal.[85] The descending hypothalamic input runs through the lateral part of the pontine and medullary brainstem tegmentum, where it is vulnerable to interruption by brainstem injury.[7] Electrical stimulation of the descending sympathoexcitatory tract in cats demonstrates that it runs in a superficial position along the surface of the ventrolateral medulla, just dorsolateral to the inferior olivary nucleus.[86] Experience with patients with lateral medullary infarction supports a similar localization in humans. Such patients have a *central Horner's syndrome,* which includes not only miosis and ptosis, but also loss of sweating on the entire ipsilateral side of the body. Thus, the sympathoexcitatory pathway remains ipsilateral from the hypothalamus all the way to the spinal cord.

Other brainstem pathways also contribute to pupillodilation. Inputs to the C8-T2 sympathetic preganglionic column arise from a number of brainstem sites, including the Kölliker-Fuse nucleus, A5 noradrenergic neurons, C1 adrenergic neurons, medullary raphe serotoninergic neurons, and other populations in the rostral ventrolateral medulla that have not been chemically characterized in detail.[8] Ascending pain afferents from the spinal cord terminate both in these sites as well as in the periaqueductal gray matter. Brainstem sympathoexcitatory neurons can cause pupillodilation in response to painful stimuli (the *ciliospinal reflex*).[10] They also provide ascending inhibitory inputs to the pupilloconstrictor neurons in the midbrain. As a result, lesions of the pontine tegmentum, which destroy both these ascending inhibitory inputs to the pupilloconstrictor system and the descending excitatory inputs to the pupillodilator system, cause the most severely constricted pupils seen in humans.

Preganglionic *parasympathetic* neurons are located in the Edinger-Westphal nucleus in primates.[87,88] This complex cell group also contains peptidergic neurons that mainly provide descending projections to the spinal cord. In rodents and cats, most of the pupilloconstrictor neurons are located outside the Edinger-Westphal nucleus, and the nucleus itself mainly consists of the spinally projecting population, so that extrapolation from nonprimate species (where the anatomy and physiology of the system has been most carefully studied) is difficult.

The main input to the Edinger-Westphal nucleus of clinical interest is the afferent limb of the pupillary light reflex. The retinal ganglion cells that contribute to this pathway belong to a special class of irradiance detectors, most of which contain the photopigment melanopsin.[89] The same population of retinal ganglion cells that drives the pupillary light reflex also provides inputs to the suprachiasmatic nucleus in the circadian system, and in many cases individual ganglion cells send axonal branches to both systems. Although these ganglion cells are activated by the traditional pathways from rods and cones, they also are directly light sensitive, and as a consequence pupillary light reflexes are preserved in animals and humans with retinal degeneration who lack rods and cones (i.e., are functionally blind). This is in contrast to acute onset of blindness, in which preservation of the pupillary light reflex implies damage to the visual system beyond the optic tracts, usually at the level of the visual cortex.

The brightness-responsive retinal ganglion cells innervate the olivary pretectal nucleus. Neurons in the olivary pretectal nucleus then send their axons through the posterior commissure to the Edinger-Westphal nucleus of both sides.[90] The Edinger-Westphal nucleus in humans, as in other species, lies very close to the midline, just dorsal to the main body of the oculomotor nucleus. As a result, lesions that involve the posterior commissure disrupt the light reflex pathway from both eyes, resulting in fixed, slightly large pupils.

Descending cortical inputs can cause either pupillary constriction or dilation, and can either be ipsilateral, contralateral, or bilateral.[91] Sites that may produce pupillary responses are found in both the lateral and medial frontal lobes, the occipital lobe, and the temporal lobe. Unilateral pupillodilation has also been reported in patients during epileptic seizures. However, the pupillary response can be either ipsilateral or contralateral to the presumed origin of the seizures. Because so little is known about descending inputs to the pupillomotor system from the cortex and their physiologic role, it is not possible at this point to use pupillary responses during seizure activity to determine the lateralization, let alone localization, of the seizure onset. However, brief, reversible changes in pupillary size may be due to seizure activity rather than structural brainstem injury. We have also seen reversible and asymmetric changes in pupillary diameter in patients with oculomotor dysfunction due to tuberculous meningitis and with severe cases of Guillain-Barré syndrome that cause autonomic denervation.

Localizing Value of Abnormal Pupillary Responses in Patients in Coma

Characteristic pupillary responses are seen with lesions at specific sites in the neuraxis (Figure 2–7).

Diencephalic injuries typically result in small, reactive pupils. Bilateral, small, reactive pupils are typically seen when there is bilateral diencephalic injury or compression, but also are seen in almost all types of metabolic encephalopathy, and therefore this finding is also of limited value in identifying structural causes of coma.

A unilateral, small, reactive pupil accompanied by ipsilateral ptosis is often of great diagnostic value. If there is no associated loss of sweating in the face or the body (even after the patient is placed under a heating lamp that causes sweating of the contralateral face), then the lesion is likely to be along the course of the internal carotid artery or in the cavernous sinus, superior orbital fissure, or the orbit itself (*Raeder's paratrigeminal syndrome*, although in some cases the Horner's syndrome is merely incomplete). If there is a sweating defect confined to the face (*peripheral Horner's syndrome*), the defect must be extracranial (from the T1–2 spinal level to the carotid bifurcation). However, if the loss of sweating involves the entire side of the body (*central Horner's syndrome*), it indicates a lesion involving the pathway between the hypothalamus and the spinal cord on the ipsilateral side. Although hypothalamic unilateral injury can produce this finding, lesions of the lateral brainstem tegmentum are a more common cause.

Midbrain injuries may cause a wide range of pupillary abnormalities, depending on the

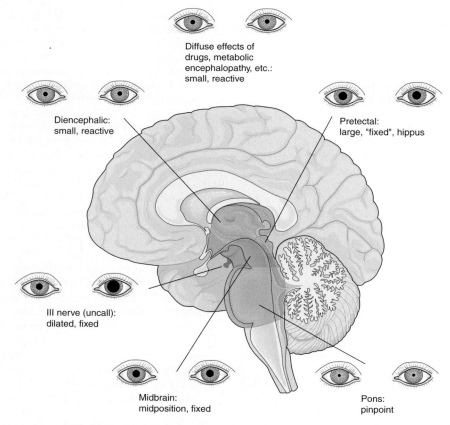

Diffuse effects of
drugs, metabolic
encephalopathy, etc.:
small, reactive

Diencephalic:
small, reactive

Pretectal:
large, "fixed", hippus

III nerve (uncall):
dilated, fixed

Midbrain:
midposition, fixed

Pons:
pinpoint

Figure 2–7. Summary of changes in pupils in patients with lesions at different levels of the brain that cause coma. (From Saper, C. Brain stem modulation of sensation, movement, and consciousness. Chapter 45 in: Kandel, ER, Schwartz, JH, Jessel, TM. *Principles of Neural Science*. 4th ed. McGraw-Hill, New York, 2000, pp. 871–909. By permission of McGraw-Hill.)

nature of the insult. Bilateral midbrain tegmental infarction, involving the oculomotor nerves or nuclei bilaterally, results in fixed pupils, which are either large (if the descending sympathetic tracts are preserved) or midposition (if they are not). However, pupils that are fixed due to midbrain injury may dilate with the ciliospinal reflex. This response distinguishes midbrain pupils from cases of brain death. It is often thought that pupils become fixed and dilated in death, but this is only true if there is a terminal release of adrenal catecholamines. The dilated pupils found immediately after death resolve over a few hours to the midposition, as are seen in patients who are brain dead or who have midbrain infarction.

More distal injury, after the *oculomotor nerve* leaves the brainstem, is typically unilateral. The oculomotor nerve's course makes it susceptible to damage by either the uncus of the temporal lobe as it herniates through the tentorial opening (see *supratentorial causes of coma*, page 103) or an aneurysm of the posterior communicating artery. Either of these lesions may compress the oculomotor nerve from the dorsal direction. Because the pupilloconstrictor fibers lie superficially on the dorsomedial surface of the nerve at this level,[92] the first sign of impending disaster may be a unilateral enlarged and poorly reactive pupil. These conditions are discussed in detail in Chapter 3.

Pontine tegmental injury typically results in pinpoint pupils. The pupils can often be seen under magnification to respond to bright light. However, the simultaneous injury to both the descending and ascending pupillodilator pathways causes near maximal pupillary constriction.[86] The most common cause is pontine hemorrhage.

Lesions involving the lateral *medullary* tegmentum, such as Wallenberg's lateral medullary infarction, may cause an ipsilateral central Horner's syndrome.

Metabolic and Pharmacologic Causes of Abnormal Pupillary Response

Although the foregoing discussion illustrates the importance of the pupillary light response in diagnosing structural causes of coma, it is critical to be able to distinguish structural causes from metabolic and pharmacologic causes of pupillary abnormalities. Nearly any metabolic encephalopathy that causes a sleepy state may result in small, reactive pupils that are difficult to differentiate from pupillary responses caused by diencephalic injuries. However, the pupillary light reflex is one of the most resistant brain responses during metabolic encephalopathy. Hence, a comatose patient who shows other signs of midbrain depression (e.g., loss of other oculomotor responses) yet retains the pupillary light reflex is likely to have a metabolic disturbance causing the coma.

During or following seizures, one or both pupils may transiently (usually for 15 to 20 minutes, and rarely as long as an hour) be large or react poorly to light. During hypoxia or global ischemia of the brain such as during a cardiac arrest, the pupils typically become large and fixed, due to a combination of systemic catecholamine release at the onset of the ischemia or hypoxia and lack of response by the metabolically depleted brain. If resuscitation is successful, the pupils usually return to a small, reactive state. Pupils that remain enlarged and nonreactive for more than a few minutes after otherwise successful resuscitation are indicative of profound brain ischemia and a poor prognostic sign (see discussion of outcomes from hypoxic/ischemic coma in Chapter 9).

Although most drugs that impair consciousness cause small, reactive pupils, a few produce quite different responses that may help to identify the cause of the coma. Opiates, for example, typically produce pinpoint pupils that resemble those seen in pontine hemorrhage. However, administration of an opioid antagonist such as naloxone results in rapid reversal of both the pupillary abnormality and the impairment of consciousness (naloxone must be given carefully to an opioid-intoxicated patient, because if the patient is opioid dependent, the drug may precipitate acute withdrawal). Chapter 7 discusses the use of naloxone. Muscarinic cholinergic antagonist drugs that cross the blood-brain barrier, such as scopolamine, may cause a confused, delirious state, in combination with large, poorly reactive pupils. Lack of response to pilocarpine eye drops (see above) demonstrates the muscarinic blockade. Glutethimide, a sedative-hypnotic drug that was popular in the 1960s, was notorious for causing large and poorly reactive pupils. Fortunately, it is rarely used anymore.

OCULOMOTOR RESPONSES

The brainstem nuclei and pathways that control eye movements lie in close association with the ascending arousal system. Hence, it is unusual for a patient with a structural cause of coma to have entirely normal eye movements, and the type of oculomotor abnormality often identifies the site of the lesion that causes coma. A key clinical tenet of the coma examination is that, with rare exception (e.g., a comatose patient with a congenital strabismus), *asymmetric oculomotor function typically identifies a patient with a structural rather than metabolic cause of coma.*

Functional Anatomy of the Peripheral Oculomotor System

Eye movements are due to the complex and simultaneous contractions of six extraocular muscles controlling each globe. In addition, the muscles of the iris (see above), the lens accommodation system, and the eyelid receive input from some of the same central cell groups and cranial nerves. Each of these can be used to identify the cause of an ocular motor disturbance, and may shed light on the origin of coma (Figure 2–8).[93]

Lateral movement of the globes is caused by the lateral rectus muscle, which in turn is un-

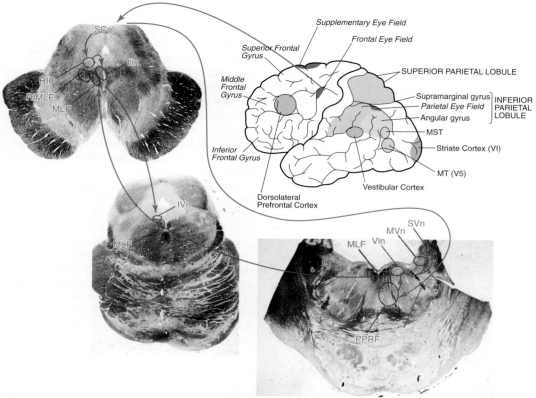

Figure 2–8. A summary diagram showing the major pathways responsible for eye movements. The frontal eye fields (A) provide input to the superior colliculus (SCol) to program saccadic eye movements. The superior colliculus then provides input to a premotor area for causing horizontal saccades (the paramedian pontine reticular formation [PPRF]), which in turn contacts neurons in the abducens nucleus. Abducens neurons (VIn) send axons across to the opposite medial longitudinal fasciculus (MLF) and to the opposite oculomotor nucleus (IIIn) to activate medial rectus motor neurons for the opposite eye. Vertical saccades are controlled by inputs from the superior colliculus to the rostral interstitial nucleus of the MLF (RIMLF) and rostral interstitial nucleus of Cajal (RIC), which act as a premotor area to instruct the neurons in the oculomotor and trochlear (IVn) nuclei to perform a vertical saccade. Vestibular and gaze-holding inputs come to the same ocular motor nuclei from the medial (MVN) and superior (SVN) vestibular nucleus. Note the intimate relationship of these cell groups and pathways with the ascending arousal system.

der the control of the abducens or sixth cranial nerve. The superior oblique muscle and trochlear or fourth cranial nerve have more complex actions. Because the trochlear muscle loops through a pulley, or trochleus, it attaches behind the equator of the globe and pulls it forward rather than back. When the eye turns medially, the action of this muscle is to pull the eye down and in. When the eye is turned laterally, however, the action of the muscle is to intort the eye (rotate it on its axis with the top of the iris moving medially). All of the other extraocular muscles receive their innervation through the oculomotor or third cranial nerve. These include the medial rectus, whose action is to turn the eye inward; the superior rectus, which pulls the eye up and out; and the inferior rectus and oblique, which turn the eye down and out and up and in, respectively. It should be clear from the above that, whereas impairment of mediolateral movements of the eyes mainly indicates imbalance of the two cognate rectus muscles, disturbances of upward or downward movement are far more complex to work out, as they result from dysfunction of the complex set of balanced contractions of the other four muscles. This situation is reflected in the central control of these movements, as will be reviewed below.

The oculomotor nerve exits the brainstem through the medial part of the cerebral peduncle, then travels anteriorly between the superior cerebellar and posterior cerebral arteries. It passes through the tentorial opening and runs adjacent to the posterior communicating artery, where it is subject to injury by posterior communicating artery aneurysms. The nerve then runs through the cavernous sinus and superior orbital fissure to the orbit, where it divides into superior and inferior branches. The superior branch innervates the superior rectus muscle and the levator palpebrae superioris, which raises the eyelid, and the inferior branch supplies the medial and inferior rectus and inferior oblique muscles as well as the ciliary ganglion. The abducens nerve exits from the base of the pons, near the midline. This slender nerve, which is often avulsed when the brain is removed at autopsy, runs along the clivus, through the tentorial opening, into the cavernous sinus and superior orbital fissure, on its way to the lateral rectus muscle. The trochlear nerve is a crossed nerve (i.e., it consists of axons whose cell bodies are on the other side of

the brainstem) and it is the only cranial nerve that exits from the dorsal side of the brainstem. The axons emerge from the anterior medullary velum just behind the inferior colliculi, then wrap around the brainstem, pass through the tentorial opening, enter the cavernous sinus, and travel through the superior orbital fissure to innervate the superior oblique muscle.

Unilateral or even bilateral abducens palsy is commonly seen as a false localizing sign in patients with increased intracranial pressure. Although the long intracranial course of the nerve is often cited as the cause of its predisposition to injury, the trochlear nerve (which is rarely injured by diffusely increased intracranial pressure) is actually longer,[94] and the sharp bend of the abducens nerve as it enters the cavernous sinus may play a more decisive role. From a clinical point of view, however, it is important to remember that isolated unilateral or bilateral abducens palsy does not necessarily indicate a site of injury. The emergence of the trochlear nerve from the dorsal midbrain just behind the inferior colliculus makes it prone to injury by the tentorial edge (which runs along the adjacent superior surface of the cerebellum) in cases of severe head trauma. Thus, trochlear nerve palsy after head trauma does not necessarily represent a focal brainstem injury (although the dorsal brainstem at this level may be damaged by the same process).

The course of all three ocular motor nerves through the cavernous sinus and superior orbital fissure means that they are often damaged in combination by lesions at these sites. Thus, a lesion of all three of these nerves unilaterally indicates injury in the cavernous sinus or superior orbital fissure rather than the brainstem. Head trauma causing a blowout fracture of the orbit may trap the eye muscles, resulting in abnormalities of ocular motility unrelated to any underlying brain injury. The entrapment of the eye muscles is determined by forced duction (i.e., resistance to physically moving the globe) as described below in the examination.

Functional Anatomy of the Central Oculomotor System

The oculomotor nuclei receive and integrate a large number of inputs that control their activity and coordinate eye muscle movement to produce normal, conjugate gaze. These afferents arise from cortical, tectal, and tegmental oculomotor systems, as well as directly from the vestibular system and vestibulocerebellum. In principle, these classes of afferents are not greatly different from the types of inputs that control alpha-motor neurons concerned with striated muscles, except the oculomotor muscles do not contain muscle spindles and hence there is no somesthetic feedback.

The oculomotor nuclei are surrounded by areas of the brainstem tegmentum containing premotor cell groups that coordinate eye movements.[93,95,96] The premotor area for regulating lateral saccades consists of the paramedian pontine reticular formation (PPRF), which is just ventral to the abducens nucleus. The PPRF contains several different classes of neurons with bursting and pausing activities related temporally to horizontal saccades.[97] Their main effect is to allow conjugate lateral saccades to the ipsilateral side of space, and when neurons in this area are inactivated by injection of local anesthetic, ipsilateral saccades are slowed or eliminated. In addition, neurons in the dorsal pontine nuclei relay smooth pursuit signals to the flocculus, and the medial vestibular nucleus and flocculus are both important for holding eccentric gaze.[98] Inputs from these systems converge on the abducens nucleus, which contains two classes of neurons: those that directly innervate the lateral rectus muscle (motor neurons) and those that project through the medial longitudinal fasciculus (MLF) to the opposite medial rectus motor neurons in the oculomotor nucleus. Axons from these latter neurons cross the midline at the level of the abducens nucleus and ascend on the contralateral side of the brainstem to allow conjugate lateral gaze. Thus, pontine tegmental lesions typically result in the inability to move the eyes to the ipsilateral side of space (lateral gaze palsy). Similarly, the premotor area for vertical saccades and gaze holding, respectively, are found in the rostral interstitial nucleus of the MLF and rostral interstitial nucleus of Cajal, which surround the oculomotor nucleus laterally. A premotor area for vergence eye movements is found at the rostral tip of this region, near the midbrain-diencephalic junction. Unilateral lesions of the rostral interstitial nuclei typically reduce vertical saccades as well as causing torsional nystagmus.[99,100] Compression of the midbrain from the tectal surface (e.g., by a pineal tumor) causes loss of vertical eye movements, usually beginning with upgaze.

The PPRF and rostral interstitial nuclei are under the control of descending inputs from the superior colliculus. Each superior colliculus contains a map of the visual world on the contralateral side of space, and electrical stimulation of a specific point in this visual map will command a saccade to the corresponding point in space. In nonmammalian vertebrates, such as frogs, this area is called the optic tectum and is the principal site for directing eye movement; in mammals, it comes largely under the control of the cortical system for directing eye movements.

The cortical descending inputs to the ocular motor system are complex.[101] The frontal eye fields (area 8) direct saccadic eye movements to explore behaviorally relevant features of the contralateral side of space. However, it would be incorrect to think of this area as a motor cortex. Unlike neurons in the primary motor cortex, which fire in relation to movements of the limbs in particular directions at particular joints, recordings from area 8 neurons in awake, behaving monkeys indicate that they do not fire during most random saccadic eye movements. However, they are engaged during tasks that require a saccade to a particular part of space only when the saccadic eye movement is part of a behavioral sequence that is rewarded. In this respect, neurons in area 8 are more similar to those in areas of the prefrontal cortex that are involved in planning movements toward the opposite side of space. Area 8 projects widely to both the superior colliculus as well as the premotor areas for vertical and lateral eye movements, and to the ocular motor nuclei themselves.[102] Descending axons from area 8 mainly run through the internal medullary lamina of the thalamus to enter the region of the rostral interstitial nucleus of the MLF. They then cross the midline to descend along with the MLF to the contralateral PPRF and abducens nucleus.

In the posterior part of the hemisphere, in the ventrolateral cortex near the occipitoparietal junction, is an area of visual cortex, sometimes called area V5 or area MT, that is important in judging movement of objects in contralateral space.[101,103] Cortex in this region plays a critical role in following movements originating in that space, including movements toward the ipsilateral space. Thus, following an object that travels from the left to the right engages the right parietal cortex (area 7) to fix attention on the object, the right area 8 to produce a saccade to pick it up, the right occipital cortex to follow the object to the right, and ultimately the left occipital cortex as well to see the object as it enters the right side of space. Thus, following moving stripes to the right, as in testing optokinetic nystagmus, engages a number of important cortical as well as brainstem pathways necessary to produce eye movements. Hence, although the test is fairly sensitive for picking up oculomotor problems at a cortical and brainstem level, the interpretation of failure of optokinetic nystagmus is a complex process.

In addition to these motor inputs, the ocular motor neurons also receive sensory inputs to guide them. Although there are no spindles in the ocular motor muscles to provide somatic sensory feedback, the ocular motor nuclei depend on two different types of sensory feedback. First, visual feedback allows the rapid correction of errors in gaze. Second, the ocular motor nuclei receive direct and relayed inputs from the vestibular system.[104] Because the eyes must respond to changes in head position very quickly to stabilize the visual image on the retina, the direct vestibular input, which identifies angular or linear acceleration of the head, is integrated to providing a signal for rapid correction of eye position. The abducens nucleus is located at the same level as the vestibular complex, and it receives inputs from the medial and superior vestibular nuclei. Additional axons from these nuclei cross the midline and ascend in the contralateral MLF to reach the trochlear and oculomotor nuclei. These inputs from the vestibular system allow both horizontal and vertical eye movements (vestibulo-ocular reflexes) in response to vestibular stimulation.

Another sensory input necessary for the brain to calculate its position in space is head position and movement. Ascending somatosensory afferents, particularly from the neck muscles and vertebral joint receptors, arise from the C2–4 levels of the spinal cord. They ascend through the MLF to reach the vestibular nuclei and cerebellum, where they are integrated with vestibular sensory inputs.

The vestibulocerebellum, including the flocculus, paraflocculus, and nodulus, receives extensive vestibular input as well as somatosensory and visual afferents.[101] The output from the flocculus ensures the accuracy of saccadic eye movements and contributes to pursuit eye movements and the ability to hold an eccentric position of gaze. The vestibulocerebellum is also critical in learning new relationships between eye movements and visual displacement (e.g., when wearing prism or magnification glasses). Lesions of the vestibulocerebellum cause ocular dysmetria (inability to perform accurate saccades), ocular flutter (rapid to-and-fro eye movements), and opsoclonus (chaotic eye movements).[105] It may be difficult to distinguish less severe cases of vestibulocerebellar function from vestibular dysfunction.

Because the MLF conveys so many classes of input from the pontine level to the midbrain, lesions of the MLF have profound effects on eye movements. After a unilateral MLF lesion, the eye ipsilateral to the lesion cannot follow the contralateral eye in conjugate lateral gaze to the other side of space (an *internuclear ophthalmoplegia*, a condition that occurs quite commonly in multiple sclerosis and brainstem lacunar infarcts). The abducting eye shows horizontal gaze-evoked nystagmus (slow phase toward the midline, rapid jerks laterally), while the adducting eye stops in the midline (if the lesion is complete) or fails to fully adduct (if it is partial). Bilateral injury to the MLF caudal to the oculomotor complex not only causes a bilateral internuclear ophthalmoplegia, but also prevents vertical vestibulo-ocular responses or pursuit. Vertical saccades, however, are implemented by the superior colliculus inputs to the rostral interstitial nucleus of Cajal, and are intact. Similarly, vergence eye movements are intact after caudal lesions of the MLF, which allows the paresis of adduction to be distinguished from a medial rectus palsy. More rostral MLF lesions, however, may also damage the closely associated preoculomotor areas for vertical or vergence eye movements.

The Ocular Motor Examination

The examination of the ocular motor system in awake, alert subjects involves testing both voluntary and reflex eye movements. In patients with stupor or coma, testing of reflex eyelid and ocular movements must suffice.[99]

EYELIDS AND CORNEAL RESPONSES

Begin by noting the position of the eyes and eyelids at rest and observing for spontaneous eye movements. The eyelids at rest in coma, as in sleep, are maintained in a closed position by tonic contraction of the orbicularis oculi muscles. (Patients with long-term impairment of consciousness who enter a persistent vegetative state have alternating cycles of eyes opening and closing; see Chapter 9.) Next, gently raise and then release the eyelids, noting their tone. The eyelids of a comatose patient close smoothly and gradually, a movement that cannot be duplicated by an awake individual simulating unconsciousness. Absence of tone or failure to close either eyelid can indicate facial motor weakness. Blepharospasm, or strong resistance to eyelid opening and then rapid closure, is usually voluntary, suggesting that the patient is not truly comatose. However, lethargic patients with either metabolic or structural lesions may resist eye opening, as do some patients with a nondominant parietal lobe infarct. In awake patients, ptosis may result from either brainstem or hemispheric injury. In patients with unilateral forebrain infarcts, the ptosis is often ipsilateral to hemiparesis.[106] In cases of brainstem injury, the ptosis may be part of a Horner's syndrome (i.e., accompanied by pupilloconstriction), due to injury to the lateral tegmentum, or it may be due to an injury to the oculomotor complex or nerve, in which case it is typically accompanied by pupillodilation. Tonically retracted eyelids (Collier's sign) may be found in patients with dorsal midbrain or, occasionally, pontine damage.

Spontaneous blinking usually is lost in coma as a function of the depressed level of consciousness and concomitant eye closure. However, in persistent vegetative state, it may return during cycles of eye opening (Chapter 9). Blinking in response to a loud sound or a bright light implies that the afferent sensory pathways are intact to the brainstem, but does not necessarily mean that they are active at a forebrain level. Even patients with complete destruction of the visual cortex may recover reflex blink responses to light,[107] but not to threat.[108] A unilateral impairment of the speed or depth of the eyelid excursion during blinking occurs in patients with ipsilateral facial paresis.

The corneal reflex can be performed by approaching the eye from the side with a wisp of cotton that is then gently applied to the sclera and pulled across it to touch the corneal surface.[109] Eliciting the corneal reflex in coma may require more vigorous stimulation than in an awake subject, but it is important not to touch the cornea with any material that might scratch its delicate surface. Corneal trauma can be completely avoided by testing the corneal reflex with sterile saline. Two to three drops of sterile saline are dropped on the cornea from a height of 4 to 6 inches.[109] Reflex closure of both eyelids and elevation of both eyes (Bell's phenomenon) indicates that the reflex pathways, from the trigeminal nerve and spinal trigeminal nucleus through the lateral brainstem tegmentum to the oculomotor and facial nuclei, remain intact. However, some patients who wear contact lenses may have permanent suppression of the corneal reflex. In other patients with an acute lesion of the descending corticofacial pathways, the blink reflex may be suppressed, but Bell's phenomenon should still occur. A structural lesion at the midbrain level may result in loss of Bell's phenomenon, but an intact blink response. A lesion at the midpontine level may not only impair Bell's phenomenon, but also cause the jaw to deviate to the opposite side (corneal-mandibular reflex), a phenomenon that may also occur with eye blink.[110]

EXAMINATION OF OCULAR MOTILITY

Hold the eyelids gently in an open position to observe eye position and movements in a comatose patient. A small flashlight or bright ophthalmoscope held about 50 cm from the face and shined toward the eyes of the patient should reflect off the same point in the cornea of each eye if the gaze is conjugate. Most patients with impaired consciousness demonstrate a slight exophoria. If it is possible to obtain a history, ask about eye movements, as a congenital strabismus may be misinterpreted as dysconjugate eye movements due to a brainstem lesion. Observe for a few moments for spontaneous eye movements. Slowly roving eye movements are typical of metabolic encephalopathy, and if conjugate, they imply an intact ocular motor system.

The vestibulo-ocular responses are then tested by rotating the patient's head (*oculocephalic reflexes*).[99] In patients who may have suffered trauma, it is important first to rule out the possibility of a fracture or dislocation of the cervical spine; until this is done, it may be necessary to skip ahead to caloric testing (see below). The head is rotated first in a lateral direction to either side while holding the eyelids open. This can be done by grasping the head on either side with both hands and using the thumbs to reach across to the eyelids and hold them open. The head movements should be brisk, and when the head position is held at each extreme for a few seconds, the eyes should gradually come back to midposition. Moving the head back to the opposite side then produces a maximal stimulus. The eye movements should be smooth and conjugate. The head is then rotated in a vertical plane (as in head nodding) and the eyes are observed for vertical conjugate movement. During downward head movement, the eyelids may also open (the doll's head phenomenon).[111]

The normal response generated by the vestibular input to the ocular motor system is for the eyes to rotate counter to the direction of the examiner's movement (i.e., turning the head to the right should cause the eyes to deviate to the left). In an awake patient, the voluntary control of gaze overcomes this reflex response. However, in patients with impaired consciousness, the oculocephalic reflex should predominate. This response is often colloquially called the *doll's eye response*,[111] and normal responses in both horizontal and vertical directions imply intact brainstem pathways from the vestibular nuclei through the lower pontine tegmentum and thence the upper pontine and midbrain paramedian tegmentum (i.e., along the course of the MLF; see below). There may also be a small contribution from proprioceptive afferents from the neck,[112] which also travel through the medial longitudinal fasciculus. Because these pathways overlap extensively with the ascending arousal system (see Figure 2–8), it is quite unusual for patients with structural causes of coma to have a normal oculocephalic examination. In contrast, patients with metabolic encephalopathy, particularly due to hepatic failure, may have exaggerated or very brisk oculocephalic responses.

Eye movements in patients who are deeply comatose may respond sluggishly or not at all to oculocephalic stimulation. In such cases, more intense vestibular stimulation may be obtained by testing *caloric vestibulo-ocular responses*. With appropriate equipment, vestibulo-ocular monitoring can be done using galvanic stimulation and video-oculography.[113] However, at the bedside, caloric stimuli and visual inspection are generally used (see Figure 2–9). The ear canal is first examined and, if necessary, cerumen is removed to allow clear visualization that the tympanic membrane is intact. The head of the bed is then raised to about 30 degrees to bring the horizontal semicircular canal into a vertical position so that the response is maximal. If the patient is merely sleepy, the canal may be irrigated with cool water (15°C to 20°C); this usually induces a brisk response and may occasionally cause nausea and vomiting. Fortunately, in practice, it is rarely necessary to use caloric stimulation in such patients. If the patient is deeply comatose, a maximal stimulus is obtained by using ice water. A large (50 mL) syringe is used, attached to a plastic IV catheter, which is gently advanced until it is near the tympanic membrane. An emesis basin can be placed below the ear, seated on an absorbent pad, to catch the effluent. The ice water is infused at a rate of about 10 mL/minute for 5 minutes, or until a response is obtained. After a response is obtained, it is necessary to wait at least 5 minutes for the response to dissipate before testing the opposite ear. To test vertical eye movements, both external auditory canals are irrigated simultaneously with cold water (causing the eyes to deviate downward) or warm water (causing upward deviation).

The cold water induces a downward convection current, away from the ampulla, in the endolymph within the horizontal semicircular canal. The effect of the current upon the hair cells in the ampulla is to reduce tonic discharge of the vestibular neurons. Because the vestibular neurons associated with the horizontal canal fire fastest when the head is turning toward that side (and thus push the eyes to the opposite side), the result of cold water stimulation is to produce a stimulus as if the head were turning to the opposite side, thus activating the ipsilateral lateral rectus and contralateral medial rectus muscles to drive the

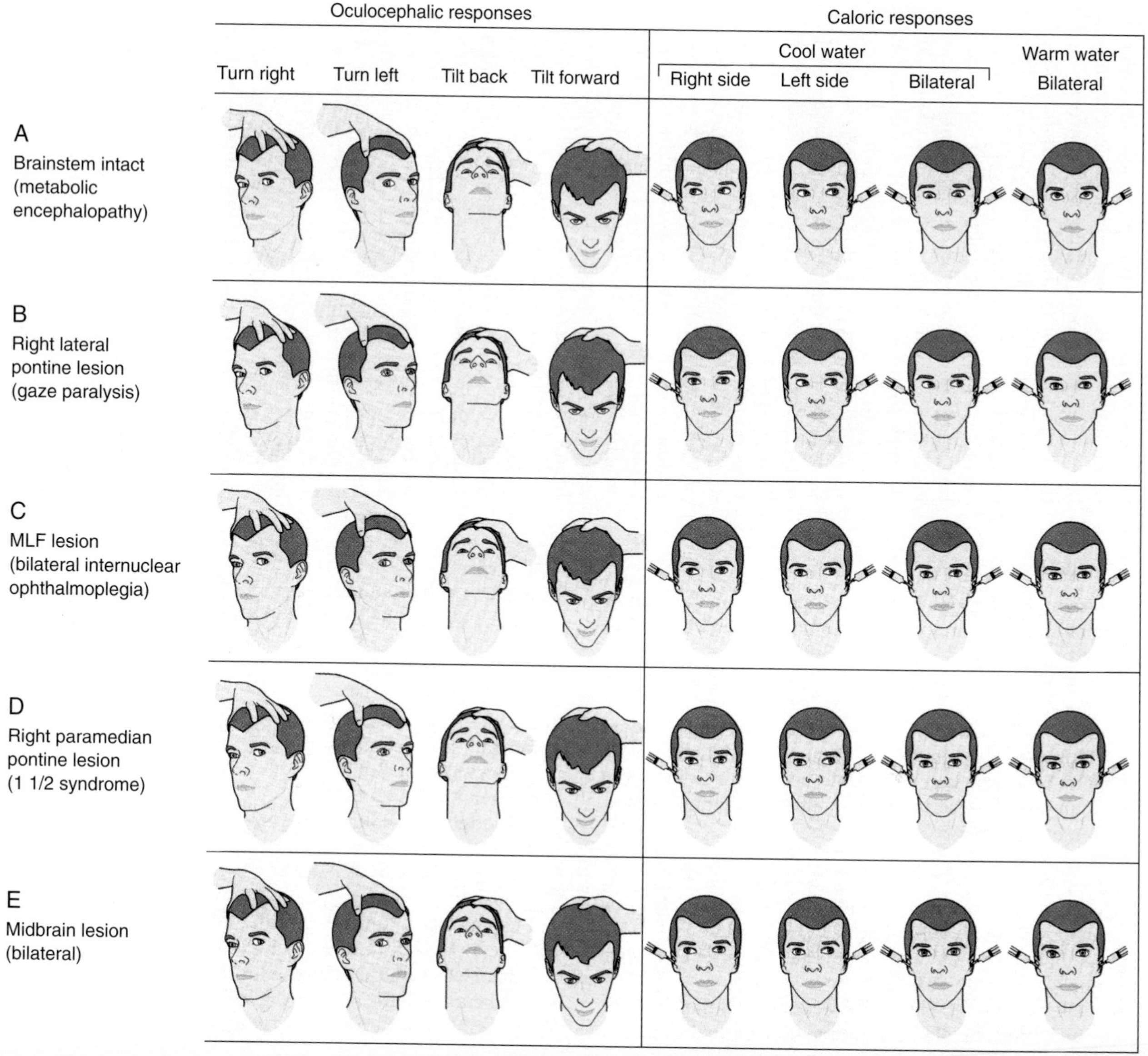

Oculocephalic responses

Caloric responses

	Turn right	Turn left	Tilt back	Tilt forward		Cool water Right side	Cool water Left side	Bilateral	Warm water Bilateral

A
Brainstem intact
(metabolic
encephalopathy)

B
Right lateral
pontine lesion
(gaze paralysis)

C
MLF lesion
(bilateral internuclear
ophthalmoplegia)

D
Right paramedian
pontine lesion
(1 1/2 syndrome)

E
Midbrain lesion
(bilateral)

Figure 2–9. Ocular reflexes in unconscious patients. The left-hand side shows the responses to oculocephalic maneuvers (which should only be done after the possibility of cervical spine injury has been eliminated). The right-hand side shows responses to caloric stimulation with cold or warm water (see text for explanation). Normal brainstem reflexes in a patient with metabolic encephalopathy are illustrated in row (A). The patient shown in row (B) has a lesion of the right side of the pons (see Figure 2–8), causing a paralysis of gaze to that side with either eye. Row (C) shows the result of a lesion involving the medial longitudinal fasciculus (MLF) bilaterally (bilateral internuclear ophthalmoplegia). Only abducens responses with each eye persist. The patient in row (D) has a lesion involving both MLFs and the right abducens nucleus (one and a half syndrome). Only left eye abduction is retained. Row (E) illustrates a patient with a midbrain infarction eliminating both the oculomotor and trochlear responses, leaving only bilateral abduction responses. Note that the extraocular responses are identical to (C), in which there is a bilateral lesion of the MLF. However, pupillary light responses would be preserved in the latter case. (From Saper, C. Brain stem modulation of sensation, movement, and consciousness. Chapter 45 in: Kandel, ER, Schwartz, JH, Jessel, TM. *Principles of Neural Science.* 4th ed. McGraw-Hill, New York, 2000, pp. 871–909. By permission of McGraw-Hill.)

eyes toward the side of cold water stimulation. Any activation of the anterior canal (which activates the ipsilateral superior rectus and the contralateral inferior oblique muscles) and the posterior canal (which activates the ipsilateral superior oblique and contralateral inferior rectus muscles) by caloric stimulation cancel each other out.

When caloric stimulation is done in an awake patient who is trying to maintain fixation (e.g., in the vestibular testing laboratory), cool water (about 30°C) causes a slow drift toward the side of stimulation, with a compensatory rapid saccade back to the midline (the direction of nystagmus is the direction of the fast component). Warm stimulation (about 44°C) induces the opposite response. The traditional mnemonic for remembering these movements is "COWS" (cold opposite, warm same), which refers to the direction of nystagmus in an awake patient. This mnemonic can be confusing for inexperienced examiners, as the responses seen in a comatose patient with an intact brainstem are the opposite: cold water induces only tonic deviation (there is no little or no corrective nystagmus), so the eyes deviate toward the ear that is irrigated. The presence of typical vestibular nystagmus in a patient who is unresponsive indicates a psychogenic cause of unresponsiveness (i.e., the patient is actually awake). The absence of a response to caloric stimulation does not always imply brainstem dysfunction. Bilateral vestibular failure occurs with phenytoin or tricyclic antidepressant toxicity. Aminoglycoside vestibular toxicity may obliterate the vestibular response, but oculocephalic responses may persist, the neck muscles supplying the afferent information.[112]

On the other hand, because the oculomotor pathways are spatially so close to those involved in producing wakefulness, it is rare for a patient to have acute damage to the oculomotor control system without a change in consciousness.

Patient 2–1

A 56-year-old man with a 20-year history of poorly controlled hypertension came to the emergency department with a complaint of sudden onset of severe dizziness. On examination, he was fully awake and conversant. Pupils were 2.5 mm and constricted to 2.0 mm with light in either eye. The patient could not follow a moving light to either side or up or down. Hearing was intact, as were facial, oropharyngeal, and tongue motor and sensory responses. Motor and sensory examination was also normal, tendon reflexes were symmetric, and toes were downgoing.

The patient was sent for computed tomography (CT) scan, which showed a hemorrhage into the periventricular gray matter in the floor of the fourth ventricle at a pontine level, which tracked rostrally into the midbrain. During the CT scan the patient lapsed into coma. At that point, the pupils were pinpoint and the patient was unresponsive with flaccid limbs. He subsequently died, but autopsy was not permitted.

Comment. The sudden onset of bilateral impairment of eye movements on the background of clear consciousness is rare, and raised the possibility of a brainstem injury even without unconsciousness. Although the CT scan demonstrated a focal hemorrhage selectively destroying the abducens nuclei and medial longitudinal fasciculi, the proximity of these structures to the ascending arousal system was demonstrated by the loss of consciousness over the next few minutes.

Finally, if there has been head trauma, one or more eye muscles may become trapped by a blowout fracture of the orbit. It is important to distinguish this cause of abnormal eye movements from damage to neural structures, either peripherally or centrally. This is generally done by an ophthalmologist, who applies topical anesthetics to the globe and uses a fine, toothed forceps to tug on the sclera to attempt to move the globe (*forced duction*). Inability to move the globe through a full range of movements may indicate a trapped muscle and requires evaluation for orbital fracture.

Interpretation of Abnormal Ocular Movements

A wide range of eye movements may be seen, both at rest and during vestibular stimulation. Each presents clues about the nature of the insult that is causing the impairment of consciousness.

RESTING AND SPONTANEOUS EYE MOVEMENTS

A great deal of information may be gained by carefully noting the position of the eyes and any movements that occur without stimulation. Table 2–3 lists some of the spontaneous eye movements that may be observed in unconscious patients. Detailed descriptions are given in the paragraphs below. Most individuals have a mild degree of exophoria when drowsy and not maintaining active fixation. However, other individuals have varying types of strabismus, which may worsen as they become less responsive and no longer attempt to maintain conjugate gaze. Hence, it is very difficult to determine the meaning of dysconjugate gaze in a stuporous or comatose patient if nothing is known about the presence of baseline strabismus.

On the other hand, certain types of dysconjugate eye movements raise suspicion of brainstem injury that may require further examination for confirmation. For example, injury to the oculomotor nucleus or nerve produces exodeviation of the involved eye. Unilateral abducens injury causes the involved eye to deviate inward. In skew deviation,[114] in which one eye is deviated upward and the other downward, there typically is an injury to the brainstem (see below).

CONJUGATE LATERAL DEVIATION OF THE EYES

This is typically seen with destructive or irritative lesions, as compressive or metabolic disorders generally do not affect the supranuclear ocular motor pathways asymmetrically. A destructive lesion involving the frontal eye fields causes the eyes to deviate toward the side of the lesion (away from the side of the associated hemiparesis). This typically lasts for a few days after the onset of the lesion. An irritative lesion may cause deviation of the eyes away from the side of the lesion. These eye movements represent seizure activity, and often there is some evidence of quick, nystagmoid jerks toward the side of eye deviation indicative of continuing seizure activity. If seizure activity abates, there may be a Todd's paralysis of gaze for several hours, causing lateral gaze deviation toward the side of the affected cortex (i.e., opposite to the direction caused by the seizures). Hemorrhage into the thalamus may also produce "wrong-way eyes," which deviate away from the side of the lesion.[115,116]

Table 2–3 Spontaneous Eye Movements Occurring in Unconscious Patients

Term	Description	Significance
Ocular bobbing	Rapid, conjugate, downward movement; slow return to primary position	Pontine strokes; other structural, metabolic, or toxic disorders
Ocular dipping or inverse ocular bobbing	Slow downward movement; rapid return to primary position	Unreliable for localization; follows hypoxic-ischemic insult or metabolic disorder
Reverse ocular bobbing	Rapid upward movement; slow return to primary position	Unreliable for localization; may occur with metabolic disorders
Reverse ocular dipping or converse bobbing	Slow upward movement; rapid return to primary position	Unreliable for localization; pontine infarction and with AIDS
Ping-pong gaze	Horizontal conjugate deviation of the eyes, alternating every few seconds	Bilateral cerebral hemispheric dysfunction; toxic ingestion
Periodic alternating gaze deviation	Horizontal conjugate deviation of the eyes, alternating every 2 minutes	Hepatic encephalopathy; disorders causing periodic alternating nystagmus and unconsciousness or vegetative state
Vertical "myoclonus"	Vertical pendular oscillations (2–3 Hz)	Pontine strokes
Monocular movements	Small, intermittent, rapid monocular horizontal, vertical, or torsional movements	Pontine or midbrain destructive lesions, perhaps with coexistent seizures

From Leigh and Zee,[93] with permission.

This may be due to interruption of descending corticobulbar pathways for gaze control, which pass through the thalamic internal medullary lamina, rather than the internal capsule. Damage to the lateral pons, on the other hand, may cause loss of eye movements toward that side (gaze palsy, Figure 2–9). The lateral gaze deviation in such patients cannot be overcome by vestibular stimulation, whereas vigorous oculocephalic or caloric stimulation usually overcomes lateral gaze deviation due to a cortical gaze paresis.

CONJUGATE VERTICAL DEVIATION OF THE EYES

Pressure on the tectal plate, such as occurs with a pineal mass or sometimes with a thalamic hemorrhage, may cause conjugate downward deviation of the eyes.[117,118] Oculogyric crises may cause conjugate upward deviation. The classical cause of oculogyric crises was postencephalitic parkinsonism.[119] Few of these patients still survive, but a similar condition is frequently seen with dystonic crises in patients exposed to neuroleptics[120] and occasionally in patients with acute bilateral injury of the basal ganglia.

NONCONJUGATE EYE DEVIATION

Whereas nonconjugate eye position may be due to an old baseline strabismus, failure of one eye to follow its mate during spontaneous or evoked eye movements is typically highly informative. Absence of abduction of a single eye suggests injury to the abducens nerve either within the brainstem or along its course to the orbit. However, either increased intracranial pressure or decreased pressure, as occurs with cerebral spinal fluid leaks,[121] can cause either a unilateral or bilateral abducens palsy, so the presence of an isolated abducens palsy may be misleading. Isolated loss of adduction of the eye contralateral to the head movement implies an injury to the medial longitudinal fasciculus (i.e., near the midline tegmentum) on that side between the abducens and oculomotor nuclei (Figure 2–9). Bilateral lesions of the medial longitudinal fasciculus impair adduction of both eyes as well as vertical oculocephalic and vestibulo-ocular eye movements, a condition that is distinguished from bilateral oculomotor nucleus or nerve injury in the comatose patient by preservation of the pupillary light responses. (Voluntary vergence and vertical eye movements remain intact, but require wakeful cooperation.)

Combined loss of adduction and vertical movements in one eye indicates an oculomotor nerve impairment. Typically, there may also be severe ptosis on that side (so that if the patient is awake, he or she may not be aware of diplopia). In rare cases with a lesion of the oculomotor *nucleus*, the weakness of the superior rectus will be on the side *opposite* the other third nerve muscles (as these fibers are crossed) and ptosis will be bilateral (but not very severe). Occasionally, oculomotor palsy may spare the pupillary fibers. This occurs most often when the paresis is due to ischemia of the oculomotor nerve (the smaller pupilloconstrictor fibers are more resistant to ischemia), such as in diabetic occlusion of the vasa nervorum. Such patients are also typically awake and alert, whereas third nerve paresis due to brainstem injury or compression of the oculomotor nerve by uncal herniation results in impairment of consciousness and early pupillodilation.

Trochlear nerve impairment causes a hyperopia of the involved eye, often with some exodeviation. If awake, the patient typically attempts to compensate by tilting the head toward that shoulder. Because the trochlear nerve is crossed, a trochlear palsy in a comatose patient suggests damage to the trochlear nucleus on the opposite side of the brainstem.

SKEW DEVIATION

Skew deviation refers to vertical dysconjugate gaze, with one eye displaced downward compared to the other. In some cases, the eye that is elevated may alternate from side to side depending on whether the patient is looking to the left or the right.[95,122] Skew deviation is due either to a lesion in the lateral rostral medulla or lower pons, vestibular system, or vestibulocerebellum on the side of the inferior eye, or in the MLF on the side of the superior eye.[123–125]

ROVING EYE MOVEMENTS

These are slow, random deviations of eye position that are similar to the eye movements seen in normal individuals during light sleep. As in sleeping individuals who typically have some degree of exophoria, the eye positions may not be quite conjugate, but the ocular excursions should be conjugate. Most roving eye movements are predominantly horizontal, although some vertical movements may also occur. Most patients with roving eye movements have a metabolic encephalopathy, and oculocephalic and caloric vestibulo-ocular responses are typically preserved or even hyperactive. The roving eye movements may disappear as the coma deepens, although they may persist in quite severe hepatic coma. Roving eye movements cannot be duplicated by patients who are awake, and hence their presence indicates that unresponsiveness is not psychogenic. A variant of roving eye movements is periodic alternating or "ping-pong" gaze,[126] in which repetitive, rhythmic, and conjugate horizontal eye movements occur in a comatose or stuporous patient. The eyes move conjugately to the extremes of gaze, hold the position for 2 to 3 seconds, and then rotate back again. The episodic movements of the eyes may continue uninterrupted for several hours to days. Periodic alternating eye movements have been reported in patients with a variety of structural injuries to the brainstem or even bilateral cerebral infarcts that leave the oculomotor system largely intact, but are most common during metabolic encephalopathies.

NYSTAGMUS

Nystagmus refers to repetitive rapid (saccadic) eye movements, often alternating with a slow drift in the opposite direction. Spontaneous nystagmus is uncommon in coma because the quick, saccadic phase is generally a corrective movement generated by the voluntary saccade system when the visual image drifts from the point of intended fixation. However, continuous seizure activity with versive eye movements may give the appearance of nystagmus. In addition, several unusual forms of nystagmoid eye movement do occur in comatose patients.

Retractory nystagmus consists of irregular jerks of both globes back into the orbit, sometimes occurring spontaneously but other times on attempted upgaze. Electromyography during retractory nystagmus shows that the retractions consist of simultaneous contractions of all six extraocular muscles.[127] Retractory nystagmus is typically seen with dorsal midbrain compression or destructive lesions[117] and is thought to be due to impairment of descending inputs that relax the opposing eye muscles when a movement is made, so that all six muscles contract when attempts are made to activate any one of them.

Convergence nystagmus often accompanies retractory nystagmus and also is typically seen in patients with dorsal midbrain lesions.[128] The eyes diverge slowly, and this is followed by a quick convergent jerk.

OCULAR BOBBING AND DIPPING

Fischer[129] first described movements in which the eyes make a brisk, conjugate downward movement, then "bob" back up more slowly to primary position. The patients were comatose and the movements were not affected by caloric vestibular stimulation. The initially described patients had caudal pontine injuries or compression, although later reports described similar eye movements in patients with obstructive hydrocephalus, uncal herniation, or even metabolic encephalopathy. A variety of related eye movements have been described including inverse bobbing (rapid elevation of the eyes, with bobbing downward back to primary position) and both dipping (downward slow movements with rapid and smooth return to primary position) and inverse dipping (slow upward movements with rapid return to primary position).[130,131] The implications of these unusual eye movements are similar to those of ocular bobbing: a lower brainstem injury or compression of normal vestibulo-ocular inputs.

Seesaw nystagmus describes a rapid, pendular, disjunctive movement of the eyes in which one eye rises and intorts while the other descends and extorts.[132] This is followed by reversal of the movements. It is most commonly seen during visual fixation in an awake patient who has severe visual field defects or impairment of visual acuity, and hence is not in a coma. Seesaw nystagmus appears to be due in most cases to lesions near the rostral end of the periaqueductal gray matter, perhaps involving the rostral interstitial nucleus of Cajal.[133] It may occasionally be seen also in comatose patients, sometimes accompanied by ocular bobbing, and in such a setting may indicate severe, diffuse brainstem damage.[134]

Nystagmoid jerks of a single eye may occur in a lateral, vertical, or rotational direction in patients with pontine injury. It may be associated with skew deviation and if bilateral, the eyes may rotate in the opposite direction.

MOTOR RESPONSES

The motor examination in a stuporous or comatose patient is, of necessity, quite different from the patient who is awake and cooperative. Rather than testing power in specific muscles, it is focused on assessing the overall responsiveness of the patient (as measured by motor response), the motor tone, and reflexes, and identifying abnormal motor patterns, such as hemiplegia or abnormal posturing.

Motor Tone

Assessment of *motor tone* is of greatest value in patients who are drowsy but responsive to voice. It may be assessed by gently grasping the patient's hand as if you were shaking hands and lifting the arm while intermittently turning the wrist back and forth. Tone can also be assessed in the neck by gently grasping the head with two hands and moving it back and forth or up and down, and in the lower extremities by grasping each leg at the knee and gently lifting it from the bed or shaking it from side to side. Normal muscle tone provides mild resistance that is constant or nearly so throughout the movement arc and of similar intensity regardless of the initial position of the body part. Spastic rigidity, on the other hand, increases with more rapid movements and generally has a clasp-knife quality or a spastic catch, so that the movement is slowed to a near stop by the resistance, at which point the resistance collapses and the movement proceeds again. Parkinsonian rigidity remains equally intense despite the movement of the examiner (lead-pipe rigidity), but is usually diminished when the patient is asleep or there is impairment of consciousness. In contrast, during diffuse metabolic encephalopathies, many otherwise normal patients develop paratonic rigidity, also called gegenhalten. Paratonic rigidity is characterized by irregular resistance to passive movement that increases in intensity as the speed of the movement increases, as if the patient were willfully resisting the examiner. If the patient is drowsy but responsive to voice, urging him or her to "relax" may result in increased tone.

Paratonia is often seen in patients with dementia and is normally found in infants between the second and eighth weeks of life, suggesting that it represents a state of disinhibition of forebrain control as the level of consciousness becomes depressed. As patients become more deeply stuporous, muscle tone tends to decrease and these pathologic forms of rigidity are less apparent.

Motor Reflexes

Muscle stretch reflexes (sometimes erroneously referred to as "deep tendon reflexes") may be brisk or hyperactive in patients who are drowsy or confused and have increased motor tone. As the level of consciousness becomes further depressed, however, the muscle stretch reflexes tend to diminish in activity, until in patients who are deeply comatose they may be unobtainable.

Cutaneous reflexes such as the abdominal or cremasteric reflex typically become depressed as the level of consciousness wanes. On the other hand, in patients who are drowsy or confused, some abnormal cutaneous reflexes may be released. These may include extensor plantar responses. If the extensor plantar response is bilateral, this may signify nothing more than a depressed level of consciousness, but if it is asymmetric or unilateral, this implies injury to the descending corticospinal tract.

Prefrontal cutaneous reflexes, sometimes called "frontal release reflexes" or primitive reflexes,[135] may also emerge in drowsy patients with diffuse forebrain impairment. Rooting, glabellar, snout, palmomental, and other reflexes are often seen in such patients. However, these responses become increasingly common with advancing age in patients without cognitive impairment, so they are of limited value in elderly individuals.[136] On the other hand, the grasp reflex is generally seen only in patients who have some degree of bilateral prefrontal impairment.[137] It is elicited by gently stroking the palm of the patient with the examiner's fingers. The patient may grasp the examiner's fingers, as if grasping a branch of a tree. The pull reflex is a variant in which the examiner curls his or her fingers under the patient's as the patient attempts to grasp. The grasp is often so strong that it is possible to pull the patient from the bed. Many elderly patients with normal cognitive function will have a mild tendency to grasp the first time the reflex is attempted, but a request not to grasp the examiner quickly abolishes the response. Patients who are unable to inhibit the reflex invariably have prefrontal pathology. The grasp reflex may be asymmetric if the prefrontal injury is greater on one side, but probably requires some impairment of both hemispheres, as small, unilateral lesions rarely cause grasping.[137] Grasping disappears when the lesion involves the motor cortex and causes hemiparesis. It is of greatest value in a sleepy patient who can cooperate with the exam; it disappears as the patient becomes more drowsy.

Like paratonia, prefrontal reflexes are normally present in young infants, but disappear as the forebrain matures.[135]

Motor Responses

After assessing muscle tone, the examiner next tests the patient for best motor response to sensory stimulation (Figure 2–10). If the patient does not respond to voice or gentle shaking, arousability and motor responses are tested by painful stimuli. The maneuvers used to provide adequate stimuli without inducing actual tissue damage are shown in Figure 2–1.

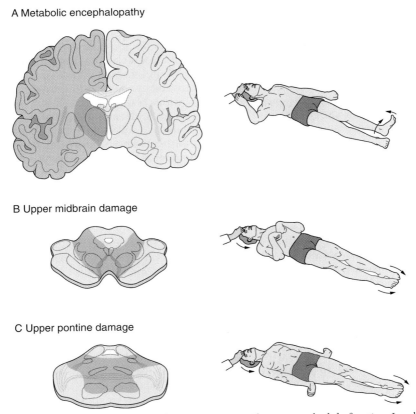

A Metabolic encephalopathy

B Upper midbrain damage

C Upper pontine damage

Figure 2–10. Motor responses to noxious stimulation in patients with acute cerebral dysfunction. Levels of associated brain dysfunction are roughly indicated at left. Patients with forebrain or diencephalic lesions often have a hemiparesis (note lack of motor response with left arm, externally rotated left foot, and left extensor plantar response), but can generally make purposeful movements with the opposite side. Lesions involving the junction of the diencephalon and the midbrain may show decorticate posturing, including flexion of the upper extremities and extension of the lower extremities. As the lesion progresses into the midbrain, there is generally a shift to decerebrate posturing (C), in which there is extensor posturing of both upper and lower extremities. (From Saper, C. Brain stem modulation of sensation, movement, and consciousness. Chapter 45 in: Kandel, ER, Schwartz, JH, Jessel, TM. *Principles of Neural Science*. 4th ed. McGraw-Hill, New York, 2000, pp. 871–909. By permission of McGraw-Hill.)

Responses are graded as appropriate, inappropriate, or no response. An appropriate response is one that attempts to escape the stimulus, such as pushing the stimulus away or attempting to avoid the stimulus. The motor response may be accompanied by a facial grimace or generalized increase in movement. It is necessary to distinguish an attempt to avoid the stimulus, which indicates intact sensory and motor connections within the spinal cord and brainstem, from a stereotyped withdrawal response, such as a triple flexion withdrawal of the lower extremity or flexion at the fingers, wrist, and elbow. The stereotyped withdrawal response is not responsive to the nature of the stimulus (e.g., if the pain is supplied over the dorsum of the toe, the foot will withdraw into, rather than away from, the stimulus) and thus is not appropriate to the stimulus that is applied. These spinal level motor patterns may occur in patients with severe brain injuries or even brain death. It is also important to assess asymmetries of response. Failure to withdraw on one side may indicate either a sensory or a motor impairment, but if there is evidence of facial grimacing, an increase in blood pressure or pupillary dilation, or movement of the contralateral side, the defect is motor. Failure to withdraw on both sides, accompanied by facial grimacing, may indicate bilateral motor impairment below the level of the pons.

Posturing responses include several stereotyped postures of the trunk and extremities. Most appear only in response to noxious stimuli or are greatly exaggerated by such stimuli. Seemingly spontaneous posturing most often represents the response to endogenous stimuli, ranging from meningeal irritation to an occult bodily injury to an overdistended bladder. The nature of the posturing ranges from flexor spasms to extensor spasms to rigidity, and may vary according to the site and severity of the brain injury and the site at which the noxious stimulation is applied. In addition, the two sides of the body may show different patterns of response, reflecting the distribution of injury to the brain.

Clinical tradition has transferred the terms *decorticate rigidity* and *decerebrate rigidity* from experimental physiology to certain patterns of motor abnormality seen in humans. This custom is unfortunate for two reasons. First, these terms imply more than we really know about the site of the underlying neuro-

logic impairment. Even in experimental animals, these patterns of motor response may be produced by brain lesions of several different kinds and locations and the patterns of motor response in an individual to any one of these lesions may vary across time. In humans, both types of responses can be produced by supratentorial lesions, although they imply at least incipient brainstem injury. There is a tendency for lesions that cause decorticate rigidity to be more rostral and less severe than those causing decerebrate rigidity. In general, there is much greater agreement among observers if they simply describe the movements that are seen rather than attempt to fit them to complex patterns.

Flexor posturing of the upper extremities and extension of the lower extremities corresponds to the pattern of movement also called decorticate posturing. The fully developed response consists of a relatively slow (as opposed to quick withdrawal) flexion of the arm, wrist, and fingers with adduction in the upper extremity and extension, internal rotation, and vigorous plantar flexion of the lower extremity. However, decorticate posturing is often fragmentary or asymmetric, and it may consist of as little as flexion posturing of one arm. Such fragmentary patterns have the same localizing significance as the fully developed postural change, but often reflect either a less irritating or smaller central lesion.

The decorticate pattern is generally produced by extensive lesions involving dysfunction of the forebrain down to the level of the rostral midbrain. Such patients typically have normal ocular motility. A similar pattern of motor response may be seen in patients with a variety of metabolic disorders or intoxications.[138] However, the presence of decorticate posturing in cases of brain injury is ominous. For example, in the series of Jennett and Teasdale, after head trauma only 37% of comatose patients with decorticate posturing recovered.[139]

Even more ominous is the presence of *extensor posturing of both the upper and lower extremities*, often called decerebrate posturing. The arms are held in adduction and extension with the wrists fully pronated. Some patients assume an opisthotonic posture, with teeth clenched and arching of the spine. Tonic neck reflexes (rotation of the head causes hyperextension of the arm on the side toward which the nose is turned and flexion of the other arm; extension of the head may cause extension of the arms and relaxation of the legs, while flexion of the head leads to the opposite response) can usually be elicited. As with decorticate posturing, fragments of decerebrate posturing are sometimes seen. These tend to indicate a lesser degree of injury, but in the same anatomic distribution as the full pattern. It may also be asymmetric, indicating the asymmetry of dysfunction of the brainstem.

Although decerebrate posturing usually is seen with noxious stimulation, in some patients it may occur spontaneously, often associated with waves of shivering and hyperpnea. Decerebrate posturing in experimental animals usually results from a transecting lesion at the level between the superior and inferior colliculi.[140] It is believed to be due to the release of vestibulospinal postural reflexes from forebrain control. The level of brainstem dysfunction that produces this response in humans may be similar, as in most cases decerebrate posturing is associated with disturbances of ocular motility. However, electrophysiologic, radiologic, or even postmortem examination sometimes reveals pathology that is largely confined to the forebrain and diencephalon. Thus, decerebrate rigidity is a clinical finding that probably represents dysfunction, although not necessarily destruction extending into the upper brainstem. Nevertheless, it represents a more severe finding than decorticate posturing; for example, in the Jennett and Teasdale series, only 10% of comatose patients with head injury who demonstrated decerebrate posturing recovered.[139] Most patients with decerebrate rigidity have either massive and bilateral forebrain lesions causing rostrocaudal deterioration of the brainstem as diencephalic dysfunction evolves into midbrain dysfunction (see Chapter 3), or a posterior fossa lesion that compresses or damages the midbrain and rostral pons. However, the same pattern may occasionally be seen in patients with diffuse, but fully reversible, metabolic disorders, such as hepatic coma, hypoglycemia, or sedative drug ingestion.[138,141,142]

Extensor posturing of the arms with flaccid or weak flexor responses in the legs is typically seen in patients with injury to the lower brainstem, at roughly the level of the vestibular nuclei. This pattern was described in the 1972 edition of this monograph, and has since been repeatedly confirmed. The physiologic basis of this motor pattern is not understood, but it may represent the transition from the extensor posturing seen with lower midbrain and high pontine injuries to the spinal shock (flaccidity) or even flexor responses seen from stimulating the isolated spinal cord.

FALSE LOCALIZING SIGNS IN PATIENTS WITH METABOLIC COMA

The main purpose of the foregoing review of the examination of a comatose patient is to distinguish patients with structural lesions of the brain from those with metabolic lesions. Most patients with structural lesions require urgent imaging. Patients with metabolic lesions often require an extensive laboratory evaluation to define the cause. When focal neurologic findings are observed, it becomes imperative to determine whether there is a destructive or compressive process that may become life threatening or irreversibly damage the brain within a matter of minutes. On the other hand, even when there is no focal or lateralizing finding to suggest a structural lesion, it is important to know which signs point to specific metabolic causes, such as hypoglycemia or sepsis, that must be sought urgently. Therefore, the physician should become familiar with the few focal neurologic findings that are seen in patients with diffuse metabolic causes of coma, and understand their implications for the diagnosis of the metabolic problem.

Respiratory Responses

The range of normal respiratory responses includes the Cheyne-Stokes pattern of breathing, which is seen in many cognitively normal people with cardiac or respiratory disorders, particularly during sleep.[43–45] Sleep apnea must also be distinguished from pathologic breathing patterns. Patients with severe sleep apnea may stop breathing for 10 seconds or so every minute or two. Their color may become dusky during the oxygen desaturation that accompanies each period of apnea.

Kussmaul breathing, in which there are deep but slow rhythmic breaths, is seen in patients with coma due to an acidotic condition (e.g., diabetic ketoacidosis or intoxication with ethylene glycol). The low blood pH drives the deep respiratory efforts, which reduce the PCO_2 in the blood, thus producing a compensatory respiratory alkalosis. This must be distinguished from sepsis, hepatic encephalopathy, or cardiac dysfunction, conditions that often cause a primary respiratory alkalosis, with compensatory metabolic acidosis.[143–145] The nature of the primary insult is determined by whether the blood pH is low (metabolic acidosis with respiratory compensation) or high (primary respiratory alkalosis).

Pupillary Responses

A key problem with interpreting pupillary responses is that either metabolic coma or diencephalic level dysfunction may cause bilaterally small and symmetric, reactive pupils. Thus, a patient with small pupils and little in the way of focal neurologic impairment may still have impairment that can be attributed to either a diencephalic lesion or to symmetric forebrain compression (e.g., by bilateral subdural hematomas). As a result, it is generally necessary to do an imaging study (see below) within the first few hours in most comatose patients, even if the cause is believed to be metabolic.

Very small pupils may be indicative of pontine level dysfunction, often indicating an acute destructive lesion such as a hemorrhage. However, similar pinpoint but reactive pupils may be seen in opiate intoxication. Hence, in patients who present with pinpoint pupils and coma, it is necessary to administer an opiate antagonist such as naloxone to reverse potential opiate overdose. (Because an opioid antagonist can elicit severe withdrawal symptoms in a physically dependent patient, the drug should be diluted and delivered slowly, stopping as soon as one notes the pupils to enlarge and the patient to arouse. See Chapter 7 for details.)

Unreactive pupils usually indicate structural disease of the nervous system, but pupils may become unreactive briefly after a seizure. When a patient is seen who may have had an unobserved seizure within the past 30 minutes or so, it is necessary to re-examine the patient 15 to 30 minutes later to make sure that the lack of pupillary responses persists. Signs of major motor seizure, such as tongue biting or incontinence, or a transient metabolic acidosis are helpful in alerting the examiner to the possibility of a recent seizure. In addition, because the seizure usually results in the release of adrenalin, the pupils typically are large after a seizure.

Very deep coma due to sedative intoxication may suppress all brainstem responses, including pupillary light reactions, and simulate brain death (see Chapter 6). For this reason, it is critical to do urinary and blood toxic and drug screening on any patient who is so deeply comatose as to lack pupillary responses.

Ocular Motor Responses

Typical oculocephalic responses, as seen in a comatose patient with an intact brainstem, are not seen in awake subjects, whose voluntary eye movements supersede the brainstem vestibular responses. In fact, brainstem oculocephalic responses (as if the eyes were fixed on a point in the distance) are nearly impossible for an awake patient to simulate voluntarily, and therefore are a useful differential point in identifying psychogenic unresponsiveness. On the other hand, oculocephalic responses may become particularly brisk in patients with hepatic coma.

Certain drugs may eliminate oculocephalic and even caloric vestibulo-ocular responses. Acute administration of phenytoin quite often has this effect, which may persist for 6 to 12 hours.[146] Occasionally, patients who have ingested an overdose of various tricyclic antidepressants may also have absence of vestibulo-ocular responses.[147] Patients in very deep metabolic coma, particularly with sedative drugs, may also eventually lose oculovestibular responses.

Ophthalmoplegia is also seen in combination with areflexia and ataxia in the Miller Fisher variant of Guillain-Barré syndrome. While such patients usually do not have impairment of consciousness, the Miller Fisher syndrome occasionally occurs in patients who also have autoimmune brainstem encephalitis (Bickerstaff's encephalitis), with impairment of consciousness, and GQ1b autoantibodies.[148] In such cases, the relationship of the loss of eye movements to the impairment of consciousness may be confusing, and the prognosis may be much better than would be indicated by the lack of these brainstem reflexes, particularly if the patient receives early plasmapheresis or intravenous immune globulin. If breathing is also affected by the Guillain-Barré syndrome, the picture may even simulate brain death.[149] This condition must be considered among the reversible causes of coma that require exclusion before brain death is declared (see Chapter 8).

Isolated unilateral or bilateral abducens palsy may be seen in some patients with increased intracranial pressure, even due to nonfocal causes such as pseudotumor cerebri.[150] It may also occur with low CSF pressure, with a spontaneous leak, or after lumbar puncture.[151] In rare cases the trochlear nerve may also be involved.[152]

Motor Responses

Patients with metabolic coma may have paratonia and/or extensor plantar responses. However, spastic rigidity should not be present. Rarely, patients with metabolic causes of coma, particularly hypoglycemia,[153] will present with asymmetric motor responses or even hemiplegia (see Chapter 5). Some have suggested that the focal signs represent the unmasking of subclinical neurologic impairment. It is true that most metabolic causes of coma may exacerbate a pre-existing neurologic focal finding, but the presence and even the distribution of focal findings in patients with hypoglycemia may vary from one episode to the next, so that the evidence for a structural cause is not convincing. Furthermore, focal signs caused by hypoglycemia are more common in children than adults, again suggesting the absence of an underlying structural lesion. Similarly, focal deficits are observed with hypertensive encephalopathy, but in this case imaging usually identifies brain edema consistent with these focal neurologic deficits. Cortical blindness is the most common of these deficits; edema of the occipital white matter is seen on magnetic resonance images, the so-called posterior leukoencephalopathy syndrome.[154] A number of severe metabolic causes of coma, especially hepatic coma, may also cause either decerebrate or decorticate posturing. In general, although it is important to be alert to the pos-

sibility of false localizing signs in patients with metabolic causes of coma, unless a structural lesion can be ruled out, it is still usually necessary to proceed as if the coma has a structural cause, until proven otherwise.

MAJOR LABORATORY DIAGNOSTIC AIDS

The neurologic examination, as described above, is the cornerstone for the diagnosis of stupor and coma. It can be done at the bedside within a matter of a few minutes, and it provides critical diagnostic clues to determine the tempo of the further evaluation. If focal findings are seen, it may be necessary to institute treatment even before the remainder of the diagnostic testing can be completed. The same may be true for some types of metabolic coma, such as meningitis or hypoglycemia. On the other hand, if the evidence from a nonfocal examination points toward a diffuse metabolic encephalopathy, the examiner usually has time to employ additional diagnostic tools.

Blood and Urine Testing

Because of the propensity for some metabolic comas to cause focal neurologic signs, it is important to perform basic blood and urine testing on virtually every patient who presents with coma. It is important to draw blood for glucose and electrolytes, and to do toxic and drug screening almost immediately. The blood should not be drawn in a limb with a running intravenous line, as this may alter the glucose or electrolytes. Blood gases should be drawn if there is any suspicion of respiratory insufficiency or acid-base abnormality. Urine can then be collected for urinalysis and screening for toxic substances or drugs (which may no longer be detectable in the bloodstream). In a woman of reproductive age, pregnancy testing should also be done as this may affect the evaluation (e.g., MRI scan may be preferable to CT, if there is a choice). A bedside measurement of blood glucose is sufficiently accurate to rule out hypoglycemia and obviate the need for giving glucose. However, if glucose is given, 100 mg of thiamine should be given as well to prevent precipitating Wernicke encephalopathy (see Chapter 5).

Computed Tomography Imaging and Angiography

CT scanning is now ubiquitous, and it should be applied to any patient who does not have an immediately obvious source of coma (e.g., a hypoglycemic patient who arouses with injection of IV glucose). However, it is still necessary to complete the examination first, as a patient who is in incipient uncal herniation, or whose fourth ventricle is compressed by a mass lesion, may die even during the few minutes it takes to get a scan, and may need to be treated emergently first. Similarly, for comatose patients in whom meningitis is suspected, it is now standard practice to give IV antibiotics first, before taking the patient for a CT scan, to rule out a mass lesion prior to doing a lumbar puncture (but see discussion on lumbar puncture below and on meningitis in Chapters 4 and 5).

Emergency CT scans done for diagnostic purposes in patients with a depressed level of consciousness may appear to be simple to interpret. This is certainly the case for large, acute hemorrhages or extensive infarcts. However, subacute infarction may become isodense with brain during the second week, and hemorrhage may be isodense during the third week after onset. Acute infarcts may be difficult to identify, and if there is bilateral edema, it may be quite difficult to distinguish from "hypernormal brain" (i.e., small ventricles and general decrease in prominence of the sulci, which may be seen in young normal brains, particularly if the scan is not of good quality).

In such cases, it may be useful either to obtain a CT scan with contrast, or to have an MRI scan done (see below). Current-generation CT scanners are fast enough that it is rarely necessary to sedate a patient to eliminate motion artifact. However, many MRI examinations still take significantly longer, and they may be compromised if the patient moves. Such patients may be sedated with a short-acting benzodiazepine, which can be reversed if necessary with flumazenil. However, conscious sedation should only be done under the continuous supervision of a physician who is capable of intubating the patient if respirations are depressed or compromised.

Computed tomography angiography (CTA) involves reconstruction of images of the intracranial circulation from images acquired during an intravenous bolus injection of contrast dye. Perfusion CT may also identify areas of decreased perfusion, even in cases where the plain CT does not yet show an infarct (see Figure 2–11). CTA is highly accurate for demonstrating occlusions or stenoses of intracranial vessels, but does not give the resolution of conventional direct imaging angiography. The images can be acquired quickly and the method is applicable to patients (see below) who may not be eligible for magnetic resonance angiography (MRA). However, extracting the vascular images currently requires more user interaction and takes longer than MRA. The use of large amounts of contrast dye can also be a drawback if the patient's history of dye reaction and renal function are not available.

Magnetic Resonance Imaging and Angiography

MRI scans take substantially longer than CT scans, and they are often less available for emergency scanning. Hence, they are less often used for primary scanning of patients with coma. However, in many cases, it is necessary to obtain an MRI scan if a significant question remains about the origin of the coma after the CT imaging. Diffusion-weighted imaging may demonstrate an infarct that otherwise cannot be documented acutely. Additional sequences that measure the apparent diffusion coefficient of water in the brain (ADC mapping) and perfusion with blood can be used in cases where the standard diffusion imaging is confounded by background T2 bright lesions. This in turn may lead to a lifesaving intervention (e.g., intra-arterial tPA in the case of basilar artery occlusion). MRA may also demonstrate arterial occlusion noninvasively, and MR venography may identify a dural sinus thrombosis. While T1 and T2 MRI sequences are not as sensitive as CT scanning for identifying acute blood, the combination of fluid-attenuated inversion recovery (FLAIR) and gradient echo T2* sequences is at least as sensitive in acute subarachnoid hemorrhage and may be more sensitive if the bleeding is subacute.[155]

On the other hand, MR scanning has significant limitations for its use in many comatose patients. Because MRI scanners use a

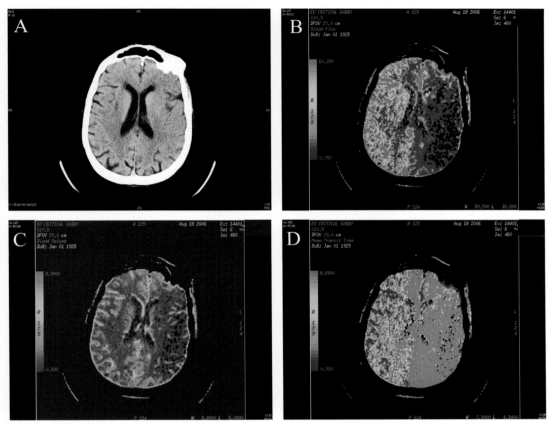

Figure 2–11. A series of computed tomography (CT) scans through the brain of a patient with a left internal carotid occlusion. Note that in the noncontrast CT scan in panel (A), there is loss of the gray-white differentiation and effacement of the sulci over the middle cerebral artery distribution on the left. Panel (B) shows the perfusion blood flow map, indicating that there is very low flow within the left middle cerebral artery distribution, but that there is also impairment of blood flow in both anterior cerebral arteries, consistent with loss of the contribution from the left internal carotid artery. Although the blood volume (C) is relatively normal in these areas, mean transit time (D) is also abnormal, indicating that tissue in the anterior cerebral distributions is at risk of infarction.

high magnetic field, they are not compatible with certain types of implants in patients, including cardiac pacemakers and deep brain stimulators. Patients who require mechanical ventilation must either be ventilated by hand during the scan or placed on a specialized MR-compatible ventilator. In addition, most sequences take substantially longer than CT scans, so that clear images require that the patient not move.

MRA can reveal most stenoses or occlusions of cerebral blood vessels. It requires only a few additional minutes during a conventional MRI scanning session, and the images are extracted by computer and therefore can be recovered very quickly. However, the MRA is very flow dependent, and tends to exaggerate the degree of stenosis in areas of slow flow.

Magnetic Resonance Spectroscopy

Magnetic resonance spectroscopy (MRS)[156] is becoming increasingly important in the diagnosis and prognosis of patients with a variety of illnesses that cause delirium, stupor, or coma (Figure 5–7). The technique identifies neurochemicals in regions of both normal and abnormal brain. Although special techniques allow the identification of as many as 80 brain metabolites, most clinical centers using standard MRI machines perform proton (^{1}H) MRS that can identify about 13 brain metabolites (see Figure 5–7, page 226).

Myo-inositol (mI) is a sugar-like molecule present in astrocytes. It helps to regulate cell volume. Its presence serves as a marker of astrocytes. The metabolite is elevated in a number of disorders including hyperosmolar states, progressive multifocal leukoencephalopathy, renal failure, and diabetes. Levels are decreased in hyponatremia, chronic hepatic encephalopathy, tumor, and stroke.

Creatine (Cr) is actually the sum of creatine and phosphocreatine, a reliable marker of energy metabolism in both neurons and astrocytes. The total creatine peak remains constant, allowing other peaks to be calculated as ratios to the height of the creatine peak.

N-Acetylaspartate (NAA) is an amino acid derivative synthesized in neurons and transported down axons. It marks the presence of viable neurons, axons, and dendrites. Its levels may be increased in hyperosmolar states and are decreased in almost any disease that causes destruction of neurons or their processes.

The choline (Cho) peak represents several membrane components, primarily phosphocholine and glycerophosphocholine. Choline is found in higher concentration in glial cells and is thus higher in white matter than gray matter. It is increased in tumors (particularly relative to NAA), strokes, and hyperosmolar states. It is decreased in liver disease and hyponatremia.

Glutamate/glutamine (Glx) represents a mixture of amino acids and amines involved in excitatory and inhibitory transmission as well as products of the Krebs cycle and mitochondrial redox systems. The peak is elevated in hypoxic encephalopathy and in hyperosmolar states; it is diminished in hyponatremia.

Lactate (Lac), not visible in normal brain, is a product of anaerobic glycolysis and is thus increased in hypoxic/ischemic encephalopathy, diabetic acidosis, stroke, and recovery from cardiac arrest. It is also increased in highly aggressive tumors.

A lipid peak is not present in normal brain but is identified in areas of brain necrosis, particularly in rapidly growing tumors. Cerebral fat embolism (see Chapter 5) can also cause a lipid peak.[157]

The clinical use of some of these spectra in stuporous or comatose patients is discussed in Chapter 5.

Neurosonography

Intracranial Doppler sonography identifies flow of blood in arteries, particularly the middle cerebral artery. The absence of flow in the brain has been used to confirm brain death, particularly in patients who have received sedative drugs that may alter some of the clinical findings (see Chapter 8).[158,159] The technique is also useful for following patients with strokes, head injuries, and hypoxic/ischemic encephalopathy.[160,161] The injection of gas-filled microbubbles enhances the sonographic echo and provides better delineation of blood flow, occlusions, pseudo-occlusions, stenosis, and collateral circulation.[162]

Doppler studies of the extracranial carotid circulation are frequently done as a routine part of stroke evaluation at many centers. However, this is rarely helpful for patients in coma. If the coma is due to a reversible stenosis or occlusion of a single vessel, it almost always will be in the vertebrobasilar, not the carotid, circulation. If the patient is going to receive an MRI scan, the MRA of the cervical vessels, which examines both the carotid and the vertebrobasilar circulation, is generally more revealing.

Lumbar Puncture

Although often overlooked in the technologic era, the examination of the CSF still plays a central role in neurologic diagnosis, particularly in patients with a depressed level of consciousness. Once an imaging study has been performed, it is necessary to proceed with lumbar puncture as soon as possible for patients with no clear diagnosis. Rare patients in whom subarachnoid hemorrhage was not detected on imaging may demonstrate blood in the CSF. Similarly, occasional patients with bacterial meningitis or viral encephalitis may present with a depressed level of consciousness (sometimes after a missed seizure), and may not yet have sufficient meningismus to make the diagnosis of meningitis clear from examination. This may be particularly difficult to determine in patients who have underlying rigidity of the cervical spine (evidenced by resistance to lateral as well as flexion movements of the neck). Nevertheless, it is imperative to identify infection as early as possible to allow the administration of antibiotics or antiviral agents.

Patient 2–2

A 73-year-old woman who was on 10 mg/day of prednisone for her ulcerative colitis had a 2-day history of presumed gastroenteritis, with fever, nausea, and vomiting. She awoke on the third day and found it difficult to walk to the bathroom. By the afternoon she had difficulty swallowing, her voice was hoarse, and her left limbs were clumsy. She was brought to the hospital by ambulance, and examination in the emergency department disclosed a lethargic patient who could be easily wakened. Pupils were equal and constricted from 3 to 2 mm with light, but the left eye was lower than the right, she complained of skewed diplopia, and there was difficulty maintaining gaze to the left. There was left-sided facial numbness and lower motor neuron facial weakness. Hearing was intact, but her voice was hoarse. The tongue deviated to the right and there was distal weakness in her arms, and the left limbs were clumsy on fine motor tasks and showed dysmetria.

MRI scan showed a left pontomedullary lesion surrounded by edema, which was bright on diffusion-weighted imaging, and she was diagnosed as having a brainstem infarct. However, despite normal MRA of the vertebrobasilar system, her deficits progressed over the next day. A senior neuroradiologist noticed some enhancement at the periphery of the lesion on review of the MRI scan, and suggested an abscess. Lumbar puncture disclosed 47 white blood cells/mm^3 and elevated protein, and she recovered after being treated for *Listeria monocytogenes*. An MRI scan much later in her course, disclosing a multioculated abscess, is shown in Figure 4–13.

Comment. This case demonstrates the importance of examining the spinal fluid, even when a presumptive diagnosis of vascular disease is entertained. This is particularly true in patients with fever, elevated white blood cell count, or stiff neck, where infectious disease is a consideration. However, every patient with an undetermined cause of coma requires lumbar puncture as part of the routine evaluation.

The timing of lumbar puncture with respect to CT scanning is discussed in Chapters 4 and 5. However, in some circumstances, scanning may not be not immediately available. In these cases it is common to give antibiotics immediately and then do imaging and lumbar puncture up to a few hours later. However, once the antibiotics have penetrated the CSF, the ability to grow a bacterial pathogen and identify its susceptibilities may be permanently compromised. Hence, deferring lumbar puncture in such cases until after the scanning procedure may do the patient harm. For this reason, when the evidence for meningitis is compelling, it may be necessary to do the lumbar puncture without benefit of prior imaging. As discussed in Chapters 4 and 5, the danger of this procedure is greatly overestimated. If the examination is nonfocal, and there is no evidence of papilledema on funduscopy, it is extremely rare to precipitate brain herniation by lumbar puncture. The benefit of establishing the exact microbial diagnosis far outweighs the risk of herniation.

A critical but often overlooked component of the lumbar puncture is to measure and record the opening pressure. Elevated pressure may be a key sign that leads to diagnosis of venous sinus thrombosis, cerebral edema, or other serious conditions that can cause coma. In addition to the routine cell count, protein, and glucose, CSF should be obtained for full cultures, including tuberculosis and fungal agents; serology and polymerase chain reaction (PCR) for specific agents such as syphilis, Lyme disease, and herpes encephalitis; and cytology, as cancer or leukemia sometimes may present with meningeal and subarachnoid infiltration. It is a good practice to set aside several milliliters of refrigerated CSF in case additional studies become necessary. This entire group of tests typically requires about 20 mL of CSF, an amount that the choroid plexus in the brain restores within about an hour.

One common problem is that the lumbar tap may be traumatic, yielding bloody CSF. This may make it difficult to determine the underlying numbers of both red and white blood cells in the CSF. If the cells come from the blood (rather than the white cells being elevated within the CSF, e.g., due to infection), the proportion of the red and white cells should remain the same as in the blood (usually

500 to 1,000 red cells per one white cell). If the tap is bloody, many clinicians send fluid from both tubes 1 and 4 for cell count. A falling count indicates that the tap was traumatic, but it does not tell you what the underlying CSF counts were compared with the count in tube 4. Nor does lack of a falling cell count indicate that the blood was there before the tap (the tip of the needle may be partially within or adjacent to a bleeding vein). An alternative approach is to examine the CSF for xanthochromia. However, CSF may be stained yellow due to high protein or bilirubin. Examination of the red blood cells under the microscope immediately after the tap may be helpful. Fresh red cells have the typical doughnut-shaped morphology, whereas crenelated cells indicate that they have been in the extravascular space for some time. Similarly, if the CSF sample is spun in a centrifuge until there are no red blood cells in the supernatant, the fluid can be tested for blood products with a urine dipstick. A positive test indicates breakdown of red blood cells, which typically takes at least 6 hours to occur after a subarachnoid hemorrhage, and demonstrates that the blood was there before the tap.

Electroencephalography and Evoked Potentials

Electroencephalography (EEG) is useful as an objective electrophysiologic assay of cortical function in patients who do not respond to normal sensory stimuli. A typical waking EEG is dominated anteriorly by low-voltage beta activity (faster than 13 Hz). During periods of quiet wakefulness, the EEG may slow into the alpha range (8 to 13 Hz) and the wave activity may be more rhythmic and symmetric. As the patient becomes more drowsy, higher voltage theta rhythms (4 to 7 Hz) become dominant; delta activity (1 to 3 Hz) predominates in patients who are deeply asleep or comatose. The EEG provides a rough but fairly accurate estimate of the degree to which a patient who is unresponsive may be simply uncooperative.

On the other hand, occasional patients with coma due to brainstem injury show an alpha EEG pattern. The alpha activity in such patients is usually more regular and less variable than in an awake patient, and it is not inhibited by opening the eyes.[163] It may be possible to

drive the EEG by photic stimulation in alpha coma. Certain types of metabolic encephalopathy may also have characteristic EEG changes. For example, triphasic waves are often seen in patients with hepatic encephalopathy, but can be seen in other metabolic disorders that cause coma.[163,164]

The EEG is most helpful in diagnosing impairment of consciousness due to nonconvulsive status epilepticus.[165] Such patients may lack the usual behavioral signs of complex partial seizures, such as lip smacking or blinking, and may present as merely confused, drowsy, or even stuporous or comatose. Some patients may demonstrate twitching movements of the eyelids or extremities, but others give no external sign of epileptic activity. In one series, 8% of comatose patients were found to be suffering from nonconvulsive status epilepticus.[166] When the EEG shows continuous epileptic activity, the diagnosis is easy and anticonvulsants are required. However, nonconvulsive status epilepticus may occur in patients without characteristic EEG changes,[167] probably because the seizure activity is mainly in areas such as the medial temporal lobes that are not sampled by the surface electrodes. Accordingly, if one suspects that the patient's loss of consciousness is a result of nonconvulsive status epilepticus, it is probably wise to administer a short-acting benzodiazepine and observe the patient's response. If the patient improves, antiepileptic drugs should be administered. Unfortunately, some patients with a clinical and electroencephalographic diagnosis of nonconvulsive status epilepticus do not respond to anticonvulsant drugs, because the underlying process causing the seizure activity is too severe to be suppressed by routine doses of drugs. Such patients are sometimes treated by large intravenous doses of gamma-aminobutyric acid agonist drugs, such as barbiturates or propofol, which at sufficiently high dosage can suppress all brain activity. However, unless the underlying brain process can be reversed, the prognosis of patients with nonconvulsive status epilepticus who do not awaken after anticonvulsant treatment is poor[168] (see also *Seizures* in Chapter 5).

Evoked potentials may also be used to test the integrity of brainstem and forebrain pathways in comatose patients. Although they do not provide reliable information on the location of a lesion in the brainstem, both auditory- and somatosensory-evoked potentials, and cortical event-related potentials, can provide information on the prognosis of patients in coma.[169] This use will be discussed in greater detail in Chapter 8.

REFERENCES

1. Dunn C, Held JL, Spitz J, et al. Coma blisters: report and review. Cutis 45 (6), 423–426, 1990.
2. Teasdale G, Jennett B. Assessment and prognosis of coma after head injury. Acta Neurochir (Wien) 34 (1–4), 45–55, 1976.
3. Gill MR, Reiley DG, Green SM. Interrater reliability of Glasgow Coma Scale scores in the emergency department. Ann Emerg Med 43, 215–223, 2004.
4. McNarry AF, Goldhill DR. Simple bedside assessment of level of consciousness: comparison of two simple assessment scales with the Glasgow Coma scale. Anaesthesia 59, 34–37, 2004.
5. Servadei F. Coma scales. Lancet 367 (9510), 548–549, 2006.
6. Ropper AH, O'Rourke D, Kennedy SK. Head position, intracranial pressure, and compliance. Neurology 32 (11), 1288–1291, 1982.
7. Saper CB, Loewy AD, Swanson LW, et al. Direct hypothalamo-autonomic connections. Brain Res 117 (2), 305–312, 1976.
8. Saper CB. Central autonomic system. In Paxinos G. ed. The Rat Nervous System. Elsevier Academic Press, San Diego, pp 761–796, 2004.
9. Rossetti AO, Reichhart MD Bogousslavsky J. Central Horner's syndrome with contralateral ataxic hemiparesis: a diencephalic alternate syndrome. Neurology 61 (3), 334–338, 2003.
10. Reeves AG, Posner JB. The ciliospinal response in man. Neurology 19, 1145–1152, 1969.
11. Vassend O, Knardahl S. Cardiovascular responsiveness to brief cognitive challenges and pain sensitivity in women. Eur J Pain 8 (4), 315–324, 2004.
12. Zidan AH, Girvin JP. Effect on the Cushing response of different rates of expansion of a supratentorial mass. J Neurosurg 49 (1), 61–70, 1978.
13. Kawahara E, Ikeda S, Miyahara Y, et al. Role of autonomic nervous dysfunction in electrocardio-graphic abnormalities and cardiac injury in patients with acute subarachnoid hemorrhage. Circ J 67 (9), 753–756, 2003.
14. Lorsheyd A, Simmers TA Robles De Medina EO. The relationship between electrocardiographic abnormalities and location of the intracranial aneurysm in subarachnoid hemorrhage. Pacing Clin Electrophysiol 26 (8), 1722–1728, 2003.
15. McLaughlin N, Bojanowski MW, Girard F, et al. Pulmonary edema and cardiac dysfunction following subarachnoid hemorrhage. Can J Neurol Sci 32 (2), 178–185, 2005.
16. Ferrante L, Artico M, Nardacci B, Fraioli B, Cosentino F, Fortuna A. Glossopharyngeal neuralgia with cardiac syncope. Neurosurgery 36, 58–63, 1995.
17. Cole CR, Zuckerman J Levine BD. Carotid sinus "irritability" rather than hypersensitivity: a new name for an old syndrome? Clin Auton Res 11(2), 109–113, 2001.

18. Paulson OB, Strandgaard S Edvinsson L. Cerebral autoregulation. Cerebrovasc Brain Metab Rev 2(2), 161–192, 1990.
19. Strandgaard S, Paulson OB. Regulation of cerebral blood flow in health and disease. J Cardiovasc Pharmacol 19 (Suppl 6), S89–S93, 1992.
20. Wahl M, Schilling L. Regulation of cerebral blood flow—a brief review. Acta Neurochir Suppl (Wien) 59, 3–10, 1993.
21. Schondorf R, Benoit J, Stein R. Cerebral autoregulation in orthostatic intolerance. Ann N Y Acad Sci 940, 514–526, 2001.
22. Sato A, Sato Y, Uchida S. Regulation of cerebral cortical blood flow by the basal forebrain cholinergic fibers and aging. Auton Neurosci 96 (1), 13–19, 2002.
23. Bieger D, Hopkins DA. Viscerotopic representation of the upper alimentary tract in the medulla oblongata in the rat: the nucleus ambiguus. J Comp Neurol 262 (4), 546–562, 1987.
24. Ross CA, Ruggiero DA, Park DH, et al. Tonic vasomotor control by the rostral ventrolateral medulla: effect of electrical or chemical stimulation of the area containing C1 adrenaline neurons on arterial pressure, heart rate, and plasma catecholamines and vasopressin. J Neurosci 4(2), 474–494, 1984.
25. Panneton WM, Loewy AD. Projections of the carotid sinus nerve to the nucleus of the solitary tract in the cat. Brain Res 191 (1), 239–244, 1980.
26. Ciriello J. Brainstem projections of aortic baroreceptor afferent fibers in the rat. Neurosci Lett 36 (1), 37–42, 1983.
27. Ross CA, Ruggiero DA, Reis DJ. Projections from the nucleus tractus solitarii to the rostral ventrolateral medulla. J Comp Neurol 242 (4), 511–534, 1985.
28. Blessing WW, Reis DJ. Inhibitory cardiovascular function of neurons in the caudal ventrolateral medulla of the rabbit: relationship to the area containing A1 noradrenergic cells. Brain Res 253 (1–2), 161–171, 1982.
29. Smith JC, Ellenberger HH, Ballanyi K, et al. Pre-Botzinger complex: a brainstem region that may generate respiratory rhythm in mammals. Science 254 (5032), 726–729, 1991.
30. Gray PA, Janczewski WA, Mellen N, et al. Normal breathing requires preBotzinger complex neurokinin-1 receptor-expressing neurons. Nat Neurosci 4, 927–930, 2001.
31. Wallach JH, Loewy AD. Projections of the aortic nerve to the nucleus tractus solitarius in the rabbit. Brain Res 188 (1), 247–251, 1980.
32. Torrealba F, Claps A. The carotid sinus connections: a WGA-HRP study in the cat. Brain Res 455 (1), 134–143, 1988.
33. Kalia M, Richter D. Rapidly adapting pulmonary receptor afferents: I. Arborization in the nucleus of the tractus solitarius. J Comp Neurol 274 (4), 560–573, 1988.
34. Feldman JL, Ellenberger HH. Central coordination of respiratory and cardiovascular control in mammals. Annu Rev Physiol 50, 593–606, 1988.
35. Weston MC, Stornetta RL, Guyenet PG. Glutamatergic neuronal projections from the marginal

layer of the rostral ventral medulla to the respiratory centers in rats. J Comp Neurol 473 (1), 73–85, 2004.

36. Richerson GB. Serotonergic neurons as carbon dioxide sensors that maintain pH homeostasis. Nat Rev Neurosci 5(6), 449–461, 2004.

37. Chamberlin NL, Saper CB. Topographic organization of respiratory responses to glutamate microstimulation of the parabrachial nucleus in the rat. J Neurosci 14 (11 Pt 1), 6500–6510, 1994.

38. Chamberlin NL, Saper CB. A brainstem network mediating apneic reflexes in the rat. J Neurosci 18 (15), 6048–6056, 1998.

39. Meah MS, Gardner WN. Post-hyperventilation apnoea in conscious humans. J Physiol 477 (Pt 3), 527–538, 1994.

40. Jennett S, Ashbridge K, North JB. Post-hyperventilation apnoea in patients with brain damage. J Neurol Neurosurg Psychiatry 37 (3), 288–296, 1974.

41. Cherniack NS, Longobardo G, Evangelista CJ. Causes of Cheyne-Stokes respiration. Neurocrit Care 3(3), 271–279, 2005.

42. Lange RL, Hecht HH. The mechanism of Cheyne-Stokes respiration. J Clin Invest 41, 42–52, 1962.

43. Murdock DK, Lawless CE, Loeb HS, et al. The effect of heart transplantation on Cheyne-Stokes respiration associated with congestive heart failure. J Heart Transplant 5(4), 336–337, 1986.

44. Hudgel DW, Devadatta P, Quadri M, et al. Mechanism of sleep-induced periodic breathing in convalescing stroke patients and healthy elderly subjects. Chest 104 (5), 1503–1510, 1993.

45. Rubin AE, Gottlieb SH, Gold AR, et al. Elimination of central sleep apnoea by mitral valvuloplasty: the role of feedback delay in periodic breathing. Thorax 59 (2), 174–176, 2004.

46. Vespa PM, Bleck TP. Neurogenic pulmonary edema and other mechanisms of impaired oxygenation after aneurysmal subarachnoid hemorrhage. Neurocrit Care 1(2), 157–170, 2004.

47. Simon RP. Neurogenic pulmonary edema. Neurol Clin 11(2), 309–323, 1993.

48. Tarulli AW, Lim C, Bui JD, et al. Central neurogenic hyperventilation: a case report and discussion of pathophysiology. Arch Neurol 62 (10), 1632–1634, 2005.

49. Shams PN, Waldman A, Plant GT. B cell lymphoma of the brain stem masquerading as myasthenia. J Neurol Neurosurg Psychiatry 72, 271–273, 2002.

50. Rodriguez M, Baele PL, Marsh HM, et al. Central neurogenic hyperventilation in an awake patient with brainstem astrocytoma. Ann Neurol 11, 625–628, 1982.

51. Siderowf AD, Balcer LJ, Kenyon LC, et al. Central neurogenic hyperventilation in an awake patient with a pontine glioma. Neurology 46, 1160–1162, 1996.

52. Hilaire G, Pasaro R. Genesis and control of the respiratory rhythm in adult mammals. News Physiol Sci 18, 23–28, 2003.

53. El Khatib MF, Kiwan RA, Jamaleddine GW. Buspirone treatment for apneustic breathing in brain stem infarct. Respir Care 48, 956–958, 2003.

54. Bassetti C, Aldrich MS, Quint D. Sleep-disordered breathing in patients with acute supra- and infra-

tentorial strokes. A prospective study of 39 patients. Stroke 28, 1765–1772, 1997.

55. Pang KP, Terris DJ. Screening for obstructive sleep apnea: an evidence-based analysis. Am J Otolaryngol 27 (2), 112–118, 2006.

56. Iber C. Sleep-related breathing disorders. Neurol Clin 23(4), 1045–1057, 2005.

57. Schlaefke ME, Kille JF, Loeschcke HH. Elimination of central chemosensitivity by coagulation of a bilateral area on the ventral medullary surface in awake cats. Pflugers Arch 378 (3), 231–241, 1979.

58. Fodstad H. Pacing of the diaphragm to control breathing in patients with paralysis of central nervous system origin. Stereotact Funct Neurosurg 53 (4), 209–222, 1989.

59. Bogousslavsky J, Khurana R, Deruaz JP, et al. Respiratory failure and unilateral caudal brainstem infarction. Ann Neurol 28 (5), 668–673, 1990.

60. Auer RN, Rowlands CG, Perry SF, et al. Multiple sclerosis with medullary plaques and fatal sleep apnea (Ondine's curse). Clin Neuropathol 15 (2), 101–105, 1996.

61. Manconi M, Mondini S, Fabiani A, et al. Anterior spinal artery syndrome complicated by the Ondine curse. Arch Neurol 60 (12), 1787–1790, 2003.

62. Polatty RC, Cooper KR. Respiratory failure after percutaneous cordotomy. South Med J 79 (7), 897–899, 1986.

63. Amiel J, Laudier B, ttie-Bitach T, et al. Polyalanine expansion and frameshift mutations of the paired-like homeobox gene PHOX2B in congenital central hypoventilation syndrome. Nat Genet 33 (4), 459–461, 2003.

64. Stankiewicz JA, Pazevic JP. Acquired Ondine's curse. Otolaryngol Head Neck Surg 101 (5), 611–613, 1989.

65. Ezure K, Tanaka I. Convergence of central respiratory and locomotor rhythms onto single neurons of the lateral reticular nucleus. Exp Brain Res 113 (2), 230–242, 1997.

66. Daquin G, Micallef J, Blin O. Yawning. Sleep Med Rev 5(4), 299–312, 2001.

67. Argiolas A, Melis MR. The neuropharmacology of yawning. Eur J Pharmacol 343 (1), 1–16, 1998.

68. Launois S, Bizec JL, Whitelaw WA, et al. Hiccup in adults: an overview. Eur Respir J 6, 563–575, 1993.

69. Straus C, Vasilakos K, Wilson RJ, et al. A phylogenetic hypothesis for the origin of hiccough. Bioessays 25, 182–188, 2003.

70. Cersosimo RJ, Brophy MT. Hiccups with high dose dexamethasone administration—a case report. Cancer 82, 412–414, 1998.

71. LeWitt PA, Barton NW, Posner JB. Hiccup with dexamethasone therapy. Letter to the editor. Ann Neurol 12, 405–406, 1982.

72. Souadjian JV, Cain JC. Intractable hiccup. Etiologic factors in 220 cases. Postgrad Med 43, 72–77, 1968.

73. Walker P, Watanabe S, Bruera E. Baclofen, a treatment for chronic hiccup. J Pain Symptom Manage 16, 125–132, 1998.

74. Friedman NL. Hiccups: a treatment review. Pharmacotherapy 16, 986–995, 1996.

75. Furukawa N, Hatano M, Fukuda H. Glutaminergic vagal afferents may mediate both retching and gastric

adaptive relaxation in dogs. Auton Neurosci 93 (1–2), 21–30, 2001.

76. Balaban CD. Vestibular autonomic regulation (including motion sickness and the mechanism of vomiting). Curr Opin Neurol 12 (1), 29–33, 1999.

77. Hornby PJ. Central neurocircuitry associated with emesis. Am J Med 111 (Suppl 8A), 106S–112S, 2001.

78. Yamamoto H, Kishi T, Lee CE, et al. Glucagon-like peptide-1-responsive catecholamine neurons in the area postrema link peripheral glucagon-like peptide-1 with central autonomic control sites. J Neurosci 23(7), 2939–2946, 2003.

79. Chen CJ, Scheufele M, Sheth M, et al. Isolated relative afferent pupillary defect secondary to contralateral midbrain compression. Arch Neurol 61, 1451–1453, 2004.

80. Hornblass A. Pupillary dilatation in fractures of the floor of the orbit. Ophthalmic Surg 10(11), 44–46, 1979.

81. Antonio-Santos AA, Santo RN, Eggenberger ER. Pharmacological testing of anisocoria. Expert Opin Pharmacother 6 (12), 2007–2013, 2005.

82. McLeod JG, Tuck RR. Disorders of the autonomic nervous system: part 2. Investigation and treatment. Ann Neurol 21(6), 519–529, 1987.

83. Zhang YH, Lu J, Elmquist JK, et al. Lipopolysaccharide activates specific populations of hypothalamic and brainstem neurons that project to the spinal cord. J Neurosci 20 (17), 6578–6586, 2000.

84. Llewellyn-Smith IJ, Martin CL, Marcus JN, et al. Orexin-immunoreactive inputs to rat sympathetic preganglionic neurons. Neurosci Lett 351 (2), 115–119, 2003.

85. Estabrooke IV, McCarthy MT, Ko E, et al. Fos expression in orexin neurons varies with behavioral state. J Neurosci 21(5), 1656–1662, 2001.

86. Loewy AD, Araujo JC, Kerr FW. Pupillodilator pathways in the brain stem of the cat: anatomical and electrophysiological identification of a central autonomic pathway. Brain Res 60 (1), 65–91, 1973.

87. Burde RM, Loewy AD. Central origin of oculomotor parasympathetic neurons in the monkey. Brain Res 198 (2), 434–439, 1980.

88. Burde RM. Disparate visceral neuronal pools subserve spinal cord and ciliary ganglion in the monkey: a double labeling approach. Brain Res 440 (1), 177–180, 1988.

89. Gooley JJ, Lu J, Fischer D, et al. A broad role for melanopsin in nonvisual photoreception. J Neurosci 23(18), 7093–7106, 2003.

90. Buttner-Ennever JA, Cohen B, Horn AK, et al. Pretectal projections to the oculomotor complex of the monkey and their role in eye movements. J Comp Neurol 366 (2), 348–359, 1996.

91. Jampel RS. Convergence, divergence, pupillary reactions and accommodation of the eyes from faradic stimulation of the macaque brain. J Comp Neurol 115, 371–399, 1960.

92. Kerr FW, Hallowell OW. Location of the pupillomotor and accommodation fibers in the oculomotor nerve: experimental observations on paralytic mydriasis. J Neurol Neurosurg Psychiatry 27, 473–481, 1964.

93. Leigh RJ, Zee DS. The Neurology of Eye Movements, 4th ed. New York: Oxford University Press, 2006.

94. Hanson RA, Ghosh S, Gonzalez-Gomez I, et al. Abducens length and vulnerability? Neurology 62 (1), 33–36, 2004.

95. Zee DS. Brain stem and cerebellar deficits in eye movement control. Trans Ophthalmol Soc U K 105 (Pt 5), 599–605, 1986.

96. Henn V. Pathophysiology of rapid eye movements in the horizontal, vertical and torsional directions. Baillieres Clin Neurol 1(2), 373–391, 1992.

97. Sparks DL, Mays LE. Signal transformations required for the generation of saccadic eye movements. Annu Rev Neurosci 13, 309–336, 1990.

98. Lewis RF, Zee DS. Ocular motor disorders associated with cerebellar lesions: pathophysiology and topical localization. Rev Neurol (Paris) 149 (11), 665–677, 1993.

99. Buettner UW, Zee DS. Vestibular testing in comatose patients. Arch Neurol 46 (5), 561–563, 1989.

100. Helmchen C, Rambold H, Kempermann U, et al. Localizing value of torsional nystagmus in small midbrain lesions. Neurology 59 (12), 1956–1964, 2002.

101. Krauzlis RJ. Recasting the smooth pursuit eye movement system. J Neurophysiol 91 (2), 591–603, 2004.

102. Leichnetz GR. An anterogradely-labeled prefrontal cortico-oculomotor pathway in the monkey demonstrated with HRP gel and TMB neurohistochemistry. Brain Res 198 (2), 440–445, 1980.

103. Barton JJ, Simpson T, Kiriakopoulos E, et al. Functional MRI of lateral occipitotemporal cortex during pursuit and motion perception. Ann Neurol 40 (3), 387–398, 1996.

104. Goldberg ME. The control of gaze. In: Kandel ER, Schwartz JH, Jessel JH, eds. Principles of Neuroscience, 4th ed. New York: McGraw Hill, pp 782–800, 2000.

105. Cogan DG, Chu FC, Reingold DB. Ocular signs of cerebellar disease. Arch Ophthalmol 100 (5), 755–760, 1982.

106. Caplan LR. Ptosis. J Neurol Neurosurg Psychiatry 37 (1), 1–7, 1974.

107. Hackley SA, Johnson LN. Distinct early and late subcomponents of the photic blink reflex: response characteristics in patients with retrogeniculate lesions. Psychophysiology 33, 239–251, 1996.

108. Liu GT, Ronthal M. Reflex blink to visual threat. J Clin Neuroophthalmol 12, 47–56, 1992.

109. Wijdicks EF, Bamlet WR, Maramattom BV, et al. Validation of a new coma scale: the FOUR score. Ann Neurol 58 (4), 585–593, 2005.

110. Pullicino PM, Jacobs L, McCall WD Jr, et al. Spontaneous palpebromandibular synkinesia: a localizing clinical sign. Ann Neurol 35 (2), 222–228, 1994.

111. Roberts TA, Jenkyn LR, Reeves AG. On the notion of doll's eyes. Arch Neurol 41, 1242–1243, 1984.

112. Schubert MC, Das V, Tusa RJ, et al. Cervico-ocular reflex in normal subjects and patients with unilateral vestibular hypofunction. Otol Neurotol 25 (1), 65–71, 2004.

113. Schlosser HG, Unterberg A, Clarke A. Using video-oculography for galvanic evoked vestibulo-ocular monitoring in comatose patients. J Neurosci Methods 145 (1–2), 127–131, 2005.

114. Brandt TH, Dieterich M. Different types of skew deviation. J Neurol Neurosurg Psychiatry 54, 549–550, 1991.

115. Fisher CM. Some neuro-ophthalmological observations. J Neurol Neurosurg Psychiatry 30 (5), 383–392, 1967.

116. Chung CS, Caplan LR, Yamamoto Y, et al. Striatocapsular haemorrhage. Brain 123 (Pt 9), 1850–1862, 2000.

117. Baloh RW, Furman JM, Yee RD. Dorsal midbrain syndrome: clinical and oculographic findings. Neurology 35 (1), 54–60, 1985.

118. Choi KD, Jung DS, Kim JS. Specificity of "peering at the tip of the nose" for a diagnosis of thalamic hemorrhage. Arch Neurol 61, 417–422, 2004.

119. Litvan I, Jankovic J, Goetz CG, et al. Accuracy of the clinical diagnosis of postencephalitic parkinsonism: a clinicopathologic study. Eur J Neurol 5 (5), 451–457, 1998.

120. Jhee SS, Zarotsky V, Mohaupt SM, et al. Delayed onset of oculogyric crisis and torticollis with intramuscular haloperidol. Ann Pharmacother 37 (10), 1434–1437, 2003.

121. Pannullo SC, Reich JB, Krol G, et al. MRI changes in intracranial hypotension. Neurology 43, 919–926, 1993.

122. Keane JR. Alternating skew deviation: 47 patients. Neurology 35 (5), 725–728, 1985.

123. Brandt TH, Dieterich M. Different types of skew deviation. J Neurol Neurosurg Psychiatry 54 (6), 549–550, 1991.

124. Keane JR. Ocular skew deviation. Analysis of 100 cases. Arch Neurol 32 (3), 185–190, 1975.

125. Smith JL, David NJ, Klintworth G. Skew deviation. Neurology 14, 96–105, 1964.

126. Johkura K, Komiyama A, Tobita M, et al. Saccadic ping-pong gaze. J Neuroophthalmol 18, 43–46, 1998.

127. Daroff RB, Hoyt WF. Supranuclear disorders of ocular control systems in man: clinical, anatomical and physiological correlations. In: Bach-y-Rita P, Collins CC, Hyde JE, eds. The Control of Eye Movements. New York: Academic Press, pp 175–235, 1971.

128. Ochs AL, Stark L, Hoyt WF, et al. Opposed adducting saccades in convergence-retraction nystagmus: a patient with sylvian aqueduct syndrome. Brain 102 (3), 497–508, 1979.

129. Fischer CM. Ocular bobbing. Arch Neurol 11, 543–546, 1964.

130. Rosenberg ML. Spontaneous vertical eye movements in coma. Ann Neurol 20 (5), 635–637, 1986.

131. Herishanu YO, Abarbanel JM, Frisher S, et al. Spontaneous vertical eye movements associated with pontine lesions. Isr J Med Sci 27 (6), 320–324, 1991.

132. Lourie H. Seesaw nystagmus. Case report elucidating the mechanism. Arch Neurol 9, 531–533, 1963.

133. Sano K, Sekino H, Tsukamoto Y, et al. Stimulation and destruction of the region of the interstitial nucleus in cases of torticollis and see-saw nystagmus. Confin Neurol 34 (5), 331–338, 1972.

134. Keane JR. Intermittent see-saw eye movements. Report of a patient in coma after hyperextension head injury. Arch Neurol 35 (3), 173–174, 1978.

135. Schott JM, Rossor MN. The grasp and other primitive reflexes. J Neurol Neurosurg Psychiatry 74 (5), 558–560, 2003.

136. Jacobs L, Gossman MD. Three primitive reflexes in normal adults. Neurology 30 (2), 184–188, 1980.

137. De RE, Barbieri C. The incidence of the grasp reflex following hemispheric lesion and its relation to frontal damage. Brain 115 (Pt 1), 293–313, 1992.

138. Greenberg DA, Simon RP. Flexor and extensor postures in sedative drug-induced coma. Neurology 32 (4), 448–451, 1982.

139. Jennett B, Teasdale G. Aspects of coma after severe head injury. Lancet 1(8017), 878–881, 1977.

140. Sherrington CS. Cataleptoid reflexes in the monkey. Proc Royal Soc Lond 60, 411–414, 1897.

141. Kirk MM, Hoogwerf BJ, Stoller JK. Reversible decerebrate posturing after profound and prolonged hypoglycemia. Cleve Clin J Med 58 (4), 361–363, 1991.

142. Conomy JP, Swash M. Reversible decerebrate and decorticate postures in hepatic coma. N Engl J Med 278 (16), 876–879, 1968.

143. Strauss GI, Moller K, Larsen FS, et al. Cerebral glucose and oxygen metabolism in patients with fulminant hepatic failure. Liver Transpl 9 (12), 1244–1252, 2003.

144. Kosaka Y, Tanaka K, Sawa H, et al. Acid-base disturbance in patients with fulminant hepatic failure. Gastroenterol Jpn 14(1), 24–30, 1979.

145. Krapf R, Caduff P, Wagdi P, et al. Plasma potassium response to acute respiratory alkalosis. Kidney Int 47 (1), 217–224, 1995.

146. Spector RH, Davidoff RA, Schwartzman RJ. Phenytoin-induced ophthalmoplegia. Neurology 26 (11), 1031–1034, 1976.

147. Pulst SM, Lombroso CT. External ophthalmoplegia, alpha and spindle coma in imipramine overdose: case report and review of the literature. Ann Neurol 14(5), 587–590, 1983.

148. Odaka M, Yuki N, Yamada M, et al. Bickerstaff's brainstem encephalitis: clinical features of 62 cases and a subgroup associated with Guillain-Barre syndrome. Brain 126 (Pt 10), 2279–2290, 2003.

149. Ragosta K. Miller Fisher syndrome, a brainstem encephalitis, mimics brain death. Clin Pediatr (Phila) 32 (11), 685–687, 1993.

150. Dhiravibulya K, Ouvrier R, Johnston I, et al. Benign intracranial hypertension in childhood: a review of 23 patients. J Paediatr Child Health 27 (5), 304–307, 1991.

151. Thomke F, Mika-Gruttner A, Visbeck A, et al. The risk of abducens palsy after diagnostic lumbar puncture. Neurology 54 (3), 768–769, 2000.

152. Speer C, Pearlman J, Phillips PH, et al. Fourth cranial nerve palsy in pediatric patients with pseudotumor cerebri. Am J Ophthalmol 127 (2), 236–237, 1999.

153. Malouf R, Brust JC. Hypoglycemia: causes, neurological manifestations, and outcome. Ann Neurol 17(5), 421–430, 1985.

154. Vaughan CJ, Delanty N. Hypertensive emergencies. Lancet 356 (9227), 411–417, 2000.

155. Mitchell P, Wilkinson ID, Hoggard N, et al. Detection of subarachnoid haemorrhage with magnetic resonance imaging. J Neurol Neurosurg Psychiatry 70, 205–211, 2001.

156. Lin A, Ross BD, Harris K, et al. Efficacy of proton magnetic resonance spectroscopy in neurological diagnosis and neurotherapeutic decision making. NeuroRx 2(2), 197–214, 2005.

157. Guillevin R, Vallee JN, Demeret S, et al. Cerebral fat embolism: Usefulness of magnetic resonance spectroscopy. Ann Neurol 57, 434–439, 2005.

158. Schoning M, Scheel P, Holzer M, et al. Volume measurement of cerebral blood flow: assessment of cerebral circulatory arrest. Transplantation 80 (3), 326–331, 2005.

159. Dominguez-Roldan JM, Garcia-Alfaro C, Jimenez-Gonzalez PI, et al. Brain death due to supratentorial masses: diagnosis using transcranial Doppler sonography. Transplant Proc 36 (10), 2898–2900, 2004.

160. Wojner-Alexandrov AW, Alexandrov AV, Rodriguez D, et al. Houston paramedic and emergency stroke treatment and outcomes study (HoPSTO). Stroke 36 (7), 1512–1518, 2005.

161. Panerai RB, Kerins V, Fan L, et al. Association between dynamic cerebral autoregulation and mortality in severe head injury. Br J Neurosurg 18 (5), 471–479, 2004.

162. Droste DW, Metz RJ. Clinical utility of echocontrast agents in neurosonology. Neurol Res 26 (7), 754–759, 2004.

163. Brenner RP. The interpretation of the EEG in stupor and coma. Neurologist 11(5), 271–284, 2005.

164. Kaplan PW. Assessing the outcomes in patients with nonconvulsive status epilepticus: nonconvulsive status epilepticus is underdiagnosed, potentially overtreated, and confounded by comorbidity. J Clin Neurophysiol 16 (4), 341–352, discussion 353, 1999.

165. Brenner RP. Is it status? Epilepsia 43 (Suppl 3), 103–113, 2002.

166. Towne AR, Waterhouse EJ, Boggs JG, et al. Prevalence of nonconvulsive status epilepticus in comatose patients. Neurology 54, 340–345, 2000.

167. Burneo JG, Knowlton RC, Gomez C, et al. Confirmation of nonconvulsive limbic status epilepticus with the sodium amytal test. Epilepsia 44, 1122–1126, 2003.

168. Kaplan PW. The clinical features, diagnosis, and prognosis of nonconvulsive status epilepticus. Neurologist 11(6), 348–361, 2005.

169. Fischer C, Luauté J, Adeleine P, et al. Predictive value of sensory and cognitive evoked potentials for awakening from coma. Neurology 63, 669–673, 2004.

Chapter 3

Structural Causes of Stupor and Coma

Two major classes of structural brain injuries cause coma (Table 3–1): (1) *Compressive lesions* may impair consciousness either by directly compressing the ascending arousal system or by distorting brain tissue so that it moves out of position and secondarily compresses components of the ascending arousal system or its forebrain targets (see *herniation syndromes*, page 95). These processes include a wide range of space-occupying lesions such as tumor, hematoma, and abscess. (2) *Destructive lesions*

cause coma by direct damage to the ascending arousal system or its forebrain targets. To cause coma, lesions of the diencephalon or brainstem must be bilateral, but can be quite focal if they damage the ascending activating system near the midline in the midbrain or caudal diencephalon; cortical or subcortical damage must be both bilateral and diffuse. Processes that may cause these changes include tumor, hemorrhage, infarct, trauma, or infection. Both destructive and compressive lesions may cause

Table 3–1 **Sites and Representative Causes of Structural Lesions That Can Cause Coma**

Compressive	Destructive
Cerebral	*Cerebral hemisphere*
Bilateral subdural hematomas	Cortex (e.g., acute anoxic injury)
	Subcortical white matter
Diencephalon	(e.g., delayed anoxic injury)
Thalamus (e.g., hemorrhage)	
Hypothalamus (e.g., pituitary tumor)	*Diencephalon*
	Thalamus (e.g., infarct)
Brainstem	
Midbrain (e.g., uncal herniation)	*Brainstem*
Cerebellum (e.g., tumor,	Midbrain, pons (e.g., infarct)
hemorrhage, abscess)	

additional compression by producing brain edema.

Most compressive lesions are treated surgically, whereas destructive lesions are generally treated medically. This chapter describes the pathophysiology and general approach to patients with structural lesions of the brain, first considering compressive and then destructive lesions. Chapter 4 deals with some of the specific causes of coma outlined in Table 3–1.

Chapter 2 has described some of the physical findings that distinguish structural from nonstructural causes of stupor and coma. The physician must first decide whether the patient is indeed stuporous or comatose, distinguishing those patients who are not in coma but suffer from abulia, akinetic mutism, psychologic unresponsiveness, or the locked-in state from those truly stuporous or comatose (see Chapter 1). This is usually relatively easily done during the course of the initial examination. More difficult is distinguishing structural from metabolic causes of stupor or coma. As indicated in Chapter 2, if the structural cause of coma involves the ascending arousal system in the brainstem, the presence of focal findings usually makes the distinction between metabolic and structural coma easy. However, when the structural disease involves the cerebral cortex diffusely or the diencephalon bilaterally, focal signs are often absent and it may be difficult to distinguish structural from metabolic coma. Compressive lesions that initially do not cause focal signs eventually do so, but by then coma

may be irreversible. Thus, if there is any question about the distinction between structural and metabolic coma, immediately after stabilizing the patient, an imaging study (usually a computed tomography [CT] scan but, if available, a magnetic resonance imaging [MRI] scan) must be obtained to rule out a mass lesion that may be surgically remediable. Identifying surgically remediable lesions that have not yet caused focal findings gives the physician time to stabilize the patient and investigate other additional nonstructural causes of coma. The time, however, is short and should be counted in minutes rather than hours or days. If focal findings are already present, efforts to decrease intracranial pressure (ICP), including hyperventilation and hyperosmolar agents and often administration of corticosteroids (Chapter 7), should be instituted before sending the patient for imaging.

COMPRESSIVE LESIONS AS A CAUSE OF COMA

Compressive lesions may impair consciousness in a number of critical ways: (1) by directly distorting the arousal system or its forebrain targets; (2) by increasing ICP diffusely to the point of impairing global cerebral blood flow; (3) by distorting tissue to the point of causing local ischemia; (4) by causing edema, thus further distorting neural tissue; or (5) by causing tissue shifts (herniations). Understanding the anatomy and pathophysiology of each of these processes is critical in evaluating patients in coma.

COMPRESSIVE LESIONS MAY DIRECTLY DISTORT THE AROUSAL SYSTEM

Compression at key levels of the brain may cause coma by exerting pressure upon the structures of the arousal system. The mechanism by which local pressure may impair neuronal function is not entirely understood. However, neurons are dependent upon axonal transport to supply critical proteins and mitochondria to their terminals, and to transport used or damaged cellular components back to the cell body for destruction and disposal. Even a loose ligature around an axon causes damming of axon contents on both sides of the stricture, due to impairment of both anterograde and retrograde axonal flow, and results in impairment of axonal function. Perhaps the clearest example of this relationship is provided by the optic nerve in patients with papilledema (see section on *increased ICP,* page 91). When a compressive lesion results in displacement of the structures of the arousal system, consciousness may become impaired, as described in the sections below.

Compression at Different Levels of the Central Nervous System Presents in Distinct Ways

When a *cerebral hemisphere is compressed by a lesion* such as a subdural hematoma, tumor, or abscess that grows slowly over a long period of time, it may reach a relatively large size with little in the way of local signs that can help identify the diagnosis. The tissue in the cerebral hemispheres can absorb a surprising amount of distortion and stretching, as long as the growth of the mass can be compensated for by displacing cerebrospinal fluid (CSF) from the ventricles in that hemisphere. However, when there is no further room in the hemisphere to expand, even a small amount of growth can only be accommodated by compressing the diencephalon and midbrain either laterally across the midline or downward. In such patients, the impairment of consciousness correlates with the displacement of the diencephalon and upper brainstem in a lateral or caudal direction.[1] Hence, when a patient with a hemispheric lesion reaches the point of impairment of consciousness, there is very little time left to intervene before the brain is irreparably injured.

The *diencephalon may also be compressed* by a mass lesion in the thalamus itself (generally a tumor or a hemorrhage) or a mass in the suprasellar cistern (typically a craniopharyngioma, a germ cell tumor, or suprasellar extension of a pituitary adenoma; see Chapter 4). In addition to causing impairment of consciousness, suprasellar tumors typically cause visual field deficits, classically a bitemporal hemianopsia, although a wide range of optic nerve or tract injuries may also occur. If a suprasellar tumor extends into the cavernous sinus, there may be injury to the cranial nerves that supply the ocular muscles (III, IV, VI) and the ophthalmic division of the trigeminal nerve (V1). On occasion, these tumors may also cause endocrine dysfunction. If they damage the pituitary stalk, they may cause diabetes insipidus or panhypopituitarism. In women, the presence of a pituitary tumor is often heralded by galactorrhea and amenorrhea, as prolactin is the sole anterior pituitary hormone under negative regulation, and it is typically elevated when the pituitary stalk is damaged.

The *dorsal midbrain* may be compressed by a tumor in the pineal region. Pineal mass lesions may be suprasellar germinomas or other germ cell tumors (embryonal cell carcinoma, teratocarcinoma) that occur along the midline, or pineal masses including pinealcytoma or pineal astrocytoma. Pineal masses compress the pretectal area as well. Thus, in addition to causing impairment of consciousness, they produce diagnostic neuro-ophthalmologic signs including fixed, slightly enlarged pupils; impairment of voluntary vertical eye movements (typically elevation is impaired earlier and more severely than depression) and convergence; and convergence nystagmus and sometimes retractory nystagmus (Parinaud's syndrome; see page 110).[2] Hemorrhage into the pulvinar of the thalamus, which overlies the pretectal area and dorsal midbrain, may sometimes produce a similar constellation of signs.

Posterior fossa compressive lesions most often originate in the cerebellum, including tumors, hemorrhages, infarctions, or abscesses, although occasionally extra-axial lesions, such as a subdural or epidural hematoma, may have a similar effect. Tumors of the cerebellum include the full range of primary and metastatic brain tumors (Chapter 4), as well as juvenile pilocytic astrocytomas and medulloblastomas in children and hemangioblastoma in patients with von Hippel-Lindau syndrome.

A cerebellar mass causes coma by direct compression of the brainstem, which may also cause the brainstem to herniate upward through the tentorial notch. As the patient loses consciousness, there is a pattern of pontine level dysfunction, with small reactive pupils, impairment of vestibulo-ocular responses (which may be asymmetric), and decerebrate motor responses.[3,4] Because the base of the pons is farthest from the cerebellum, motor signs (e.g., upgoing toes) are usually a relatively late finding, and suggest instead an intrinsic brainstem mass. With upward pressure on the midbrain, the pupils become asymmetric or unreactive. If vestibulo-ocular responses were not previously impaired by pontine compression, vertical eye movements may be lost.

Cerebellar mass lesions may also cause coma by compressing the fourth ventricle to the point where it impairs flow of CSF. This causes acute hydrocephalus and rapidly increasing ICP (see page 147). The onset of obstruction of the fourth ventricle is typically heralded by nausea and sometimes sudden, projectile vomiting. There may also be a history of ataxia, vertigo, neck stiffness, and eventually respiratory arrest as the cerebellar tonsils are impacted upon the lip of the foramen magnum. If the compression develops slowly (i.e., over more than 12 hours), there may also be papilledema. Because cerebellar masses may cause acute obstruction of the fourth ventricle by expanding by only a few millimeters in diameter, they are potentially very dangerous.

On occasion, impairment of consciousness may occur as a result of *a mass lesion directly compressing the brainstem*. These are more commonly intrinsic masses, such as an abscess or a hemorrhage, in which case it is difficult to determine how much of the impairment is due to compression as opposed to destruction. Occasionally, a mass lesion of the cerebellopontine angle, such as a vestibular schwannoma, meningioma, or cholesteatoma, may compress the brainstem. However, these are usually slow processes and the mass may reach a very large

size and often causes signs of local injury before consciousness is impaired.

The Role of Increased Intracranial Pressure in Coma

A key and often misunderstood point is that increases in ICP are withstood remarkably well by the brain, as long as they progress relatively slowly. In patients with chronic elevation of CSF pressure, such as those with pseudotumor cerebri, there is little evidence of brain dysfunction, even when CSF pressures reach 600 mm of water or greater. The chief problems induced by increased ICP are papilledema and headache, until the pressure gets high enough to impair cerebral blood flow.

Papilledema is due to the pressure differential applied to the optic nerve by the increase in ICP. Retinal ganglion cells within the eye are subject to intraocular pressure, typically in the same range as normal CSF pressure. Their axons leave the eye through the optic disk and travel to the brain via the optic nerve. Axoplasm flows from the retinal ganglion cell bodies in the eye, down the axon and through the optic disc. Similarly, the retinal veins within the eye are subject to intraocular pressure. They also leave through the optic disc and run along the optic nerve. The optic nerve in turn is surrounded by a dural and arachnoid sleeve, which contains CSF that communicates with the CSF in the subarachnoid space around the brain.[5] The optic disk itself is composed of a dense fibrous network forming a cribriform (from the Latin for *sieve*) plate that acts as a pressure fitting, so that the optic nerve and retinal vein are exposed to intraocular pressure on one side of the disk and to ICP on the other side.

Normally, axonal transport proceeds unimpeded and the retinal veins show normal venous pulsations, as there is little, if any, pressure differential between the two compartments. As ICP rises above systemic venous pressure, retinal venous pulsations are damped or eliminated as an early feature of papilledema. The retinal veins become larger and more numerous appearing, because increased venous pressure causes smaller veins to become more noticeable on funduscopy. Thus, the presence of retinal venous pulsations is a good but not invariable sign of normal ICP, and engorgement of retinal veins is a reliable early sign of increased ICP.[6,7] A second consequence of increased ICP is that axoplasmic flow is impaired (as if a loose ligature had been tied around the nerve), and there is buildup of axoplasm on the retinal side of the disk. The swollen optic axons obscure the disk margins, beginning at the superior and inferior poles, then extending laterally and finally medially.[8] The size of the optic disk increases, and this can be mapped as a larger "blind spot" in the visual field. Some patients even complain of a visual scotoma in this area. If ICP is increased sufficiently, the ganglion cells begin to fail from the periphery of the retina in toward the macula. This results in a concentric loss of vision.

Because papilledema reflects the back-pressure on the optic nerves from increased ICP, it is virtually always bilateral. A rare exception occurs when the optic nerve on one side is itself compressed by a mass lesion (such as an olfactory groove meningioma), thus resulting in optic atrophy in one eye and papilledema in the other eye (the Foster Kennedy syndrome). On the other hand, optic nerve injury at the level of the optic disk, either due to demyelinating disease or vascular infarct of the vasa nervorum (anterior ischemic optic neuropathy), can also block axonal transport and venous return, due to retrobulbar swelling of the optic nerve.[9] The resulting papillitis can look identical to papilledema but is typically unilateral, or at least does not involve the optic nerves simultaneously. In addition, papillitis is usually accompanied by the relatively rapid onset of visual loss, particularly focal loss called a scotoma, so the clinical distinction is usually clear.

The origin of *headache* in patients with increased ICP is not understood. CSF normally leaves the subarachnoid compartment mainly by resorption at the arachnoid villi.[10] These structures are located along the surface of the superior sagittal sinus, and they consist of invaginations of the arachnoid membrane into the wall of the sinus. CSF is taken up from the subarachnoid space by endocytosis into vesicles, the vesicles are transported across the arachnoid epithelial cells, and then their contents are released by exocytosis into the venous sinus. Imbalance in the process of secretion and resorption of CSF occurs in cases of CSF-secreting tumors as well as in pseudotumor cerebri. In both conditions, very high levels of CSF pressure, in excess of 600 mm of water, may be achieved, but rather little in the way of brain dysfunction occurs, other than headache. Experimental infusion of artificial CSF into the subarachnoid space, to pressures as high as 800 or even 1,000 mm of water, also does not cause cerebral dysfunction and, curiously, often does not cause headache.[11,12] However, conditions that cause diffusely increased ICP such as pseudotumor cerebri usually do cause headache,[13] suggesting that they must cause some subtle distortion of pain receptors in the cerebral blood vessels or the meninges.[14]

On the other hand, when there is *obstruction of the cerebral venous system*, increased ICP is often associated with signs of brain dysfunction as well as severe headache. The headache is localized to the venous sinus that is obstructed (superior sagittal sinus headache is typically at the vertex of the skull, whereas lateral sinus headache is usually behind the ear on the affected side). The headache in these conditions is thought to be due to irritation and local distortion of the sinus itself. Brain dysfunction is produced by back-pressure on the draining veins that feed into the sinus, thus reducing the perfusion pressure of the adjacent areas of the brain, to the point of precipitating venous infarction (see page 154). Small capillaries may be damaged, producing local hemorrhage and focal or generalized seizures. Superior sagittal sinus thrombosis produces parasagittal ischemia in the hemispheres, causing lower extremity paresis. Lateral sinus thrombosis typically causes infarction in the inferior lateral temporal lobe, which may produce little in the way of signs, other than seizures.

The most important mechanism by which diffusely raised ICP can cause symptoms is by *impairment of the cerebral arterial supply*. The brain usually compensates for the increased ICP by regulating its blood supply as described in Chapter 2. However, as ICP reaches and exceeds 600 mm of water, the back-pressure on cerebral perfusion reaches 45 to 50 mm Hg, which becomes a major hemodynamic challenge. Typically, this is seen in severe acute liver failure,[15] with vasomotor paralysis following head injury, or occasionally in acute encephalitis. When perfusion pressure falls below the lower limit required for brain function, neurons fail to maintain their ionic gradients due to energy failure, resulting in additional swelling, which further increases ICP and results in a downward spiral of reduced perfusion and further brain infarction.

Decreased perfusion pressure can also occur when systemic blood pressure drops, such as when assuming a standing position. Some patients with increased ICP develop brief bilateral visual loss when they stand, called *visual obscurations*, presumably due to failure to autoregulate the posterior cerebral blood flow. Failure of perfusion pressure can also occur focally (i.e., in a patient with an otherwise asymptomatic carotid occlusion who develops symptoms in the ipsilateral carotid distribution on standing because of the resulting small drop in blood pressure). If the patient has bilateral chronic carotid occlusions, transient loss of consciousness may result.[16]

Patients with elevated ICP from mass lesions often suffer sudden rises in ICP precipitated by changes in posture, coughing, sneezing, or straining, or even during tracheal suctioning (plateau waves).[17] The sudden rises in ICP can reduce cerebral perfusion and produce a variety of neurologic symptoms including confusion, stupor, and coma[18] (Table 3–2). In general, the symptoms last only a few minutes and then resolve, leading some observers to confuse these with seizures.

Finally, the *loss of compliance of the intracranial system to further increases in volume and the rate of change in ICP* plays an important role in the response of the brain to increased ICP. Compliance is the change in pressure caused by an increase in volume. In a normal brain, increases in brain volume (e.g., due to a small intracerebral hemorrhage) can be compensated by displacement of an equal volume of CSF from the compartment. However, when a mass has increased in size to the point where there is little remaining CSF in the compartment, even a small further increase in volume can produce a large increase in compartmental pressure. This loss of compliance in cases where diffuse brain edema has caused a critical increase in ICP can lead to the development of *plateau waves*. These are large, sustained increases in ICP, which may approach the mean arterial blood pressure, and which occur at intervals as often as every 15 to 30 minutes.[19,20] They are thought to be due to episodic arterial vasodilation, which is due to systemic vasomotor rhythms, but a sudden increase in vascular volume in a compartment with no compliance, even if very small, can dramatically increase ICP.[21] These sudden increases in ICP can thus cause a wide range of neurologic paroxysmal symptoms (see Table 3–2). When pressure in neighboring compartments is lower, this imbalance can cause herniation (see below).[22]

Table 3–2 **Paroxysmal Symptoms That May Result From a Sudden Increase in Intracranial Pressure**

Impairment of consciousness	Opisthotonus, trismus
Trancelike state	Rigidity and tonic extension/flexion of the arms and legs
Unreality/warmth	
Confusion, disorientation	Bilateral extensor plantar responses
Restlessness, agitation	Sluggish/absent deep tendon reflexes
Disorganized motor activity, carphologia	Generalized muscular weakness
Sense of suffocation, air hunger	Facial twitching
Cardiovascular/respiratory disturbances	Clonic movements of the arms and legs
Headache	Facial/limb paresthesias
Pain in the neck and shoulders	Rise in temperature
Nasal itch	Nausea, vomiting
Blurring of vision, amaurosis	Facial flushing
Mydriasis, pupillary areflexia	Pallor, cyanosis
Nystagmus	Sweating
Oculomotor/abducens paresis	Shivering and "goose flesh"
Conjugate deviation of the eyes	Thirst
External ophthalmoplegia	Salivation
Dysphagia, dysarthria	Yawning, hiccoughing
Nuchal rigidity	Urinary and fecal urgency/incontinence
Retroflexion of the neck	

Adapted from Ingvar.[18]

Conversely, when a patient shows early signs of herniation, it is often possible to reverse the situation by restoring a small margin of compliance to the compartment containing the mass lesion. Hyperventilation causes a fall in arterial pCO$_2$, resulting in arterial and venous vasoconstriction. The small reduction in intracranial blood volume may reverse the herniation syndrome dramatically in just a few minutes.

The Role of Vascular Factors and Cerebral Edema in Mass Lesions

As indicated above, an important mechanism by which compressive lesions may cause symp-

toms is by inducing local tissue ischemia. Even in the absence of a diffuse impairment of cerebral blood flow, local increases in pressure and tissue distortion in the vicinity of a mass lesion may stretch small arteries and reduce their caliber to the point where they are no longer able to supply sufficient blood to their targets.

Many mass lesions, including tumors, inflammatory lesions, and the capsules of subdural hematomas, are able to induce the growth of new blood vessels (angiogenesis).[23] These blood vessels do not have the features that characterize normal cerebral capillaries (i.e., lack of fenestrations and tight junctions between endothelial cells) that are the basis for the blood-brain barrier. Thus, the vessels leak; the leakage of

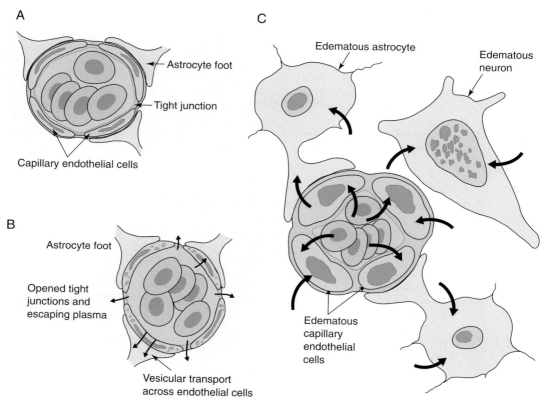

Figure 3–1. A schematic drawing illustrating cytotoxic versus vasogenic edema. (A) Under normal circumstances, the brain is protected from the circulation by a blood-brain barrier, consisting of tight junctions between cerebral capillary endothelial cells that do not permit small molecules to penetrate the brain, as well as a basal lamina surrounded by astrocytic end-feet. (B) When the blood-brain barrier is breached (e.g., by neovascularization in a tumor or the membranes of subdural hematoma), fluid transudates from fenestrated blood vessels into the brain. This results in an increase in fluid in the extracellular compartment, vasogenic edema. Vasogenic edema can usually be reduced by corticosteroids, which decrease capillary permeability. (C) When neurons are injured, they can no longer maintain ion gradients. The increased intracellular sodium causes a shift of fluid from the extracellular to the intracellular compartment, resulting in cytotoxic edema. Cytotoxic edema is not affected by corticosteroids. (From Fishman, RA. Brain edema. *N Engl J Med* 293 (14):706–11, 1975. By permission of Massachusetts Medical Society.)

contrast dyes during CT or MRI scanning provides the basis for contrast enhancement of a lesion that lacks a blood-brain barrier. The vascular leak results in the extravasation of fluid into the extracellular space and *vasogenic edema*[24,25] (see Figure 3–1B). This edema further displaces surrounding tissues that are pushed progressively farther from the source of their own feeding arteries. Because the large arteries are tethered to the circle of Willis and small ones are tethered to the pial vascular system, they may not be able to be displaced as freely as the brain tissue they supply. Hence, the distensibility of the blood supply becomes the limiting factor to tissue perfusion and, in many cases, tissue survival.

Ischemia and consequent energy failure cause loss of the electrolyte gradient across the neuronal membranes. Neurons depolarize but are no longer able to repolarize and so fail. As neurons take on more sodium, they swell (*cytotoxic edema*), thus further increasing the mass effect on adjacent sites (see Figure 3–1C). Increased intracellular calcium meanwhile results in the activation of apoptotic programs for neuronal cell death. This vicious cycle of swelling produces ischemia of adjacent tissue, which in turn causes further tissue swelling. *Cytotoxic edema* may cause a patient with a chronic and slowly growing mass lesion to decompensate quite suddenly,[24,25] with rapid onset of brain failure and coma when the lesion reaches a critical limit.

HERNIATION SYNDROMES: INTRACRANIAL SHIFTS IN THE PATHOGENESIS OF COMA

The Monro-Kellie doctrine hypothesizes that because the contents of the skull are not compressible and are contained within an unyielding case of bone, the sum of the volume of the brain, CSF, and intracranial blood is constant at all times.[26] A corollary is that these same restrictions apply to each compartment (right vs. left supratentorial space, infratentorial space, spinal subarachnoid space). In a normal brain, increases in the size of a growing mass lesion can be compensated for by the displacement of an equal volume of CSF from the compartment. The displacement of CSF, and in some cases blood volume, by the mass lesion raises ICP. As the mass grows, there is less CSF to be

displaced, and hence *the compliance of the intracranial contents decreases as the size of the compressive lesion increases*. When a mass has increased in size to the point where there is little remaining CSF in the compartment, even a small further increase in volume can produce a large increase in compartmental pressure. When pressure in neighboring compartments is lower, this imbalance causes herniation. Thus, intracranial shifts are of key concern in the diagnosis of coma due to supratentorial mass lesions (Figure 3–2).

The pathogenesis of signs and symptoms of an expanding mass lesion that causes coma is rarely a function of the increase in ICP itself, but usually results from imbalances of pressure between different compartments leading to tissue herniation.

To understand herniation syndromes, it is first necessary to review briefly the structure of the intracranial compartments between which herniations occur.

Anatomy of the Intracranial Compartments

The cranial sutures of babies close at about 18 months, encasing the intracranial contents in a nondistensible box of finite volume. The intracranial contents include the brain tissue (approximately 87%, of which 77% is water), CSF (approximately 9%), blood vessels (approximately 4%), and the meninges (dura, arachnoid, and pia that occupy a negligible volume). The dural septa that divide the intracranial space into compartments play a key role in the herniation syndromes caused by supratentorial mass lesions.

The falx cerebri (Figures 3–2 and 3–3) separates the two cerebral hemispheres by a dense dural leaf that is tethered to the superior sagittal sinus along the midline of the cranial vault. The falx contains the inferior sagittal sinus along its free edge. The free edge of the falx normally rests just above the corpus callosum. One result is that severe head injury can cause a contusion of the corpus callosum by violent upward displacement of the brain against the free edge of the falx.[33] The pericallosal branches of the anterior cerebral artery also run in close proximity to the free edge of the falx. Hence, displacement of the cingulate gyrus under the falx by a hemispheric mass may compress the pericallosal artery and result in ischemia or infarction of

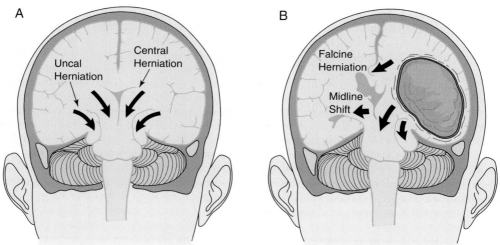

Figure 3–2. A schematic drawing to illustrate the different herniation syndromes seen with intracranial mass effect. When the increased mass is symmetric in the two hemispheres (A), there may be central herniation, as well as herniation of either or both medial temporal lobes, through the tentorial opening. Asymmetric compression (B), from a unilateral mass lesion, may cause herniation of the ipsilateral cingulate gyrus under the falx (falcine herniation). This type of compression may cause distortion of the diencephalon by either downward herniation or midline shift. The depression of consciousness is more closely related to the degree and rate of shift, rather than the direction. Finally, the medial temporal lobe (uncus) may herniate early in the clinical course.

the cingulate gyrus (see *falcine herniation*, page 100).

The tentorium cerebelli (Figure 3–3) separates the cerebral hemispheres (supratentorial compartment) from the brainstem and cerebellum (infratentorial compartment/posterior fossa). The tentorium is less flexible than the falx, because its fibrous dural lamina is stretched across the surface of the middle fossa and is tethered in position for about three-quarters of its extent (see Figure 3–3). It attaches anteriorly at the petrous ridges and posterior clinoid processes and laterally to the occipital bone along the lateral sinus. Extending posteriorly into the center of the tentorium from the posterior clinoid processes is a large semioval opening, the incisura or tentorial notch, whose diameter is usually between 25 and 40 mm mediolaterally and 50 to 70 mm rostrocaudally.[34] The tentorium cerebelli also plays a key role in the pathophysiology of supratentorial mass lesions, as when the tissue volume of the supratentorial compartments exceeds that compartment's capacity, there is no alternative but for tissue to herniate through the tentorial opening (see *uncal herniation*, page 100).

Tissue shifts in any direction can damage structures occupying the tentorial opening. The midbrain, with its exiting oculomotor nerves,

traverses the opening from the posterior fossa to attach to the diencephalon. The superior portion of the cerebellar vermis is typically applied closely to the surface of the midbrain and occupies the posterior portion of the tentorial opening. The quadrigeminal cistern, above the tectal plate of the midbrain, and the peduncular and interpeduncular cisterns along the base of the midbrain provide flexibility; there may be considerable tissue shift before symptoms are produced if a mass lesion expands slowly (Figure 3–2).

The basilar artery lies along the ventral surface of the midbrain. As it nears the tentorial opening, it gives off superior cerebellar arteries bilaterally, then branches into the posterior cerebral arteries (Figure 3–4). The posterior cerebral arteries give off a range of thalamoperforating branches that supply the posterior thalamus and pretectal area, followed by the posterior communicating arteries.[35] Each posterior cerebral artery then wraps around the lateral surface of the upper midbrain and reaches the ventral surface of the hippocampal gyrus, where it gives off a posterior choroidal artery.[36] The posterior choroidal artery anastomoses with the anterior choroidal artery, a branch of the internal carotid artery that runs between the dentate gyrus and the free lateral edge of the tentorium. The

Box 3–1 Historical View of the Pathophysiology of Brain Herniation

In the 19th century, many neurologists thought that supratentorial lesions caused stupor or coma by impairing function of the cortical mantle, although the mechanism was not understood. Cushing proposed that the increase in ICP caused impairment of blood flow, especially to the medulla.[27] He was able to show that translation of pressure waves from the supratentorial compartments to the lower brainstem may occur in experimental animals. Similarly, in young children, a supratentorial pressure wave may compress the medulla, causing an increase in blood pressure and fall in heart rate (the Cushing reflex). Such responses are rare in adults, who almost always show symptoms of more rostral brainstem failure before developing symptoms of lower brainstem dysfunction.

The role of temporal lobe herniation through the tentorial notch was appreciated by MacEwen in the 1880s, who froze and then serially cut sections through the heads of patients who died from temporal lobe abscesses.[28] His careful descriptions demonstrated that the displaced medial surface of the temporal uncus compressed the oculomotor nerve, causing a dilated pupil. In the 1920s, Meyer[29] pointed out the importance of temporal lobe herniation into the tentorial gap in patients with brain tumors; Kernohan and Woltman[30] demonstrated the lateral compression of the brainstem produced by this process. They noted that lateral shift of the midbrain compressed the cerebral peduncle on the side opposite the tumor against the opposite tentorial edge, resulting in ipsilateral hemiparesis. In the following decade, the major features of the syndrome of temporal lobe herniation were clarified, and the role of the tentorial pressure cone was widely appreciated as a cause of symptoms in patients with coma.

More recently, the role of lateral displacement of the diencephalon and upper brainstem versus downward displacement of the same structures in causing coma has received considerable attention.[31,32] Careful studies of the displacement of midline structures, such as the pineal gland, in patients with coma due to forebrain mass lesions demonstrate that the symptoms are due to distortion of the structures at the mesodiencephalic junction, with the rate of displacement being more important than the absolute value or direction of the movement.

posterior cerebral artery then runs caudally along the medial surface of the occipital lobe to supply the visual cortex. Either one or both posterior cerebral arteries are vulnerable to compression when tissue herniates through the tentorium. Unilateral compression causes a homonymous hemianopia; bilateral compression causes cortical blindness (see Patient 3–1).

The oculomotor nerves leave the ventral surface of the midbrain between the superior cerebellar arteries and the diverging posterior cerebral arteries (Figure 3–3). The oculomotor nerves cross the posterior cerebral artery and run along the posterior communicating artery to penetrate through the dural edge at the petroclinoid ligament and enter the cavernous sinus. Along this course, the oculomotor nerves run along the medial edge of the temporal lobe (Figure 3–5). The uncus, which represents the bulging medial surface of the amygdala within the medial temporal lobe, usually sits over the tentorial opening, and its medial surface may even be grooved by the tentorium.

A key relationship in the pathophysiology of supratentorial mass lesions is the close proximity of the oculomotor nerve to the posterior

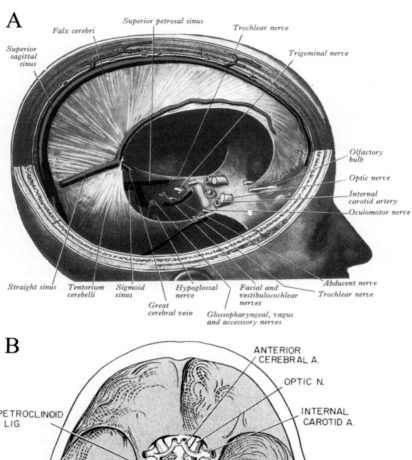

A

Superior
sagittal
sinus

Falx cerebri

Superior petrosal sinus

Trochlear nerve

Trigeminal nerve

Olfactory
bulb

Optic nerve

Internal
carotid artery

Oculomotor nerve

Straight sinus   Tentorium   Sigmoid   Hypoglossal   Facial and   Abducent nerve
                 cerebelli   sinus   nerve   vestibulocochlear   Trochlear nerve
                                                      nerves
                 Great   Glossopharyngeal, vagus
                 cerebral vein   and accessory nerves

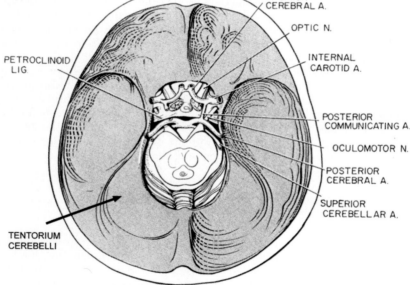

B

ANTERIOR
CEREBRAL A.

OPTIC N.

INTERNAL
CAROTID A.

PETROCLINOID
LIG.

POSTERIOR
COMMUNICATING A.

OCULOMOTOR N.

POSTERIOR
CEREBRAL A.

SUPERIOR
CEREBELLAR A.

TENTORIUM
CEREBELLI

Figure 3–3. The intracranial compartments are separated by tough dural leaflets. (A) The falx cerebri separates the two cerebral hemispheres into separate compartments. Excess mass in one compartment can lead to herniation of the cingulate gyrus under the falx. (From Williams, PL, and Warwick, R. *Functional Neuroanatomy of Man.* WB Saunders, Philadelphia, 1975, p. 986. By permission of Elsevier B.V.) (B) The midbrain occupies most of the tentorial opening, which separates the supratentorial from the infratentorial (posterior fossa) space. Note the vulnerability of the oculomotor nerve to both herniation of the medial temporal lobe and aneurysm of the posterior communicating artery.

Arteries of Brain (basal views)

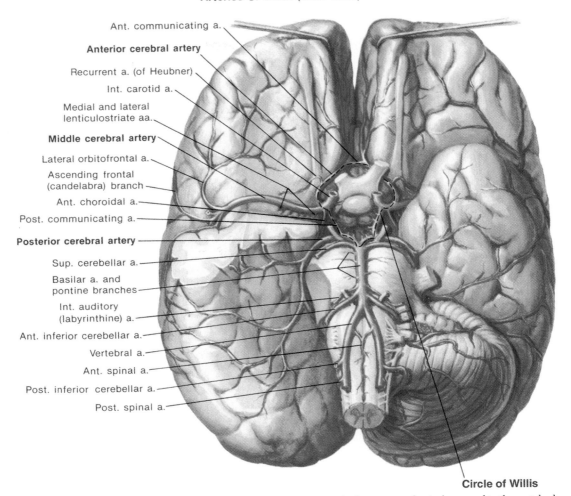

Ant. communicating a.
Anterior cerebral artery
Recurrent a. (of Heubner)
Int. carotid a.
Medial and lateral lenticulostriate aa.
Middle cerebral artery
Lateral orbitofrontal a.
Ascending frontal (candelabra) branch
Ant. choroidal a.
Post. communicating a.
Posterior cerebral artery
Sup. cerebellar a.
Basilar a. and pontine branches
Int. auditory (labyrinthine) a.
Ant. inferior cerebellar a.
Vertebral a.
Ant. spinal a.
Post. inferior cerebellar a.
Post. spinal a.

Circle of Willis

Figure 3–4. The basilar artery is tethered at the top to the posterior cerebral arteries, and at its lower end to the vertebral arteries. As a result, either upward or downward herniation of the brainstem puts at stretch the paramedian feeding vessels that leave the basilar at a right angle and supply the paramedian midbrain and pons. The posterior cerebral arteries can be compressed by the medial temporal lobes when they herniate through the tentorial notch. (From Netter, FH. *The CIBA Collection of Medical Illustrations*. CIBA Pharmaceuticals, New Jersey, 1983, p. 46. By permission of CIBA Pharmaceuticals.)

communicating artery (Figure 3–4) and the medial temporal lobe (Figure 3–5). Compression of the oculomotor nerve by either of these structures results in early injury to the pupillodilator fibers that run along its dorsal surface[37]; hence, a unilateral dilated pupil frequently heralds a neurologic catastrophe.

The other ocular motor nerves are generally not involved in early transtentorial herniation. The trochlear nerves emerge from the dorsal surface of the midbrain just caudal to the inferior colliculi. These slender fiber bundles wrap around the lateral surface of the midbrain and follow the third nerve through the petroclinoid ligament into the cavernous sinus. Because the free edge of the tentorium sits over the posterior edge of the inferior colliculi, severe trauma that displaces the brainstem back into the unyielding edge of the tentorium may result in hemorrhage into the superior cerebellar peduncles and the surrounding parabrachial nuclei.[38,39] The trochlear nerves may also be injured in this way.[40]

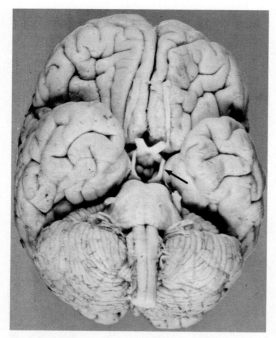

Figure 3–5. Relationship of the oculomotor nerve to the medial temporal lobe. Note that the course of the oculomotor nerve takes it along the medial aspect of the temporal lobe where uncal herniation can compress its dorsal surface. (From Williams, PL, and Warwick, R. *Functional Neuroanatomy of Man*. WB Saunders, Philadelphia, 1975, p. 929. By permission of Elsevier B.V.)

The abducens nerves emerge from the ventral surface of the pons and run along the ventral surface of the midbrain to enter the cavernous sinus as well. Abducens paralysis is often a nonspecific sign of increased[41] or decreased[42] (e.g., after a lumbar puncture or CSF leak) ICP. However, the abducens nerves are rarely damaged by supratentorial or infratentorial mass lesions unless they invade the cavernous sinus or displace the entire brainstem downward.

The foramen magnum, at the lower end of the posterior fossa, is the only means by which brain tissue may exit from the skull. Hence, just as progressive enlargement of a supratentorial mass lesion inevitably results in herniation through the tentorial opening, continued downward displacement either from an expanding supratentorial or infratentorial mass lesion ultimately causes herniation of the cerebellum and the brainstem through the foramen magnum.[43] Here the medulla, the cerebellar tonsils, and the vertebral arteries are

juxtaposed. Usually, a small portion of the cerebellar tonsils protrudes into the aperture (and may even be grooved by the posterior lip of the foramen magnum). However, when the cerebellar tonsils are compressed against the foramen magnum during tonsillar herniation, compression of the tissue may compromise its blood supply, causing tissue infarction and further swelling.

Patterns of Brain Shifts That Contribute to Coma

There are seven major patterns of brain shift: falcine herniation, lateral displacement of the diencephalon, uncal herniation, central transtentorial herniation, rostrocaudal brainstem deterioration, tonsillar herniation, and upward brainstem herniation. The first five patterns are caused by supratentorial mass lesions, whereas tonsillar herniation and upward brainstem herniation usually result from infratentorial mass lesions, as described below.

Falcine herniation occurs when an expanding lesion presses the cerebral hemisphere medially against the falx (Figure 3–2A). The cingulate gyrus and the pericallosal and callosomarginal arteries are compressed against the falx and may be displaced under it. The compression of the pericallosal and callosomarginal arteries causes ischemia in the medial wall of the cerebral hemisphere that swells and further increases the compression. Eventually, the ischemia may advance to frank infarction, which increases the cerebral mass effect further.[44]

Lateral displacement of the diencephalon occurs when an expanding mass lesion, such as a basal ganglionic hemorrhage, pushes the diencephalon laterally (Figure 3–2B). This process may be monitored by displacement of the calcified pineal gland, whose position with respect to the midline is easily seen on plain CT scanning.[45] This lateral displacement is roughly correlated with the degree of impairment of consciousness: 0 to 3 mm is associated with alertness, 3 to 5 mm with drowsiness, 6 to 8 mm with stupor, and 9 to 13 mm with coma.[1]

Uncal herniation occurs when an expanding mass lesion usually located laterally in one cerebral hemisphere forces the medial edge of the temporal lobe to herniate medially and downward over the free tentorial edge into the tentorial notch (Figure 3–2). In contrast to central herniation, in which the first signs are mainly those of diencephalic dysfunction, in uncal herniation the most prominent signs are due to pressure of the herniating temporal lobe on the structures that occupy the tentorial notch.

The key sign associated with uncal herniation is an ipsilateral fixed and dilated pupil due to compression of the dorsal surface of the oculomotor nerve. There is usually also evidence of some impairment of ocular motility by this stage, but it may be less apparent to the examiner as the patient may not be sufficiently awake either to complain about it or to follow commands on examination (i.e., to look to the side or up or down), and some degree of exophoria is present in most people when they are not completely awake. However, examining oculocephalic responses by rotating the head usually will disclose eye movement problems associated with third nerve compression.

A second key feature of uncal herniation that is sufficient to cause pupillary dilation is impaired level of consciousness. This may be due to the distortion of the ascending arousal systems as they pass through the midbrain, distortion of the adjacent diencephalon, or perhaps stretching of blood vessels perfusing the midbrain, thus causing parenchymal ischemia. Nevertheless, the impairment of arousal is so prominent a sign that in a patient with a unilateral fixed and dilated pupil and normal level of consciousness, the examiner must look for another cause of pupillodilation. Pupillary dilation from uncal herniation with a preserved level of consciousness is rare enough to be the subject of case reports.[46]

Hemiparesis may also occur due to compression of the cerebral peduncle by the uncus. The paresis may be contralateral to the herniation (if the advancing uncus impinges upon the adjacent cerebral peduncle) or ipsilateral (if the uncus pushes the midbrain so that the opposite cerebral peduncle is compressed against the incisural edge of Kernohan's notch,[47] but see [48]). Hence, the side of paresis is not helpful in localizing the lesion, but the side of the enlarged pupil accurately identifies the side of the herniation over 90% of the time.[49]

An additional problem in many patients with uncal herniation is compression of the posterior cerebral artery in the tentorial notch, which may give rise to infarction in the territory of its distribution.[50] Often this is overlooked at the time of the herniation, when the impairment of consciousness may make it impossible to test visual fields, but emerges as a concern after the crisis is past when the patient is unable to see on the side of space opposite the herniation. Bilateral compression of the posterior cerebral arteries results in bilateral visual field infarction and cortical blindness (see Patient 3–1, Figure 3–6).[51]

Patient 3–1

A 30-year-old woman in the seventh month of pregnancy began to develop right frontal headaches. The headaches became more severe, and toward the end of the eighth month she sought medical assistance. An MRI revealed a large right frontal mass. Her physicians planned to admit her to hospital, perform an elective cesarean section, and then operate on the tumor. She was admitted to the hospital the day before the surgery. During the night she complained of a more severe headache and rapidly became lethargic and then stuporous. An emergency CT scan disclosed hemorrhage into the tumor and transtentorial herniation, and at craniotomy a right frontal hemorrhagic oligodendroglioma was removed, and she rapidly recovered consciousness. Upon awakening she complained that she was unable to see. Examination revealed complete loss of vision including ability to appreciate light but with retained pupillary light reflexes. Repeat MRI scan showed an evolving infarct involving the occipital lobes bilaterally (see Figure 3–6). Over the following week she gradually regained some central vision, after which it became clear that she had severe prosopagnosia (difficulty recognizing faces).[52] Many months after recovery of vision she was able to get around and read, but she was unable to recognize her own face in the mirror and could only distinguish between her husband and her brother by the fact that her brother was taller.

Central transtentorial herniation is due to pressure from an expanding mass lesion on the diencephalon. If the mass effect is medially located, the displacement may be primarily downward, in turn pressing downward on the midbrain, although the mass may also have a substantial lateral component shifting the diencephalon in the lateral direction.[31] The diencephalon is mainly supplied by small penetrating endarteries that arise directly from the

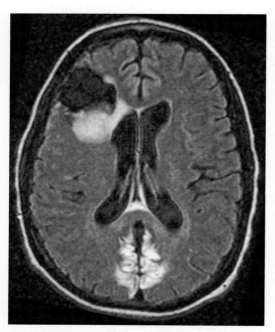

Figure 3–6. Bilateral occipital infarction in Patient 3–1. Hemorrhage into a large frontal lobe tumor caused transtentorial herniation, compressing both posterior cerebral arteries. The patient underwent emergency craniotomy to remove the tumor, but when she recovered from surgery she was cortically blind.

vessels of the circle of Willis. Hence, even small degrees of displacement may stretch and compress important feeding vessels and reduce blood flow. In addition to accounting for the pathogenesis of coma (due to impairment of the ascending arousal system at the diencephalic level), the ischemia causes local swelling and eventually infarction, which causes further edema, thus contributing to gradually progressive displacement of the diencephalon. In severe cases, the pituitary stalk may even become partially avulsed, causing diabetes insipidus, and the diencephalon may buckle against the midbrain. The earliest and most subtle signs of impending central herniation tend to begin with compression of the diencephalon.

Less commonly, the midbrain may be forced downward through the tentorial opening by a mass lesion impinging upon it from the dorsal surface. Pressure from this direction produces the characteristic dorsal midbrain or Parinaud's syndrome (loss of upgaze and convergence, retractory nystagmus; see below).

Rostrocaudal deterioration of the brainstem may occur when the distortion of the brainstem

compromises its vascular supply. Downward displacement of the midbrain or pons stretches the medial perforating branches of the basilar artery, which itself is tethered to the circle of Willis and cannot shift downward (Figure 3–4). Paramedian ischemia may contribute to loss of consciousness, and postmortem injection of the basilar artery demonstrates that the paramedian arteries are at risk of necrosis and extravasation. The characteristic slit-like hemorrhages seen in the area of brainstem displacement postmortem are called Duret hemorrhages[53] (Figure 3–7). Such hemorrhages can be replicated experimentally in animals.[54] It is also possible for the venous drainage of the brainstem to be compromised by compression of the great vein of Galen, which runs along the midline on the dorsal surface of the midbrain. However, in postmortem series, venous infarction is a rare contributor to brainstem injury.[55]

Tonsillar herniation occurs in cases in which the pressure gradient across the foramen magnum impacts the cerebellar tonsils against the foramen magnum, closing off the fourth ventricular outflow and compressing the medulla (Figures 3–7 and 3–8). This may occur quite suddenly, as in cases of subarachnoid hemorrhage, when a large pressure wave drives the cerebellar tonsils against the foramen magnum, compressing the caudal medulla. The patient suddenly stops breathing, and blood pressure rapidly increases as the vascular reflex pathways in the lower brainstem attempt to perfuse the lower medulla against the intense local pressure. A similar syndrome is sometimes seen when lumbar puncture is performed on a patient whose intracranial mass lesion has exhausted the intracranial compliance.[56] In patients with sustained tonsillar herniation, the cerebellar tonsils are typically found to be necrotic due to their impaction against the unyielding edge of the foramen magnum. This problem is discussed further below.

Upward brainstem herniation may also occur through the tentorial notch in the presence of a rapidly expanding posterior fossa lesion.[3] The superior surface of the cerebellar vermis and the midbrain are pushed upward, compressing the dorsal mesencephalon as well as the adjacent blood vessels and the cerebral aqueduct (Figure 3–8).

The dorsal midbrain compression results in impairment of vertical eye movements as well as consciousness. The pineal gland is typically

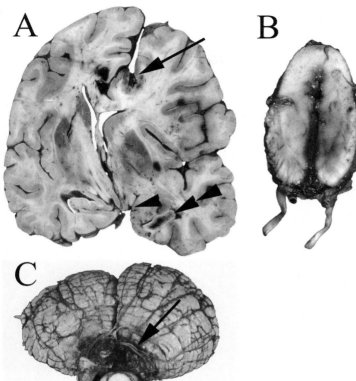

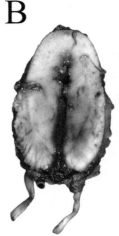

Figure 3–7. Neuropathology of herniation due to a large brain tumor. A large, right hemisphere brain tumor caused subfalcine herniation (arrow in A) and pushed the temporal lobe against the diencephalon (arrowhead). Herniation of the uncus caused hemorrhage into the hippocampus (double arrowhead). Downward displacement of the brainstem caused elongation of the brainstem and midline Duret hemorrhages (B). Downward displacement of the cerebellum impacted the cerebellar tonsils against the foramen magnum, infarcting the tonsillar tissue (arrow in C).

displaced upward on CT scan.[57] The compression of the cerebral aqueduct can cause acute hydrocephalus, and the superior cerebellar artery may be trapped against the tentorial edge, resulting in infarction and edema of the superior cerebellum and increasing the upward pressure.

Clinical Findings in Uncal Herniation Syndrome

EARLY THIRD NERVE STAGE

The proximity of the dorsal surface of the oculomotor nerve to the medial edge of the temporal lobe (Figure 3–5) means that the earliest and most subtle sign of uncal herniation is often an increase in the diameter of the ipsilateral pupil. The pupil may respond sluggishly to light, and typically it dilates progressively as the herniation continues. Early on, there may be no other impairment of oculomotor func-

tion (i.e., no ptosis or ocular motor signs). Once the herniation advances to the point where the function of the brainstem is compromised, signs of brainstem deterioration may proceed rapidly, and the patient may slip from full consciousness to deep coma over a matter of minutes (Figure 3–9).

Patient 3–2

A 22-year-old woman was admitted to the emergency room with the complaint of erratic behavior "since her boyfriend had hit her on the head with a gun." She was awake but behaved erratically in the emergency room, and was sent for CT scanning while a neurology consult was called. The neurologist found the patient in the x-ray department and the technician noted that she had initially been uncooperative, but for the previous 10 minutes she had lain still while the study was completed.

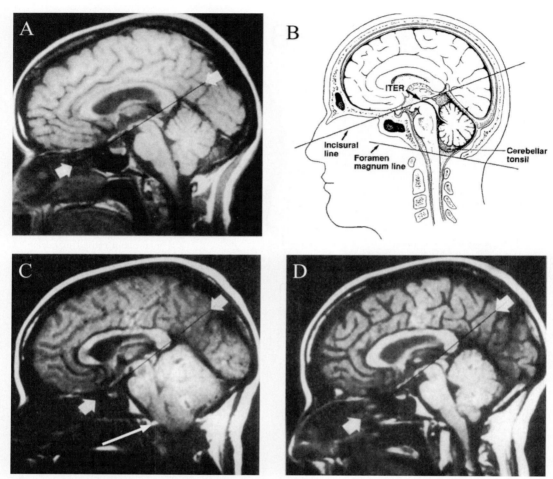

Figure 3–8. Herniation due to a cerebellar mass lesion. The incisural line (A, B) is defined by a line connecting the dorsum sellae with the inferior point of the confluence of the inferior sagittal and straight sinuses with the great vein of Galen, in a midline sagittal magnetic resonance imaging (MRI) scan, shown by a line in each panel. The iter, or anterior tip of the cerebral aqueduct, should lie along this line; upward herniation of the brainstem is defined by the iter being displaced above the line. The cerebellar tonsils should be above the foramen magnum line (B), connecting the most inferior tip of the clivus and the inferior tip of the occiput, in the midline sagittal plane. Panel (C) shows the MRI of a 31-year-old woman with metastatic thymoma to the cerebellum who developed stupor and loss of upgaze after placement of a ventriculoperitoneal shunt. The cerebellum is swollen, the fourth ventricle is effaced, and the brainstem is compressed. The iter is displaced 4.8 mm above the incisural line, and the anterior tip of the base of the pons is displaced upward toward the mammillary body, which also lies along the incisural line. The cerebellar tonsils have also been forced 11.1 mm below the foramen magnum line (demarcated by thin, long white arrow). Following treatment, the cerebellum and metastases shrank (C), and the iter returned to its normal location, although the cerebellar tonsils remained somewhat displaced. (Modified from Reich et al.,[59] with permission.)

Immediate examination on the radiology table showed that breathing was slow and regular and she was unresponsive except to deep pain, with localizing movements of the right but not the left extremities. The right pupil was 8 mm and unreactive to light, and there was no adduction, elevation, or depression of the right eye on oculocephalic testing. Muscle tone was increased on the left compared to the right, and the left plantar response was extensor.

She was immediately treated with hyperventilation and mannitol and awakened. The radiologist reported that there were fragments of metal embedded in the skull over the right frontal lobe.

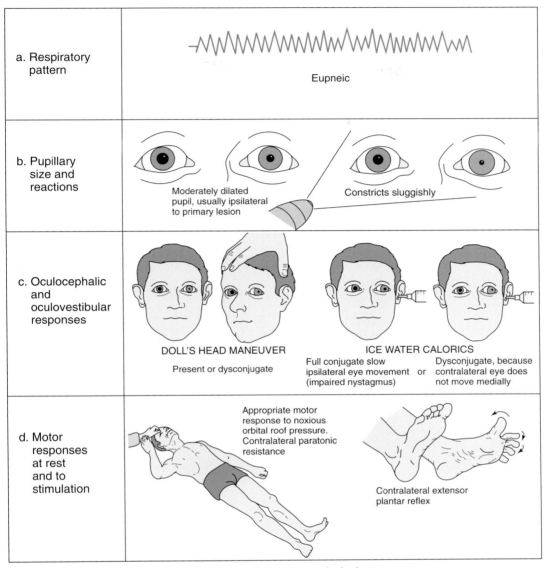

a. Respiratory pattern	Eupneic
b. Pupillary size and reactions	Moderately dilated pupil, usually ipsilateral to primary lesion — Constricts sluggishly
c. Oculocephalic and oculovestibular responses	DOLL'S HEAD MANEUVER — Present or dysconjugate — ICE WATER CALORICS — Full conjugate slow ipsilateral eye movement (impaired nystagmus) or Dysconjugate, because contralateral eye does not move medially
d. Motor responses at rest and to stimulation	Appropriate motor response to noxious orbital roof pressure. Contralateral paratonic resistance — Contralateral extensor plantar reflex

Figure 3–9. Signs of uncal herniation, early third nerve stage.

The patient confirmed that the boyfriend had actually tried to shoot her, but that the bullet had struck her skull with only a glancing blow where it apparently had fragmented. The right frontal lobe was contused and swollen and downward pressure had caused transtentorial herniation of the uncus. Following right frontal lobectomy to decompress her brain, she improved and was discharged.

LATE THIRD NERVE STAGE

As the foregoing case illustrates, the signs of the late third nerve stage are due to more complete impairment of the oculomotor nerve as well as compression of the midbrain. Pupillary dilation becomes complete and the pupil no longer reacts to light. Adduction, elevation, and depression of the affected eye are lost, and there is usually ptosis (if indeed the patient opens the eyes at all).

The lapse into coma may take place over just a few minutes, as in the patient above who was uncooperative with the x-ray technician and 10 minutes later was found by the neurologist to be deeply comatose. Hemiparesis may be ipsilateral to the herniation (if the midbrain is compressed against the opposite tentorial edge) or may be contralateral (if the paresis is due to the lesion damaging the descending corti-cospinal tract or to a herniating temporal lobe compressing the ipsilateral cerebral peduncle). Breathing is typically normal, or the patient may lapse into a Cheyne-Stokes pattern of respiration (Figure 3–10).

MIDBRAIN-UPPER PONTINE STAGE

If treatment is delayed or unsuccessful, signs of midbrain damage appear and progress caudally, as in central herniation (see below). Both pupils

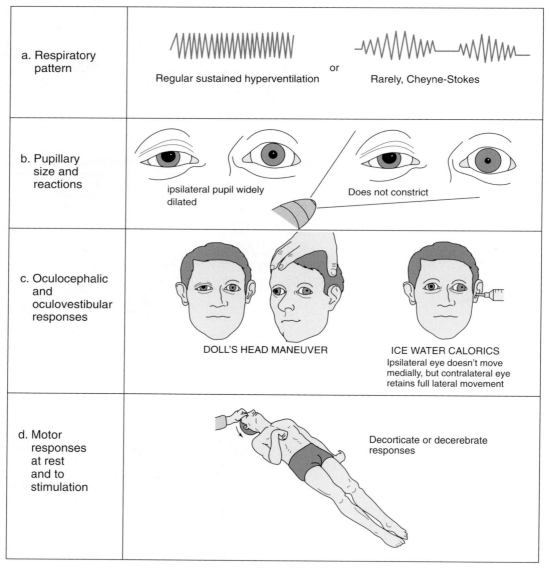

Figure 3–10. Signs of uncal herniation, late third nerve stage.

may fix at midposition, and neither eye elevates, depresses, or turns medially with oculocephalic or caloric vestibular testing. Either decorticate or decerebrate posturing may be seen.

Clinical Findings in Central Herniation Syndrome

DIENCEPHALIC STAGE

The first evidence that a supratentorial mass is beginning to impair the diencephalon is usually a change in alertness and behavior. Initially, subjects might find it difficult to concentrate and may be unable to retain the orderly details of recent events. As the compression of the diencephalon progresses, the patient lapses into torpid drowsiness, and finally stupor and coma.

Respiration in the *early diencephalic stage* of central herniation is commonly interrupted by sighs, yawns, and occasional pauses (Figure 3–11). As the sleepiness deepens, many patients lapse into the periodic breathing of Cheyne-Stokes respiration. The pupils are typically small (1 to 3 mm), and it may be difficult to identify their reaction to light without a bright light source or a magnifying glass. However, the pupils typically dilate briskly in response to a pinch of the skin over the neck (ciliospinal reflex).[58] The eyes are typically conjugate or slightly divergent if the patient is not awake, and there may be roving eye movements, with slow to-and-fro rolling conjugate displacement. Oculocephalic testing typically demonstrates brisk, normal responses. There is typically a diffuse, waxy increase in motor tone (paratonia or gegenhalten), and the toe signs may become bilaterally extensor.

The appearance of a patient in the early diencephalic stage of central herniation is quite similar to that in metabolic encephalopathy. This is a key problem, because one would like to identify patients in the earliest phase of central herniation to institute specific therapy, and yet these patients look most like patients who have no structural cause of coma. For this reason, every patient with the clinical appearance of metabolic encephalopathy requires careful serial examinations until a structural lesion can be ruled out with an imaging study and a metabolic cause of coma can be identified and corrected.

During the *late diencephalic stage* (Figure 3–12), the clinical appearance of the patient becomes more distinctive. The patient becomes gradually more difficult to arouse, and eventually localizing motor responses to pain may disappear entirely or decorticate responses may appear. Initially, the upper extremity flexor and lower extremity extensor posturing tends to appear on the side contralateral to the lesion, and only in response to noxious stimuli. Later, the response may become bilateral, and eventually the contralateral and then ipsilateral side may progress to full extensor (decerebrate) posturing.

The mechanism for brain impairment during the diencephalic stage of central herniation is not clear. Careful quantitative studies show that the depressed level of consciousness correlates with either lateral or vertical displacement of the pineal gland, which lies along the midline at the rostral extreme of the dorsal midbrain.[59,60] The diencephalic impairment may be due to the stretching of small penetrating vessels tethered to the posterior cerebral and communicating arteries that supply the caudal thalamus and hypothalamus. There is little evidence that either increases in ICP or changes in cerebral blood flow can account for these findings. On the other hand, if patients with diencephalic signs of the central herniation syndrome worsen, they tend to pass rapidly to the stage of midbrain damage, suggesting that the same pathologic process has merely extended to the next more caudal level.

The clinical importance, therefore, of the diencephalic stage of central herniation is that it warns of a potentially reversible lesion that is about to encroach on the brainstem and create irreversible damage. If the supratentorial process can be alleviated before the signs of midbrain injury emerge, chances for a complete neurologic recovery are good. Once signs of lower diencephalic and midbrain dysfunction appear, it becomes increasingly likely that they will reflect infarction rather than compression and reversible ischemia, and the outlook for neurologic recovery rapidly becomes much poorer.

As herniation progresses to the *midbrain stage* (Figure 3–13), signs of oculomotor failure appear. The pupils become irregular, then fixed at midposition. Oculocephalic movements become more difficult to elicit, and it may be necessary to examine cold water caloric responses to determine their full extent. Typically, there is limited and slower, and finally no medial movement of the eye contralateral to the cold water stimulus, and bilateral warm or cold water irrigation

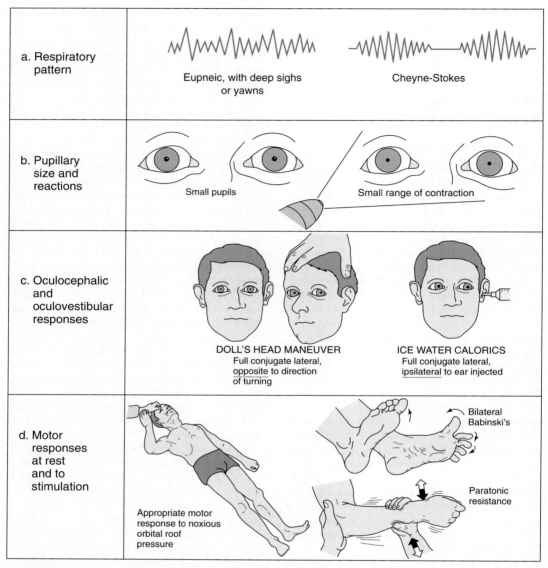

Figure 3–11. Signs of central transtentorial herniation or lateral displacement of the diencephalon, early diencephalic stage.

confirms lack of vertical eye movements. Motor responses are difficult to obtain or result in extensor posturing. In some cases, extensor posturing appears spontaneously, or in response to internal stimuli. Motor tone and tendon reflexes may be heightened, and plantar responses are extensor.

After the midbrain stage becomes complete, it is rare for patients to recover fully. Most patients in whom the herniation can be reversed suffer chronic neurologic disability.[61,62]

Hence, it is critical, if intervention is anticipated, that it begin as early as possible and that it be as vigorous as possible, as the patient's life hangs in the balance.

As the patient enters the *pontine stage* (Figure 3–14) of herniation, breathing becomes more shallow and irregular, as the upper pontine structures that modulate breathing are lost. As the damage approaches the lower pons, the lateral eye movements produced by cold water caloric stimulation are also lost. Motor tone be-

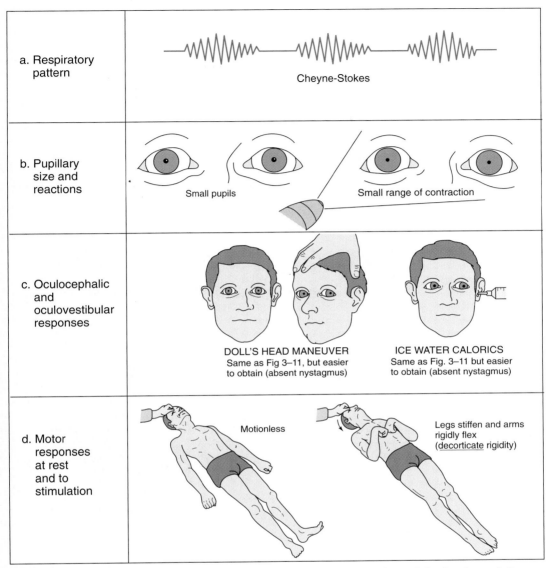

a. Respiratory pattern	Cheyne-Stokes
b. Pupillary size and reactions	Small pupils — Small range of contraction
c. Oculocephalic and oculovestibular responses	DOLL'S HEAD MANEUVER Same as Fig 3–11, but easier to obtain (absent nystagmus) — ICE WATER CALORICS Same as Fig. 3–11 but easier to obtain (absent nystagmus)
d. Motor responses at rest and to stimulation	Motionless — Legs stiffen and arms rigidly flex (decorticate rigidity)

Figure 3–12. Signs of central transtentorial herniation, or lateral displacement of the diencephalon, late diencephalic stage.

comes flaccid, tendon reflexes may be difficult to obtain, and lower extremity posturing may become flexor.

The *medullary stage* is terminal. Breathing becomes irregular and slows, often assuming a gasping quality. As breathing fails, sympathetic reflexes may cause adrenalin release, and the pupils may transiently dilate. However, as cerebral hypoxic and baroreceptor reflexes also become impaired, autonomic reflexes fail and blood pressure drops to levels seen after high spinal transection (systolic pressures of 60 to 70 mm Hg).

At this point, intervening with artificial ventilation and pressor drugs may keep the body alive, and all too often this is the reflexive response in a busy intensive care unit. It is important to recognize, however, that once herniation progresses to respiratory compromise, there is no chance of useful recovery. Therefore, it is important to discuss the situation with the family of the patient before the onset of the medullary stage,

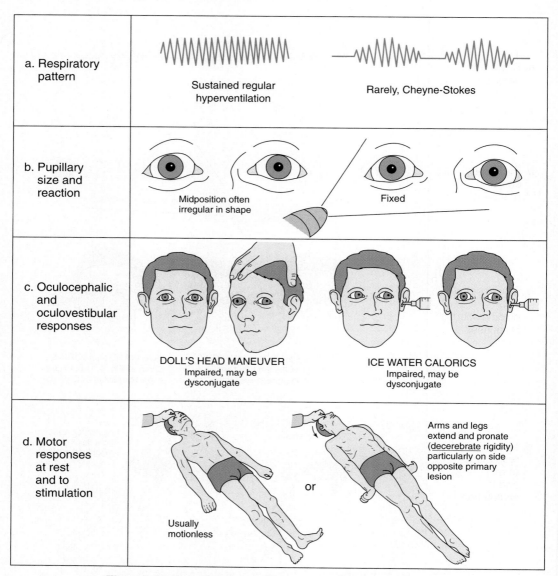

a. Respiratory pattern	Sustained regular hyperventilation	Rarely, Cheyne-Stokes
b. Pupillary size and reaction	Midposition often irregular in shape	Fixed
c. Oculocephalic and oculovestibular responses	DOLL'S HEAD MANEUVER Impaired, may be dysconjugate	ICE WATER CALORICS Impaired, may be dysconjugate
d. Motor responses at rest and to stimulation	Usually motionless	or	Arms and legs extend and pronate (decerebrate rigidity) particularly on side opposite primary lesion

Figure 3–13. Signs of transtentorial herniation, midbrain-upper pons stage.

and to make it clear that mechanical ventilation in this situation merely prolongs the process of dying.

Clinical Findings in Dorsal Midbrain Syndrome

The midbrain may be forced downward through the tentorial opening by a mass lesion impinging upon it from the dorsal surface (Figure 3–15).

The most common causes are masses in the pineal gland (pinealocytoma or germ cell line tumors) or in the posterior thalamus (tumor or hemorrhage into the pulvinar, which normally overhangs the quadrigeminal plate at the posterior opening of the tentorial notch). Pressure from this direction produces the characteristic dorsal midbrain syndrome. A similar picture may be seen during upward transtentorial herniation, which kinks the midbrain (Figure 3–8).

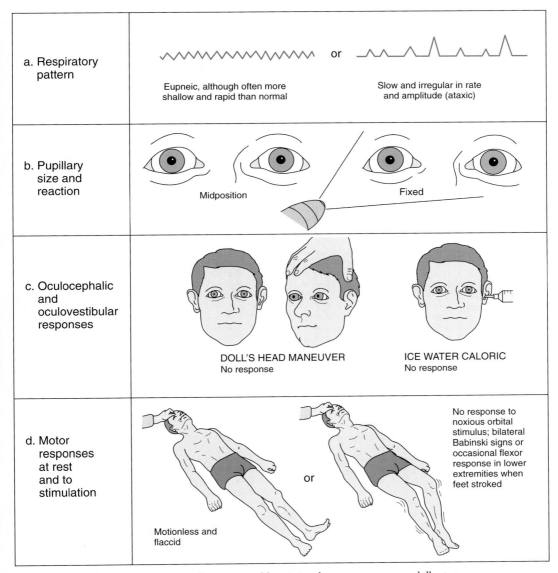

a. Respiratory pattern	Eupneic, although often more shallow and rapid than normal	or	Slow and irregular in rate and amplitude (ataxic)
b. Pupillary size and reaction	Midposition		Fixed
c. Oculocephalic and oculovestibular responses	DOLL'S HEAD MANEUVER No response		ICE WATER CALORIC No response
d. Motor responses at rest and to stimulation	Motionless and flaccid	or	No response to noxious orbital stimulus; bilateral Babinski signs or occasional flexor response in lower extremities when feet stroked

Figure 3–14. Signs of transtentorial herniation, lower pons-upper medulla stage.

Pressure on the olivary pretectal nucleus and the posterior commissure produces slightly enlarged (typically 4 to 6 mm in diameter) pupils that are fixed to light.[2] There is limitation of vertical eye movements, typically manifested first by limited upgaze. In severe cases, the eyes may be fixed in a forced, downward position. If the patient is awake, there may also be a deficit of convergent eye movements and associated pupilloconstriction. The presence of retractory nystagmus, in which all of the eye

muscles contract simultaneously to pull the globe back into the orbit, is characteristic. Retraction of the eyelids may produce a staring appearance.

Deficits of arousal are present in only about 15% of patients with pineal region tumors, but these are due to early central herniation.[63,64] If the cerebral aqueduct is compressed sufficiently to cause acute hydrocephalus, however, an acute increase in supratentorial pressure may ensue. This may cause an acute increase in

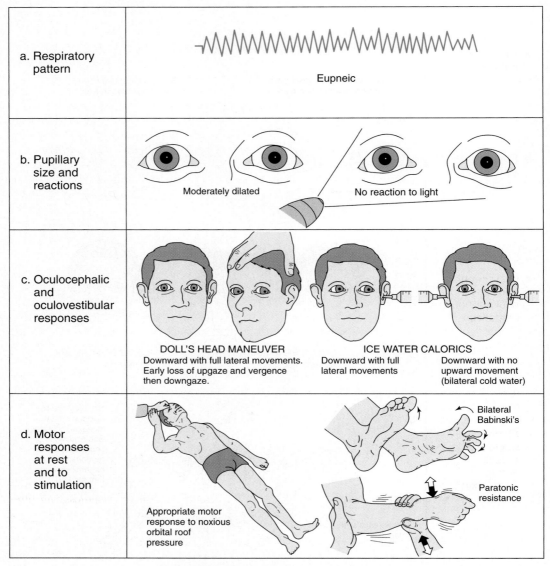

a. Respiratory pattern	Eupneic
b. Pupillary size and reactions	Moderately dilated / No reaction to light
c. Oculocephalic and oculovestibular responses	DOLL'S HEAD MANEUVER / Downward with full lateral movements. Early loss of upgaze and vergence then downgaze. / ICE WATER CALORICS / Downward with full lateral movements / Downward with no upward movement (bilateral cold water)
d. Motor responses at rest and to stimulation	Appropriate motor response to noxious orbital roof pressure / Bilateral Babinski's / Paratonic resistance

Figure 3–15. Signs of dorsal midbrain compression.

downward pressure on the midbrain, resulting in sudden lapse into deep coma.

Safety of Lumbar Puncture in Comatose Patients

A common question encountered clinically is, *"Under what circumstances is lumbar puncture safe in a patient with an intracranial mass lesion?"* There is often a large pressure gradi-

ent between the supratentorial compartment and the lumbar sac,[65] and lowering the lumbar pressure by removing CSF may increase the gradient. The actual frequency of cases in which this hypothetical risk causes transtentorial herniation is difficult to ascertain. Most available studies date to the pre-CT era, as clinicians perform a lumbar puncture only rarely after the presence of a supratentorial mass lesion of any size is identified. Several older studies examining series of patients with brain tumors who underwent lumbar puncture found complication rates in the range of 1% to 2% in patients with documented increased CSF pressure or papilledema.[66,67] On the other hand, of patients referred to a neurosurgical service because of complications following lumbar puncture, Duffy reported that 22 had focal neurologic signs before the lumbar puncture, but only one-half had increased CSF pressure and one-third had papilledema.[56] The experience of the authors supports the view that although lumbar puncture rarely precipitates transtentorial (or foramen magnum) herniation, even in patients who may be predisposed by an existing supratentorial mass lesion, neither the physical examination nor the evaluation of CSF pressure at lumbar puncture is sufficient to predict which patients will suffer complications. Hence, before any patient undergoes lumbar puncture, it is wise to obtain a CT (or MRI) scan of the cranial contents. If a patient has no evidence of compartmental shift on the study, it is quite safe to obtain a lumbar puncture. On the other hand, if it is impossible to obtain an imaging study in a timely fashion and the neurologic examination shows no papilledema or focal signs, the risk of lumbar puncture is quite low (probably less than 1%). Under such circumstances, risk-benefit analysis may well favor proceeding with lumbar puncture if the study is needed to make potentially life-saving decisions about clinical care.

False Localizing Signs in the Diagnosis of Structural Coma

It is usually relatively easy for a skilled examiner to differentiate supratentorial from infratentorial signs, and the cranial nerve findings due to herniation syndromes are characteristic. However, there are a number of specific situations in which the neurologic signs may falsely cause the examiner to consider an infratentorial process or to mistake an infratentorial process for one that is supratentorial.

The most common false localizing sign is abducens palsy. This may be caused by increased ICP, or it may occur after lumbar puncture. In the latter case, the reduced CSF volume can cause the brain to lose its usual buoyant suspension in the CSF. The sagging of the brain in an upright posture is thought to cause traction on the abducens nerve. More rarely other cranial nerves, including the trochlear, oculomotor, or trigeminal nerves, may be similarly affected.

Differentiation of supratentorial from infratentorial causes of ataxia has presented a diagnostic dilemma since the earliest days of neurology.[68] In the days before imaging, despite highly developed clinical skills, it was not unusual for a neurosurgeon to explore the posterior fossa, find nothing, and then turn the patient over and remove a frontal tumor. The gait disorder that is associated with bilateral medial frontal compression or hydrocephalus can be replicated on occasion by cerebellar lesions. Similarly, unilateral ataxia of finger-nose-finger testing, which appears to be cerebellar in origin, may occasionally be seen with parietal lobe lesions.[69]

Another source of confusion is the differentiation of upper (supranuclear) versus lower motor neuron cranial nerve palsies. Although rare, acute supratentorial lesions can on occasion cause lower cranial nerve palsies (asymmetric palate, tongue weakness on one side). Bilateral supratentorial lesions can produce dysarthria, dysphagia, and bilateral facial weakness (pseudobulbar palsy, also called the opercular or Foix-Chavany-Marie syndrome[70]). Conversely, the well-known upper motor neuron facial palsy (weakness of the lower part of the face) can be seen with some posterior fossa lesions. The distinction between upper versus lower motor neuron cranial nerve weakness can often be made on the basis of reflex versus voluntary movement. For example, a patient with supranuclear bulbar weakness will often show intact, or even hyperactive, corneal or gag reflexes. A patient with an upper motor neuron facial palsy will typically show a much more symmetric smile on responding to a joke than when asked to smile voluntarily.

Fortunately, these classic problems with localization rarely intrude on interpretation of the examination of a patient with an impaired level of consciousness, as the signs associated with herniation typically develop relatively rapidly as the patient loses consciousness. If the patient displays false localizing signs while awake, the progression of new signs that occur during the herniation process generally clarifies the matter. Nearly all patients with impaired consciousness and focal brainstem signs should be treated as structural coma and receive immediate imaging studies, so that any confusion about the source of the findings should be short-lived.

DESTRUCTIVE LESIONS AS A CAUSE OF COMA

Destructive lesions of the ascending arousal system or its forebrain targets are paradoxically less of an immediate diagnostic concern for the examining neurologist. Unlike compressive lesions, which can often be reversed by removing a mass, destructive lesions typically cannot be reversed. Although it is important to recognize the hallmarks of a destructive, as opposed to a compressive, lesion, the real value comes in distinguishing patients who may benefit from immediate therapeutic intervention from those who need mainly supportive care.

DIFFUSE, BILATERAL CORTICAL DESTRUCTION

Diffuse, bilateral destruction of the cerebral cortex or its underlying white matter can occur as a result of deprivation of metabolic substrate (i.e., oxygen, glucose, or the blood that carries them) or as a consequence of certain metabolic or infectious diseases. This condition is often the consequence of prolonged cardiac arrest in a patient who is eventually resuscitated, but it may also occur in patients who have diffuse hypoxia due to pulmonary failure or occasionally in patients with severe and prolonged hypoglycemia. The lack of metabolic substrate causes neurons in layers III and V of the cerebral cortex, and in the CA1 and CA3 fields of the hippocampal formation, to be damaged,[71,72] presumably as a result of excitatory amino acid toxicity (see Figure 1–10). During periods of metabolic deprivation, there is rundown of the ion gradients that support normal membrane polarization, resulting in depolarization of neurons and release of their neurotransmitters. Excess excitatory transmitter, particularly acting on N-methyl-D-aspartate (NMDA) receptors that allow the intracellular shift of calcium ions, results in activation of genetic neuronal death programs and the elimination of neurons that receive intense excitatory amino acid inputs.[73] Because excitatory amino acids are used extensively for corticocortical communication, the neurons that are at greatest risk are those that

receive those connections, which in turn are the ones that are most responsible for cortical output as well. The remaining neurons are essentially cut off from one another and from their outputs, and thus are unable to provide meaningful behavioral response.

Patients who have suffered from a period of hypoxia of somewhat lesser degree may appear to recover after brain oxygenation is restored. However, over the following week or so there may be a progressive degeneration of the subcortical white matter, essentially isolating the cortex from its major inputs and outputs.[74] This condition is seen most commonly after carbon monoxide poisoning (see page 30), but may occur after other sublethal episodes of hypoxia. The mechanism of white matter injury is not known, although it may be related to similar white matter injury that is seen in Leigh's disease, mitochondrial encephalopathy with "strokes," and other disorders of cerebral intermediary metabolism that leave the brain with inadequate but sublethal impairment of oxidative energy metabolism.[75]

Other metabolic leukoencephalopathies, such as metachromatic leukodystrophy and Canavan's disease, rarely occur in adults but are considerations when assessing infants or very young children. Adrenoleukodystrophy may cause mainly posterior hemispheric white matter disease, but rarely affects the level of consciousness until very late in the disease.

Infectious causes of dysfunction of the cerebral cortex or subjacent white matter include prion infections (Creutzfeldt-Jakob disease, Gerstmann-Sträussler syndrome, etc.) and progressive multifocal leukoencephalopathy. These disorders progress over a period of weeks to months, and so rarely present a diagnostic dilemma by the time global consciousness is impaired. Subacute sclerosing panencephalitis, due to slow viral infection with the measles virus, can also cause this picture, but it is rarely seen in populations in which measles vaccination is practiced.

DESTRUCTIVE DISEASE OF THE DIENCEPHALON

Bilateral destructive lesions of the *diencephalon* are a rare cause of coma, in part because the diencephalon receives its blood supply directly from feeding vessels that take off from the major arteries of the circle of Willis. Hence, although vascular disease may affect the diencephalon when any one major arterial source is compromised, it is typically unilateral and does not impair consciousness. An exception occurs when there is occlusion of the tip of the basilar artery, which supplies the posterior cerebral and communicating arteries bilaterally. The posterior thalamic penetrating arteries take their origin from these posterior components of the circle of Willis, and as a consequence there may be bilateral posterior thalamic infarction with a single site of vascular occlusion.[76] However, nearly all cases in which there is impairment of consciousness also have some midbrain ischemia as well (see *vascular causes of coma* in Chapter 4, page 152).

Occasional inflammatory and infectious disorders may have a predilection for the diencephalon. Fatal familial insomnia, a prion disorder, is reported to affect the thalamus selectively, and this has been proposed as a cause of the sleep disorder (although this produces hyperwakefulness, not coma).[77] Behçet's disease may cause sterile abscess formation in the diencephalon, which may depress the level of consciousness.[78]

Autoimmune disorders may also affect the diencephalon. In patients with anti-Ma antitumor antibodies, there are often diencephalic lesions as well as excessive sleepiness and sometimes other symptoms of narcolepsy, such as cataplexy.[79] It is now recognized that in most patients with narcolepsy, there is a progressive loss of neurons in the lateral hypothalamus that express the neurotransmitter orexin, also called hypocretin.[80,81] This selective loss of orexin neurons is believed to be autoimmune in origin, although this remains to be demonstrated definitively.[82] Loss of orexin neurons results in excessive sleepiness, but should not cause impairment of consciousness while awake.

Rarely, primary brain tumors may arise in the diencephalon. These may be either astrocytomas or primary central nervous system lymphomas, and they can cause impairment of consciousness as an early sign. Suprasellar tumors such as craniopharyngioma or suprasellar germinoma, or suprasellar extension of a large pituitary adenoma, can compress the diencephalon, but does not usually cause destruction unless attempts at surgical excision cause local vasospasm.[83]

DESTRUCTIVE LESIONS OF THE BRAINSTEM

In destructive disorders of the brainstem, acute loss of consciousness is typically accompanied by a distinctive pattern of pupillary, oculomotor, motor, and respiratory signs that indicate the level of the brainstem that has been damaged. Unlike rostrocaudal deterioration, however, in which all functions of the brainstem above the level are lost, tegmental lesions of the brainstem often are accompanied by more limited findings that pinpoint the level of the lesion.

Destructive lesions at the level of the *midbrain* tegmentum typically destroy the oculomotor nuclei bilaterally, resulting in fixed midposition pupils and paresis of adduction, elevation, and depression of the eyes. At the same time, the abduction of the eyes with oculocephalic maneuvers is preserved. If the cerebral peduncles are also damaged, as with a basilar artery occlusion, there is bilateral flaccid paralysis.

A destructive lesion of the *rostral pontine* tegmentum spares the oculomotor nuclei, so that the pupils remain reactive to light. If the lateral pontine tegmentum is involved, the descending sympathetic and ascending pupillodilator pathways are both damaged, resulting in tiny pupils whose reaction to light may be discernible only by using a magnifying glass. Damage to the medial longitudinal fasciculus causes loss of adduction, elevation, and depression in response to vestibular stimulation, but abduction is preserved, as are behaviorally directed vertical and vergence eye movements. If the lesion extends somewhat caudally into the midpons, there may be gaze paresis toward the side of the lesion or slow vertical eye movements, called ocular bobbing, or its variants (Table 2–3). When the lesion involves the base of the pons, there may be bilateral flaccid paralysis. However, this is not necessarily seen if the lesion is confined to the pontine tegmentum. Facial or trigeminal lower motor neuron paralysis can also be seen if the lesion extends into the more caudal pons. Involvement of the pons may also produce apneustic or ataxic breathing.

On the other hand, destructive lesions that are confined to the lower pons or medulla do not cause loss of consciousness.[84] Such patients may, however, have sufficient damage to the descending motor systems that they are locked in (i.e., have quadriplegia and supranuclear impairment of facial and oropharyngeal motor function).[85] Motor responses may be limited to vertical eye movements and blinking.

Destructive lesions of the brainstem may occur as a result of vascular disease, tumor, infection, or trauma. The most common cause of brainstem destructive lesions is the occlusion of the vertebral or basilar arteries. Such occlusions typically produce signs that pinpoint the level of the infarction. Hemorrhagic lesions of the brainstem are most commonly intraparenchymal hemorrhages into the base of the pons, although arteriovenous malformations may occur at any level. Infections that have a predilection for the brainstem include *Listeria monocytogenes*, which tends to cause rhombencephalic abscesses[86] (see Figure 4–13). Trauma that penetrates the brainstem is usually not a problem diagnostically, as it is almost always immediately fatal.

REFERENCES

1. Ropper AH. A preliminary MRI study of the geometry of brain displacement and level of consciousness with acute intracranial masses. Neurology 39 (5), 622–627, 1989.
2. Baloh RW, Furman JM, Yee RD. Dorsal midbrain syndrome: clinical and oculographic findings. Neurology 35 (1), 54–60, 1985.
3. Cuneo RA, Caronna JJ, Pitts L, et al. Upward transtentorial herniation: seven cases and a literature review. Arch Neurol 36, 618–623, 1979.
4. van Loon J, Van Calenbergh F, Goffin J, et al. Controversies in the management of spontaneous cerebellar haemorrhage. A consecutive series of 49 cases and review of the literature. Acta Neurochir (Wien) 122, 187–193, 1993.
5. Hayreh SS The sheath of the optic nerve. Ophthalmologica 189 (1–2), 54–63, 1984.
6. Jacks AS, Miller NR. Spontaneous retinal venous pulsation: aetiology and significance. J Neurol Neurosurg Psychiatry 74, 7–9, 2003.
7. Van Uitert RL, Eisenstadt ML. Venous pulsations not always indicative of normal intracranial pressure. Letter to the editor. Arch Neurol 35, 550–550, 1978.
8. Hayreh SS. Optic disc edema in raised intracranial pressure. V. Pathogenesis. Arch Ophthalmol 95 (9), 1553–1565, 1977.
9. Hayreh SS. Anterior ischemic optic neuropathy. V. Optic disc edema an early sign. Arch Ophthalmol 99 (6), 1030–1040, 1981.
10. d'Avella D, Baroni A, Mingrino S, et al. An electron microscope study of human arachnoid villi. Surg Neurol 14(1), 41–47, 1980.
11. Browder J, Meyers R. Behavior of the systemic blood pressure, pulse rate and spinal fluid pressure associated with acute changes in intracranial pressure artificially produced. Arch Surg 36, 1–19, 1938.
12. Schumacher GA, Wolfe HG. Experimental studies on headache of. Arch Neurol Psychiat 45, 199–214, 1941.
13. Galvin JA, Van Stavern GP. Clinical characterization of idiopathic intracranial hypertension at the Detroit Medical Center. J Neurol Sci 223 (2), 157–160, 2004.
14. Goodwin J. Recent developments in idiopathic intracranial hypertension (IIH). Semin Ophthalmol 18 (4), 181–189, 2003.
15. Ranjan P, Mishra AM, Kale R, et al. Cytotoxic edema is responsible for raised intracranial pressure in fulminant hepatic failure: in vivo demonstration using diffusion-weighted MRI in human subjects. Metab Brain Dis 20 (3), 181–192, 2005.
16. Yanagihara T, Klass DW, Piepgras DG, et al. Brief loss of consciousness in bilateral carotid occlusive disease. Arch Neurol 46 (8), 858–861, 1989.
17. Magnaes B. Body position and cerebrospinal fluid pressure. Part I: clinical studies on the effect of rapid postural changes. J Neurosurg 44, 687–697, 1976.
18. Ingvar DH, Lundberg N. Paroxysmal systems in intracranial hypertension, studied with ventricular fluid pressure recording and electroencephalography. Brain 84, 446–459, 1961.
19. Lundberg N. Continuous recording and control of ventricular fluid pressure in neurosurgical practice. Acta Neurol Scand Supp 149, 1–193, 1960.
20. Ethelberg S, Jensen VA. Obscurations and further time-related paroxysmal disorders in intracranial tumors: syndrome of initial herniation of parts of the brain through the tentorial incisure. J Neurol Psychiatry 68, 130–149, 1952.
21. Lemaire JJ. [Slow pressure waves during intracranial hypertension]. Ann Fr Anesth Reanim 16 (4), 394–398, 1997.
22. Sullivan HC. Fatal tonsillar herniation in pseudotumor cerebri. Neurology 41, 1142–1144, 1991.
23. Greenberg DA, Jin K. From angiogenesis to neuropathology. Nature 438 (7070), 954–959, 2005.
24. Fishman RA. Cerebrospinal Fluid in Diseases of the Nervous System, 2nd ed. 1992.
25. Fishman RA. Brain edema. N Engl J Med 293 (14), 706–711, 1975.
26. Mokri B. The Monro-Kellie hypothesis—applications in CSF volume depletion. Neurology 56, 1746–1748, 2001.
27. Cushing H. Some experimental and clinical observations concerning states of increased intracranial tension. Am J Med Sci 124, 375–400, 1902.
28. MacEwen W. Pyrogenic Infective Diseases of the Brain and Spinal Cord. Glasgow: James Maclehose, 1893.
29. Meyer A. Herniation of the brain. Arch Neurol Psychiatry 4, 387–400, 1920.
30. Kernohan JW. Incisura of the crus due to contralateral brain tumor. Arch Neurol Psychiatry 21, 274–287, 1929.
31. Ropper AH. Lateral displacement of the brain and level of consciousness in patients with an acute hemispheral mass. N Engl J Med 314, 953–958, 1986.
32. Fisher CM. Brain herniation: a revision of classical concepts. Can J Neurol Sci 22 (2), 83–91, 1995.

33. Gadda D, Carmignani L, Vannucchi L, et al. Traumatic lesions of corpus callosum: early multidetector CT findings. Neuroradiology 46 (10), 812–816, 2004.

34. Adler DE, Milhorat TH. The tentorial notch: anatomical variation, morphometric analysis, and classification in 100 human autopsy cases. J Neurosurg 96, 1103–1112, 2002.

35. Bogousslavsky J, Regli F, Uske A. Thalamic infarcts: clinical syndromes, etiology, and prognosis. Neurology 38 (6), 837–848, 1988.

36. Neau JP, Bogousslavsky J. The syndrome of posterior choroidal artery territory infarction. Ann Neurol 39 (6), 779–788, 1996.

37. Kerr FW, Hallowell OW. Localization of the pupillomotor and accommodation fibers in the oculomotor nerve: experimental observations on paralytic mydriasis. J Neurol Neurosurg Psychiatry 27, 473–481, 1964.

38. Adams JH, Graham DI, Murray LS, et al. Diffuse axonal injury due to nonmissile head injury in humans: an analysis of 45 cases. Ann Neurol 12 (6), 557–563, 1982.

39. Adams JH, Graham DI, Gennarelli TA, et al. Diffuse axonal injury in non-missile head injury. J Neurol Neurosurg Psychiatry 54 (6), 481–483, 1991.

40. Burgerman RS, Wolf AL, Kelman SE, et al. Traumatic trochlear nerve palsy diagnosed by magnetic resonance imaging: case report and review of the literature. Neurosurgery 25 (6), 978–981, 1989.

41. Giuseffi V, Wall M, Siegel PZ, et al. Symptoms and disease associations in idiopathic intracranial hypertension (pseudotumor cerebri): a case-control study. Neurology 41, 239–244, 1991.

42. Nishio I, Williams BA, Williams JP. Diplopia: a complication of dural puncture. Anesthesiology 100, 158–164, 2004.

43. Simonetti F, Pergami P, Ceroni M, et al. About the original description of cerebellar tonsil herniation by Pierre Marie. J Neurol Neurosurg Psychiatry 63 (3), 412, 1997.

44. Rothfus WE, Goldberg AL, Tabas JH, et al. Callosomarginal infarction secondary to transfalcial herniation. AJNR Am J Neuroradiol 8, 1073–1076, 1987.

45. Ropper AH. Lateral displacement of the brain and level of consciousness in patients with an acute hemispheral mass. N Engl J Med 314, 953–958, 1986.

46. Weiner LP, Porro RS. Total third nerve paralysis: a case with hemorrhage in the oculomotor nerve in subdural hematoma. Neurology 15, 87–90, 1965.

47. Binder DK, Lyon R, Manley GT. Transcranial motor evoked potential recording in a case of Kernohan's notch syndrome: case report. Neurosurgery 54, 999–1002, 2004.

48. Derakhsan I. Kernohan notch. J Neurosurg 100, 741–742, 2004.

49. Marshman LA, Polkey CE, Penney CC. Unilateral fixed dilation of the pupil as a false-localizing sign with intracranial hemorrhage: case report and literature review. Neurosurgery 49, 1251–1255, 2001.

50. Sato M, Tanaka S, Kohama A, et al. Occipital lobe infarction caused by tentorial herniation. Neurosurgery 18 (3), 300–305, 1986.

51. Keane JR. Blindness following tentorial herniation. Ann Neurol 8, 186–190, 1980.

52. Barton JJ. Disorders of face perception and recognition. Neurol Clin 21(2), 521–548, 2003.

53. Parizel PM, Makkat S, Jorens PG, et al. Brainstem hemorrhage in descending transtentorial herniation (Duret hemorrhage). Intensive Care Med 28 (1), 85–88, 2002.

54. Klintworth GK. The pathogenesis of secondary brainstem hemorrhages as studied in an experimental model. Am J Pathol 47 (4), 525–536, 1965.

55. Friede RL, Roessmann U. The pathogenesis of secondary midbrain hemorrhages. Neurology 16 (12), 1210–1216, 1966.

56. Duffy GP. Lumbar puncture in the presence of raised intracranial pressure. BMJ 1, 407–409, 1969.

57. Osborn AG, Heaston DK, Wing SD. Diagnosis of ascending transtentorial herniation by cranial computed tomography. AJR Am J Roentgenol 130 (4), 755–760, 1978.

58. Reeves AG, Posner JB. The ciliospinal response in man. Neurology 19 (12), 1145–1182, 1969.

59. Reich JB, Sierra J, Camp W, et al. Magnetic resonance imaging measurements and clinical changes accompanying transtentorial and foramen magnum brain herniation. Ann Neurol 33, 159–170, 1993.

60. Wijdicks EFM, Miller GM. MR imaging of progressive downward herniation of the diencephalon. Neurology 48, 1456–1459, 1997.

61. Zervas NT, Hedley-Whyte J. Successful treatment of cerebral herniation in five patients. N Engl J Med 286 (20), 1075–1077, 1972.

62. Brendler SJ, Selverstone B. Recovery from decerebration. Brain 93 (2), 381–392, 1970.

63. Schild SE, Scheithauer BW, Schomberg PJ, et al. Pineal parenchymal tumors. Clinical, pathologic, and therapeutic aspects. Cancer 72, 870–880, 1993.

64. Kretschmar CS. Germ cell tumors of the brain in children: a review of current literature and new advances in therapy. Cancer Invest 15, 187–198, 1997.

65. Kaufmann GE, Clark K. Continuous simultaneous monitoring of intraventricular and cervical subarachnoid cerebrospinal fluid pressure to indicate development of cerebral or tonsillar herniation. J Neurosurg 33 (2), 145–150, 1970.

66. Lubic LG, Marotta JT. Brain tumor and lumbar puncture. AMA Arch Neurol Psychiatry 72 (5), 568–572, 1954.

67. Korein J, Cravioto H, Leicach M. Reevaluation of lumbar puncture; a study of 129 patients with papilledema or intracranial hypertension. Neurology 9 (4), 290–297, 1959.

68. Grant FC. Cerebellar symptoms produced by supratentorial tumors: a further report. Arch Neurol Psychiat 20, 292–308, 1928.

69. Battaglia-Mayer A, Caminiti R. Optic ataxia as a result of the breakdown of the global tuning fields of parietal neurones 2. Brain 125, 225–237, 2002.

70. Weller M. Anterior opercular cortex lesions cause dissociated lower cranial nerve palsies and anarthria but no aphasia: Foix-Chavany-Marie syndrome and "automatic voluntary dissociation" revisited. J Neurol 240 (4), 199–208, 1993.

71. Adams JH. Hypoxic brain damage. Br J Anaesth 47 (2), 121–129, 1975.

72. Zola-Morgan S, Squire LR, Amaral DG. Human amnesia and the medial temporal region: enduring memory impairment following a bilateral lesion limited to

field CA1 of the hippocampus. J Neurosci 6 (10), 2950–2967, 1986.

73. Snider BJ, Gottron FJ, Choi DW. Apoptosis and necrosis in cerebrovascular disease. Ann N Y Acad Sci 893, 243–253, 1999.

74. Peter L, Nighoghossian N, Jouvet A, et al. [Delayed post-anoxic leukoencephalopathy]. Rev Neurol (Paris) 160 (11), 1085–1088, 2004.

75. Lerman-Sagie T, Leshinsky-Silver E, Watemberg N, et al. White matter involvement in mitochondrial diseases. Mol Genet Metab 84 (2), 127–136, 2005.

76. Caplan LR. "Top of the basilar" syndrome. Neurology 30, 72–79, 1980.

77. Montagna P, Gambetti P, Cortelli P, et al. Familial and sporadic fatal insomnia. Lancet Neurol 2(3), 167–176, 2003.

78. Akman-Demir G, Bahar S, Coban O, et al. Cranial MRI in Behcet's disease: 134 examinations of 98 patients. Neuroradiology 45 (12), 851–859, 2003.

79. Rosenfeld MR, Eichen JG, Wade DF, et al. Molecular and clinical diversity in paraneoplastic immunity to Ma proteins. Ann Neurol 50, 339–348, 2001.

80. Peyron C, Faraco J, Rogers W, et al. A mutation in a case of early onset narcolepsy and a generalized absence of hypocretin peptides in human narcoleptic brains. Nat Med 6, 991–997, 2000.

81. Thannickal TC, Moore RY, Nienhuis R, et al. Reduced number of hypocretin neurons in human narcolepsy. Neuron 27, 469–474, 2000.

82. Scammell TE. The neurobiology, diagnosis, and treatment of narcolepsy. Ann Neurol 53 (2), 154–166, 2003.

83. Scammell TE, Nishino S, Mignot E, et al. Narcolepsy and low CSF orexin (hypocretin) concentration after a diencephalic stroke. Neurology 56 (12), 1751–1753, 2001.

84. Parvizi J, Damasio AR. Neuroanatomical correlates of brainstem coma. Brain 126, 1524–1536, 2003.

85. Levy DE, Sidtis JJ, Rottenberg DA, et al. Differences in cerebral blood flow and glucose utilization in vegetative versus locked-in patients. Ann Neurol 22 (6), 673–682, 1987.

86. Armstrong RW, Fung PC. Brainstem encephalitis (rhombencephalitis) due to Listeria monocytogenes: case report and review. Clin Infect Dis 16, 689–702, 1993.

Chapter 4

Specific Causes of Structural Coma

BRAINSTEM VASCULAR DESTRUCTIVE
DISORDERS
Brainstem Hemorrhage
Basilar Migraine
Posterior Reversible Leukoencephalopathy
Syndrome

INFRATENTORIAL INFLAMMATORY
DISORDERS

INFRATENTORIAL TUMORS

CENTRAL PONTINE MYELINOLYSIS

INTRODUCTION

The previous chapter divided structural lesions causing coma into compressive and destructive lesions. It further indicated that lesions could be supratentorial, compressing or destroying the diencephalon and upper midbrain, or infratentorial, directly affecting the pons and cerebellum. A physician attempting to determine the cause of coma resulting from a structural lesion must establish first the site of the lesion, determining whether the lesion is supratentorial or infratentorial, and second whether the lesion is causing its symptoms by compression or destruction or both. Those considerations were the focus of Chapter 3. This chapter discusses, in turn, the specific causes of supratentorial and infratentorial compressive and destructive lesions that cause coma.

Although these designations are useful for rapid bedside diagnosis, it is of course possible for a lesion such as an intracerebral hemorrhage both to destroy and to compress normal tissues. Extracerebral mass lesions can also cause sufficient compression to lead to infarction (i.e., tissue destruction). Thus, in some instances, the division is arbitrary. However, the types of conditions that cause the compression versus destruction of neural tissue tend to be distinct, and often they have distinct clinical presentations as well. The guide provided in this chapter, while not exhaustive, is meant to cover the most commonly encountered causes and ones where understanding their pathophysiology can influence diagnosis and treatment (Table 4–1).

When any structural process impairs consciousness, the physician must find a way to halt the progression promptly or the patient will run the risk of irreversible brain damage or death. Beyond that generality, different structural lesions have distinct clinical properties that govern the rate of progression, hint at the diagnosis, and may dictate the treatment.

Structural causes of unconsciousness often cause focal signs that help localize the lesion, particularly when the lesion develops acutely. However, if the lesion has developed slowly, over a period of many weeks or even months, it may attain a remarkably large size without causing focal neurologic signs. In those cases, the first evidence of a space-occupying lesion may be signs of increased intracranial pressure (e.g., headache, nausea) or even herniation itself (see Patient 3–2).

SUPRATENTORIAL COMPRESSIVE LESIONS

The supratentorial compartments are dominated by the cerebral hemispheres. However, many of the most dangerous and difficult lesions to diagnose involve the overlying meninges. Within the hemisphere, a compressive lesion may originate in the gray matter or the white matter of the hemisphere, and it may directly compress the diencephalon from above or laterally (central herniation) or compress the midbrain by herniation of the temporal lobe through the tentorial notch (uncal herniation). In addition, there are a number of compressive lesions that affect mainly the diencephalon.

EPIDURAL, DURAL, AND SUBDURAL MASSES

Tumors, infections, and hematomas can occupy the epidural, dural, and subdural spaces to eventually cause herniation. Most epidural tumors result from extensions of skull lesions that grow into the epidural space. Their growth is relatively slow; they mostly occur in patients with known cancer and are usually discovered long before they affect consciousness. Dural tumors, by contrast, are usually primary tumors of the meninges, or occasionally metastases.

Table 4–1 **Examples of Structural Causes of Coma**

Compressive Lesions	Destructive Lesions
Cerebral hemispheres	*Cerebral hemispheres*
Epidural and subdural hematomas, tumors, and abscesses	Hypoxia-ischemia
Subarachnoid hemorrhages, infections (meningitis), and tumors (leptomeningeal neoplasms)°	Hypoglycemia
	Vasculitis
	Encephalitis
	Leukoencephalopathy
Intracerebral hemorrhages, infarcts, tumors, and abscesses	Prion diseases
	Progressive multifocal leukoencephalopathy
Diencephalon	*Diencephalon*
Basal ganglia hemorrhages, tumors, infarcts, and abscesses°	Thalamic infarct
	Encephalitis
Pituitary tumor	Fatal familial insomnia
Pineal tumor	Paraneoplastic syndrome
	Tumor
Brainstem	*Brainstem*
Cerebellar tumor	Infarct
Cerebellar hemorrhage	Hemorrhage
Cerebellar abscess	Infection

°Both compressive and destructive.

Epidural Hematoma

Because the external leaf of the dura mater forms the periosteum of the inner table of the skull, the space between the dura and the skull is a potential space that accumulates blood only when there has been an injury to the skull itself. Epidural hematomas typically result from head trauma with a skull fracture that crosses a groove in the bone containing a meningeal vessel (see Figure 4–1). The ruptured vessel may be either arterial or venous; venous bleeding usually develops slowly and often is self-limiting, having a course more similar to subdural hematomas, which are discussed below. On rare occasions, epidural hematomas may result from bleeding into skull lesions such as eosinophilic granuloma,[1] metastatic skull or dural tumors,[2] or craniofacial infections such as sinusitis.[3]

Arterial bleeding is usually under high pressure with the result that the vessel may not seal and blood continues to accumulate. Thus, in-

Epidural or subdural hematomas, on the other hand, may develop acutely or subacutely and can be a diagnostic problem.

stead of causing symptoms that develop slowly or wax and wane over days or weeks, a patient with an epidural hematoma may pass from having only a headache to impairment of consciousness and signs of herniation within a few hours after the initial trauma.

Although epidural hematomas can occur frontally, occipitally, at the vertex,[4] or even on the side opposite the side of trauma (contrecoup),[5] the most common site is in the lateral temporal area as a result of laceration of the middle meningeal artery. Trauma sufficient to cause such a fracture may also fracture the skull base. For this reason, it is necessary for the examiner to be alert to signs of basal skull fracture on examination, such as blood behind the tympanic membrane or ecchymosis of the skin behind the ear (Battle's sign) or around the eyes (raccoon eyes). The epidural hemorrhage pushes the brain medially, and in so doing stretches and tears pain-sensitive meninges and blood vessels at the base of the middle fossa, causing headache. However, the headache is often attributed to the original head injury, and unless the lesion causes sufficiently increased intracranial pressure (ICP) to produce nausea and vomiting, the condition may

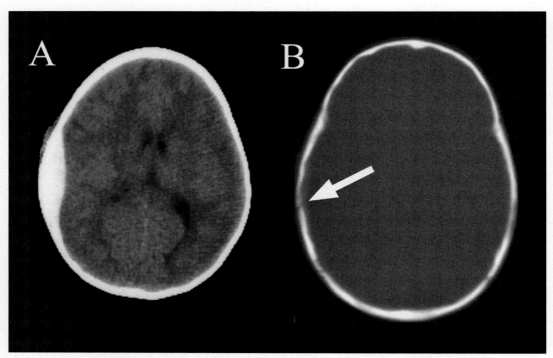

Figure 4–1. A pair of computed tomography scans showing an epidural hematoma. The image in (A) shows the lens-shaped (biconvex), bright mass along the inner surface of the skull. In (B), the skull is imaged with bone windows, showing a fracture at the white arrow, crossing the middle meningeal groove.

not be recognized. Subsequently, the hematoma compresses the adjacent temporal lobe and causes uncal herniation with gradual impairment of consciousness. Early dilation of the ipsilateral pupil is often seen followed by complete ophthalmoparesis and then impairment of the opposite third nerve as the herniation progresses.[6] Motor signs often occur late in such cases.

In many patients the degree of head trauma is less than one might expect to cause a fracture. In Jamieson and Yelland's series, for example, of 167 patients with epidural hematoma, nearly one-half had no initial loss of consciousness,[7] and in Gallagher and Browder's equally large series, two-thirds of such patients had an initial injury too mild to command hospital attention.[8] This is particularly true in children, one-half of whom have suffered a fall of less than one-half meter, and many of whom complained of nonspecific symptoms.[9] Only 15% to 20% of patients had the "classic" history of traumatic loss of consciousness, followed by a lucid interval and then a relapse into coma (patients who "talk and die").[10] Thus,

even though most epidural hematomas are identified by computed tomography (CT) scans performed acutely in emergency departments on trauma patients by using current evidence-based decision paradigms,[11,12] the examiner must remain alert to the possibility of an epidural hematoma that develops or rapidly enlarges after an apparently negative CT. It is therefore important to review the CT scan of trauma patients with attention directed to whether there is a skull fracture that crosses the middle meningeal groove. The hematoma appears as a hyperdense, lens-shaped mass between the skull and the brain (i.e., the hematoma is convex on both surfaces; subdural hematomas, by comparison, are concave on the surface facing the brain; see Figure 4–1). A vertex hematoma may be missed on a routine axial CT scan,[13] but a coronal reconstruction should identify the lesion.[4] A magnetic resonance imaging (MRI) scan is not required for evaluation of an epidural hematoma, but may be necessary to evaluate contusions and edema in the underlying brain. In addition, mass lesions outside the brain may cause hyperdensity of subarachnoid cisterns that may be mistaken for subarachnoid hemorrhage on CT, but is probably an artifact of partial volume averaging.[14] In these instances, MRI helps rule out subarachnoid hemorrhage.

In those circumstances where CT scan is not readily available, a plain skull film can often identify the fracture. Certainly, all patients with head trauma should be cautioned that it is important to remain under the supervision of a family member or friend for at least 24 hours; the patient must be returned to the hospital immediately if a lapse of consciousness occurs. Careful follow-up is required even in patients in whom the original CT was negative, as occasionally the development of the hematoma is delayed.[15]

In comatose patients with epidural hematomas, the treatment is surgical evacuation. The surgery is an emergency, as the duration from time of injury to treatment is an important determinant of the prognosis.[16] Other factors in determining outcome are age, depth of coma, degree of midline shift, and size of the hematoma.[17] Most patients operated on promptly recover, even those whose pupils are dilated and fixed before surgery.[18] Rarely, acute epidural hematomas resolve spontaneously, probably a result of tamponade of the bleeding vessel by underlying edematous brain.[19]

Subdural Hematoma

The unique anatomy of the subdural space also can produce much slower, chronic subdural hematomas in patients in whom the history of head trauma is remote or trivial. The potential space between the inner leaf of the dura mater and the arachnoid membrane (subdural space) is traversed by numerous small draining veins that bring venous blood from the brain to the dural sinus system that runs between the two leaves of the dura. These veins can be damaged with minimal head trauma, particularly in elderly individuals with cerebral atrophy in whom the veins are subject to considerable movement of the hemisphere that may occur with acceleration-deceleration injury. When focal signs are absent, these cases can be quite difficult to diagnose. A useful rule when faced with a comatose patient is that "it could always be a subdural," and hence imaging is needed even in cases where focal signs are absent.

Subdural bleeding is usually under low pressure, and it typically tamponades early unless there is a defect in coagulation. Acute subdural bleeding is particularly dangerous in patients who take anticoagulants for vascular thrombotic disease. Continued venous leakage over several hours can cause a mass large enough to produce herniation. Warfarin inhibits the synthesis of vitamin K-dependent clotting factors II, VII, IX, and X and the anticoagulant proteins C and S. The conventional treatment includes administering fresh frozen plasma and vitamin K. However, these measures take hours to days to become effective and are too slow to stop subdural bleeding. Hence, in the case of a subdural (or epidural) bleed in a patient on warfarin, it is important to administer pooled cryoprecipitate of factors II, VII, IX, and X immediately. Recombinant factor VII has also been used,[20] but data are lacking as to its effectiveness.

Acute subdural hematomas, which are usually the result of a severe head injury, are often associated with underlying cerebral contusions. Rarely, acute subdural hematomas may occur without substantial trauma, particularly in patients on anticoagulants. Rupture of an aneurysm into the subdural space, sparing the subarachnoid space, can also cause an acute subdural hematoma. The mass accumulates rapidly, causing underlying brain edema and herniation. Ischemic brain edema results when herniation compresses the anterior or posterior cerebral arteries and causes ischemic brain damage.[21] Patients with acute subdural hematomas usually present with coma, and such cases are surgical emergencies. Early evacuation of the mass probably improves outcome, but because of underlying brain damage, mortality remains significant. Prognostic factors include age, time from injury to treatment, presence of pupillary abnormalities, immediate and persisting coma as opposed to the presence of a lucid interval, and volume of the mass.[22]

Chronic subdural hematomas usually occur in elderly patients or those on anticoagulants. Chronic alcoholism, hemodialysis, and intracranial hypotension are also risk factors. A history of trauma can be elicited in only about one-half of patients, and then the trauma is usually minor. The pathogenesis of chronic subdural hematomas is controversial. One hypothesis is that minor trauma to an atrophic brain causes a small amount of bleeding. A membrane forms around the blood. Vessels of the membrane are quite friable and this, plus an increase of fibrinolytic products in the fluid, leads to repetitive bleeding, causing an enlarging hematoma.[23] Another hypothesis is that minor trauma leads to the accumulation of either serum or cerebrospinal fluid (CSF) in the subdural space. This subdural hygroma also causes membrane formation that leads to repetitive bleeding and an eventual mass lesion.[24] If the hemorrhage is small and no additional bleeding occurs, the hematoma may resorb spontaneously. However, if the hematoma is larger or it is enlarged gradually by recurrent bleeds, it may swell as the breakdown of the blood into small molecules causes the hematoma to take on additional water, thus further compressing the adjacent brain.[24] In addition, the membrane surrounding the hematoma contains luxuriant neovascularization that lacks a blood-brain barrier and may cause additional edema in the underlying brain. Chronic subdural hematomas are usually unilateral, overlying the lateral cerebral cortex, but may be subtemporal. They are bilateral in about 20% of patients, and occasionally are interhemispheric (i.e., within the falx cerebri), sometimes causing bilateral leg weakness by compression of the medial frontal lobes.

Table 4–2 lists the clinical features of the typical patient with a chronic subdural hematoma who presents with a fluctuating level of consciousness.

A majority of patients, but no more than 70%, complain of headache. A fluctuating level of consciousness is common.[23,25,26] There may be tenderness to percussion of the skull at the site of the hematoma. About 15% to 30% of patients present with parenchymal signs such as seizures, hemiparesis, or visual field defects. Unusual focal signs such as parkinsonism, dystonia,[27] or chorea occasionally confuse the clinical picture. Focal signs such as hemiparesis or aphasia may fluctuate, giving an appearance similar to transient ischemic attacks.[28] Occasionally patients may have unilateral asterixis. Because subdural hematoma can appear identical to a metabolic encephalopathy (Chapter 5), imaging is required in any patient without an obvious cause of the impairment of consciousness.

The symptoms of subdural hematoma have a remarkable tendency to fluctuate from day to day or even from hour to hour, which may

Table 4–2 Diagnostic Features of 73 Patients With Fluctuating Level of Consciousness Due to Subdural Hematoma

Unilateral hematoma	62
Bilateral hematomas	11
Mortality	14
	(3 unoperated)
Number of patients in stupor or coma	27
Principal clinical diagnosis before hematoma discovered	
Intracranial mass lesion or subdural hematoma	24
Cerebral vascular disease, but subdural hematoma possible	17
Cerebral infarction or arteriosclerosis	12
Cerebral atrophy	5
Encephalitis	8
Meningitis	3
Metabolic encephalopathy secondary to systemic illness	3
Psychosis	1

suggest the diagnosis. The pathophysiology of fluctuations is not clear. Some may reflect increases in ICP associated with plateau waves,[29] and careful clinical observations suggest that the level of consciousness reflects the patient moving in and out of diencephalic or uncal herniation. Given the breakdown in the blood-brain barrier along the margin of the hematoma, this fluctuation may be due to fluid shifts into and out of the brain, a situation from which the brain is normally protected. When the brain is critically balanced on the edge of herniation, such fluid shifts may rapidly make the difference between full consciousness and an obtunded state. Cerebral blood flow in the hemisphere underlying a subdural hematoma is reduced, perhaps accounting for some of the unusual clinical symptoms.[30]

In favor of the vasogenic edema hypothesis is the observation that oral administration of corticosteroids rapidly and effectively reverses the symptoms in subdural hematoma.[31] Corticosteroids reduce the leakage of fluid from capillaries,[32] and they are quite effective in minimizing the cerebral edema associated with subdural hematomas.

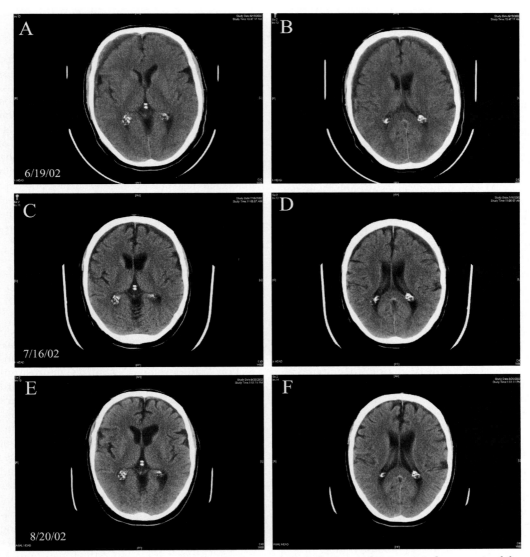

Figure 4–2. A series of magnetic resonance imaging scans through the brain of Patient 4–1 demonstrating bilateral subdural hematomas and their evolution over time. In the initial scan from 6/19/02 (A, B), there is an isodense subdural hematoma of 11.5 mm thickness on the right (left side of image) and 8 mm thickness on the left. The patient was treated conservatively with oral prednisone, and by the time of the second scan 1 month later (C, D), the subdural hematomas were smaller and hypodense and the underlying brain was less edematous. By the end of the second month (E, F), the subdural hematomas had been almost completely resorbed.

Subdural hematoma can usually be diagnosed by CT scanning. Depending on the age of the bleeding, the contents of the mass between the dura and the brain may be either hyperdense or isodense (Figure 4–2). Acute subdural hematomas are hyperdense, with the rare exception of those occurring in extremely anemic patients and those in whom CSF has entered the subdural space, diluting the blood. Although the hematoma may become isodense with brain after 2 to 3 weeks, it may still contain areas of hyperdense fresh blood, assisting with the diagnosis. However, if the entire mass is isodense and contrast is not given, the subdural hematoma may be difficult to distinguish from brain tissue, particularly if the hematomas are bilaterally symmetric and do not cause the brain to shift. The lack of definable sulci in the area of the hematoma and a "supraphysiologic"-appearing brain in an elderly individual (i.e., a brain that lacks atrophy and deep sulci, usually seen with aging) are clues to the presence of bilateral isodense subdural hematomas. Chronic subdurals may become hypodense. A CT scan with contrast clearly defines the hematoma as the membranes, with a luxuriant, leaky vascular supply, enhance profusely. MRI scanning can also define the hematoma, but the density is a complex function of the sequence used and age of the hemorrhage.

Lumbar puncture is potentially dangerous in a patient with a subdural hematoma. If the brain is balanced on the edge of herniation, the sudden relief of subarachnoid pressure from below may further enhance the pressure cone and lead to frank herniation. In such patients, the CSF pressure may be low, due to the blockage at the foramen magnum, leading to a false sense of security. Hence, all patients who have an impaired level of consciousness require an imaging study of the brain prior to lumbar puncture, even if meningitis is a consideration.[33] This issue is discussed further in the section on meningitis on page 133.

The treatment of subdural hematomas has traditionally been surgical.[34] Three surgical procedures, twist drill drainage, burr hole drainage, and craniotomy with excision of membranes, are used.[34,35] The procedure chosen depends on whether the subdural hematoma has developed membranes, requiring more extensive drainage, or is complex and compartmentalized, requiring excision of the membranes. The outcome of treatment varies in different series and probably reflects differences in the patient population.[34]

Although there have been no randomized clinical trials of medical treatment of subdural hematomas, many patients who have modest-sized subdural hematomas with minimal symptoms (typically only a headache) and considerable ventricular and cisternal space, so there is no danger of herniation, can be treated conservatively with corticosteroids for several months until the hematoma resorbs.[31,36] However, subdural hematomas have a tendency to recur after both medical and surgical therapy, and patients must be followed carefully for the first several months after apparently successful treatment.

Patient 4–1

A 73-year-old professor of art history developed chronic bifrontal, dull headache. He had no history of head trauma, but was taking 81 mg of aspirin daily for cardiovascular prophylaxis. He felt mentally dulled, but his neurologic examination was normal. CT scan of the brain disclosed bilateral chronic (low density) subdural hematomas of 8 mm depth on the left and 11.5 mm on the right. He was started on 20 mg/day of prednisone with immediate resolution of the headaches, and over a period of 2 months serial CT scans showed that the hematoma resolved spontaneously (see Figure 4–2). Repeat scan 3 months later showed no recurrence.

Epidural Abscess/Empyema

In developing countries, epidural infections are a feared complication of mastoid or sinus infection.[37] In developed countries, neurosurgical procedures,[38] particularly second or third craniotomies in the same area, and trauma are more likely causes.[39] Sinusitis and otitis, if inadequately treated, may extend into the epidural space, either along the base of the temporal lobe or along the surface of the frontal lobe. The causative organisms are usually aerobic and anaerobic streptococci if the lesion originates from the ear or the sinuses, and *Staphylococcus aureus* if from trauma or surgery. The patient typically has local pain and fever. Vomiting is common[37]; focal skull tenderness and meningism suggest infection rather than hemorrhage. The pathophysiology of impairment of consciousness is similar to that of an epidural hematoma, except that epidural empyema typically has a much slower course and is not associated with acute trauma. CT scan is characterized by a crescentic or lentiform mass between the skull and the brain with an enhanced rim. Diffusion is restricted on diffusion-weighted MRI, distinguishing it from hematomas or effusions where diffusion is normal or increased.[40,41] Antibiotics and surgical drainage are effective treatments.[38] The causal organisms can usually be cultured to allow appropriate selection of antibiotics. Some children whose epidural abscess originates from the sinuses can be treated conservatively with antibiotics and drainage of the sinus rather than the epidural mass.[42]

Dural and Subdural Tumors

A number of tumors and other mass lesions may invade the dura and compress the brain. These lesions include dural metastases,[43] primary tumors such as hemangiopericytoma,[44] hematopoietic neoplasms (plasmacytoma, leukemia, lymphoma), and inflammatory diseases such as sarcoidosis.[44] These are often mistaken for the most common dural tumor, meningioma.[45]

Meningiomas can occur anywhere along the dural lining of the anterior and middle cranial fossas. The most common locations are over the convexities, along the falx, or along the base of the skull at the sphenoid wing or olfactory tubercle. The tumors typically present by compression of local structures. In some cases, this produces seizures, but over the convexity there may be hemiparesis. Falcine meningiomas may present with hemiparesis and upper motor neuron signs in the contralateral lower extremity; the "textbook presentation" of paraparesis is quite rare. If the tumor occurs near the frontal pole, it may compress the medial prefrontal cortex, causing lapses in judgment, inconsistent behavior, and, in some cases, an apathetic, abulic state. Meningioma underlying the orbitofrontal cortex may similarly compress both frontal lobes and present with behavioral and cognitive dysfunction. When the tumor arises from the olfactory tubercle, ipsilateral loss of smell is a clue to the nature of the problem. Meningiomas of the sphenoid wing may invade the cavernous sinus and cause impairment of the oculomotor (III), trochlear (IV), and abducens nerves (VI) as well as the first division of the trigeminal nerve (V$_1$).

On rare occasions, a meningioma may first present symptoms of increased intracranial pressure or even impaired level of consciousness. Acute presentation with impairment of consciousness may also occur with hemorrhage into a meningioma. Fortunately, this condition is rare, involving only 1% to 2% of meningiomas, and may suggest a more malignant phenotype.[46] In such cases, the tumor typically has reached sufficient size to cause diencephalic compression or herniation. There is often considerable edema of the adjacent brain, which may be due in part to the leakage of blood ves-

sels in the tumor or to production by the tumor of angiogenic factors.[47] Treatment with corticosteroids reduces the edema and may be life-saving while awaiting a definitive surgical procedure.

On CT scanning, meningiomas are typically isodense with brain, although they may have areas of calcification. On MRI scan, a typical meningioma is hypointense or isointense on T1-weighted MRI and usually hypointense on T2. In either imaging mode, the tumor uniformly and intensely enhances with contrast unless it is heavily calcified, a situation where the CT scan may give more accurate information. The CT scan may also help in identifying bone erosion or hyperostosis, the latter rather characteristic of meningiomas. Meningiomas typically have an enhancing dural tail that spreads from the body of the tumor along the dura, a finding less common in other dural tumors. The dural tail is not tumor, but a hypervascular response of the dura to the tumor.[48]

Dural malignant metastases and hematopoietic tumors grow more rapidly than meningiomas and cause more underlying brain edema. Thus, they are more likely to cause alterations of consciousness and, if not detected and treated early enough, cerebral herniation. Breast and prostate cancer and M4-type acute myelomonocytic leukemia have a particular predilection for the dura, and that may be the only site of metastasis in an otherwise successfully treated patient. CT and MRI scans may be similar to those of meningioma, the diagnosis being established only by surgery.

PITUITARY TUMORS

Tumors of the pituitary fossa are outside the brain and its coverings, separated from the subarachnoid space by the diaphragma sellae, a portion of the dura that covers the pituitary fossa but that contains an opening for the pituitary stalk. Pituitary tumors may cause alterations of consciousness, either by causing endocrine failure (see Chapter 5) or by hemorrhage into the pituitary tumor, so-called *pituitary apoplexy.*[49]

Pituitary adenomas typically cause symptoms by growing out of the pituitary fossa. Because the optic chiasm overlies the pituitary fossa, the most common finding is bitemporal hemianopsia. If the tumor extends laterally through the wall of the sella turcica into the cavernous sinus, there may be impairment of cranial nerves III, IV, VI, or V1. In some cases, pituitary tumors may achieve a very large size by suprasellar extension. These tumors compress the overlying hypothalamus and basal forebrain and may extend up between the frontal lobes or backward down the clivus. Such tumors may present primarily with prefrontal signs, or signs of increased ICP, but they occasionally present with impairment of consciousness.

The most common endocrine presentation in women is amenorrhea and in some galactorrhea due to high prolactin secretion. Prolactin is the only pituitary hormone under inhibitory control; if a pituitary tumor damages the pituitary stalk, other pituitary hormones fall to basal levels, but prolactin levels rise. Most pituitary adenomas are nonsecreting tumors, but some pituitary tumors may secrete anterior pituitary hormones, resulting in Cushing's syndrome (if the tumor secretes adrenocorticotropic hormone [ACTH]), hyperthyroidism (if it secretes thyroid-stimulating hormone [TSH]), galactorrhea/amenorrhea (if it secretes prolactin), or acromegaly (if it secretes growth hormone).

Pituitary adenomas may outgrow their blood supply and undergo spontaneous infarction or hemorrhage. Pituitary apoplexy[49] presents with the sudden onset of severe headache, signs of local compression of the optic chiasm, and sometimes the nerves of the cavernous sinus.[50,51]

There may be subarachnoid blood and there often is impairment of consciousness. It is not clear if the depressed level of consciousness is due to the compression of the overlying hypothalamus, the release of subarachnoid blood (see below), or the increase in intracranial pressure. If there are cranial nerve signs, pituitary apoplexy is often sufficiently characteristic to be diagnosed clinically, but if the main symptoms are due to subarachnoid hemorrhage, it may be confused with meningitis or meningoencephalitis[52]; the correct diagnosis is easily confirmed by MRI or CT scan (Figure 4–3). If the tumor is large, it typically requires surgical intervention. However, subarachnoid hemorrhage can be treated conservatively. The hemorrhage may destroy the tumor; careful follow-up will determine whether there is remaining tumor that continues to endanger the patient.

Craniopharyngiomas are epithelial neoplasms that are thought to arise from a remnant of Rathke's pouch, the embryologic origin of the anterior pituitary gland.[53] The typical presentation is similar to that of a pituitary tumor, but craniopharyngiomas are often cystic and may rupture, releasing thick fluid into the subarachnoid space that may cause a chemical meningitis (see below). Craniopharyngiomas are more common in childhood, but there is a second peak in the seventh decade of life.[54]

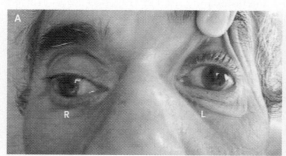
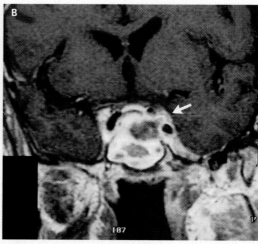

Figure 4–3. Images from a patient with pituitary apoplexy. This 63-year-old man had a severe headache with sudden onset of left III and IV nerve palsies. In A, the examiner is holding the left eye open because of ptosis, and the patient is trying to look to his right. An MRI scan, B, shows a hemorrhage (bright white on T1 imaging) into a large pituitary tumor that is invading the left cavernous sinus (arrow). The tumor abuts the optic chiasm. In pituitary apoplexy, there may be sudden visual loss in either or both eyes if the optic nerves are compressed, or in a bitemporal pattern if the chiasm is compressed, as well as impairment of some combination of cranial nerves III, IV, VI, and V_1.

PINEAL TUMORS

The pineal gland is technically outside the brain, sitting in the subdural space overlying the pretectal area and rostral midbrain. Tumors of the pineal gland commonly compress the dorsal surface of the midbrain, causing Parinaud's syndrome (loss of upward gaze, large poorly reactive pupils, and retractory convergence nystagmus), which points to the diagnosis. The tumor may also compress the cerebral aqueduct, causing hydrocephalus; typically this only alters consciousness when increased intracranial pressure from hydrocephalus causes plateau waves (see page 93) or if there is sudden hemorrhage into the pineal tumor (pineal apoplexy).[55] CT or MRI will demonstrate both the tumor and the hydrocephalus and can detect hemorrhage into the tumor.

SUBARACHNOID LESIONS

Like epidural, dural, and subdural lesions, subarachnoid lesions are outside of the brain itself. Unlike epidural or dural lesions, alterations of consciousness resulting from subarachnoid lesions are not usually the result of a mass effect, but occur when hemorrhage, tumor, or infection either compress, infiltrate, or cause inflammation of blood vessels in the subarachnoid space that supply the brain, or alter CSF absorptive pathways, thus causing hydrocephalus. Thus, strictly speaking, in some cases the damage done by these lesions may be more "metabolic" than structural. On the other hand, subarachnoid hemorrhage and bacterial meningitis are among the most acute emergencies encountered in evaluating comatose patients, and for that reason this class of disorders is considered here.

Subarachnoid Hemorrhage

Subarachnoid hemorrhage, in which there is little if any intraparenchymal component, is usually due to a rupture of a saccular aneurysm, although it can also occur when a superficial arteriovenous malformation ruptures. Saccular aneurysms occur throughout life, generally at branch points of large cerebral arteries, such as the origin of the anterior communicating artery from the anterior cerebral artery; the origin of the posterior communicating artery from

the posterior cerebral artery; the origin of the posterior cerebral artery from the basilar artery; or the origin of the middle cerebral artery from the internal carotid artery. Microscopic examination discloses an incomplete elastic media, which results in an aneurysmal dilation that may enlarge with time. Aneurysms are found with increasing frequency with age.

Aneurysms are typically silent until they hemorrhage. Some ruptures are presaged by a severe headache, a so-called sentinel headache,[56,57] presumably resulting from sudden dilation or leakage of blood from the aneurysm. The frequency of sentinel headaches varies in different series from 0% to 40%. Giant aneurysms of the internal carotid artery sometimes occur in the region of the cavernous sinus, and these may present as a mass lesion causing impairment of the cranial nerves of the cavernous sinus (III, IV, VI, and V_1) or by compressing the frontal lobes. Occasionally an aneurysm of the posterior communicating artery compresses the adjacent third nerve causing ipsilateral pupillary dilation. For this reason, new onset of anisocoria even in an awake patient is considered a medical emergency until the possibility of a posterior communicating artery aneurysm is eliminated.

Unfortunately, most aneurysms are not apparent until they bleed. The classic presentation of a subarachnoid hemorrhage is the sudden onset of the worst headache of the patient's life. However, many other types of headaches may present in this way (e.g., "thunderclap headache"),[58] so it is often necessary to rule out subarachnoid hemorrhage in the emergency department. If the hemorrhage is sufficiently large, the sudden pressure wave, as intracranial pressure approximates arterial pressure, may result in impaired cerebral blood flow and loss of consciousness. About 12% of patients with subarachnoid hemorrhage die before reaching medical care.[59] At the other end of the spectrum, if the leak is small or seals rapidly, there may be little in the way of neurologic signs. The most important finding is impairment of consciousness. The symptoms may vary from mild dullness to confusion to stupor or coma. The cause of the behavioral impairment after subarachnoid hemorrhage is not well understood. It is believed that the blood excites an inflammatory response with cytokine expression that may diffusely impair brain metabolism as well as cause brain edema. Parenchymal signs are

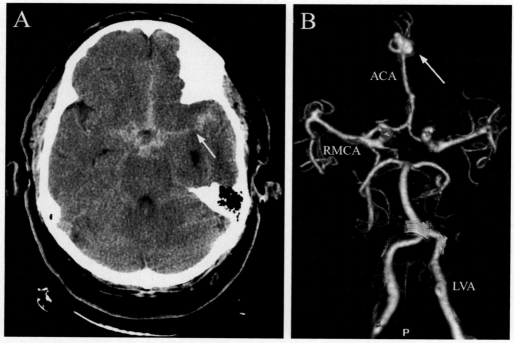

Figure 4–4. A 66-year-old man was brought to the Emergency Department after sudden onset of a severe global headache with nausea and vomiting. His legs collapsed under him. CT scan (A) showed blood in the cisterns surrounding the circle of Willis at the base of the brain, with blood extending into the interhemispheric fissure at the midline, and the right Sylvian fissure (arrow). A CT angiogram (B) showed that the anterior cerebral arteries were fused from the anterior communicating artery up to a bifurcation point, at which a large saccular aneurysm was noted (arrow). ACA, anterior cerebral artery; LVA, left vertebral artery; RMCA, right middle cerebral artery.

often lacking unless a jet of blood from the ruptured aneurysm has damaged the brain.

Patient 4–2

An 18-year-old woman was brought to the emergency department by her sister because she had been confused and forgetful for 2 days. She did not offer a history of headache, but upon being asked, the patient did admit that she had one. On examination the neck was stiff, but the neurologic examination showed only lethargy and inattention. A CT scan disclosed a subarachnoid hemorrhage, with blood collection around the circle of Willis on the right side. Lumbar puncture yielded bloody fluid, with 23,000 red blood cells and 500 white blood cells. Cultures were negative. A cerebral angiogram demonstrated a saccular aneurysm at the junction of the internal carotid and middle cerebral arteries on the right.

CT scans are highly sensitive to subarachnoid blood, making the diagnosis in more than 95% of cases if done within 12 hours[60] (Figure 4–4). MRI fluid-attenuated inversion recovery (FLAIR) sequences may be more sensitive,[61,62] but in a patient with a suspected subarachnoid hemorrhage if the CT is negative, a lumbar puncture is mandatory.[57,62,63] As lumbar puncture itself may introduce blood into the CSF, the analysis of blood in the CSF is of great importance. Signs that suggest that the blood was present before the tap include the persistence of the same number of red cells in tubes 1 and 4, or the presence of crenated red blood cells and/or xanthochromia if the hemorrhage is at least several hours old. Spectrophotometry of CSF is available in some institutions.[64] Another alternative is to centrifuge the CSF and test the supernate with a urine dipstick for blood. If the bleeding preceded the tap by at least 6 hours, it is likely that there will be blood breakdown products in the CSF, which can be visualized on the dipstick.

Even in those patients who are not comatose on admission, alterations of consciousness may develop in the ensuing days. Deterioration may occur due to rebleeding, which is particularly common in the first 24 to 48 hours. About 3 to 7 days after the hemorrhage, cerebral vasospasm may occur.[65] Vasospasm typically develops first and is most intense in the area of the greatest amount of extracerebral clot. This delayed cerebral ischemia may result in brain infarction and further edema, thus exacerbating the impairment of consciousness. Acutely developing hydrocephalus[66] from obstruction of spinal fluid pathways may also impair consciousness. The patient should be observed carefully for these complications and appropriate treatment applied.[65,66]

Subarachnoid Tumors

Both benign and malignant tumors may invade the subarachnoid space, infiltrating the leptomeninges either diffusely or focally and sometimes invading roots, or growing down the Virchow-Robin spaces to invade the brain. Leptomeningeal tumors include lymphomas and leukemias and solid tumors such as breast, renal cell, and lung cancers, as well as medulloblastomas and glial tumors.[67-69] The hallmark of meningeal neoplasms is multilevel dysfunction of the nervous system, including signs of damage to cranial or spinal nerves, spinal cord, brainstem, or cerebral hemispheres. Many patients with meningeal carcinoma have impairment of consciousness that is difficult to explain on the basis of the distribution of the tumor cells. The cause of the depressed level of consciousness in these patients is not clear. Explanations have included hydrocephalus from obstruction of spinal fluid pathways,[70,71] invasion of the brain along the Virchow-Robin spaces of penetrating pial vessels (the so-called encephalitic form of metastatic carcinoma),[72] nonconvulsive status epilepticus,[73] interference by the tumor with cortical metabolism,[74,75] or an immunologic response to the tumor[76] with production of cytokines and prostaglandins; most patients also have some white blood cells in their CSF as well as tumor cells.

The diagnosis of subarachnoid tumor is challenging, particularly when the multilevel dysfunctions of the nervous system are the first signs of the tumor. The MRI scan may show tumor implants in the leptomeninges or on the surface of the brain, or it may demonstrate thickening of cranial nerve or spinal roots (Figure 4–5). If the scan is negative, the diagnosis is established by the presence of tumor cells[77] or tumor markers[78] in the spinal fluid. However, the clinician must think of the diagnosis to perform these tests. Fortunately, there are nearly always other abnormalities in the CSF (lymphocytes, low glucose, elevated protein), which may lead to repeat examination if the first cytology is negative, as CSF cytology has a low degree of sensitivity. Wasserstrom and colleagues found that in patients with pathologically demonstrated meningeal carcinoma or lymphoma, only 40% of the first CSF samples contained malignant cells.[79]

Although the diagnosis of meningeal cancer generally indicates a poor prognosis, there are occasional patients with leukemia, lymphoma, or breast cancer in whom vigorous treatment of the meningeal tumor may result in marked improvement or even complete remission. Treatment usually includes high-dose intravenous[80] or intraventricular chemotherapy, as well as irradiation of areas of focal central nervous system (CNS) dysfunction (but not the entire neuraxis).[81]

Subarachnoid Infection

Subarachnoid infection (i.e., meningitis) is a common cause of impaired consciousness. Meningitis can be either acute or chronic and can be caused by a variety of different organisms including bacteria, fungi, rickettsiae, and viruses. Neurologic signs and symptoms caused by meningitis vary depending on the acuity of the infection and the nature of the infecting organisms, but certain aspects are common to all. For organisms to cause meningitis, they must first invade the meninges. This is usually done via the bloodstream, and for this reason blood cultures will often identify the organism. Less commonly, meningitis is a result of spread of organisms from structures adjacent to the brain (sinusitis, otitis). Meningitis can also occur in the absence of sepsis if there is communication between the meninges and the surface (CSF fistula, head injury, neurosurgery). Once in the meninges, organisms multiply, inducing the macrophage system that lines the meninges and superficial blood vessels in the brain

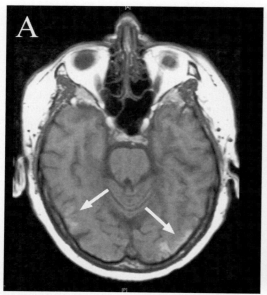
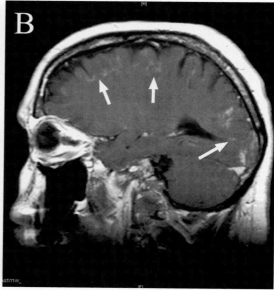

Figure 4–5. A pair of images from a magnetic resonance imaging (MRI) scan with contrast in a patient with meningeal lymphoma. This 52-year-old man presented with bilateral visual distortion and some left leg weakness. Both chronic lymphocytic leukemia and a non-Hodgkin's lymphoma had recently been diagnosed. The MRI scan showed superficial enhancement outlining the cortical sulci (arrows).

to produce a variety of cytokines and other proinflammatory molecules that in turn attract other white cells to the meninges. The inflammatory reaction can disrupt the blood-brain barrier; obstruct spinal fluid absorptive pathways, causing hydrocephalus and cellular swelling; or cause a vasculitis of subarachnoid or penetrating cortical blood vessels with resulting cerebral ischemia or infarction. Inflammatory reactions also cause metabolic disturbances that lower the pH, promoting vasodilation and increasing cerebral blood volume, leading to increased ICP.[82] Thus, although the infection itself does not cause a supratentorial mass, the combination of vasogenic and cytotoxic edema caused by the inflammatory response may produce enough diffuse mass effect to cause herniation. Both transtentorial and tonsillar herniation may occur, although both are rare.

The major causes of community-acquired bacterial meningitis include *Streptococcus pneumoniae* (51%) and *Neisseria meninigitis* (37%).[83] In immunocompromised patients, *Listeria monocytogenes* meningitis accounts for about 4% of cases.[84–86] Listeria meningitis may be noticeably slower in its course but has a tendency to cause brainstem abscesses. *Staphylococcus aureus* and, since a vaccine became

available, *Haemophilus influenzae* are uncommon causes of community-acquired meningitis.[83]

Acute bacterial meningitis is a medical emergency, as treated patients can die within hours of onset. Viral meningitis may clinically mimic bacterial meningitis, but in most cases are self-limiting. The clinical signs of acute bacterial meningitis are headache, fever, stiff neck, photophobia, and an alteration of mental status. Focal neurologic signs can occur either from ischemia of underlying brain or from damage to cranial nerves as they pass through the subarachnoid space. In a series of adults with acute bacterial meningitis,[87] 97% of patients had fever, 87% nuchal rigidity, and 84% headache. Nausea or vomiting was present in 55%, confusion in 56%, and a decreased level of consciousness in 51%. Papilledema was identified in only 2% of patients, although it was not tested in almost half. Seizure activity occurred in 25% of patients, but was always within 24 hours of the clinical diagnosis of acute meningitis. Over 40% of the patients had been partially treated before the diagnosis was established, so that in 30% of patients neither Gram stain nor cultures were positive. Eighteen percent of the patients died (Table 4–3).

Table 4–3 **Clinical Findings in 103 Patients With Acute Bacterial Meningitis**

Symptom	%
Fever	97*
Nuchal rigidity	87
Headache	66
Nausea/vomiting	55
Confusion	56
Altered consciousness	51
Seizures	25
Focal signs	23
Papilledema	2

*Not all patients were examined for each finding.

Data from Hussein and Shafran.[87]

In a series of 62 adults with community-acquired acute bacterial meningitis admitted to an intensive care unit, 95% had impaired consciousness.

However, the classic triad of fever, nuchal rigidity, and alteration of mental status was present in only 44% of patients in a large series of community-acquired meningitis.[83] Focal neurologic signs were present in one-third and included cranial nerve palsies, aphasia, and hemiparesis; papilledema was found in only 3%.

Subacute or chronic meningitis runs an indolent course and may be accompanied by the same symptoms, but also may occur in the absence of fever in debilitated or immune-suppressed patients. Both acute and chronic meningitis may be characterized only by lethargy, stupor, or coma in the absence of the other common signs. Chronic meningitis (e.g., with tuberculosis or cryptococcus) can also cause a local arteritis, resulting in cranial nerve dysfunction and focal areas of CNS infarction.[88] Aspergillus meningitis, which is typically seen only in patients who have been immune suppressed, causes a hemorrhagic arteritis, which may produce a combination of focal findings and impaired consciousness. However, the impairment of consciousness in each of these cases is primarily due to the immunologic processes concerned with the infection rather than structural causes (see Chapter 5).

The examination should include careful evaluation of nuchal rigidity even in patients who are stuporous. Attempting to flex the neck in a patient with meningitis may lead to grimacing and a rapid flexion of knees and hips (Brudzinski sign). Lateral movement of the neck, such as in eliciting the doll's head/eye signs, is not resisted. If one flexes the thigh to the right angle with the axis of the trunk, the patient grimaces and resists extension of the leg on the thigh (Kernig sign). Pain with jolt accentuation (the patient turns the head horizontally at two to three cycles per second) is a very sensitive sign of meningismus (positive in 97% of patients with meningitis) if the patient is sufficiently awake to cooperate, but is nonspecific (positive in 40% of patients with suspected meningitis, but no pleocytosis in the CSF).[89] Examination of the nose and ears for CSF discharge, and of the back for a CSF-to-skin sinus tract, may aid in the diagnosis. CSF can be distinguished from other clear fluid discharges at the bedside by its containing glucose. Measurement of beta-trace protein in the blood and discharge fluid is more accurate.[90]

Meningitis, particularly in children, can cause acute brain edema with transtentorial herniation as the initial sign. Clinically, such children rapidly lose consciousness and develop hyperpnea disproportionate to the degree of fever. The pupils dilate, at first moderately and then widely, then fix, and the child develops decerebrate motor signs. Urea, mannitol, or other hyperosmotic agents, if used properly, can prevent or reverse the full development of the ominous changes that are otherwise rapidly fatal.

In elderly patients, bacterial meningitis sometimes presents as insidiously developing stupor or coma in which there may be focal neurologic signs but little evidence of severe systemic illness or stiff neck. In one series, 50% of such patients with meningitis were admitted to the hospital with another and incorrect diagnosis.[91,92] Such patients can be regarded incorrectly as having suffered a stroke, but this error is readily avoided by accurate spinal fluid examinations.

If meningitis is suspected, a lumbar puncture is essential. Whether it should be performed before or after a CT scan is controversial.[33,93,94] Some observers believe that the diagnostic value warrants the small but definite risk. Many physicians believe that a CT scan cannot determine the safety of a lumbar puncture. Many patients with either supratentorial or infratentorial mass lesions tolerate lumbar puncture without complication; conversely, some patients with apparently normal CT may herniate. Most who want to perform CT first argue that when there is a strong suspicion of acute bacterial meningitis, one can begin antibiotics before the CT scan if the tap is done promptly after an emergent CT; Gram stain and cultures may still be positive. They further argue that the presence of a mass lesion suggests that the neurologic signs are not a result of meningitis alone and that lumbar puncture is probably unnecessary. Finally, even in the absence of a mass lesion, obliteration of the perimesencephalic cisterns or descent of the tonsils below the foramen magnum is a major risk factor for the development of herniation after a lumbar puncture. In such cases, lumbar puncture should be deferred until hyperosmolar agents (see Chapter 7) decrease the ICP. Regardless of which approach is taken, it is critical for the diagnostic evaluation not to prevent the immediate drawing of blood cultures, followed by administration of appropriate antibiotics.

In acute bacterial meningitis, CSF pressure at lumbar puncture is usually elevated. A normal or low pressure raises the question of whether there has already been partial herniation of the cerebellar tonsils. The cell count and protein are elevated, and glucose may be depressed or normal. Examination for bacterial antigens sometimes is diagnostic in the absence of a positive culture. Examination of the spinal fluid helps one differentiate acute bacterial meningitis from acute aseptic meningitis (Table 4–4). Because S. pneumoniae and N. meningitidis are the most common causal organisms, empiric therapy in adults should include either ceftriaxone (4 g/day in divided doses every 12 hours), cefotaxime (up to 8 to 12 g/day in divided doses every 4 to 6 hours), or cefepime (4 to 6 g/day in divided doses every 8 to 12 hours); vancomycin should be added until the results of antimicrobial susceptibility testing are known. In elderly patients and those who are immune suppressed, L. monocytogenes and H. influenzae play a role, and ampicillin should be added to those drugs. Meropenem may turn out to be an attractive candidate for monotherapy in elderly patients. In a setting where Rocky Mountain spotted fever or ehrlichiosis are possible infectious organisms, the addition of doxycycline is prudent.

Whether corticosteroids should be used is controversial. Adjuvant dexamethasone is recommended for children and adults with haemophilus meningitis or pneumococcal meningitis but is not currently recommended for the treatment of Gram-negative meningitis.

Table 4–4 Typical Cerebrospinal Fluid (CSF) Findings in Bacterial Versus Aseptic Meningitis

CSF Parameter	Bacterial Meningitis	Aseptic Meningitis
Opening pressure	>180 mm H_2O	Normal or slightly elevated
Glucose	<40 mg/dL	<45 mg/dL
CSF-to-serum glucose ratio	<0.31	>0.6
Protein	>50 mg/dL	Normal or elevated
White blood cells	>10 to <10,000/mm^3—neutrophils predominate	50–2,000/mm^3—lymphocytes predominate
Gram stain	Positive in 70%–90% of untreated cases	Negative
Lactate	≥3.8 mmol/L	Normal
C-reactive protein	>100 ng/mL	Minimal
Limulus lysate assay	Positive indicates Gram-negative meningitis	Negative
Latex agglutination	Specific for antigens of Streptococcus pneumoniae, Neisseria meningitidis (not serogroup B), and Hib	Negative
Coagglutination	Same as above	Negative
Counterimmunoelectrophoresis	Same as above	Negative

From Roos et al.,[95] with permission

Nevertheless, if prompt antibiotic therapy is begun and the patient shows any signs of increased ICP, it is probably wise to use dexamethasone.[96]

CT scans may show pus in the subarachnoid space as hypodense CSF with enlargement of sulci, but in the absence of prior scans in the same patient, this is often difficult to interpret. Meningeal enhancement usually does not occur until several days after the onset of infection. Cortical infarction, which may be due to inflammation and occlusion either of penetrating arteries or cortical veins, also tends to occur late. The MRI scan is much more sensitive for showing the changes indicated above but may be entirely normal in patients with acute meningitis (Table 4–5).[97]

INTRACEREBRAL MASSES

Intracerebral masses by nature tend to include both destructive and compressive elements. However, in many cases, the damage from the mass effect far exceeds the damage from disruption of local neurons and white matter. Hence, we have included this class of lesions with compressive processes.

Intracerebral Hemorrhage

Intracerebral hemorrhage may result from a variety of pathologic processes that affect the blood vessels. These include rupture of deep

Table 4–5 Imaging Findings in Acute Meningitis

Finding	CT*	MR*	Sensitivity
Sulcal dilation	Hypodense CSF; enlargement of sulci	T1WI: Hypointense CSF in sulci T2WI: Hyperintense CSF in sulci	MR > CT
Leptomeningeal enhancement	CE: Increase in density of subarachnoid space	T1WI, CE: Marked increase in signal intensity	MR > CT
Ischemic cortical infarction secondary to vasculitis	Hypodense cortical mass effect CE: Subacute increase in density (enhancement)	T1WI: Hypointense cortex; mass effect T2WI: Hyperintense cortex, mass effect FLAIR: Hyperintense cortex, mass effect CE: Subacute enhancement; hyperintense on T1WI DWI: Bright (white) ADC: Dark (black)	MR > CT
Subdural collections	Hypodense peripheral CSF plus density collection CE: Hygroma, no; empyema, yes	T1WI: Hypointense peripheral collection T2WI: Hyperintense peripheral collection FLAIR: hygroma, hypointense; empyema, variable CE: Hygroma, no; empyema, yes DWI: Hydroma, dark; empyema, bright ADC: Hygroma, bright; empyema, dark	MR > CT

ADC, apparent diffusion coefficient map; CE, contrast enhanced; CSF, cerebrospinal fluid; CT, computed tomography; DWI, diffusion-weighted imaging; FLAIR, fluid-attenuated inversion recovery; MR, magnetic resonance; T1WI, T1-weighted image; T2WI, T2-weighted image.
*Intensity relative to normal brain ±.

From Zimmerman et al.,[98] with permission.

cerebral end arteries, trauma, rupture of an arteriovenous malformation, rupture of a mycotic aneurysm, amyloid angiopathy, or hemorrhage into a tumor. Rupture of a saccular aneurysm can also cause an intraparenchymal hematoma, but the picture is generally dominated by the presence of subarachnoid blood. In contrast, despite their differing pathophysiology, the signs and symptoms of primary intracerebral hemorrhages are due to the compressive effects of the hematoma, and thus are more alike than different, depending more on location than on the underlying pathologic process. Spontaneous supratentorial intracerebral hemorrhages are therefore usually classified as lobar or deep, with the latter sometimes extending intraventricularly.

Lobar hemorrhages can occur anywhere in the cerebral hemispheres, and may involve one or multiple lobes (Figure 4–6A). As compared to deeper hemorrhages, patients with lobar hemorrhages are older, less likely to be male, and less likely to be hypertensive. Severe headache is a characteristic of lobar hemorrhages. Focal neurologic deficits occur in almost 90% of patients and vary somewhat depending on the site of the hemorrhage. About half the patients have a decreased level of consciousness and 20% are in a coma when admitted.[99] Seizures are a common occurrence and may be nonconvulsive (see page 281), so that electroencephalographic (EEG) evaluation is valuable if there is impairment of consciousness.

Deep hemorrhages in the supratentorial region include those into the basal ganglia, internal capsule, and thalamus. Hemorrhages into the pons and cerebellum are discussed in the section on infratentorial hemorrhages. Chung and colleagues divided patients with striatocapsular hemorrhages into six groups with varying clinical findings and prognoses.[100] These included posterolateral (33%), affecting primarily the posterior portion of the putamen; massive (24%), involving the entire striatal capsular region but occasionally sparing the caudate nucleus and the anterior rim of the internal capsule; lateral (21%), located between the external capsule and insular cortex; anterior (11%), involving the caudate nucleus; middle (7%), involving the globus pallidus in the middle portion of the medial putamen; and posterior medial (4%), localized to the anterior half of the posterior rim of the internal capsule. Consciousness was only rarely impaired in anterior and posterior medial lesions, but was impaired in about one-third of patients

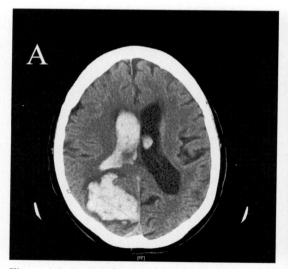 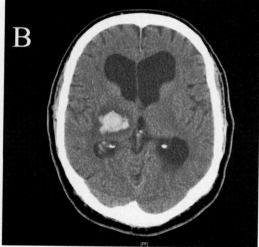

Figure 4–6. Computed tomography scans from two patients with intracerebral hemorrhages. (A) shows a large hemorrhage into the right parieto-occipital lobe in a 77-year-old woman who was previously healthy and presented with difficulty walking and a headache. Examination showed left-sided neglect. She took 325 mg aspirin at home on the advice of her primary care doctor because she suspected a stroke. The hematoma ruptured into the lateral ventricle. (B) shows a right thalamocapsular hemorrhage in a 60-year-old man with a history of hypertension who was not being treated at the time of the hemorrhage. He presented with headache, left-sided weakness and sensory loss, and some left-sided inattention.

with middle lesions. About half the patients with posterolateral lesions were drowsy, but not comatose, as were about one-half the patients with the lateral lesions who rarely become comatose. However, massive lesions usually cause severe impairment of consciousness including coma. Hemiparesis is common in posterolateral and massive lesions. Sensory deficits are relatively frequent in posterior and medial lesions. Prognosis is fair to good in patients with all of the lesions save the massive ones, where the fatality rate is about 50%. Eye deviation occurs usually toward the lesion site, but may be "wrong way" in those with posterolateral and massive lesions.

Thalamic hemorrhages can be categorized by size (smaller or larger than 2 cm in diameter) and by location (posterolateral, anterolateral, medial, and dorsal; Figure 4–6B). About one-fifth of patients with thalamic hemorrhages are stuporous or comatose at presentation.[101] The loss of consciousness is usually accompanied by ocular signs including skew deviation (the lower eye on the side of the lesion); gaze preference, which may either be toward or away (wrong-way eyes) from the side of the lesion; loss of vertical gaze; and miotic pupils. "Peering at the tip of the nose" is an almost pathognomonic sign.[102] Sensory and motor disturbances depend on the site and size of the lesion. About 25% of patients die,[101] and the outcome is related to the initial consciousness, nuchal rigidity, size of the hemorrhage, and whether the hemorrhage dissects into the lateral ventricle or causes hydrocephalus.[101]

Intraventricular hemorrhages may be either primary or result from extension of an intracerebral hemorrhage. Intraventricular hemorrhages were once thought to be uniformly fatal, but since the advent of CT scanning, have been shown to run the gamut of symptoms from simple headache to coma and death.[103] *Primary intraventricular hemorrhages* can result from vascular anomalies within the ventricle, surgical procedures, or bleeding abnormalities.[104] Clinical findings include sudden onset of headache and vomiting sometimes followed by collapse and coma. If the hemorrhage finds its way into the subarachnoid space, nuchal rigidity occurs. The clinical findings of *secondary intraventricular hemorrhage* depend on the initial site of bleeding. Hemorrhage into the ventricle from a primary intracerebral hemorrhage worsens the prognosis.

The treatment of intraventricular hemorrhage is aimed at controlling intracranial pressure. Ventricular drainage may help, but the catheter often becomes occluded by the blood. Injection of fibrinolytic agents (such as t-PA) has been recommended by some.[104]

The treatment of an intracerebral hemorrhage is controversial. Early surgery to evacuate the hematoma has not been associated with better outcome.[105] However, treatment with hemostatic drugs, such as recombinant factor VIIa, which limit hematoma size, are associated with improved outcomes.[106] Most patients who have relatively small lesions and do not die make good recoveries; those with massive lesions typically either die or are left devastated. Herniation should be treated vigorously in patients with relatively small hematomas because of the potential for good recovery.

Despite these similarities, the clinical setting in which one sees patients with intracerebral hemorrhage depends on the pathologic process involved. These include rupture of a deep cerebral endartery, amyloid angiopathy, mycotic aneurysm, arteriovenous malformation, or hemorrhage into a tumor, and each requires a different clinical approach.

Box 4–1 summarizes the major points that differentiate clinically between acute cerebral vascular lesions potentially causing stupor or coma.

Rupture of deep cerebral end arteries usually occurs in patients with long-term, poorly treated hypertension; it can also complicate diabetes or other forms of atherosclerotic arteriopathy. The blood vessels that are most likely to hemorrhage are the same ones that cause lacunar strokes (i.e., end arteries that arise at a right angle from a major cerebral artery): the *striatocapsular arteries*, which give rise to *capsular and basal ganglionic bleeds*; the *thalamic perforating arteries*, which give rise to *thalamic hemorrhages*; the midline *perforating arteries of the pons*, which give rise to *pontine hemorrhages*; and the *penetrating branches of the cerebellar long circumferential arteries*, which cause *cerebellar hemorrhages*. We will deal with the first two, which cause supratentorial masses, in this section, and the latter two in the section on infratentorial masses.

The focal neurologic findings in each case are characteristic of the part of the brain that is injured. Capsular or basal ganglionic hemorrhages typically present with the acute onset of

Box 4–1 Typical Clinical Profiles of Acute Cerebrovascular Lesions Affecting Consciousness

Acute massive cerebral infarction with or without hypotension

Distribution: Internal carotid-proximal middle cerebral artery or middle cerebral plus anterior cerebral arteries. Onset during wakefulness or sleep. Massive hemiplegia with aphasia, hemisensory defect. Obtundation from the start or within hours, progressing to stupor in 12 to 24 hours, coma usually in 36 to 96 hours. Convulsions rare. Pupils small and reactive, or constricted ipsilateral to lesion (Horner's), or moderately dilated ipsilateral to lesion (III nerve). Conjugate gaze paresis to side of motor weakness; contralateral oculovestibulars can be suppressed for 12 hours or so. Contralateral hemiplegia, usually with extensor plantar response and paratonia ipsilateral to lesion. Cheyne-Stokes breathing 10% to 20%. Signs of progressive rostral caudal deterioration begin in 12 to 24 hours. Spinal fluid usually unremarkable or with mildly elevated pressure and cells.

Frontoparietal hemorrhage

Onset during wakefulness. Sudden-onset headache, followed by more or less rapidly evolving aphasia, hemiparesis to hemiplegia, conjugate ocular deviation away from hemiparesis. Convulsions at onset in approximately one-fifth. Pupils small and reactive, or ipsilateral Horner's with excessive contralateral sweating, or stupor to coma and bilateral motor signs within hours of onset. Bloody spinal fluid.

Thalamic hemorrhage

Hypertensive, onset during wakefulness. Clinical picture similar to frontoparietal hemorrhage but seizures rare, vomiting frequent, eyes characteristically deviated down and laterally to either side. Pupils small and reactive. Conscious state ranges from awake to coma. Bloody spinal fluid.

Bilateral thalamic infarction in the paramedian regions

Sudden onset of coma, akinetic mutism, hypersomnolence or altered mental status may accompany bland infarcts of the paramedian thalamus arising bilaterally as a result of a "top of the basilar" syndrome or a branch occlusion of a thalamoperduncular artery (Percheron's artery) providing vascular supply to both thalami and often the tegmental mesencephalon.

Pontine hemorrhage

Hypertensive. Sudden onset of coma or speechlessness, pinpoint pupils, ophthalmoplegia with absent or impaired oculovestibular responses, quadriplegia, irregular breathing, hyperthermia. Bloody spinal fluid.

Cerebellar hemorrhage

Hypertensive and awake at onset. Acute and rapid onset and worsening within hours of occipital headache, nausea and vomiting, dizziness or vertigo, unsteadiness, dysarthria, and drowsiness. Small and reactive pupils, nystagmus or horizontal gaze paralysis toward the side of the lesion. Midline and ipsilateral ataxia,

(continued)

ipsilateral peripheral facial palsy, and contralateral extensor plantar response. Occasionally, course may proceed for 1 to 2 weeks. Spinal fluid bloody.

Acute cerebellar infarction

Mostly hypertensive, mostly males. Onset at any time. Vertigo, ataxia, nausea, dull headache, nystagmus, dysarthria, ipsilateral dysmetria; 24 to 96 hours later: drowsiness, miosis, ipsilateral gaze paresis and facial paresis, worsening ataxia, extensor plantar responses. Coma, quadriplegia, and death may follow if not decompressed. Spinal fluid sometimes microscopically bloody.

Acute subarachnoid hemorrhage

Awake at onset, sometimes hypertensive, sudden headache, often followed within minutes by unconsciousness. Pupils small or unilaterally dilated. Subhyaloid hemorrhages, hemiparesis or aphasia may or may not be present, hemisensory changes rare. Neck stiff within 24 hours. Bloody spinal fluid.

hemiplegia. Thalamic hemorrhage may present with sensory phenomena, but often the hemorrhage compresses ascending arousal systems early so that loss of consciousness is the primary presentation.[101] When the hemorrhage is into the caudal part of the thalamus, such as the putamen, which overlies the posterior commissure, the initial signs may be due to dorsal midbrain compression or injury[102] (see page 110), with some combination of forced downgaze and convergence ("peering at the tip of the nose"), fixed pupils, and retractory nystagmus. Another neuro-ophthalmologic presentation of thalamic hemorrhage was described by Miller Fisher as "wrong-way eyes."[107] Whereas frontal lobe insults usually result in deviation of the eyes toward the side of the lesion (i.e., paresis of gaze to the opposite side of space), after thalamic hemorrhage (or occasionally deep intraparenchymal hemorrhage that damages the same pathways[108]) there may be a paresis of gaze toward the side of the lesion (see Chapter 3).

PATHOPHYSIOLOGY

Hemorrhages of the end artery type are often called hypertensive hemorrhages, although they may occur in other clinical settings. The reason for the predilection of this class of artery for both occlusion (lacunar infarction) and hemorrhage is not known. Miller Fisher attempted to identify the arteries that had caused lacunar infarctions in postmortem examination of the brain.[109] He found an eosinophilic degeneration of the wall of small penetrating arteries in the region of the infarct and proposed that this "lipohyalinosis" was the cause of the infarction. However, this description was based on a small number of samples and did not give any insight into the nature of the pathologic process. Given the fact that such vessels typically take off at a right angle from large cerebral arteries, one might expect high sheering forces at the vessel origin, so that high blood pressure or other atherosclerotic risk factors might cause earlier or more severe damage. However, the mechanism for this phenomenon remains unclear.

End artery hemorrhages typically produce a large hematoma with considerable local tissue destruction and edema. Because much of the clinical appearance is due to the mass effect, which eventually is resorbed, the patient may initially to be much more neurologically impaired than would be caused by a comparably sized infarct. However, if the patient can be supported through the initial event, recovery is often much greater than might be initially anticipated, and the hematoma is resorbed, leaving a slit-like defect in the brain.

Amyloid angiopathy results from deposition of beta-amyloid peptide in the walls of cerebral blood vessels.[110] These deposits disrupt the arterial elastic media resulting in predisposition to bleeding. Because amyloid deposits occur along blood vessels as they penetrate the cerebral cortex, the hemorrhages are typically lobar (i.e., into a specific lobe of the cerebral cortex).[111] The arteries that hemorrhage tend to be small vessels, which seal spontaneously, so that the patient usually survives but may have multiple recurrences in later years.[112] Acute onset of focal hemispheric signs and a headache are the most common presentation. As with end artery hemorrhages, the severity of the initial presentation often is misleading, and as the hemorrhage is resorbed, there may be much greater return of function than in a patient with a similarly placed infarction. Gradient echo MRI may reveal additional areas of small, subclinical cortical and subcortical hemorrhage.[113]

Mycotic aneurysms are typically seen in the setting of a patient who has subacute bacterial endocarditis.[114] Infected emboli that reach the brain lodge in small penetrating arteries in the white matter just deep to the cerebral cortex. The wall of the blood vessel is colonized by bacteria, resulting in aneurysmal dilation several millimeters in diameter. These aneurysms, which may be visualized on cerebral angiography, may be multiple. Because there may be multiple mycotic aneurysms, and to eliminate an arteriovenous malformation or saccular aneurysm as the source, an angiogram is generally necessary. Unruptured mycotic aneurysms are treated by antibiotics, but ruptured aneurysms may require endovascular or open surgical intervention.[115]

Vascular malformations may occur in any location in the brain. They range from small cavernous angiomas to large arteriovenous malformations that are life threatening. MRI identifies many more cavernous angiomas than are seen on conventional arteriography or CT scanning. The abnormal vessels in these malformations are thin-walled, low-pressure and low-flow venous channels. As a result, cavernous angiomas bleed easily, but rarely are life threatening. Cavernous angiomas of the brainstem may cause coma if they hemorrhage and have a tendency to rebleed.[116] They can often be removed successfully.[117] Radiosurgery may also reduce the risk of hemorrhage, but can cause local edema or even hemorrhage acutely.[118,119]

Complex arteriovenous malformations (AVMs) contain large arterial feeding vessels and are often devastating when they bleed.[120] Although somewhat less likely to cause immediate death than are saccular aneurysms, arteriovenous malformations may be much harder to treat and bleeding may recur multiple times with gradually worsening outcome. AVMs may also cause symptoms by inducing epilepsy, or by causing a vascular steal from surrounding brain. AVMs that come to attention without hemorrhage have about a 2% to 4% per year chance of bleeding, but those that have previously bled have a much higher risk. AVMs are typically treated by a combination of endovascular occlusion of the arterial supply followed, if necessary, by surgery, although radiosurgery may also shrink AVMs in inaccessible regions.

Hemorrhage into a tumor typically occurs in the setting of a patient with known metastatic cancer. However, in some cases, the hemorrhage may be the first sign of the tumor. A higher percentage of metastatic melanoma, thyroid carcinoma, renal cell carcinoma, and germ cell tumors hemorrhage than is true for other tumor types, but lung cancer is so much more common than these tumors that it is the single most common cause of hemorrhage into a tumor.[121] Primary brain tumors, particularly oligodendrogliomas, may also present with a hemorrhage into the tumor. Because it is often difficult to see contrast enhancement of the tumor amidst the initial blood on MRI or CT scan, it is generally necessary to reimage the brain several weeks later, when the acute blood has been resorbed, if no cause of the hemorrhage is seen on initial imaging.

Intracerebral Tumors

Both primary and metastatic tumors may invade the brain, resulting in impairment of consciousness.[121,122] Primary tumors are typically either gliomas or primary CNS lymphomas, whereas metastatic tumors may come from many types of systemic cancer. Certain principles apply broadly across these classes of tumors.

Gliomas include both astrocytic tumors and oligodendrogliomas.[122] Astrocytic tumors typically invade the substance of the brain, and in extreme cases (gliomatosis cerebri), may diffusely infiltrate the entire brain.[123] Oligodendrogliomas typically are slower growing, and may contain calcifications visible on CT or MRI.

They more often present as seizures than as mass lesions.[124] Astrocytomas typically present either with seizures or as a mass lesion, with headache and increased intracranial pressure. In other cases, the patients may present with focal or multifocal signs of cerebral dysfunction. As they enlarge, astrocytomas may outgrow their blood supply, resulting in internal areas of necrosis or hemorrhage and formation of cystic components. Impairment of consciousness is usually due to compression or infiltration of the diencephalon or herniation. Surprisingly, primary brainstem astrocytomas, which are typically seen in adolescents and young adults, cause mainly impairment of cranial motor nerves while leaving sensory function and consciousness intact until very late in the course.

Primary CNS lymphoma (PCNSL) was once considered to be a rare tumor that was seen mainly in patients who were immune suppressed; however, PCNSL has increased in frequency in recent years in patients who are not immune compromised.[123,125] The reason for the increased incidence is not known. PCNSL behaves quite differently from systemic lymphomas.[122] The tumors invade the brain much like astrocytic tumors. They often occur along the ventricular surfaces and may infiltrate along white matter tracts. In this respect, primary CNS lymphomas present in ways that are similar to astrocytic tumors. However, it is unusual for a primary CNS lymphoma to reach so large a size, or to present by impairment of consciousness, unless it begins in the diencephalon.

Metastatic tumors are most often from lung, breast, or renal cell cancers or melanoma.[121] Tumors arising below the diaphragm usually do not invade the brain unless they first cause pulmonary metastases. Unlike primary brain tumors, metastases rarely infiltrate the brain, and can often be shelled out at surgery. Metastatic tumors usually present either as seizures or as mass lesions, and often enlarge quite rapidly. This tendency also results in tumors outgrowing their blood supply, resulting in infarction and hemorrhage (see previous section).

The ease of removing metastatic brain tumors has led to some controversy over the optimal treatment. Patients who have solitary metastatic tumors removed on average survive longer than patients who are treated with corticosteroids and radiation.[126] Occasional patients with lung cancer may have long-term survival and even apparent cure has been reported after removal of a single brain metastasis as well as the lung primary tumor. Patients with brain tumors frequently suffer from seizures, but prophylactic administration of anticonvulsants has not been found to be of value.[127] Small, surgically inaccessible metastases can be treated by stereotactic radiosurgery.[128]

Brain Abscess and Granuloma

A wide range of microorganisms, including viruses, bacteria, fungi, and parasites, can invade the brain parenchyma, producing an acute destructive encephalitis (see page 156). However, if the immune response is successful in containing the invader, a more chronic abscess or granuloma may result, which may act more as a compressive mass.

A brain abscess is a focal collection of pus within the parenchyma of the brain. The infective agents reach the brain hematogenously or by direct extension from an infected contiguous organ (paranasal sinus, middle ear).[129] Most bacterial brain abscesses occur in the cerebral hemispheres, particularly in the frontal or temporal lobes. In many countries in Central and South America, cysticercosis is the most common cause of infectious mass lesions in the cerebral hemispheres. However, cysticercosis typically presents as seizures, and only occasionally as a mass lesion.[130] In countries in which sheep herding is a major activity, echinococcal (hydatid) cyst must also be considered, although these can usually be recognized because they are more cystic in appearance than abscesses on CT or MRI scan.[131] Patients with HIV infection present a special challenge in the diagnosis of coma, as they may have a much wider array of cerebral infectious lesions and are also disposed to primary CNS lymphoma. However, toxoplasmosis is so common in this group of patients that most clinicians begin with 2 weeks of therapy for that organism.[132] When the appearance on scan is unusual, though, early biopsy is often indicated to establish the cause of the lesion(s) and optimal mode of treatment.

Other organisms may cause chronic infection resulting in formation of granulomas that

Table 4–6 **Presenting Signs and Symptoms in 968 Patients With Brain Abscess**

Sign or Symptom	Frequency Range	Mean
Headache	55%–97%	77%
Depressed consciousness	28%–91%	53%
Fever	32%–62%	53%
Nausea with vomiting	35%–85%	51%
Papilledema	9%–56%	39%
Hemiparesis	23%–44%	36%
Seizures	13%–35%	24%
Neck stiffness	5%–41%	23%

From Kastenbauer et al.,[133] with permission.

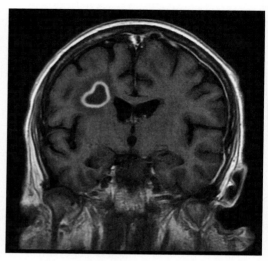

Figure 4–7. A 49-year-old man with AIDS was admitted for evaluation of headache, nausea, and bilateral weakness and intermittent focal motor seizures. MRI showed multiple ring-enhancing lesions. Note that the smooth, contrast-enhancing wall of this right parietal lesion is typical of an abscess. He was treated with broad spectrum antibiotics and improved.

may reach sufficient size to act as a mass lesion. These include tuberculomas in tuberculosis, torulomas in cryptococcal infection, and gummas in syphilis.

Because the symptoms are mainly due to brain compression, the clinical symptoms of brain abscess are similar to those of brain neoplasms, except they usually evolve more rapidly (Table 4–6).

Headache, focal neurologic signs, and seizures are relatively common. Fever and nuchal rigidity are generally present only during the early encephalitic phase of the infection, and are uncommon in encapsulated brain abscesses. The diagnosis may be suspected in a patient with a known source of infection or an immunosuppressed patient.

On imaging with either CT or MRI, the enhanced rim of an abscess is usually thinner and more regular than that of a tumor and may be very thin where it abuts the ventricle, sometimes leading to ventricular rupture (Figure 4–7). The infective nidus is often surrounded by more vasogenic edema than usually surrounds brain neoplasms. Diffusion-weighted images indicate restricted diffusion within the abscess, which can be distinguished from the cystic areas within tumors, which represent areas of infarction. The presence of higher levels of amino acids within the abscess on magnetic resonance spectroscopy (MRS) may also be helpful in differentiating the pathologies (Table 4–7).

If the lesion is small and the organism can be identified, antibiotics can treat the abscess successfully. Larger lesions require drainage or excision.

INFRATENTORIAL COMPRESSIVE LESIONS

The same mass lesions that affect the supratentorial space can also occur infratentorially (i.e., in the posterior fossa). Hence, while both the focal symptoms caused by posterior fossa masses and the symptoms of herniation differ substantially from those of supratentorial masses, the pathophysiologic mechanisms are similar. For that reason, we will focus in this section on the ways in which posterior fossa compressive lesions differ from those that occur supratentorially. Depending on the site of the lesion, compressive lesions of the posterior fossa are more likely to cause cerebellar signs and eye movement disorders and less likely to cause isolated hemiplegia. Herniation may be either downward as the cerebellar tonsils are forced through the foramen magnum or upward as the cerebellar vermis pushes the up-

Table 4–7 **Imaging Findings in Brain Abscess**

Finding	CT	MR*	Sensitivity
Capsule	Isodense	T1WI: Isointense to hyperintense Enhances T2WI: Hypointense to hyperintense	Plain: MR>CT CE: MR>CT
Vasogenic edema	Hypodense	T1WI: Hypointense T2WI: Hyperintense	Plain: MR>CT
Abscess contents	Hypodense	T1WI: Hypointense T2WI: Hyperintense MRS: Amino acid, lactate, acetate, succinate, and pyruvate peaks DWI: Bright (white) ADC: Dark (black)	Plain: MR=CT

ADC, apparent diffusion coefficient map; CE, contrast enhanced; CT, computed tomography; DWI, diffusion-weighted image; MR, magnetic resonance spectroscopy; T1WI, T1-weighted image; T2WI, T2-weighted image.
*Intensity relative to normal brain.

From Zimmerman et al.,[98] with permission.

per brainstem through the tentorium, or usually both.

EPIDURAL AND DURAL MASSES

Epidural Hematoma

Epidural hematomas of the posterior fossa are much less common than their supratentorial counterparts, representing about 10% of all epidural hematomas.[134] Posterior fossa epidural hematomas typically follow fracture of the occipital bone; they are usually arterial, but may occasionally result from venous bleeding.[135] The hematomas are bilateral in about one-third of cases.[134]

Patients present with headache, nausea and vomiting, and loss of consciousness.[136,137] Neuro-ophthalmologic signs are relatively uncommon, usually consisting of abducens paresis due to the increased intracranial pressure. Occasionally a stiff neck is seen as an early sign of tonsillar herniation.

A typical lucid interval occurs in only a minority of patients[138]: after initial injury, those patients either continue to be alert or rapidly recover after a brief loss of consciousness only to subsequently, after minutes to days, first become lethargic and then lapse into coma. Without treatment death ensues from acute respi-

ratory failure (tonsillar herniation). Even those patients with a lucid interval suffer headache and often cerebellar ataxia after the injury. If not treated, symptoms progress to vertigo, stiff neck, ataxia, nausea, and drowsiness.

It is important to identify an occipital fracture even in the absence of a hematoma because of the possibility of delayed development of an epidural hematoma.[134] If a fracture crosses the transverse sinus, it may cause thrombosis of that vessel, causing a supratentorial hemorrhagic infarct or increased ICP. Because of the small amount of space in the posterior fossa and the narrow exit foramina of CSF (Sylvian aqueduct and fourth ventricle), obstructive hydrocephalus is often an early problem that may require emergent therapy.[139] About one-half of patients have evidence of other injury, such as cerebellar hemorrhage or supratentorial bleeding.[140]

Most patients with posterior fossa epidural hematomas are treated surgically,[134] although alert patients with small lesions may be treated conservatively.[141] A hematoma with a volume under 10 mL, a thickness under 15 mm, and a midline shift of no more than 5 mm may be treated conservatively but requires careful watching for increase in the size of the lesion. In the supratentorial space, epidural hematomas with volumes up to 30 mL may be treated conservatively.[141] The availability of rapid imaging has substantially reduced the mortality from about 25% in older series[142] to about 5% in more modern series.[134] Most current mortality and morbidity is related not to the hematoma, but to other brain injuries sustained in the trauma.

Epidural Abscess

Epidural abscesses in the posterior fossa are rare, representing only nine out of almost 4,000 patients with intracranial infections in one series.[143] Most were complications of ear infections and mastoiditis. Unlike epidural hematomas, fever and meningismus, as well as evidence of a chronic draining ear, are common. Focal neurologic signs are similar to those of epidural hematomas, but develop over days to weeks rather than hours. Cerebellar signs occur in a minority of patients. The CT scan demonstrates a hypodense or isodense extraaxial mass with a contrast-enhancing rim. Hydrocephalus is common. Diffusion-weighted MRI identifies restricted diffusion, as in supratentorial empyemas and abscesses.[41] The prognosis is generally good with evacuation of the abscess and treatment with antimicrobials, except in those patients suffering venous sinus thrombosis as a result of the infection.

Dural and Epidural Tumors

As with supratentorial lesions, both primary and metastatic tumors can involve the dura of the posterior fossa. *Meningioma* is the most common primary tumor.[144] Meningiomas usually arise from the tentorium or other dural structures, but can occur in the posterior fossa without dural attachment.[145] Meningiomas produce their symptoms both by direct compression and by causing hydrocephalus. However, because they grow slowly, focal neurologic symptoms are common and the diagnosis is generally made long before they cause alterations of consciousness. Dural *metastases* from myelocytic leukemia, so-called chloromas or granulocytic sarcomas,[146] have a particular predilection for the posterior fossa. Although more rapidly growing than primary tumors, these tumors rarely cause alterations of consciousness. Other metastatic tumors to the posterior fossa meninges may cause symptoms by involving cranial nerves.

SUBDURAL POSTERIOR FOSSA COMPRESSIVE LESIONS

Subdural hematomas of the posterior fossa are rare. Only 1% of traumatic acute subdural hematomas are found in the posterior fossa.[147] Chronic subdural hematomas in the posterior fossa, without a clear history of head trauma, are even rarer. A review in 2002 reported only 15 previous cases, including those patients taking anticoagulants.[148] Patients with acute subdural hematomas can be divided into those who are stuporous or comatose on admission and those who are alert. Patients with chronic subdural hematomas, many of whom had been on anticoagulation therapy or have sustained very mild head trauma, usually present with headache, vomiting, and cerebellar signs. The diagnosis is made by CT or MRI and treatment is usually surgical. Stupor or coma portends a poor outcome, as do the CT findings of obliterated basal cisterns and fourth ventricle with resultant hydrocephalus.[147]

Subdural Empyema

Posterior fossa subdural empyemas are rare.[149] They constitute less than 2% of all subdural empyemas.[143] Like their epidural counterparts, ear infections and mastoiditis are the major cause. Headache, lethargy, and meningismus are common symptoms. Ataxia and nystagmus are less common.[143] The diagnosis is made by CT, which reveals a hypo- or isodense extraaxial collection with enhancement. On MRI, diffusion is restricted,[41] unlike tumors or hemorrhage. Treatment with drainage and antibiotics is usually successful.

Subdural Tumors

Isolated subdural tumors are exceedingly rare. Meningioma and other tumors of the dura may invade the subdural space. Subdural metastases from leukemia or solid tumors rarely occur in isolation. They can be differentiated from hematomas and infection on scans by their uniform contrast enhancement.

SUBARACHNOID POSTERIOR FOSSA LESIONS

Subarachnoid blood, infection, or tumor usually occurs in the posterior fossa in association with similar supratentorial lesions. Exceptions include subdural or parenchymal posterior fossa lesions that rupture into the subarachnoid space and posterior fossa subarachnoid hemorrhage.[150] *Posterior fossa subarachnoid hemorrhages* are caused either by aneurysms or dissection of vertebral or basilar arteries or their branches. Unruptured aneurysms of the basilar and vertebral arteries sometimes grow to a size of several centimeters and act like posterior fossa extramedullary tumors. However, they generally do not cause coma unless they rupture. When a vertebrobasilar aneurysm ruptures, the event is characteristically abrupt and frequently is marked by the complaint of sudden weak legs, collapse, and coma. Most patients also have sudden occipital headache, but in contrast with anterior fossa aneurysms in which the history of coma, if present, is usually clear cut, it sometimes is difficult to be certain whether a patient with a ruptured posterior fossa aneurysm had briefly lost consciousness or merely collapsed because of paralysis of the lower extremities. Ruptured vertebrobasilar aneurysms are often reported as presenting few clinical signs that clearly localize the source of the subarachnoid bleeding to the posterior fossa. In Logue's 12 patients,[151] four had unilateral sixth nerve weakness (which can occur with any subarachnoid hemorrhage), one had bilateral sixth nerve weakness, and only two had other cranial nerve abnormalities to signify a posterior fossa localization. Duvoisin and Yahr[152] reported that only about one-half of their patients with ruptured posterior fossa aneurysms had signs that suggested the origin of their bleeding. Jamieson reported 19 cases with even fewer localizing signs: five patients suffered third nerve weakness and two had sixth nerve palsies.[153]

Our own experience differs somewhat from the above. We have had eight patients with ruptured vertebrobasilar aneurysms confirmed at arteriography or autopsy, and six had pupillary, motor, or oculomotor signs indicating a posterior fossa lesion (Table 4–8).

The diagnosis is usually obvious on CT. Blood isolated to the fourth ventricle suggests

Table 4–8 Localizing Signs in Six Cases of Ruptured Vertebrobasilar Aneurysms

Occipital headache	5
Skew deviation of the eyes	3
Third nerve paralysis	2
Cerebellar signs	3
Acute paraplegia before loss of consciousness	2

a ruptured posterior inferior cerebellar artery aneurysm.[150] Perimesencephalic hemorrhage is characterized by subarachnoid blood accumulating around the midbrain. While this often presents with a headache and loss of consciousness, it has a relatively benign prognosis.[154] Unlike most subarachnoid hemorrhage, the bleeding is usually venous in origin[155]; cerebral angiograms are negative and bleeding rarely recurs.

INTRAPARENCHYMAL POSTERIOR FOSSA MASS LESIONS

Intraparenchymal mass lesions in the posterior fossa that cause coma usually are located in the cerebellum. In part this is because the cerebellum occupies a large portion of this compartment, but in part because the brainstem is so small that an expanding mass lesion often does more damage by tissue destruction than as a compressive lesion.

Cerebellar Hemorrhage

About 10% of intraparenchymal intracranial hemorrhages occur in the cerebellum. A cerebellar hemorrhage can cause coma and death by compressing the brainstem. Increasing numbers of reports in recent years indicate that if the diagnosis is made promptly, many patients can be treated successfully by evacuating the clot or removing an associated angioma.[156,157] However, for those patients who are comatose, mortality is high despite prompt surgical intervention.[156,158] Approximately three-quarters of patients with cerebellar hemorrhage have hypertension; most of the remaining ones have cerebellar angiomas or are receiving anticoagulant drugs. In elderly patients, amyloid angiopathy may be the culprit.[159] On rare occasions, a cerebellar hemorrhage may follow a supratentorial craniotomy.[160] Among our own 28 patients,[161] five had posterior fossa arteriovenous vascular malformations, one had thrombocytopenic purpura, three were normotensive but receiving anticoagulants, and the remainder, who ranged between 39 and 83 years of age, had hypertensive vascular disease. Hemorrhages in hypertensive patients arise in the neighborhood of the dentate nuclei; those coming from angiomas tend to lie more superficially. Both types usually rupture into the subarachnoid space or fourth ventricle and cause coma chiefly by compressing the brainstem.

Fisher's paper in 1965[162] did much to stimulate efforts at clinical diagnosis and encouraged attempts at successful treatment. Subsequent reports from several large centers have increasingly emphasized that early diagnosis is critical for satisfactory treatment of cerebellar hemorrhage, and that once patients become stuporous or comatose, surgical drainage is a near-hopeless exercise.[156] The most common initial symptoms of cerebellar hemorrhage are headaches (most often occipital), nausea and vomiting, dizziness or vertiginous sensations, unsteadiness or an inability to walk, dysarthria, and, less often, drowsiness. Messert and associates described two patients who had unilateral eyelid closure contralateral to the cerebellar hemorrhage, apparently as an attempt to prevent diplopia.[163] Patient 4–3, below, is a typical example.

Patient 4–3

A 55-year-old man with hypertension and a history of poor medication compliance had sudden onset of severe occipital headache and nausea when sitting down with his family to Christmas dinner. He noticed that he was uncoordinated when he tried to carve the turkey. When he arrived in the hospital emergency department he was unable to sit or stand unaided, and had severe bilateral ataxia in both upper extremities. He was a bit drowsy but had full eye movements with end gaze nystagmus to either side. There was no weakness or change in muscle tone, but tendon reflexes were brisk, and toes were downgoing. He was sent for a CT scan, but by the time the scan was finished the CT technician could no longer arouse him.

The CT scan showed a 5-cm egg-shaped hemorrhage into the left cerebellar hemisphere, compressing the fourth ventricle, with hydrocephalus. By the time the patient returned to the emergency department he had no oculocephalic responses, and breathing was ataxic. Shortly afterward, he had a respiratory arrest and died before the neurosurgical team could take him to the operating room.

Table 4–9 Presenting Clinical Findings in 72 Patients With Cerebellar Hemorrhage

Symptoms	No. Patients (%)	Signs	No. Patients (%)
Vomiting	58 (81)	Anisocoria	10 (14)
Headache	48 (67)	Pinpoint pupils	4 (6)
Dizziness/vertigo	43 (60)	Abnormal OCR or EOM	23 (32)
Truncal/gait ataxia	40 (56)	Skew deviation	6 (8)
Dysarthria	30 (42)	Nystagmus	24 (33)
Drowsiness	30 (42)	Absent/asymmetric CR	9 (13)
Confusion	8 (11)	Facial paresis	13 (18)
		Dysarthria	18 (25)
		Limb ataxia	32 (44)
		Hemiparesis	8 (11)
		Babinski sign	36 (50)

CR, corneal reflex; EOM, extraocular movements; OCR, oculocephalic reflex.

Modified from Fisher et al.[162]

Table 4–9 lists the most frequent early physical signs as recorded in a series of 72 patients.[164]

As Patient 4–3 illustrates, deterioration from alertness or drowsiness to stupor often comes over a few minutes, and even brief delays to carry out radiographic procedures can prove fatal. Mutism, a finding encountered in children after operations that split the inferior vermis of the cerebellum, occasionally occurs in adults with cerebellar hemorrhage.[165] Although usually not tested during the rush of the initial examination, cognitive dysfunction, including impairment of executive functions, difficulty with spatial cognition, and language deficits, as well as affective disorders including blunting of affect or disinhibited or inappropriate behavior, called the "cerebellar cognitive affective syndrome,"[166] are sometimes present (see also page 306, Chapter 6). Similar abnormalities may persist if there is damage to the posterior hemisphere of the cerebellum, even following successful treatment of cerebellar mass lesions.[167]

All patients who present to the emergency room with acute cerebellar signs, particularly when associated with headache and vomiting, require an urgent CT. The scan identifies the hemorrhage and permits assessment of the degree of compression of the fourth ventricle and whether there is any complicating hydrocephalus. Our experience with acute cerebellar hemorrhage points to a gradation in severity that can be divided roughly into four relatively distinct clinical patterns. The least serious form occurs with small hemorrhages, usually less than 1.5 to 2 cm in diameter by CT, and includes self-limited, acute unilateral cerebellar dysfunction accompanied by headache. Without imaging, this disorder undoubtedly would go undiagnosed. With larger hematomas, occipital headache is more prominent and signs of cerebellar or oculomotor dysfunction develop gradually or episodically over 1 to several days. There may be some associated drowsiness or lethargy. Patients with this degree of impairment have been reported to recover spontaneously, particularly from hemorrhages measuring less than 3 cm in diameter by CT. However, the condition requires extremely careful observation until one is sure that there is no progression due to edema formation, as patients almost always do poorly if one waits until coma develops to initiate surgical treatment. The most characteristic and therapeutically important syndrome of cerebellar hemorrhages occurs in individuals who develop acute or subacute occipital headache, vomiting, and progressive neurologic impairment including ipsilateral ataxia, nausea, vertigo, and nystagmus. Parenchymal brainstem signs, such as gaze paresis or facial weakness on the side of the hematoma, or pyramidal motor signs develop as a result of brainstem compression, and hence usually are not seen until after drowsiness or obtundation is apparent. The appearance of impairment of consciousness mandates emergency intervention and surgical decompression that can be lifesaving. About one-fifth of patients with cerebellar hemorrhage develop early pontine compression with sudden loss of consciousness, respiratory irregularity, pinpoint pupils, absent oculovestibular responses, and quadriplegia; the picture is clinically indistinguishable from primary pontine hemorrhage and is almost always fatal.

Kirollos and colleagues have proposed a protocol based on CT and the patient's clinical state to help determine which patients are candidates for surgical intervention and to predict prognosis (Figure 4–8). The degree of fourth ventricular compression is divided into three grades depending on whether the fourth ventricle is normal (grade 1), is compressed (grade 2), or is completely effaced (grade 3). Grade 1 or 2 patients who are fully conscious are carefully observed for deterioration of level of consciousness. If grade 1 patients have impaired consciousness, a ventricular drain is placed. If grade 2 patients have impaired consciousness with hydrocephalus, a ventricular drain is placed. In grade 3 patients and grade 2 patients who have impaired consciousness without hydrocephalus, the hematoma is evacuated. No grade 3 patients with a Glasgow Coma Score less than 8 experienced a good outcome.[156]

Clinical predictors of neurologic deterioration are a systolic blood pressure over 200 mm Hg, pinpoint pupils, and abnormal corneal or oculocephalic reflexes. Imaging predictors are hemorrhage extending into the vermis, a hematoma greater than 3 cm in diameter, brainstem distortion, interventricular hemorrhage, upward herniation, or acute hydrocephalus. Hemorrhages in the vermis and acute hydrocephalus on admission independently predict deterioration.[164]

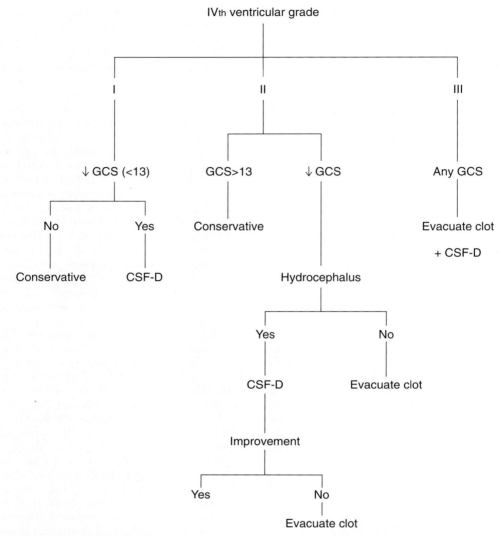

Figure 4–8. Protocol scheme for the treatment of spontaneous cerebellar hematomas. CSF-D, cerebrospinal fluid ventricular drainage or shunt; GCS, Glasglow Coma Scale. (From Kirollos et al.,[156] with permission.)

Cerebellar Infarction

Cerebellar infarction can act as a mass lesion if there is cerebellar edema. In these cases, as in cerebellar hemorrhage, the mass effect can cause stupor or coma by compression of the brainstem and death by herniation. Cerebellar infarction represents 2% of strokes.[168,169] Most victims are men. Hypertension, atrial fibrillation, hypercholesterolemia, and diabetes are important risk factors in the elderly[168]; verte-

bral artery dissection should be considered in younger patients.[169] Marijuana use has been implicated in a few patients.[170] The neurologic symptoms are similar to those of cerebellar hemorrhage, but they progress more slowly, as they are typically due to edema that develops gradually over 2 to 3 days after the onset of the infarct, rather than acutely (Table 4–10).

The onset is characteristically marked by acute or subacute dizziness, vertigo, unsteadiness, and, less often, dull headache. Most of the

Table 4–10 **Symptoms, Signs, and Consciousness Levels on Admission in 293 Patients With Cerebellar Infarction**

Symptoms	No. (%)	Signs	No. (%)	Consciousness Levels on Admission	No. (%)
Vertigo/dizziness	206 (70)	Limb ataxia	172 (59)	Clear	195 (67)
Nausea/vomiting	165 (56)	Truncal ataxia	133 (45)	Confused	73 (25)
Gait disturbance	116 (40)	Dysarthria	123 (42)	Obtunded	20 (7)
Headache	94 (32)	Nystagmus	111 (38)	Comatose	5 (2)
Dysarthria	59 (20)	Hemiparesis	59 (20)		
Tinnitus	14 (5)	Facial palsy	23 (8)		
		Anisocoria	17 (6)		
		Conjugate deviation	18 (6)		
		Horner's syndrome	15 (5)		
		Upward gaze palsy	12 (4)		
		Loss of light reflex	11 (4)		

From Tohgi et al.,[168] with permission.

patients examined within hours of onset are ataxic, have nystagmus with gaze in either direction but predominantly toward the infarct, and have dysmetria ipsilateral to the infarct. Dysarthria and dysphagia are present in some patients and presumably reflect associated lateral medullary infarction. Only a minority of patients are lethargic, stuporous, or comatose on admission, which suggests additional injury to the brainstem.[168]

Initial CT rules out a cerebellar hemorrhage, but it is often difficult to demonstrate an infarct. Even if a hypodense lesion is not seen, asymmetric compression of the fourth ventricle may indicate the development of acute edema. A diffusion-weighted MRI is usually positive on initial examination.

In most instances, further progression, if it is to occur, develops by the third day and may progress to coma within 24 hours.[171] Progression is characterized by more intense ipsilateral dysmetria followed by increasing drowsiness leading to stupor, and then miotic and poorly reactive pupils, conjugate gaze paralysis ipsilateral to the lesion, ipsilateral peripheral facial paralysis, and extensor plantar responses. Once the symptoms appear, unless surgical decompression is conducted promptly, the illness progresses rapidly to coma, quadriplegia, and death.

Only the evaluation of clinical signs can determine whether the swelling is resolving or the enlarging mass must be surgically treated

(by ventricular shunt or extirpation of infarcted tissue).[171,172] The principles of management of a patient with a space-occupying cerebellar infarct are similar to those in cerebellar hemorrhage. If the patient remains awake, he or she is observed carefully. If consciousness is impaired and there is some degree of acute hydrocephalus on scan, ventriculostomy may relieve the compression. However, if there is no acute hydrocephalus, or if the patient fails to improve after ventriculostomy, craniotomy with removal of infarcted tissue is necessary to relieve brainstem compression. Survival may follow prompt surgery, but patients may have distressing neurologic residua if they survive.

Cerebellar Abscess

About 10% of all brain abscesses occur in the cerebellum.[173] Cerebellar abscesses represent about 2% of all intracranial infections. Most arise from chronic ear infections,[174] but some occur after trauma (head injury or neurosurgery) and others are hematogenous in origin. If untreated, they enlarge, compress the brainstem, and cause herniation and death. If successfully recognized and treated, the outcome is usually good. The clinical symptoms of a cerebellar abscess differ little from those of other cerebellar masses (Table 4–11).

Headache and vomiting are very common. Patients may or may not be febrile or have nu-

Table 4–11 **Clinical Features of Cerebellar Abscesses**

	Cases Before 1975 (N = 47)*		Cases After 1975 (N = 77)†	
	No.	%	No.	%
Symptoms				
Headache	47	100	74	96
Vomiting	39	83		
Drowsiness	32	66		
Unsteadiness	23	49		
Confusion	16	34		
Ipsilateral limb weakness	6	13		
Visual disturbances	4	8		
Blackout	3	6		
Signs				
Nystagmus	35	74		
Meningismus	31	66	59	77
Cerebellar signs	27	57	40	52
Papilledema	21	45		
Fever	16	34	70	90
Sixth nerve palsy	2	4	7	15
Depressed consciousness	32	66	44	57

*Data from Shaw and Russell.[175]
†Data from Nadvi et al.[173]

chal rigidity.[175] If the patient does not have an obvious source of infection, is not febrile, and has a supple neck, a cerebellar abscess is often mistaken for a tumor, the correct diagnosis being made only by surgery. About one-half of patients have a depressed level of consciousness.[173] The diagnosis is made by imaging, scans revealing a mass with a contrast-enhancing rim and usually an impressive amount of edema. Restricted diffusion on diffusion-weighted MRI helps distinguish the abscess from tumor or hematoma. Hydrocephalus is a common complication. The treatment is surgical, either primary excision[176] or aspiration.[177] The outcome is better when patients with hydrocephalus are treated with CSF diversion or drainage.[173]

Cerebellar Tumor

Most cerebellar tumors of adults are metastases.[178] The common cerebellar primary tumors of children, medulloblastoma and pilocytic astrocytoma, are rare in adults. Cerebellar hemangioblastomas may occur in adults, but they

are uncommon.[179] The symptoms of cerebellar tumors are the same as those of any cerebellar mass, but because their growth is relatively slow, they rarely cause significant alterations of consciousness unless there is a sudden hemorrhage in the tumor. Patients present with headache, dizziness, and ataxia. Because the symptoms are rarely acute, MRI scanning can usually be obtained. The contrast-enhanced image will not only identify the enhancing cerebellar tumor, but will also inform the physician whether there are other metastatic lesions and whether hydrocephalus is present. The treatment of a single metastasis in the cerebellum is generally surgical or, in some instances, by radiosurgery.[128] Multiple metastases are treated with radiation therapy.

Pontine Hemorrhage

Although pontine hemorrhage compresses the brainstem, it causes damage as much by tissue destruction as by mass effect (Figure 4–9). Hemorrhage into the pons typically produces

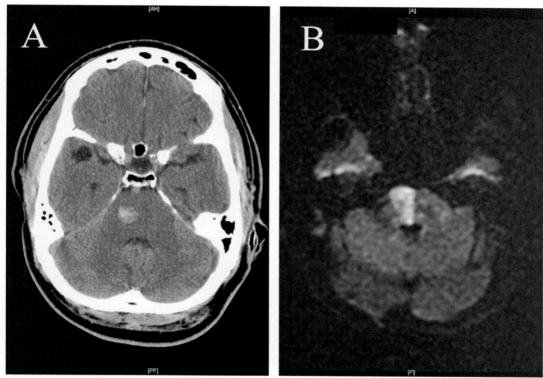

Figure 4–9. A pair of scans without contrast from two patients with pontine strokes. (A) A noncontrast computed tomography scan demonstrating a small hemorrhage into the right pontine base and tegmentum in a 55-year-old man with hypertension, who presented with left hemiparesis and dysarthria. He was treated by blood pressure control and improved markedly. (B) A diffusion-weighted magnetic resonance imaging (MRI) scan of a medial pontine infarct in a 77-year-old man with hypertension, hyperlipidemia, and prior history of coronary artery disease. He presented with left hemiparesis, dysarthria, and diplopia. On examination, there was right lateral gaze paresis and inability to adduct either eye on lateral gaze (one-and-a-half syndrome). There was extensive irregularity of the vertebrobasilar vessels on MR angiogram. He was treated with anticoagulants and improved slowly, although with significant residual diplopia and left hemiparesis at discharge.

the characteristic pattern of sudden onset of unconsciousness with tiny but reactive pupils (although it may require a magnifying glass or the plus 20 lens of the ophthalmoscope to visualize the light response). Most patients have impairment of oculocephalic responses, and eyes may show skew deviation, ocular bobbing, or one of its variants. Patients may have decerebrate rigidity, or they may demonstrate flaccid quadriplegia. We have seen one patient in whom a hematoma that dissected along the medial longitudinal fasciculus, and caused initial vertical and adduction ophthalmoparesis, was followed about an hour later by loss of consciousness (see Patient 2–1). However, in most patients, the onset of coma is so sudden that

there is not even a history of a complaint of headache.[180]

SUPRATENTORIAL DESTRUCTIVE LESIONS CAUSING COMA

The most common supratentorial destructive lesions causing coma result from either anoxia or ischemia, although the damage may occur due to trauma, infection, or the associated immune response. To cause coma, a supratentorial lesion must either involve bilateral cortical or subcortical structures multifocally or diffusely or affect the thalamus bilaterally. Following recovery from the initial insult, the coma is usually short lived, the patient either awakening, entering a persistent vegetative state within a few days or weeks, or dying (see Chapter 9).

VASCULAR CAUSES OF SUPRATENTORIAL DESTRUCTIVE LESIONS

Diffuse anoxia and ischemia, including carbon monoxide poisoning and multiple cerebral emboli from fat embolism[181] or cardiac surgery,[182] are discussed in detail in Chapter 5. We will concentrate here on focal ischemic lesions that can cause coma.

Carotid Ischemic Lesions

Unilateral hemispheric infarcts due to *carotid or middle cerebral occlusion* may cause a quiet, apathetic, or even confused appearance, as the remaining cognitive systems in the patient's functional hemisphere attempt to deal with the sudden change in cognitive perspective on the world. This appearance is also seen in patients during a Wada test, when a barbiturate is injected into one carotid artery to determine the lateralization of language function prior to surgery. The appearance of the patient may be deceptive to the uninitiated examiner; acute loss of language with a dominant hemisphere lesion may make the patient unresponsive to verbal command, and acute lesions of the nondominant hemisphere often cause an "eye-opening apraxia," in which the patient keeps his or her eyes closed, even though awake. However, a careful neurologic examination demonstrates that despite the appearance of reduced responsiveness, true coma rarely occurs in such cases.[183]

In the rare cases where unilateral carotid occlusion does cause loss of consciousness, there is nearly always an underlying vascular abnormality that explains the observation.[184,185] For example, there may be pre-existing vascular anomaly or occlusion of the contralateral carotid artery, so that both cerebral hemispheres may be supplied, across the anterior communicating artery, by one carotid. In the absence of such a situation, unilateral carotid occlusion does not cause acute loss of consciousness.

Patients with large hemispheric infarcts are nearly always hemiplegic at onset, and if in the dominant hemisphere, aphasic as well. The lesion can be differentiated from a cerebral hemorrhage by CT scan that, in the case of infarct, may initially appear normal or show only slight edema with loss of gray-white matter distinction (Figure 4–10). MRI scans, however, show marked hyperintensity on the diffusion-weighted image, indicating ischemia. Symptoms may be relieved by early use of thrombolytic agents,[186] but only if the stroke is identified and treated within a few hours of onset. There are currently no neuroprotective agents that have demonstrated effectiveness. Patients with massive infarcts should be given good supportive care to ensure adequate blood flow, oxygen, and nutrients to the brain, but hyperglycemia should be avoided as it worsens the outcome.[187,188] These patients are best treated in a stroke unit[189]; they should be watched carefully for the development of brain edema and increased ICP.

Although impairment of consciousness is rare as an immediate result of carotid occlusion, it may occur 2 to 4 days after acute infarction in the carotid territory, as edema of the infarcted hemisphere causes compression of the other hemisphere and the diencephalon, and may even result in uncal or central herniation.[186,190] This problem is presaged by increasing lethargy and pupillary changes suggesting either central or uncal herniation. Many patients who survive the initial infarct succumb during this period. The swelling does not respond to corticosteroids as it is cytotoxic in origin. It may be diminished transiently with mannitol or hypertonic saline,[191] but these agents soon equilibrate across the blood-brain barrier and cease to draw fluid out of the brain, if they ever did[192,193] (see Chapter 7). Surgical resection of the infarcted tissue may improve survival,[194,195] but this approach often results in a severely impaired outcome. Decompressive craniotomy (removing bone overlying the damaged hemisphere) may increase survival, but many of the patients have a poor neurologic outcome.[196]

Distal Basilar Occlusion

Distal basilar occlusion typically presents with a characteristic set of findings (the "top of the basilar syndrome") that can include impairment

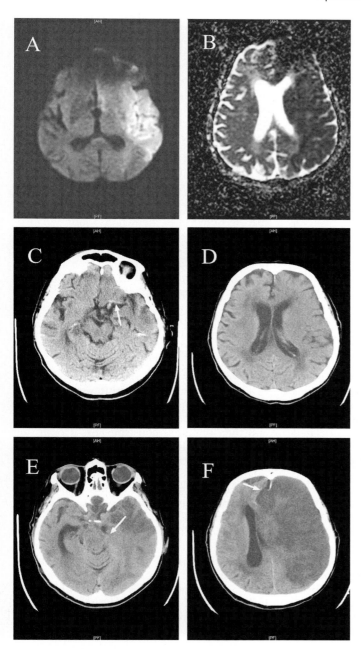

Figure 4–10. Development of cerebral edema and herniation in a patient with a left middle cerebral artery infarct. A 90-year-old woman with hypertension and diabetes had sudden onset of global aphasia, right hemiparesis, and left gaze preference. (A) A diffusion-weighted magnetic resonance imaging scan and (B) an apparent diffusion coefficient (ADC) map, which identify the area of acute infarction as including both the anterior and middle cerebral artery territories. The initial computed tomography scan (C, D) identified a dense left middle cerebral artery (arrow), indicating thrombosis, and swelling of the sulci on the left compared to the right, consistent with the region of restricted diffusion shown on the ADC map. By 48 hours after admission, there was massive left cerebral edema, with the medial temporal lobe herniation compressing the brainstem (arrow E) and subfalcine herniation of the left cingulate gyrus (arrow in F) and massive midline shift and compression of the left lateral ventricle. The patient died shortly after this scan.

of consciousness.[197] The basilar arteries give rise to the posterior cerebral arteries, which perfuse the caudal medial part of the hemispheres. The posterior cerebral arteries also give rise to posterior choroidal arteries, which perfuse the caudal part of the hippocampal formation, the globus pallidus, and the lateral geniculate nucleus.[198] In addition, thalamoperforating arteries originating from the basilar tip, posterior cerebral arteries, and posterior communicating arteries supply the caudal part of the thalamus.[199] Occlusion of the distal posterior cerebral arteries causes bilateral blindness, paresis, and memory loss. Some patients who are blind deny their condition (Anton's syndrome). However, the infarction does not cause loss of consciousness. On the other hand, more proximal occlusion of the basilar artery that reduces perfusion of the junction of the midbrain with the posterior thalamus and hypothalamus bilaterally can cause profound coma.[197,200–202]

Isolated *thalamic infarction* can cause a wide variety of cognitive problems, depending on which feeding vessels are occluded (Table 4–14). Castaigne and colleagues[203] and others[204] have provided a comprehensive analysis of clinical syndromes related to occlusion of each vessel (Table 4–12). Surprisingly, even bilateral thalamic injuries are typically not associated with a depressed level of consciousness unless there is some involvement of the paramedian mesencephalon.[205,206] Most such patients become more responsive within a few days, although the prognosis for full recovery is poor.[207]

Venous Sinus Thrombosis

The venous drainage of the brain is susceptible to thrombosis in the same way as other venous circulations.[208] Most often, this occurs during a hypercoagulable state, related either to dehydration, infection, or childbirth, or associated with a systemic neoplasm.[209,210] The thrombosis may begin in a draining cerebral vein, or it may involve mainly one or more of the dural sinuses. The most common of these conditions is thrombosis of the superior sagittal sinus.[210] Such patients complain of a vertex headache, which is usually quite severe. There is increased ICP, which may be as high as 60 cm of water on lumbar puncture and often causes papilledema. The CSF pressure may be sufficiently high to impair brain perfusion. There is also an increase in venous back-pressure in the brain (due to poor venous drainage), and so the arteriovenous pressure gradient is further reduced, and cerebral perfusion is at risk. This causes local edema and sometimes frank infarction. For example, in sagittal sinus thrombosis, the impaired venous outflow from the paramedian walls of the cerebral hemisphere may result in bilateral lower extremity hyperreflexia and extensor plantar responses, and sometimes even paraparesis. Extravasation into the infarcted tissue, due to continued high

perfusion pressure, causes local hemorrhage, hemorrhagic CSF, and seizures.

Thrombosis of the lateral sinus causes pain in the region behind the ipsilateral ear. The thrombosis may be associated with mastoiditis, in which case the pain due to the sinus thrombosis may be overlooked. If the outflow through the other lateral sinus remains patent, there may be little or no change in CSF pressure. However, the lateral sinuses are often asymmetric, and if the dominant one is occluded, there may not be sufficient venous outflow from the intracranial space. This may cause impairment of CSF outflow as well, a condition that is sometimes known as "otitic hydrocephalus." There typically is also venous stasis in the adjacent ventrolateral wall of the temporal lobe. Infarction in this area may produce little in the way of focal signs, but hemorrhage into the infarcted tissue may produce seizures.

Thrombosis of superficial cortical veins may be associated with local cortical dysfunction, but more often may present with seizures and focal headache.[211] Thrombosis of deep cerebral veins, such as the internal cerebral veins or vein of Galen, or even in the straight sinus generally presents as a rapidly progressive syndrome with headache, nausea and vomiting, and then impaired consciousness progressing to coma.[212,213] Impaired blood flow in the thalamus and upper midbrain may lead to venous infarction, hemorrhage, and coma. Venous thrombosis associated with coma generally has a poor prognosis, whereas awake and alert patients usually do well.[210]

Venous occlusion is suggested when the pattern of infarction does not match an arterial distribution, especially if the infarct contains a region of hemorrhage. However, in many cases of venous sinus thrombosis, there will be little, if any, evidence of focal brain injury. In those cases, the main clues will often be elevated pressure with or without red cells in the CSF. Sometimes lack of blood flow in the venous sinus system will be apparent even on routine CT or MRI scan, although often it is not clearly evident. Either CT or MR venogram can easily make the diagnosis, but neither is a routine study, and unless the examining physician thinks of the diagnosis and asks for the study, the diagnosis may be overlooked. Although no controlled trials prove efficacy,[214]

Table 4–12 Thalamic Arterial Supply and Principal Clinical Features of Focal Infarction

Thalamic Blood Vessel	Nuclei Irrigated	Clinical Features Reported
Tuberothalamic artery (arises from middle third of posterior communicating artery)	Reticular, intralaminar, VA, rostral VL, ventral pole of MD, anterior nuclei (AD, AM, AV), ventral internal medullary lamina, ventral amygdalofugal pathway, mamillothalamic tract	Fluctuating arousal and orientation Impaired learning, memory, autobiographic memory Superimposition of temporally unrelated information Personality changes, apathy, abulia Executive failure, perseveration True to hemisphere: language if VL involved on left; hemispatial neglect if right sided Emotional expression, acalculia, apraxia
Paramedian artery (arises from P1 segment of posterior cerebral artery)	MD, intralaminar (CM, Pf, CL), posteromedial VL, ventromedial pulvinar, paraventricular, LD, dorsal internal medullary lamina	Decreased arousal (coma vigil if bilateral) Impaired learning and memory, confabulation, temporal disorientation, poor autobiographic memory Aphasia if left sided, spatial deficits if right sided Altered social skills and personality, including apathy, aggression, agitation
Inferolateral artery (arises from P2 segment of posterior cerebral artery)		
Principal inferolateral branches	Ventroposterior complexes: VPM, VPL, VPl Ventral lateral nucleus, ventral (motor) part	Sensory loss (variable extent, all modalities) Hemiataxia Hemiparesis Postlesion pain syndrome (Dejerine-Roussy): right hemisphere predominant
Medial branches	Medial geniculate	Auditory consequences
Inferolateral pulvinar branches	Rostral and lateral pulvinar, LD nucleus	Behavioral
Posterior choroidal artery (arises from P2 segment of posterior cerebral artery)		
Lateral branches	LGN, LD, LP, inferolateral parts of pulvinar	Visual field loss (hemianopsia, quadrantanopsia)
Medial branches	MGN, posterior parts of CM and CL, pulvinar	Variable sensory loss, weakness, aphasia, memory impairment, dystonia, hand tremor

Modified from Schmahmann,[197] with permission.

Table 4–13 **Symptoms and Signs in 78 Reported Cases of Patients With Documented Central Nervous System Granulomatous Angitis**

Symptom/Sign	No. at Onset	Total No. Recorded During the Course of the Disease
Mental changes	45	61
Headache	42	42
Coma	0	42
Focal weakness	12	33
Seizure	9	18
Fever	16	16
Ataxia	7	11
Aphasia	4	10
Visual changes (diplopia, amaurosis, and blurring)	7	9
Tetraparesis	0	9
Flaccid or spastic paraparesis (with back pain, sensory level, and urinary incontinence)	7	8

From Younger et al.,[217] with permission.

anticoagulation and thrombolytic therapy are believed to be effective[210,215]; some thrombi recanalize spontaneously.

Vasculitis

Vasculitis affecting the brain either can occur as part of a systemic disorder[216] (e.g., polyarteritis nodosa, Behçet's syndrome) or can be restricted to the nervous system (e.g., CNS granulomatous angiitis).[217] The disorder can affect large or small vessels. Vasculitis causes impairment of consciousness by ischemia or infarction that either affects the hemispheres diffusely or the brainstem arousal systems. The diagnosis can be suspected in a patient with headache, fluctuating consciousness, and focal neurologic signs (Table 4–13). Granulomatous angiitis, the most common CNS vasculitis, is discussed here. Other CNS vasculopathies are discussed in Chapter 5 (see page 273).

The CSF may contain an increased number of lymphocytes or may be normal. The CT scan may likewise be normal, but MRI usually demonstrates areas of ischemia or infarction. Magnetic resonance angiography may demonstrate multifocal narrowing of small blood vessels or may be normal. High-resolution arteriography

is more likely to demonstrate small vessel abnormalities. A definitive diagnosis can be made only by biopsy. Even then, because of sampling error, biopsy may not establish the diagnosis. The treatment depends on the cause of vasculitis; most of the disorders are immune mediated and are treated by immunosuppression, usually with corticosteroids and cyclophosphamide.[218]

INFECTIONS AND INFLAMMATORY CAUSES OF SUPRATENTORIAL DESTRUCTIVE LESIONS

Viral Encephalitis

Although bacteria, fungi, and parasites can all invade the brain (encephalitis) with or without involvement of the meninges (meningoencephalitis), they tend to form localized infections. Viral encephalitis, by distinction, is often widespread and bilateral, and hence coma is a common feature. The organisms destroy tissue both by direct invasion and as a result of the immune response to the infectious agent. They may further impair neurologic function as toxins

Table 4–14 **Findings in 113 Patients With Herpes Simplex Encephalitis**

	No. (%) of Patients		No. (%) of Patients
Historic Findings		*Clinical Findings at Presentation*	
Alteration of consciousness	109/112 (97)		
Cerebrospinal fluid pleocytosis	107/110 (97)	Fever	101/110 (92)
Fever	101/112 (90)	Personality change	69/81 (85)
Headache	89/110 (81)	Dysphasia	58/76 (76)
Personality change	62/87 (71)	Autonomic dysfunction	53/88 (60)
Seizures	73/109 (67)	Ataxia	22/55 (40)
Vomiting	51/111 (46)	Hemiparesis	41/107 (38)
Hemiparesis	33/100 (33)	Seizures	43/112 (38)
Memory loss	14/59 (24)	Focal	28
Cranial nerve defects	34/105 (32)	Generalized	10
		Both	5
		Visual field loss	8/58 (14)
		Papilledema	16/111 (14)

From Whitley et al.,[220] with permission.

produced by the organisms or cytokines or prostaglandins in response to the presence of the organisms may interfere with neuronal function.

Although many different organisms can cause encephalitis, including a number of mosquito-borne viruses with regional variations in prevalence (eastern and western equine, St. Louis, Japanese, and West Nile viruses), *by far the most common and serious cause of sporadic encephalitis is herpes simplex type I*.[219] This disorder accounts for 10% to 20% of all viral infections of the CNS. Patients characteristically have fever, headache, and alteration of consciousness that culminate in coma (Table 4–14). Personality changes, memory impairment, or seizures focus attention on the medial temporal, frontal, and insular areas, where the infection usually begins and is most severe.

Routine examination of CSF is not very helpful. There is usually a pleocytosis with a white count of as many as 100 cells and a protein concentration averaging 100 mg/dL. Red cells may or may not be present. As many as 10% of patients may have a normal CSF examination when initially seen. However, polymerase chain reaction (PCR) detection of herpes simplex virus in CSF is diagnostic. The EEG may be helpful if it shows slowing or epileptiform activity arising from the temporal lobe. CT and MRI are very helpful, showing edema and then destruction predominantly in the temporal and frontal lobes, and often in the insular cortex (Figure 4–11). The destruction can initially be unilateral but usually rapidly becomes bilateral. The differential diagnosis includes other forms of encephalitis including bacteria and viruses, and even low-grade astrocytomas of the medial temporal lobe, which may present with seizures and a subtle low density lesion.

It is very important to begin treatment as early as possible with an antiviral agent such as acyclovir at 10 mg/kg every 8 hours for 10 to 14 days.[221] Most patients who are treated promptly make a full recovery, although an occasional patient is left with severe memory loss.

Acute Disseminated Encephalomyelitis

Acute disseminated encephalomyelitis (ADEM) is an allergic, presumably autoimmune, encephalitis that is seen during or after an infectious illness, but which may also be caused by vaccination. Spontaneous sporadic cases are believed to result from a subclinical infectious illness.[222,223] Patients develop multifocal neurologic symptoms, usually over a period of several days, about 1 to 2 weeks after a febrile illness. Neurologic signs may include a wide variety of sensory and motor complaints, as they do in patients with multiple sclerosis, but a

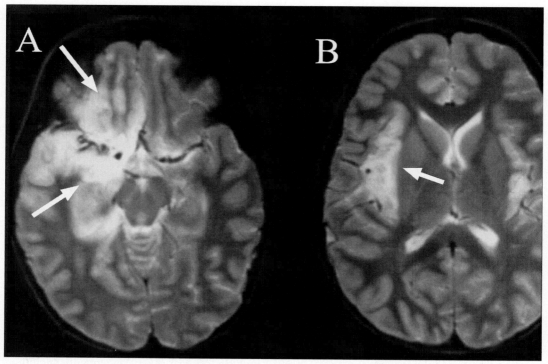

Figure 4–11. A pair of magnetic resonance images from the brain of a patient with herpes simplex 1 encephalitis. Note the preferential involvement of the medial temporal lobe and orbitofrontal cortex (arrows in A) and insular cortex (arrow in B). There is milder involvement of the contralateral side.

key differentiating point is that a much larger percentage of patients with ADEM present with behavioral disturbances, whereas this is rare early in multiple sclerosis. Occasionally patients with ADEM may become stuporous or comatose (see Patient 4–4), findings that are also rare in early multiple sclerosis. CT or MRI scan shows multifocal enhancing lesions in the white matter, but these may appear late in the illness (see Patient 4–4). Although the pathology is distinct from multiple sclerosis, showing mainly perivascular infiltration and demyelination, the appearance of the lesions on MRI scan is essentially identical in the two illnesses. CSF may show 100 or more white blood cells and an elevation of protein, but may show no changes at all; oligoclonal bands are often absent.

In most cases, it is difficult to distinguish ADEM from first onset of multiple sclerosis. The likelihood of ADEM is increased if the patient has recently had a febrile illness, if the illness is dominated by behavioral or cogni-

tive problems or impairment of consciousness, or if there are large plaques in the hemispheric white matter. However, the proof of the diagnosis is established by the course of the illness. Although ADEM can fluctuate, and new symptoms and plaques can continue to appear for up to several weeks, it is essentially a monotonic illness, whereas new lesions appearing after 1 or more months generally portend the diagnosis of multiple sclerosis. Overall, in various series approximately one-third of patients initially diagnosed with ADEM go on to develop multiple sclerosis.

Treatment of ADEM also differs from multiple sclerosis. Although there has been no randomized, controlled series, in our experience patients often improve dramatically with oral prednisone, 40 to 60 mg daily. The dose is then tapered to the lowest maintenance level that does not allow recrudescence of symptoms. However, the patient may require oral steroid treatment for months, or even a year or two.

Patient 4–4

A 42-year-old secretary had pharyngitis, fever, nausea, and vomiting, followed 3 days later by confusion and progressive leg weakness. She came to the emergency department, where she was found to have a stiff neck, left abducens palsy, and moderate leg weakness, with a sensory level at around T8 to pin. She rapidly became stuporous, then comatose, with flaccid quadriplegia.

Spinal fluid showed 81 white blood cells/mm^3, with 87% lymphocytes, protein 66 mg/dL, and glucose 66 mg/dL. An MRI scan of the brain and the spinal cord, including contrast, at the time of onset of impaired consciousness and then again 2 days later did not show any abnormalities. She required intubation and mechanical ventilation. A repeat MRI scan on day 8 demonstrated patchy, poorly marginated areas of T2 signal hyperintensity in the white matter of both cerebral hemispheres, the brainstem, and the cerebellum, consistent with ADEM. She was treated with corticosteroids and over a period of 3 months, recovered, finished rehabilitation, and was able to resume her career and playing tennis.

CONCUSSION AND OTHER TRAUMATIC BRAIN INJURIES

Traumatic brain injury, a common cause of coma, is usually easily established because there is a history or external signs of head injury at the time of presentation. Nevertheless, because so many traumatic events occur in individuals who are already impaired by drug ingestion or comorbid illnesses (e.g., hypoglycemia in a diabetic), other causes of loss of consciousness must always be considered. The nature of the traumatic intracranial process that produces impairment of consciousness requires rapid evaluation, as compressive processes such as epidural or subdural hematoma may need immediate surgical intervention. Once these have been ruled out, however, the underlying traumatic brain injury may itself be sufficient to cause coma.

Traumatic brain injury that causes coma falls into two broad classes: closed head trauma and direct brain injury as a result of penetrating head trauma. Penetrating head trauma may directly injure the ascending arousal system, or it may lead to hemorrhage or edema that further impairs brain function. These issues have been discussed in Chapter 3. An additional consideration is that trauma sufficient to cause head injury may also involve the neck, with dissection of a carotid or vertebral artery. These considerations are covered in the sections on vascular occlusions. The discussion that follows will focus primarily on the injuries that occur to the brain as a result of closed head trauma.

Mechanism of Brain Injury During Closed Head Trauma

During closed head trauma, several physical forces may act upon the brain to cause injury. If the injuring force is applied focally, the skull is briefly distorted and a shock wave is transmitted to the underlying brain. This shock wave can be particularly intense when the skull is struck a glancing blow by a high-speed projectile, such as a bullet. As demonstrated in Patient 3–2, the bullet need not penetrate the skull or even fracture the bone to transmit enough kinetic energy to injure the underlying brain.

A second mechanism of injury occurs when the initial blow causes the head to snap backward or forward, to the point where it is stopped either by the limits of neck movement or by another solid object (a wall or floor, a head restraint in a car, etc.). The initial blow causes the skull to accelerate against the underlying brain, which floats semi-independently in a pool of CSF. The brain then accelerates to the same speed as the skull, but when the skull's trajectory is suddenly stopped, the brain continues onward to strike the inner table of the skull opposite the original site of the blow (Figure 4–12). This *coup-contrecoup injury* model was first described by Courville (1950) and then documented in the pioneering studies by Gurdjian,[224] who used high-speed motion pictures to capture the brain and skull movements in monkeys in whom the calvaria had been replaced by a plastic dome. If the initial blow is occipital, frontal and temporal lobe damage may be worse than the damage at the site of the blow because of the conformation of the skull, which is smoothly curved at the occipital pole but comes to a narrow angle at

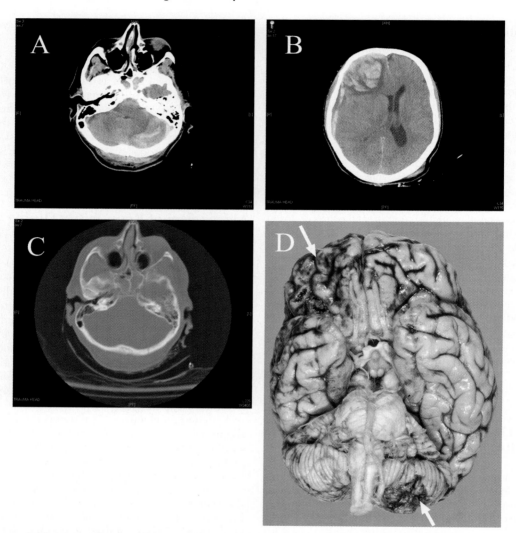

Figure 4–12. A series of computed tomography (CT) scans, and postmortem brain examination, of a 74-year-old woman who fell down a flight of stairs. She was initially alert and confused, but rapidly slipped into coma, which progressed to complete loss of brainstem reflexes by the time she arrived at the hospital. CT scan showed left cerebellar contusion (A) underlying an occipital fracture (C). There was a right frontal intraparenchymal hematoma and subdural hematoma (B). The cerebellar and frontal contusions could be seen from the surface of the brain at autopsy to demonstrate a coup (occipital injury) and contrecoup (frontal contusion from impact against the inside of the skull) injury pattern (arrows in D).

the frontal and temporal poles. As a result of this anatomy, it is not unusual for the greatest damage to the brain to occur at these poles, regardless of where the head is hit. Even in the absence of parenchymal brain damage, movement of the brain may shear off the delicate olfactory nerve fibers exiting the skull through the cribriform plate, causing anosmia.

Brain injury as a result of closed head trauma may be either a contusion (an area of brain edema visualized on CT or MRI) or focal hemorrhage. Even when no hemorrhage is seen initially on scan, it is not unusual for CSF to show some blood if a lumbar puncture is done. The hemorrhage itself is typically not large enough to cause brain injury or dysfunction. However, the blood may incite seizure activity. Seizures occurring at the time of the head injury do not necessarily herald a subsequent seizure disorder. Nevertheless, seizures themselves and the following postictal state may complicate the evaluation of the degree of brain injury.

A third mechanism of brain injury is due to shearing force on long axonal tracts. Because the long axis of the brainstem is located at about an 80-degree angle with respect to the long axis of the forebrain, the long tracts connecting the forebrain with the brainstem and spinal cord take an abrupt turn at the mesodiencephalic junction. In addition, because the head is tethered to the neck, which is not displaced by a blow to the head, there is an additional rotational displacement of the head, depending on the angle of the blow. These movements of the forebrain with respect to the brainstem produce a transverse sheering force at the mesodiencephalic juncture, resulting in diffuse axonal injury to the long tracts that run between the forebrain and brainstem.[225-228]

Mechanism of Loss of Consciousness in Concussion

The term *concussion* refers to transient alteration in mental status that may or may not involve loss of consciousness, resulting from trauma to the brain.[229-231] Although the most dramatic symptom of concussion is transient coma, the hallmarks of the disorder are amnesia and confusion; other symptoms may include headache, visual disturbances, and dizziness.

The mechanism of loss of consciousness with a blow to the head is not completely understood. However, in experiments by Gennarelli and colleagues, using an apparatus to accelerate the heads of monkeys without skull impact, rotational acceleration in the sagittal plane typically produced only brief loss of consciousness, whereas acceleration from the lateral direction caused mainly prolonged and severe coma.[227] Brief loss of consciousness, which in humans is usually not associated with any changes on CT or MRI scan, may be due to the shearing forces transiently applied to the ascending arousal system at the mesodiencephalic junction. Physiologically, the concussion causes abrupt neuronal depolarization and promotes release of excitatory neurotransmitters. There is an efflux of potassium from cells with calcium influx into cells and sequestration in mitochondria leading to impaired oxidative metabolism. There are also alterations in cerebral blood flow and glucose metabolism, all of which impair neuronal and axonal function.[231]

Longer term loss of consciousness may be due to mechanical injury to the brain, a condition that Adams and colleagues termed *diffuse axonal injury*.[225] Examination of the brains of animals with prolonged unconsciousness in the Gennarelli experiments was associated with diffuse axonal injury (axonal retraction balls and microglial clusters in the white matter, indicating a site of injury) and with hemorrhagic injury to the corpus callosum and to the dorsal surface of the mesopontine junction. These sites underlie the free edge of the falx and the tentorium, respectively. Hence, in these cases the brain displacement is presumably severe enough to hammer the free dural edges against the underlying brain with sufficient force to cause local tissue necrosis and hemorrhage. Similar pathology was seen in 45 human cases of traumatic closed head injury, all of whom died without awakening after the injury.[225,226] Contusion or hemorrhage into the corpus callosum or dorsolateral mesopontine tegmentum may be visible on MRI scan, but diffuse axonal injury generally is not. Magnetic resonance spectroscopy may be useful in evaluating patients with diffuse axonal injury, who typically have a reduction in N-acetylaspartate as well as elevation of glutamate/glutamine and choline/creatinine ratios.[232-234]

Delayed Encephalopathy After Head Injury

In some cases after an initial period of unconsciousness after a closed head injury, the patient may awaken and the CT scan may be normal, but then the patient may show cognitive deterioration and lapse into coma hours to several days later. This pattern was characterized by Reilly and colleagues as patients who "talk and die."[10,235] Repeat CT scan typically shows areas of intraparenchymal edema and perhaps hemorrhage, which may have shown only minimal injury at the time of initial presentation. However, with the evolution of brain edema over the next few hours and days, the mass effect may reach a critical level at which it impairs cerebral perfusion or causes brain herniation.

This condition occurs most commonly in children and young adults in whom the brain usually fully occupies the intracranial space, so that even minimal swelling may put the brain at risk of injury. Elderly individuals, in whom there has been some cerebral atrophy, may have enough excess intracranial capacity to avoid reaching this crossroad. On the other hand, older individuals may be more likely to deteriorate later due to subdural or epidural hemorrhage or to injuries outside the nervous system.[10] Hence, any patient with deterioration of wakefulness in the days following head injury requires repeat and urgent scanning, even if the original scan was normal.

More common is the so-called postconcussion syndrome. This disorder is characterized by headache, dizziness, irritability, and difficulty with memory and attention after mild concussion and particularly after repeated concussions.[236] Because it often follows mild head injury, psychologic factors have been imputed by some, but the syndrome clearly appears to result from mild although not anatomically identifiable brain damage.[237]

INFRATENTORIAL DESTRUCTIVE LESIONS

Infratentorial destructive lesions causing coma include hemorrhage, tumors, infections, and infarcts in the brainstem. Although hemorrhage into tumors, infections, or masses also compress normal tissue, they appear to have their major effect in the brainstem through direct destruction of arousal systems.

If the lesion is large enough, patients with destructive infratentorial lesions often lose consciousness immediately, and the ensuing coma is accompanied by distinctive patterns of respiratory, pupillary, oculovestibular, and motor signs that clearly indicate whether it is the tegmentum of the midbrain, the rostral pons, or the caudal pons that initially is most severely damaged. The brainstem arousal system lies so close to nuclei and pathways influencing the pupils, eye movements, and other major functions that primary brainstem destructive lesions that cause coma characteristically cause focal neurologic signs that can precisely localize the lesion anatomically. This restricted, discrete localization is unlike metabolic lesions causing coma, where the signs commonly indicate incomplete but symmetric dysfunction and few, if any, focal signs of brainstem dysfunction

(see Chapter 2). Primary brainstem injury also is unlike the secondary brainstem dysfunction that follows supratentorial herniation, in which *all* functions above a given brainstem level tend to be lost as the process descends from rostral to caudal along the neuraxis.

Certain combinations of signs stand out prominently in patients with infratentorial destructive lesions causing coma. At the *midbrain* level, centrally placed brainstem lesions interrupt the pathway for the pupillary light reflex and often damage the oculomotor nuclei as well. The resulting deep coma commonly is accompanied by pupils that are fixed at midposition or slightly wider, by abnormalities of eye movements due to damage to the third or fourth nerves or their nuclei, and by long-tract motor signs. These last-mentioned signs result from involvement of the cerebral peduncles and commonly are bilateral, although asymmetric.

Destructive lesions of the *rostral pons* commonly spare the oculomotor nuclei but interrupt the medial longitudinal fasciculus and the adjacent ocular sympathetic pathways. Patients typically have tiny pupils, internuclear ophthalmoplegia (only lateral movements of the eyes on vestibulo-ocular testing), and, in many instances, cranial nerve signs of trigeminal or facial dysfunction, betraying pontine destruction.

Severe *midpontine destruction* can cause a functional transection with physiologic effects that may be difficult to differentiate from metabolic coma. The pupils of such patients are miotic but may react minimally to light since midbrain parasympathetic oculomotor fibers are spared. Reflex lateral eye movements are absent because the pontine structures for lateral conjugate eye movements are destroyed. However, upward and downward ocular deviation occasionally is retained either spontaneously or in response to vestibulo-ocular testing, and if present, this dissociation between lateral and vertical movement clearly identifies pontine destruction. Ocular bobbing sometimes accompanies such acute destructive lesions and when present usually, but not always, indicates primary posterior fossa disease. The motor signs of severe pontine destruction are not the same in every patient and can include flaccid quadriplegia, less often extensor posturing, or occasionally extensor posturing responses in the arms with flexor responses or flaccidity in the legs. Respiration may show any of the patterns characteristic of low brainstem dysfunction described in Chapter 1, but cluster breathing, apneusis, gasping, and ataxic breathing are characteristic.

As discussed in Chapter 2, patients with destructive lesions confined to the lower pons or medulla do not show loss of consciousness, although they may be locked in, in which case only the preservation of voluntary vertical eye and eyelid movements may indicate the wakeful state.

BRAINSTEM VASCULAR DESTRUCTIVE DISORDERS

In contrast to the carotid circulation, occlusion of the vertebrobasilar system is frequently associated with coma. Although lesions confined to the lower brainstem do not cause coma, impairment of blood flow in the vertebral or low basilar arteries may reduce blood flow distally in the basilar artery to a level that is below the critical minimum necessary to maintain normal function. The classic presentation of ischemic coma of brainstem origin is produced by occlusion of the basilar artery. The patient falls acutely into a comatose state, and the pupils may initially be large, usually indicating intense adrenal outflow at the time of the initial onset, but eventually become either miotic (pontine level occlusion) or fixed and midposition (midbrain level occlusion). Oculovestibular eye movements may be absent, asymmetric, or skewed (pontine level), or vertical and adduction movements may be absent with preserved abduction (midbrain level). There may be hemiplegia, quadriplegia, or decerebrate posturing. Respiration may be apneustic or ataxic in pattern if the lesion also involves the pons.

Occlusion of the basilar artery either by thrombosis or embolism is a relatively common cause of coma. The occlusions are usually the result of atherosclerotic or hypertensive disease. Emboli to the basilar artery usually result from valvular heart disease or artery-to-artery embolization.[238] Cranial arteritis involving the vertebral arteries in the neck also can lead to secondary basilar artery ischemia with brainstem infarction and coma.[239] Vertebrobasilar artery dissection, either from trauma such as whiplash injury or chiropractic manipulation[240] or occurring spontaneously, is becoming increasingly recognized as a common cause of brainstem infarction, due to the ease of identifying it on MR angiography.[241]

Most patients in coma from brainstem infarction are over 50 years of age, but this is not an exclusive limit. One of our patients was only 34 years old. The onset can be sudden coma or progressive neurologic symptoms culminating in coma. In some patients, characteristic transient symptoms and signs owing to brief ischemia of the brainstem precede coma by days or weeks.[242] These transient attacks typically change from episode to episode but always reflect infratentorial CNS dysfunction and include headaches (mainly occipital), diplopia, vertigo (usually with nausea), dysarthria, dysphagia, bilateral or alternating motor or sensory symptoms, or drop attacks (sudden spontaneous falls while standing or walking, without loss of consciousness and with complete recovery in seconds). The attacks usually last for as short a period as 10 seconds or as long as several minutes. Seldom are they more prolonged, although we have seen recurrent transient attacks of otherwise unexplained akinetic coma lasting 20 to 30 minutes in a patient who later died from pontine infarction caused by basilar occlusion. Except in patients who additionally have recurrent asystole or other severe cardiac arrhythmias, transient ischemic attacks caused by vertebrobasilar artery insufficiency nearly always occur in the erect or sitting position. Some patients with a critical stenosis may have positional symptoms, which are present while sitting but improve when lying down.

Patient 4–5

A 78-year-old architect with hypertension and diabetes was returning on an airplane from Europe to the United States when he complained of dizziness, double vision, and nausea, then collapsed back into his seat unconscious. His seat was laid back and he gradually regained consciousness. A neurologist was present on the airplane and was called to his side. Limited neurologic examination found that he was drowsy, with small but reactive pupils and lateral gaze nystagmus to either side. There was dysmetria with both hands.

On taking a history, he was returning from a vacation in Germany where he had similar symptoms and had been hospitalized for several weeks.

MRI scans, which he was carrying with him back to his doctors at home, showed severe stenosis of the midportion of the basilar artery. He had been kept at bedrest with the head of the bed initially down, but gradually raised to 30 degrees while in the hospital, and then discharged when he could sit without symptoms. His chair back was kept as low as possible for the remainder of the flight, and he was taken from the airplane to a tertiary care hospital where he was treated with anticoagulants and gradual readjustment to an upright posture.

In some cases, segmental thrombi can occlude the vertebral or basilar arteries while producing only limited and temporary symptoms of brainstem dysfunction.[242] In one series, only 31 of 85 patients with angiographically proved basilar or bilateral vertebral artery occlusion were stuporous or comatose.[242] The degree of impairment of consciousness presumably depends on how much the collateral vascular supply protects the central brainstem structures contributing to the arousal system. The clinical signs of basilar artery occlusion are listed in Table 4–15. Most unconscious patients have respiratory abnormalities, which may include periodic breathing, or various types of irregular or ataxic respiration. The pupils are almost always abnormal and may be small (pontine), midposition (midbrain), or dilated (third nerve outflow in midbrain). Most patients have divergent or skewed eyes reflecting direct nuclear and internuclear damage (Table 4–15). Patients with basilar occlusion who become comatose have a nearly uniformly fatal outcome in the absence of thrombolytic or endovascular intervention.[243]

The diagnosis can usually be made on the basis of clinical signs alone, and eye movement signs are particularly helpful in determining the brainstem level of the dysfunction (Table 4–16). However, the nature of the problem must be confirmed by imaging.

Acutely, the CT scan may not reveal a parenchymal lesion. Occasionally, hyperintensity

Table 4–15 Symptoms and Signs of Basilar Artery Occlusion in 85 Patients

Symptom	No. of Patients	Long Tract Signs	No. of Patients
Vertigo, nausea	39	Hemiparesis	21
Headache, neckache	22	Tetraparesis	31
Dysarthria	23	Tetraplegia	15
Ataxia, dysdiadochokinesia	27	Locked-in syndrome	9
Cranial nerve palsy		Hemihypesthesia	11
III	13		
IV, VI, VII	30	**Supranuclear Oculomotor Disturbances**	**No. of Patients**
VIII (acoustic)	5		
IX-XII	24	Horizontal gaze paresis	22
Occipital lobe signs	11	Gaze-paretic, gaze-induced nystagmus	15
Respiration	9		
Central Horner's syndrome	4	Oculocephalic reflex lost	6
Seizures	4	Vestibular nystagmus	5
Sweating	5	Vertical gaze palsy	4
Myoclonus	6	Downbeat nystagmus	4
		Internuclear ophthalmoplegia	4
Consciousness	**No. of Patients**	Ocular bobbing	3
		One-and-a-half syndrome	2
Awake	31	Other/not classifiable	16
Psychosis, disturbed memory	5		
Somnolence	20		
Stupor	5		
Coma	26		

Modified from Ferbert et al.[242]

Table 4–16 **Eye Movement Disorders in Brainstem Infarcts**

Midbrain Syndromes	Pons Syndromes
Upper Midbrain Syndromes	**Paramedian Syndromes**

Conjugate vertical gaze palsy: upgaze palsy, downgaze, palsy, combined upgaze and downgaze palsy	Conjugate disorders
	    Ipsilateral gaze paralysis
	    Complete gaze paralysis

Dorsal midbrain syndrome	Loss of ipsilateral horizontal saccades
Slowness of smooth pursuit movements	Loss of both horizontal and vertical saccadic
Torsional nystagmus	gaze movements
Pseudoabducens palsy	Primary-position downbeating nystagmus
Convergence-retraction nystagmus	Tonic conjugate eye deviation away from lesion
Disconjugate vertical gaze palsy: monocular elevation palsy, prenuclear syndrome of the oculomotor nucleus, crossed vertical gaze paresis, and vertical one-and-a half syndrome	from lesion
	Disconjugate disorders
	Unilateral internuclear ophthalmoplegia
	Bilateral internuclear ophthalmoplegia
	Internuclear ophthalmoplegia and
Skew deviation with alternating appearance	skew deviation
Ocular tilt reaction	One-and-a-half syndrome
See-saw nystagmus	Paralytic pontine exotropia
Middle Midbrain Syndrome	Ocular bobbing: typical, atypical, and paretic
Nuclear third nerve palsy	**Lateral Pontine Syndrome**
Fascicular third nerve palsy: isolated or associated with crossed hemiplegia, ipsilateral or contralateral hemiataxia, and abnormal movements	Horizontal gaze palsy
	Horizontal and rotatory nystagmus
	Skew deviation
	Internuclear ophthalmoplegia
Lower Midbrain Syndrome	Ocular bobbing
Internuclear ophthalmoplegia: isolated or associated with fourth nerve palsy, bilateral ataxia, and dissociated vertical nystagmus	One-and-a-half syndrome
Superior oblique myokymia	

Modified from Moncayo and Bogousslavsky.[244]

within the basilar artery on CT will suggest basilar occlusion.[245] The best diagnostic test is an MRI scan with diffusion-weighted imaging (see Figure 4–9B). Early diagnosis may allow effective treatment with thrombolysis,[246] angioplasty,[247] or embolectomy.[248] The differential diagnosis of acute brainstem infarction can usually be made from clinical clues alone. With brainstem infarction, the fact that signs of midbrain or pontine damage accompany the *onset* of coma immediately places the site of the lesion as infratentorial. The illness is maximal at onset or evolves rapidly and in a series of steps, as would be expected with ischemic vascular disease. Supratentorial ischemic vascular lesions, by contrast, with rare exceptions pointed out on page 152, are not likely to cause coma at onset, and they do not begin with pupillary abnormalities or other signs of direct brainstem injury (unless the mesencephalon is also

involved, e.g., as in the top of the basilar syndrome). Pontine and cerebellar hemorrhages, since they also compress the brainstem, sometimes resemble brainstem infarction in their manifestations. However, most such hemorrhages have a distinctive picture (see above). Furthermore, they nearly always arise in hypertensive patients and often are more likely to cause occipital headache (which is unusual with infarction).

Patient 4–6

A 56-year-old woman was admitted in coma. She had been an accountant and in good health, except for known hypertension treated with hydrochlorothiazide. She suddenly collapsed at her desk and was rushed to the emergency department, where her blood pressure was 180/100 mm Hg. She had sighing respirations, which shortly changed to a Cheyne-Stokes pattern. The pupils were 4 mm in diameter and unreactive to light. The oculocephalic responses were absent, but cold caloric irrigation induced abduction of the eye only on the side being irrigated. She responded to noxious stimuli with extensor posturing and occasionally was wracked by spontaneous waves of extensor rigidity.

CT scan was initially read as normal, and she was brought to the neurology intensive care unit. The CSF pressure on lumbar puncture was 140 mm of water; the fluid was clear, without cells, and contained 35 mg/dL of protein. Two days later, the patient continued in coma with extensor responses to noxious stimulation; the pupils remained fixed in midposition, and there was no ocular response to cold caloric irrigation. Respirations were eupneic. Repeat CT scan showed lucency in the medial pons and midbrain. The next day she died and the brain was examined postmortem. The basilar artery was occluded in its midportion by a recent thrombus 1 cm in length. There was extensive infarction of the rostral portion of the base of the pons, as well as the medial pontine and midbrain tegmentum. The lower portion of the pons and the medulla were intact.

Comment: This woman suffered an acute brainstem infarction with unusually symmetric neurologic signs. She was initially diagnosed with an infarct at the midbrain level based on her clinical picture. Other considerations included a thalamic hemorrhage with sudden acute transtentorial her-niation producing a picture of acute midbrain transection. However, such rapid progression to a midbrain level almost never occurs in patients with supratentorial intracerebral hemorrhages. The CT scan and the absence of red blood cells on the lumbar puncture ruled out subarachnoid hemorrhage as well. Finally, the neurologic signs of midbrain damage in this patient remained nearly constant from onset, whereas transtentorial herniation would rapidly have produced further rostral-caudal deterioration.

Brainstem Hemorrhage

Relatively discrete brainstem hemorrhage can affect the midbrain,[249] the pons,[250] or the medulla.[251] The causes of brainstem hemorrhage include hypertension, vascular malformations, clotting disorders, or trauma. Hypertensive brainstem hemorrhages tend to lie deep within the brainstem substance, are rather diffuse, frequently rupture into the fourth ventricle, occur in elderly persons, and have a poor prognosis for recovery.[252] Brainstem hematomas caused by vascular malformations occur in younger individuals, are usually subependymal in location, tend to be more discrete, do not rupture into the ventricle, and have a good prognosis for recovery. Surgery generally does not have a place in treating brainstem hypertensive hemorrhages, but it is sometimes possible to remove a vascular malformation, particularly a cavernous angioma.

Table 4–17 **Clinical Findings in Patients With Spontaneous Midbrain Hemorrhage**

Findings	Literature Cases (N = 66)	Mayo Cases (N = 7)	Combined Series (N = 73)
Cranial nerve III or IV paresis	58	6	64
Disturbance of consciousness	33	6	39
Headache	34	4	38
Corticospinal tract deficits	32	4	36
Corticobulbar deficits	22°	2	24
Hemisensory deficits	21	3	24
Gait ataxia	22	2	24
Visual hallucinations	3	0	3
Tinnitus or hyperacusis	3	2	5

°One patient had corticobulbar deficit without a corticospinal deficit.

From Link et al.,[249] with permission.

Primary *midbrain hemorrhages*, which may be of either type, are rare. Most patients present acutely with headache, alterations of consciousness, and abnormal eye signs (Table 4–17). The diagnosis is obvious on imaging. Most patients recover completely from bleeds from cavernous angiomas; some remain with mild neurologic deficits.

Hemorrhage into the pons typically arises from the paramedian arterioles, beginning at the base of the tegmentum, and usually dissecting in all directions in a relatively symmetric fashion (Figure 4–9A). Rupture into the fourth ventricle is frequent, but dissection into the medulla is rare. Although most patients lose consciousness immediately, in a few cases (such as Patient 2–1) this is delayed, and in others when the hematoma is small, and particularly when it is confined to the base of the pons, consciousness can be retained. However, such patients often have other focal signs (e.g., a bleed into the base of the pons can present with an acute locked-in state). Such patients, however, often have considerable recovery.[254]

Coma caused by pontine hemorrhage begins abruptly, usually during the hours when patients are awake and active and often without a prodrome. When the onset is witnessed, only a few patients complain of symptoms such as sudden occipital headache, vomiting, dyscoordination, or slurred speech before losing consciousness.[255] Almost every patient with pontine hemorrhage has respiratory abnormalities of the brainstem type: Cheyne-Stokes breathing, apneustic or gasping breathing, and progressive slowing of respiration or apnea[250] (Table 4–18).

In patients who present in coma, the pupils are nearly always abnormal and usually pinpoint. The pupils are often thought to be fixed to light on initial examination, but close examination with a magnifying glass usually demonstrates further constriction. The ciliospinal response disappears. If the hemorrhage extends into the midbrain, pupils may become asymmetric or dilate to midposition. About one-third of patients suffer from oculomotor abnormalities such as skewed or lateral ocular deviations or ocular bobbing (or one of its variants), and the oculocephalic responses disappear. Motor signs vary according to the extent of the hemorrhage. Some subjects become diffusely rigid, tremble, and suffer repeated waves

of decerebrate rigidity. More frequently, however, patients are quadriplegic and flaccid with flexor responses at the hip, knee, and great toe to plantar stimulation, a reflex combination characteristic of acute low brainstem damage when it accompanies acute coma. Nearly all patients with pontine hemorrhage who survive more than a few hours develop fever with body temperatures of 38.5°C to 40°C.[256,257]

The diagnosis of pontine hemorrhage is usually straightforward. Almost no other lesion, except an occasional cerebellar hemorrhage with secondary dissection into the brainstem, produces sudden coma with periodic or ataxic breathing, pinpoint pupils, absence of oculovestibular responses, and quadriplegia. The pinpoint pupils may suggest an opiate overdose, but the other eye signs and the flaccid quadriplegia are not seen in that condition. If there is any question in an ambiguous case, naloxone can be administered to reverse any opiate intoxication.

Table 4–18 Clinical Findings in 80 Patients With Pontine Hemorrhage

Level of Consciousness	
Alert	15 (0)
Drowsy	21 (3)
Stuporous	4 (3)
Coma	40 (32)
Respiratory Disturbance	
Yes	37 (29)
Brachycardia	
Yes	34 (23)
Hyperthermia	
Yes	32 (30)
Pupils	
Normal	29 (1)
Anisocoria	29 (11)
Pinpoint	23 (17)
Mydriasis	9 (9)
Motor Disturbance	
Hemiplegia	34 (4)
Tetraplegia	22 (17)
Decerebrate posture°	16 (14)

°Number that died in parentheses.

Modified from Murata.[250]

Patient 4–7

A 54-year-old man with poorly treated hypertension was playing tennis when he suddenly collapsed on the court. The blood pressure was 170/90 mm Hg; the pulse was 84 per minute; respirations were Cheyne-Stokes in character and 16 per minute. The pupils were pinpoint but reacted equally to light; eyes were slightly dysconjugate with no spontaneous movement, and vestibulo-ocular responses were absent. The patient was flaccid with symmetric stretch reflexes of normal amplitude and bilateral flexor withdrawal responses in the lower extremities to plantar stimulation. CT scan showed a hemorrhage into the pontine tegmentum. The next morning he was still in deep coma, but now was diffusely flaccid except for flexor responses to noxious stimuli in the legs. He had slow, shallow, eupneic respiration; small, equally reactive pupils; and eyes in the neutral position. Shortly thereafter, breathing became irregular and he died. A 3-cm primary hemorrhage destroying the central pons and its tegmentum was found at autopsy.

The clinical features in Patient 4–7, including coma in the absence of motor responses, corneal reflexes, and oculocephalic responses, predicted the poor outcome.[258] In addition, if CT scanning shows a hematoma greater than 4 mL, hemorrhage in a ventral location,[259] evidence of extension into the midbrain and thalamus, or hydrocephalus on admission, the prognosis is poor.[258]

Primary *hemorrhage into the medulla* is rare.[251] Patients present with ataxia, dysphagia, nystagmus, and tongue paralysis. Respiratory and cardiovascular area may occur, leaving the patient paralyzed and unable to breathe, but not unconscious.

Basilar Migraine

Altered states of consciousness are an uncommon but distinct aspect of what Bickerstaff called basilar artery migraine,[260] associated with prodromal symptoms that suggest brainstem dysfunction. The alteration in consciousness can take any of four major forms: confusional states, brief syncope, stupor, and unarousable coma. Although not technically a destructive lesion, and with a pathophysiology that is not understood, basilar migraine clearly causes parenchymal dysfunction of the brainstem that is often mistaken for a brainstem ischemic attack.

Alterations in consciousness often last longer than the usual sensorimotor auras seen with migraine. Encephalopathy and coma in migraine occur in patients with familial hemiplegic migraine associated with mutations in a calcium channel[261] and in patients with the disorder known as cerebral autosomal dominant arteriopathy with subcortical infarcts and leukoencephalopathy (CADASIL)[262] (see page 276, Chapter 5). The former often have fixed cerebellar signs and the latter multiple hyperintensities of the white matter on MR scanning. Blood flow studies concurrent with migraine aura have demonstrated both diffuse and focal cerebral vasoconstriction, but this is an insufficient explanation for the striking focal symptoms in basilar migraine; however, some clinical lesions suggestive of infarction can be found in patients with migraine significantly more often than in controls.[263]

Selby and Lance[264] observed that among 500 consecutive patients with migraine, 6.8% had prodromal episodes of confusion, automatic behavior, or transient amnesia, while 4.6% actually fainted. The confusional and stuporous attacks can last from minutes to as long as 24 hours or, rarely, more. They range in content from quiet disorientation through agitated delirium to unresponsiveness in which the patient is barely arousable. Transient vertigo, ataxia, diplopia, hemianopsia, hemisensory changes, or hemiparesis changes may immediately precede the mental changes. During attacks, most observers have found few somatic neurologic abnormalities, although occasional patients are reported as having oculomotor palsies, pupillary dilation, or an extensor plantar response. A few patients, at least briefly, have appeared to be in unarousable coma.

Posterior Reversible Leukoencephalopathy Syndrome

Once believed to be associated only with malignant hypertension (hypertensive encephalopathy),[265] posterior reversible leukoencephalopathy syndrome (PRES) is known to be caused by several illnesses that affect endothe-

Table 4–19 **Common Differential Diagnoses of Posterior Leukoencephalopathy Syndrome**

	Posterior Leukoencephalopathy	Central Venous Thrombosis	Top of Basilar Syndrome
Predisposing factors	Eclampsia, renal failure, cytotoxic and immunosuppressive agents, hypertension	Pregnancy, puerperium, dehydration	Risk factors for stroke, cardiac disorders
Onset and progression	Acute, evolves in days	Acute, evolves in days	Sudden, evolves in hours
Clinical features	Seizures precede all other manifestations, visual aura, cortical blindness, confusion, headache, rarely focal deficit	Headaches, seizures, stupor or coma, focal neurologic deficits (monoparesis or hemiparesis), papilledema, evidence of venous thrombosis elsewhere, infrequently hypertensive	Cortical blindness, hemianopia, confusional state, brainstem signs, cerebral signs, rarely seizures
Imaging features	Predominantly white matter edema in bilateral occipital and posterior parietal regions, usually spares paramedian brain parenchyma	Hemorrhage and ischemic infarcts, small ventricles, "cord sign" caused by hyperdense thrombosed vein, evidence of major venous sinus thrombosis on MRI	Infarcts of bilateral paracalcarine cortex, thalamus, inferior medial temporal lobe, and brainstem
Prognosis	Completely resolves after rapid control of BP and removal of offending drug	Intensive management is needed; mortality high in severe cases	No recovery or only partial eventual recovery

BP, blood pressure; MRI, magnetic resonance imaging.

From Garg,[266] with permission.

lial cells, particularly in the posterior cerebral circulation.[266] Among the illnesses other than hypertension, pre-eclampsia and immunosuppressive and cytotoxic agents (e.g., cyclosporin, cisplatin) are probably the most common causes. Vasculitis, porphyria, and thrombotic thrombocytopenic purpura are also reported causes, as is occasionally migraine. Posterior leukoencephalopathy is characterized by vasogenic edema of white matter of the posterior circulation, particularly the occipital lobes, but sometimes including the brainstem. Clinically, patients acutely develop headache, confusion, seizures, and cortical blindness; coma is rare. The MRI reveals vasogenic edema primarily affecting the occipital and posterior parietal lobes. Brainstem and cerebellum may also be affected. With appropriate treatment (controlling hypertension or discontinuing drugs), symptoms resolve. In patients with pre-eclampsia who are pregnant, intravenous infusion of magnesium sulfate followed by delivery of the fetus has a similar effect. If PRES due to pre-eclampsia occurs in the postpartum period, immediate administration of magnesium sulfate followed by treatment for several weeks with verapamil is often effective, in our experience. The differential diagnosis includes posterior circulation infarction, venous thrombosis, and metabolic coma (Table 4–19 and Patient 5–8).

INFRATENTORIAL INFLAMMATORY DISORDERS

The same infective agents that affect the cerebral hemispheres can also affect the brainstem and cerebellum. Encephalitis, meningitis, and abscess formation may either be part of a more generalized infective process or be

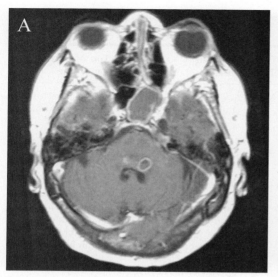 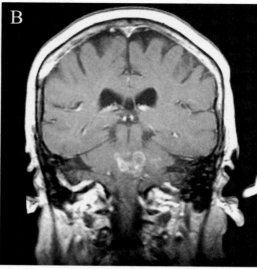

Figure 4–13. A pair of magnetic resonance images demonstrating a multiloculated pontine abscess in a 73-year-old woman (Patient 2–2) who had been taking chronic prednisone for ulcerative colitis. She developed a fever, nausea and vomiting, left facial numbness, left gaze paresis, left lower motor neuron facial weakness, and left-sided ataxia. Lumbar puncture showed 47 white blood cells/mm^3, but culture was negative. She was treated for suspected *Listeria mono-cytogenes* and recovered slowly, but had residual facial and oropharyngeal weakness requiring chronic tracheostomy.

restricted to the brainstem.[267] Organisms that have a particular predilection for the brainstem include *L. monocytogenes*, which often causes brainstem abscesses [268] (Figure 4–13). Occasionally herpes zoster or simplex infection that begins in one of the sensory cranial nerves may cause a segmental brainstem encephalitis.[269] Behçet's disease may also cause brainstem inflammatory lesions.[270] These disorders usually cause headache with or without nuchal rigidity, fever, and lethargy, but rarely coma. In a minority of instances, the CT scan may show brainstem swelling. The MR scan is usually more sensitive. CSF usually contains an increased number of cells. In bacterial infections cultures are usually positive; in viral infections PCR may establish the diagnosis. Stereotactic drainage of a brain abscess often identifies the organisms; appropriate antimicrobial therapy is usually successful.[271]

A brainstem disorder often confused with infection is Bickerstaff's brainstem encephalitis.[272] Patients with this disorder have often had a preceding systemic viral infection, then acutely develop ataxia, ophthalmoplegia, long-tract signs, and alterations of consciousness including coma. In some patients, MRI reveals brainstem swelling and increased T2 signal[273];

in others, the scan is normal. The CSF protein may be elevated, but there are no cells. The disease is believed to be autoimmune in origin related to postinfectious polyneuropathy (the Guillain-Barré syndrome) and the related Miller Fisher syndrome.[272] The diagnosis can be established by the identification of anti-GQ1b ganglioside antibodies in serum.[272] Patients recover spontaneously.

INFRATENTORIAL TUMORS

Tumors within the brainstem cause their symptoms by a combination of compression and destruction. Although relatively common in children, primary tumors of the brainstem (brainstem glioma) are rare in adults. Metastatic tumors are more common, but with both primary and metastatic tumors, slowly or subacutely evolving brainstem signs typically establish the diagnosis long before impairment of consciousness occurs. An exception is the rare instance of an acute hemorrhage into the tumor, causing the abrupt onset of paralysis and sometimes coma, in which case the signs and treatment are similar to other brainstem hemorrhages.

CENTRAL PONTINE MYELINOLYSIS

This is an uncommon disorder in which the myelin sheaths in the central basal pons are destroyed in a single confluent and symmetric lesion. Similar lesions may be found in the corpus callosum or cerebral hemispheres.[274] Lesions vary from a few millimeters across to ones that encompass almost the entire base of the pons, sparing only a rim of peripheral myelin. The typical clinical picture is one of quadriparesis, with varying degrees of supranuclear paresis of lower motor cranial nerves and impairment of oculomotor or pupillary responses. A majority of patients become "locked in." Approximately one-quarter of patients demonstrate impairment of level of consciousness, reflecting extension of the lesion into the more dorsal and rostral regions of the pons.

It is now recognized that most cases of central pontine myelinolysis are due to overly vigorous correction of hyponatremia, giving rise to the "osmotic demyelination syndrome." Since the adoption of current regimens that recommend that hyponatremia be reversed at a rate no greater than 10 mEq/day, the frequency of this once-feared complication has decreased dramatically. On the other hand, a similar syndrome is seen in patients with liver transplantation, possibly due to the use of cyclosporine.[274] As liver transplant has become more common, this population is increasing.

REFERENCES

1. Mut M, Cataltepe O, Bakar B, et al. Eosinophilic granuloma of the skull associated with epidural haematoma: a case report and review of the literature. Childs Nerv Syst 2004; 20, 765–769.
2. Simmons NE, Elias WJ, Henson SL, et al. Small cell lung carcinoma causing epidural hematoma: case report. Surg Neurol 1999; 51, 56–59.
3. Griffiths SJ, Jatavallabhula NS, Mitchell RD. Spontaneous extradural haematoma associated with craniofacial infections: case report and review of the literature. Br J Neurosurg 2002; 16, 188–191.
4. Miller DJ, Steinmetz M, McCutcheon IE. Vertex epidural hematoma: surgical versus conservative management: two case reports and review of the literature. Neurosurgery 1999; 45, 621–624.
5. Mishra A, Mohanty S. Contre-coup extradural haematoma: a short report. Neurol India 2001; 49, 94–95.
6. Sunderland S, Bradley KC. Disturbances of oculomotor function accompanying extradural haemorrhage. J Neurochem 1953; 16, 35–46.
7. Jamieson KG, Yelland JD. Extradural hematoma. Report of 167 cases. J Neurosurg 1968; 29, 13–23.
8. Gallagher JP, Browder EJ. Extradural hematoma. Experience with 167 patients. J Neurosurg 1968; 29, 1–12.
9. Browne GJ, Lam LT. Isolated extradural hematoma in children presenting to an emergency department in Australia. Pediatr Emerg Care 2002; 18, 86–90.
10. Dunn LT, Fitzpatrick MO, Beard D, et al. Patients with a head injury who "talk and die" in the 1990s. J Trauma 2003; 54, 497–502.
11. Mower WR, Hoffman JR, Herbert M, et al. Developing a decision instrument to guide computed tomographic imaging of blunt head injury patients. J Trauma 2005; 59, 954–959.
12. Stiell IG, Clement CM, Rowe BH, et al. Comparison of the Canadian CT Head Rule and the New Orleans Criteria in patients with minor head injury. JAMA 2005; 294, 1511–1518.
13. Zee CS, Go JL. CT of head trauma. Neuroimaging Clin N Am 1998; 8, 525–539.
14. Shimizu S, Endo M, Kan S, et al. Tight Sylvian cisterns associated with hyperdense areas mimicking subarachnoid hemorrhage on computed tomography—four case reports. Neurol Med Chir (Tokyo) 2001; 41, 536–540.
15. Servadei F, Teasdale G, Merry G. Defining acute mild head injury in adults: a proposal based on prognostic factors, diagnosis, and management. J Neurotrauma 2001; 18, 657–664.
16. Servadei F. Prognostic factors in severely head injured adult patients with epidural haematoma's. Acta Neurochir (Wien) 1997; 139, 273–278.
17. Servadei F, Piazza G, Seracchioli A, et al. Extradural haematomas: an analysis of the changing characteristics of patients admitted from 1980 to 1986. Diagnostic and therapeutic implications in 158 cases. Brain Inj 1988; 2, 87–100.
18. Sakas DE, Bullock MR, Teasdale GM. One-year outcome following craniotomy for traumatic hematoma in patients with fixed dilated pupils. J Neurosurg 1995; 82, 961–965.
19. Pozzati E, Tognetti F. Spontaneous resolution of acute extradural hematoma—study of twenty-five selected cases. Neurosurg Rev 1989; 12 (Suppl 1), 188–189.
20. Lin J, Hanigan WC, Tarantino M, et al. The use of recombinant activated factor VII to reverse warfarin-induced anticoagulation in patients with hemorrhages in the central nervous system: preliminary findings. J Neurosurg 2003; 98, 737–740.
21. Abe M, Udono H, Tabuchi K, et al. Analysis of ischemic brain damage in cases of acute subdural hematomas. Surg Neurol 2003; 59, 464–472.
22. Servadei F. Prognostic factors in severely head injured adult patients with acute subdural haematoma's. Acta Neurochir (Wien) 1997; 139, 279–285.
23. Adhiyaman V, Asghar M, Ganeshram KN, et al. Chronic subdural haematoma in the elderly. Postgrad Med J 2002; 78, 71–75.
24. Lee KS. Natural history of chronic subdural haematoma. Brain Inj 2004; 18, 351–358.

25. Cameron MM. Chronic subdural haematoma: a review of 114 cases. J Neurol Neurosurg Psychiatry 1978; 41, 834–839.

26. Jones S, Kafetz K. A prospective study of chronic subdural haematomas in elderly patients. Age Ageing 1999; 28, 519–521.

27. Nobbe FA, Krauss JK. Subdural hematoma as a cause of contralateral dystonia. Clin Neurol Neurosurg 1997; 99, 37–39.

28. Moster ML, Johnston DE, Reinmuth OM. Chronic subdural hematoma with transient neurological deficits: a review of 15 cases. Ann Neurol 1983; 14, 539–542.

29. Ingvar DH, Lundberg N. Paroxysmal systems in intracranial hypertension, studied with ventricular fluid pressure recording and electroencephalography. Brain 1961; 84, 446–459.

30. Inao S, Kawai T, Kabeya R, et al. Relation between brain displacement and local cerebral blood flow in patients with chronic subdural haematoma. J Neurol Neurosurg Psychiatry 2001; 71, 741–746.

31. Voelker JL. Nonoperative treatment of chronic subdural hematoma. Neurosurg Clin N Am 2000; 11, 507–513.

32. Olson JJ, Poor MM Jr, Beck DW. Methylprednisolone reduces the bulk flow of water across an in vitro blood-brain barrier. Brain Res 1988; 439, 259–265.

33. Hasbun R, Abrahams J, Jekel J, et al. Computed tomography of the head before lumbar puncture in adults with suspected meningitis. N Engl J Med 2001; 345, 1727–1733.

34. Weigel R, Schmiedek P, Krauss JK. Outcome of contemporary surgery for chronic subdural haematoma: evidence based review. J Neurol Neurosurg Psychiatry 2003; 74, 937–943.

35. Asfora WT, Schwebach L. A modified technique to treat chronic and subacute subdural hematoma: technical note. Surg Neurol 2003; 59, 329–332.

36. Pichert G, Henn V [Conservative therapy of chronic subdural hematomas]. Schweiz Med Wochenschr 1987; 117, 1856–1862.

37. Nathoo N, Nadvi SS, Van Dellen JR. Cranial extradural empyema in the era of computed tomography: a review of 82 cases. Neurosurgery 1999; 44, 748–753.

38. Hlavin ML, Kaminski HJ, Fenstermaker RA, et al. Intracranial suppuration: a modern decade of postoperative subdural empyema and epidural abscess. Neurosurgery 1994; 34, 974–980.

39. Nathoo N, Nadvi SS, Van Dellen JR. Traumatic cranial empyemas: a review of 55 patients. Br J Neurosurg 2000; 14, 326–330.

40. Tamaki T, Eguchi T, Sakamoto M, et al. Use of diffusion-weighted magnetic resonance imaging in empyema after cranioplasty. Br J Neurosurg 2004; 18, 40–44.

41. Tsuchiya K, Osawa A, Katase S, et al. Diffusion-weighted MRI of subdural and epidural empyemas. Neuroradiology 2003; 45, 220–223.

42. Heran NS, Steinbok P, Cochrane DD. Conservative neurosurgical management of intracranial epidural abscesses in children. Neurosurgery 2003; 53, 893–897.

43. Kleinschmidt-DeMasters BK. Dural metastases—a retrospective surgical and autopsy series. Arch Pathol Lab Med 2001; 125, 880–887.

44. Johnson MD, Powell SZ, Boyer PJ, et al. Dural lesions mimicking meningiomas. Hum Pathol 2002; 33, 1211–1226.

45. Whittle IR, Smith C, Navoo P, et al. Meningiomas. Lancet 2004; 363, 1535–1543.

46. Bosnjak R, Derham C, Popovic M, et al. Spontaneous intracranial meningioma bleeding: clinicopathological features and outcome. J Neurosurg 2005; 103, 473–484.

47. Pistolesi S, Fontanini G, Camacci T, et al. Meningioma-associated brain oedema: the role of angiogenic factors and pial blood supply. J Neuro-Oncol 2002; 60, 159–164.

48. Engelhard HH. Progress in the diagnosis and treatment of patients with meningiomas. Part I: diagnostic imaging, preoperative embolization. Surg Neurol 2001; 55, 89–101.

49. Wiesmann M, Gliemroth J, Kehler U, et al. Pituitary apoplexy after cardiac surgery presenting as deep coma with dilated pupils. Acta Anaesthesiol Scand 1999; 43, 236–238.

50. Sibal L, Ball SG, Connolly V, et al. Pituitary apoplexy: a review of clinical presentation, management and outcome in 45 cases. Pituitary 2004; 7, 157–163.

51. Elsasser Imboden PN, De TN, Lobrinus A, et al. Apoplexy in pituitary macroadenoma: eight patients presenting in 12 months. Medicine (Baltimore) 2005; 84, 188–196.

52. Jassal DS, McGinn G, Embil JM. Pituitary apoplexy masquerading as meningoencephalitis. Headache 2004; 44, 75–78.

53. Prabhu VC, Brown HG. The pathogenesis of craniopharyngiomas. Childs Nerv Syst 2005; 21, 622–627.

54. Haupt R, Magnani C, Pavanello M, et al. Epidemiological aspects of craniopharyngioma. J Pediatr Endocrinol Metab 2006; 1, 289–293.

55. Swaroop GR, Whittle IR. Pineal apoplexy: an occurrence with no diagnostic clinicopathological features. Br J Neurosurg 1998; 12, 274–276.

56. Polmear A. Sentinel headaches in aneurysmal subarachnoid haemorrhage: what is the true incidence? A systematic review. Cephalalgia 2003; 23, 935–941.

57. Edlow JA, Caplan LR. Avoiding pitfalls in the diagnosis of subarachnoid hemorrhage. N Engl J Med 2000; 342, 29–36.

58. Landtblom AM, Fridriksson S, Boivie J, et al. Sudden onset headache: a prospective study of features, incidence and causes. Cephalalgia 2002; 22, 354–360.

59. Schievink WI, Wijdicks EF, Parisi JE, et al. Sudden death from aneurysmal subarachnoid hemorrhage. Neurology 1995; 45, 871–874.

60. Liebenberg WA, Worth R, Firth GB, et al. Aneurysmal subarachnoid haemorrhage: guidance in making the correct diagnosis. Postgrad Med J 2005; 81, 470–473.

61. Boesiger BM, Shiber JR. Subarachnoid hemorrhage diagnosis by computed tomography and lumbar puncture: are fifth generation CT scanners better at identifying subarachnoid hemorrhage? J Emerg Med 2005; 29, 23–27.

62. Mohamed M, Heasly DC, Yagmurlu B, et al. Fluid-attenuated inversion recovery MR imaging and subarachnoid hemorrhage: not a panacea. AJNR Am J Neuroradiol 2004; 25, 545–550.

63. Edlow JA, Wyer PC. Evidence-based emergency medicine/clinical question. How good is a negative cranial computed tomographic scan result in excluding subarachnoid hemorrhage? Ann Emerg Med 2000; 36, 507–516.

64. Petzold A, Keir G, Sharpe TL. Why human color vision cannot reliably detect cerebrospinal fluid xanthochromia. Stroke 2005; 36, 1295–1297.

65. Klimo P Jr, Kestle JR, MacDonald JD, et al. Marked reduction of cerebral vasospasm with lumbar drainage of cerebrospinal fluid after subarachnoid hemorrhage. J Neurosurg 2004; 100, 215–224.

66. Klopfenstein JD, Kim LJ, Feiz-Erfan I, et al. Comparison of rapid and gradual weaning from external ventricular drainage in patients with aneurysmal subarachnoid hemorrhage: a prospective randomized trial. J Neurosurg 2004; 100, 225–229.

67. Pavlidis N. The diagnostic and therapeutic management of leptomeningeal carcinomatosis. Ann Oncol 2004; Suppl 4, iv285-iv291.

68. Grossman SA, Krabak MJ. Leptomeningeal carcinomatosis. Cancer Treat Rev 1999; 25, 103–119.

69. Yung WA, Horten BC, Shapiro WR. Meningeal gliomatosis: a review of 12 cases. Ann Neurol 1980; 8, 605–608.

70. Cinalli G, Sainte-Rose C, Lellouch-Tubiana A, et al. Hydrocephalus associated with intramedullary low-grade glioma. J Neurosurg 1995; 83, 480–485.

71. Chen HS, Shen MC, Tien HF, et al. Leptomeningeal seeding with acute hydrocephalus—unusual central nervous system presentation during chemotherapy in Ki-1- positive anaplastic large-cell lymphoma. Acta Haematol 1996; 95, 135–139.

72. Floeter MK, So YT, Ross DA, et al. Miliary metastasis to the brain: clinical and radiologic features. Neurology 1987; 37, 1817–1818.

73. Broderick JP, Cascino TL. Nonconvulsive status epilepticus in a patient with leptomeningeal cancer. Mayo Clin Proc 1987; 62, 835–837.

74. Klein P, Haley EC, Wooten GF, et al. Focal cerebral infarctions associated with perivascular tumor infiltrates in carcinomatous leptomeningeal metastases. Arch Neurol 1989; 46, 1149–1152.

75. Herman C, Kupsky WJ, Rogers L, et al. Leptomeningeal dissemination of malignant glioma simulating cerebral vasculitis—case report with angiographic and pathological studies. Stroke 1995; 26, 2366–2370.

76. Weller M, Stevens A, Sommer N, et al. Tumor cell dissemination triggers an intrathecal immune response in neoplastic meningitis. Cancer 1992; 69, 1475–1480.

77. Glantz MJ, Cole BF, Glantz LK, et al. Cerebrospinal fluid cytology in patients with cancer: minimizing false-negative results. Cancer 1998; 82, 733–739.

78. van Zanten AP, Twijnstra A, Ongerboer DE, et al. Cerebrospinal fluid tumour markers in patients treated for meningeal malignancy. J Neurol Neurosurg Psychiatry 1991; 54, 119–123.

79. Wasserstrom WR, et al. Diagnosis and treatment of leptomeningeal metastases from solid tumors: experience with 90 patients. Cancer 1982; 49, 759–772.

80. Siegal T, Lossos A, Pfeffer MR. Leptomeningeal metastases: analysis of 31 patients with sustained off-therapy response following combined-modality therapy. Neurology 1994; 44, 1463–1469.

81. DeAngelis LM, Boutros D. Leptomeningeal metastasis. Cancer Invest 2005; 23, 145–154.

82. Scheld WM, Koedel U, Nathan B, et al. Pathophysiology of bacterial meningitis: mechanism(s) of neuronal injury. J Infect Dis 2002; 186, S225–S233.

83. van de BD, De Gans J, Spanjaard L, et al. Clinical features and prognostic factors in adults with bacterial meningitis. N Engl J Med 2004; 351, 1849–1859.

84. Mylonakis E, Hohmann EL, Caderwood SB. Central nervous system infection with *Listeria monocytogenes*—33 years' experience at a general hospital and review of 776 episodes from the literature. Medicine 1998; 77, 313–336.

85. Gerner-Smidt P, Ethelberg S, Schiellerup P, et al. Invasive listeriosis in Denmark 1994–2003: a review of 299 cases with special emphasis on risk factors for mortality. Clin Microbiol Infect 2005; 11, 618–624.

86. Drevets DA, Leenen PJ, Greenfield RA. Invasion of the central nervous system by intracellular bacteria. Clin Microbiol Rev 2004; 17, 323–347.

87. Hussein AS, Shafran SD. Acute bacterial meningitis in adults. A 12-year review. Medicine (Baltimore) 2000; 79, 360–368.

88. Podlecka A, Dziewulska D, Rafalowska J. Vascular changes in tuberculous meningoencephalitis. Folia Neuropathol 1998; 36, 235–237.

89. Attia J, Hatala R, Cook DJ, et al. The rational clinical examination. Does this adult patient have acute meningitis? JAMA 1999; 282, 175–181.

90. Risch L, Lisec I, Jutzi M, et al. Rapid, accurate and non-invasive detection of cerebrospinal fluid leakage using combined determination of beta-trace protein in secretion and serum. Clin Chim Acta 2005; 351, 169–176.

91. Romer FK. Difficulties in the diagnosis of bacterial meningitis. Evaluation of antibiotic pretreatment and causes of admission to hospital. Lancet 1977; 2, 345–347.

92. Romer FK. Bacterial meningitis: a 15-year review of bacterial meningitis from departments of internal medicine. Dan Med Bull 1977; 24, 35–40.

93. Clark T, Duffell E, Stuart JM, et al. Lumbar puncture in the management of adults with suspected bacterial meningitis-a survey of practice. J Infect 2005; 52, 316–319.

94. Begg N, Cartwright KA, Cohen J, et al. Consensus statement on diagnosis, investigation, treatment and prevention of acute bacterial meningitis in immunocompetent adults. British Infection Society Working Party. J Infect 1999; 39, 1–15.

95. Roos KL, Tunkel AR, Scheld WM. Acute bacterial meningitis. In: Scheld WM, Whitley RJ, Marra CM, eds. Infections of the Central Nervous System, 3rd ed. Philadelphia: Lippincott Williams & Wilkins, pp 347–422, 2004.

96. Chaudhuri A. Adjunctive dexamethasone treatment in acute bacterial meningitis. Lancet Neurol 2004; 3, 54–62.

97. Kastrup O, Wanke I, Maschke M. Neuroimaging of infections. NeuroRx 2005; 2, 324–332.

98. Zimmerman RA, Wong AM, Girard N. Imaging of intracranial infections. In: Scheld WM, Whitley RJ, Marra CM, eds. Infections of the Central Nervous System, 3rd ed. Philadelphia: Lippincott Williams & Wilkins, pp 31–55, 2004.

99. Massaro AR, Sacco RL, Mohr JP, et al. Clinical discriminators of lobar and deep hemorrhages: the Stroke Data Bank. Neurology 1991; 41, 1881–1885.

100. Chung CS, Caplan LR, Yamamoto Y, et al. Striato-capsular haemorrhage. Brain 2000; 123, 1850–1862.

101. Kumral E, Kocaer T, Ertubey NO, et al. Thalamic hemorrhage. A prospective study of 100 patients. Stroke 1995; 26, 964–970.

102. Choi KD, Jung DS, Kim JS. Specificity of "peering at the tip of the nose" for a diagnosis of thalamic hemorrhage. Arch Neurol 2004; 61, 417–422.

103. Darby DG, Donnan GA, Saling MA, et al. Primary intraventricular hemorrhage: clinical and neuropsychological findings in a prospective stroke series. Neurology 1988; 38, 68–75.

104. Engelhard HH, Andrews CO, Slavin KV, et al. Current management of intraventricular hemorrhage. Surg Neurol 2003; 60, 15–21.

105. Mendelow AD, Gregson BA, Fernandes HM, et al. Early surgery versus initial conservative treatment in patients with spontaneous supratentorial intracerebral haematomas in the International Surgical Trial in Intracerebral Haemorrhage (STICH): a randomised trial. Lancet 2005; 365, 387–397.

106. Mayer SA, Brun NC, Begtrup K, et al. Recombinant activated factor VII for acute intracerebral hemorrhage. N Engl J Med 2005; 352, 777–785.

107. Fisher CM. Some neuro-ophthalmological observations. J Neurol Neurosurg Psychiatry 1967; 30, 383–392.

108. Pessin MS, Adelman LS, Prager RJ, et al. "Wrong-way eyes" in supratentorial hemorrhage. Ann Neurol 1981; 9, 79–81.

109. Fisher CM. Lacunes: small, deep cerebral infarcts. Neurology 1965; 15, 774–784.

110. Greenberg SM, Gurol ME, Rosand J, et al. Amyloid angiopathy-related vascular cognitive impairment. Stroke 2004; 35, 2616–2619.

111. Yamada M. Cerebral amyloid angiopathy: an overview. Neuropathology 2000; 20, 8–22.

112. Miller JH, Wardlaw JM, Lammie GA. Intracerebral haemorrhage and cerebral amyloid angiopathy: CT features with pathological correlation. Clin Radiol 1999; 54, 422–429.

113. Koennecke HC. Cerebral microbleeds on MRI: prevalence, associations, and potential clinical implications. Neurology 2006; 66, 165–171.

114. Barami K, Ko K. Ruptured mycotic aneurysm presenting as an intraparenchymal hemorrhage and non-adjacent acute subdural hematoma: case report and review of the literature. Surg Neurol 1994; 41, 290–293.

115. Chun JY, Smith W, Halbach VV, et al. Current multimodality management of infectious intracranial aneurysms. Neurosurgery 2001; 48, 1203–1213.

116. Mathiesen T, Edner G, Kihlstrom L. Deep and brainstem cavernomas: a consecutive 8-year series. J Neurosurg 2003; 99, 31–37.

117. Porter RW, Detwiler PW, Spetzler RF, et al. Cavernous malformations of the brainstem: experience with 100 patients. J Neurosurg 1999; 90, 50–58.

118. Kim MS, Pyo SY, Jeong YG, et al. Gamma knife surgery for intracranial cavernous hemangioma. J Neurosurg 2005; 102 (Suppl), 102–106.

119. Liscak R, Vladyka V, Simonova G, et al. Gamma knife surgery of brain cavernous hemangiomas. J Neurosurg 2005; 102 (Suppl), 207–213.

120. Choi JH, Mohr JP. Brain arteriovenous malformations in adults. Lancet Neurol 2005; 4, 299–308.

121. Posner JB. Neurologic Complications of Cancer. Philadelphia: F.A. Davis, 1995.

122. DeAngelis LM, Gutin PH, Leibel SA, et al. Intracranial Tumors: Diagnosis and Treatment. London: Martin Dunitz Ltd., 2002.

123. Behin A, Hoang-Xuan K, Carpentier AF, et al. Primary brain tumours in adults. Lancet 2003; 361, 323–331.

124. Engelhard HH. Current diagnosis and treatment of oligodendroglioma. Neurosurg Focus 2002; 12, E2.

125. Panageas KS, Elkin EB, DeAngelis LM, et al. Trends in survival from primary central nervous system lymphoma, 1975–1999: a population-based analysis. Cancer 2005; 104, 2466–2472.

126. Patchell RA, Tibbs PA, Walsh JW. A randomized trial of surgery in the treatment of single metastases to the brain. N Engl J Med 1990; 322, 494–500.

127. Glantz MJ, Cole BF, Forsyth PA, et al. Practice parameter: anticonvulsant prophylaxis in patients with newly diagnosed brain tumors—report of the Quality Standards Subcommittee of the American Academy of Neurology. Neurology 2000; 54, 1886–1893.

128. Fuentes R, Bonfill X, Exposito J. Surgery versus radiosurgery for patients with a solitary brain metastasis from non-small cell lung cancer. Cochrane Database Syst Rev 2006; (1), CD004840.

129. Roche M, Humphreys H, Smyth E, et al. A twelve-year review of central nervous system bacterial abscesses; presentation and aetiology. Clin Microbiol Infect 2003; 9, 803–809.

130. Garcia HH, Del Brutto OH. Neurocysticercosis: updated concepts about an old disease. Lancet Neurol 2005; 4, 653–661.

131. Tuzun Y, Kadioglu HH, Izci Y, et al. The clinical, radiological and surgical aspects of cerebral hydatid cysts in children. Pediatr Neurosurg 2004; 40, 155–160.

132. Collazos J. Opportunistic infections of the CNS in patients with AIDS: diagnosis and management. CNS Drugs 2003; 17, 869–887.

133. Kastenbauer S, Pfister H-W, Wispelwey B, et al. Brain abscess. In: Scheld WM, Whitley RJ, Marra CM, eds. Infections of the Central Nervous System, 3rd ed. Philadelphia: Lippincott Williams & Wilkins, pp 479–507, 2004.

134. Bozbuga M, Izgi N, Polat G, et al. Posterior fossa epidural hematomas: observations on a series of 73 cases. Neurosurg Rev 1999; 22, 34–40.

135. Khwaja HA, Hornbrey PJ. Posterior cranial fossa venous extradural haematoma: an uncommon form of intracranial injury. Emerg Med J 2001; 18, 496–497.

136. Berker M, Cataltepe O, Ozcan OE. Traumatic epidural haematoma of the posterior fossa in childhood: 16 new cases and a review of the literature. Br J Neurosurg 2003; 17, 226–229.

137. Bor-Seng-Shu E, Aguiar PH, de Almeida Leme RJ, et al. Epidural hematomas of the posterior cranial fossa. Neurosurg Focus 2004; 16, ECP1.

138. Parkinson D, Hunt B, Shields C. Double lucid interval in patients with extradural hematoma of the posterior fossa. J Neurosurg 1971; 34, 534–536.

139. Karasawa H, Furuya H, Naito H, et al. Acute hydrocephalus in posterior fossa injury. J Neurosurg 1997; 86, 629–632.

140. Pozzati E, Tognetti F, Cavallo M, et al. Extradural hematomas of the posterior cranial fossa. Observations on a series of 32 consecutive cases treated after the introduction of computed tomography scanning. Surg Neurol 1989; 32, 300–303.

141. Wong CW. The CT criteria for conservative treatment—but under close clinical observation—of posterior fossa epidural haematomas. Acta Neurochir (Wien) 1994; 126, 124–127.

142. Roda JM, Gimenez D, Perez-Higueras A, et al. Posterior fossa epidural hematomas: a review and synthesis. Surg Neurol 1983; 19, 419–424.

143. Nathoo N, Nadvi SS, Van Dellen JR. Infratentorial empyema: analysis of 22 cases. Neurosurgery 1997; 41, 1263–1268.

144. Roberti F, Sekhar LN, Kalavakonda C, et al. Posterior fossa meningiomas: surgical experience in 161 cases. Surg Neurol 2001; 56, 8–20.

145. Cantore G, Ciappetta P, Delfini R, et al. Meningiomas of the posterior cranial fossa without dural attachment. Surg Neurol 1986; 25, 127–130.

146. Psiachou-Leonard E, Paterakis G, Stefanaki K, et al. Cerebellar granulocytic sarcoma in an infant with CD56+ acute monoblastic leukemia. Leuk Res 2001; 25, 1019–1021.

147. d'Avella D, Servadei F, Scerrati M, et al. Traumatic acute subdural haematomas of the posterior fossa: clinicoradiological analysis of 24 patients. Acta Neurochir (Wien) 2003; 145, 1037–1044.

148. Stendel R, Schulte T, Pietila TA, et al. Spontaneous bilateral chronic subdural haematoma of the posterior fossa. Case report and review of the literature. Acta Neurochir (Wien) 2002; 144, 497–500.

149. Sahjpaul RL, Lee DH. Infratentorial subdural empyema, pituitary abscess, and septic cavernous sinus thrombophlebitis secondary to paranasal sinusitis: case report. Neurosurgery 1999; 44, 864–866.

150. Sadato N, Numaguchi Y, Rigamonti D, et al. Bleeding patterns in ruptured posterior fossa aneurysms: a CT study. J Comput Assist Tomogr 1991; 15, 612–617.

151. Logue V. Posterior fossa aneurysms. Clin Neurosurg 1964; 11, 183–219.

152. Duvoisin RC, Yahr MD. Posterior fossa aneurysms. Neurology 1965; 15, 231–241.

153. Jamieson KG. Aneurysms of the vertebrobasilar system. Further experience with nine cases. J Neurosurg 1968; 28, 544–555.

154. Flaherty ML, Haverbusch M, Kissela B, et al. Perimesencephalic subarachnoid hemorrhage: incidence, risk factors, and outcome. J Stroke Cerebrovasc Dis 2005; 14, 267–271.

155. Van der Schaap I, Velthius BK, Gouw A, Rinkel GJ. Venous drainage in perimesencephalic hemorrhage. Stroke 2004; 35, 1614–1618.

156. Kirollos RW, Tyagi AK, Ross SA, et al. Management of spontaneous cerebellar hematomas: a prospective treatment protocol. Neurosurgery 2001; 49, 1378–1386.

157. Mezzadri JJ, Otero JM, Ottino CA. Management of 50 spontaneous cerebellar haemorrhages. Importance of obstructive hydrocephalus. Acta Neurochir (Wien) 1993; 122, 39–44.

158. Da Pian R, Bazzan A, Pasqualin A. Surgical versus medical treatment of spontaneous posterior fossa haematomas: a cooperative study on 205 cases. Neurol Res 1984; 6, 145–151.

159. Itoh Y, Yamada M, Hayakawa M, et al. Cerebral amyloid angiopathy: a significant cause of cerebellar as well as lobar cerebral hemorrhage in the elderly. J Neurol Sci 1993; 116, 135–141.

160. Siu TL, Chandran KN, Siu T. Cerebellar haemorrhage following supratentorial craniotomy. J Clin Neurosci 2003; 10, 378–384.

161. Brennan RW, Bergland RM. Acute cerebellar hemorrhage. Analysis of clinical findings and outcome in 12 cases. Neurology 1977; 27, 527–532.

162. Fisher CM, Picard EH, Polak A, et al. Acute hypertensive cerebellar hemorrhage: diagnosis and surgical treatment. J Nerv Ment Dis 1965; 140, 38–57.

163. Messert B, Leppik IE, Sato S. Diplopia and involuntary eye closure in spontaneous cerebellar hemorrhage. Stroke 1976; 7, 305–307.

164. St Louis EK, Wijdicks EF, Li H. Predicting neurologic deterioration in patients with cerebellar hematomas. Neurology 1998; 51, 1364–1369.

165. Coplin WM, Kim DK, Kliot M, et al. Mutism in an adult following hypertensive cerebellar hemorrhage: nosological discussion and illustrative case. Brain Lang 1997; 59, 473–493.

166. Schmahmann JD, Sherman JC. The cerebellar cognitive affective syndrome. Brain 1998; 121, 561–579.

167. Aarsen FK, Van Dongen HR, Paquier PF, et al. Long-term sequelae in children after cerebellar astrocytoma surgery. Neurology 2004; 62, 1311–1316.

168. Tohgi H, Takahashi S, Chiba K, et al. Cerebellar infarction. Clinical and neuroimaging analysis in 293 patients. The Tohoku Cerebellar Infarction Study Group. Stroke 1993; 24, 1697–1701.

169. Barinagarrementeria F, Amaya LE, Cantu C. Causes and mechanisms of cerebellar infarction in young patients. Stroke 1997; 28, 2400–2404.

170. Geller T, Loftis L, Brink DS. Cerebellar infarction in adolescent males associated with acute marijuana use. Pediatrics 2004; 113, 365–370.

171. Hornig CR, Rust DS, Busse O, et al. Space-occupying cerebellar infarction. Clinical course and prognosis. Stroke 1994; 25, 372–374.

172. Jauss M, Krieger D, Hornig C, et al. Surgical and medical management of patients with massive cerebellar infarctions: results of the German-Austrian Cerebellar Infarction Study. J Neurol 1999; 246, 257–264.

173. Nadvi SS, Parboosing R, Van Dellen JR. Cerebellar abscess: the significance of cerebrospinal fluid diversion. Neurosurgery 1997; 41, 61–66.

174. Sennaroglu L, Sozeri B. Otogenic brain abscess: review of 41 cases. Otolaryngol Head Neck Surg 2000; 123, 751–755.

175. Shaw MD, Russell JA. Cerebellar abscess. A review of 47 cases. J Neurol Neurosurg Psychiatry 1975; 38, 429–435.

176. Agrawal D, Suri A, Mahapatra AK. Primary excision of pediatric posterior fossa abscesses—towards zero mortality? A series of nine cases and review. Pediatr Neurosurg 2003; 38, 63–67.

177. Brydon HL, Hardwidge C. The management of cerebellar abscess since the introduction of CT scanning. Br J Neurosurg 1994; 8, 447–455.

178. Fadul C, Misulis KE, Wiley RG. Cerebellar metastases: diagnostic and management considerations. J Clin Oncol 1987; 5, 1107–1115.

179. Slater A, Moore NR, Huson SM. The natural history of cerebellar hemangioblastomas in von Hippel-Lindau disease. AJNR Am J Neuroradiol 2003; 24, 1570–1574.

180. Haines SJ, Mollman HD. Primary pontine hemorrhagic events. Hemorrhage or hematoma? Surgical or conservative management? Neurosurg Clin N Am 1993; 4, 481–495.

181. Takahashi M, Suzuki R, Osakabe Y, et al. Magnetic resonance imaging findings in cerebral fat embolism: correlation with clinical manifestations. J Trauma 1999; 46, 324–327.

182. Wityk RJ, Goldsborough MA, Hillis A, et al. Diffusion- and perfusion-weighted brain magnetic resonance imaging in patients with neurologic complications after cardiac surgery. Arch Neurol 2001; 58, 571–576.

183. Meador KJ, Loring DW, Lee GP, et al. Level of consciousness and memory during the intracarotid sodium amobarbital procedure. Brain Cogn 1997; 33, 178–188.

184. Kwon SU, Lee SH, Kim JS. Sudden coma from acute bilateral internal carotid artery territory infarction. Neurology 2002; 58, 1846–1849.

185. Hagiwara N, Toyoda K, Fujimoto S, et al. Extensive bihemispheric ischemia caused by acute occlusion of three major arteries to the brain. J Neurol Sci 2003; 212, 99–101.

186. Qureshi AI, Suarez JI, Yahia AM, et al. Timing of neurologic deterioration in massive middle cerebral artery infarction: a multicenter review. Crit Care Med 2003; 31, 272–277.

187. Baird TA, Parsons MW, Phanh T, et al. Persistent poststroke hyperglycemia is independently associated with infarct expansion and worse clinical outcome. Stroke 2003; 34, 2208–2214.

188. Gray CS, Hildreth AJ, Alberti GK, et al. Poststroke hyperglycemia: natural history and immediate management. Stroke 2004; 35, 122–126.

189. Alberts MJ, Latchaw RE, Selman WR, et al. Recommendations for comprehensive stroke centers: a consensus statement from the Brain Attack Coalition. Stroke 2005; 36, 1597–1616.

190. Ayata C, Ropper AH. Ischaemic brain oedema. J Clin Neurosci 2002; 9, 113–124.

191. Schwarz S, Georgiadis D, Aschoff A, et al. Effects of hypertonic (10%) saline in patients with raised intracranial pressure after stroke. Stroke 2002; 33, 136–140.

192. Muizelaar JP, Wei EP, Kontos HA, et al. Mannitol causes compensatory cerebral vasoconstriction and vasodilation in response to blood viscosity changes. J Neurosurg 1983; 59, 822–828.

193. Burke AM, Quest DO, Chien S, et al. The effects of mannitol on blood viscosity. J Neurosurg 1981; 55, 550–553.

194. Koh MS, Goh KY, Tung MY, et al. Is decompressive craniectomy for acute cerebral infarction of any benefit? Surg Neurol 2000; 53, 225–230.

195. Gupta R, Connolly ES, Mayer S, et al. Hemicraniectomy for massive middle cerebral artery territory infarction: a systematic review. Stroke 2004; 35, 539–543.

196. Cheung A, Telaghani CK, Wang J, et al. Neurological recovery after decompressive craniectomy for massive ischemic stroke. Neurocrit Care 2005; 3, 216–223.

197. Schmahmann JD. Vascular syndromes of the thalamus. Stroke 2003; 34, 2264–2278.

198. Neau JP, Bogousslavsky J. The syndrome of posterior choroidal artery territory infarction. Ann Neurol 1996; 39, 779–788.

199. Bogousslavsky J, Regli F, Uske A. Thalamic infarcts: clinical syndromes, etiology, and prognosis. Neurology 1988; 38, 837–848.

200. Kumral E, Evyapan D, Balkir K, et al. Bilateral thalamic infarction. Clinical, etiological and MRI correlates. Acta Neurol Scand 2001; 103, 35–42.

201. Steinke W, Sacco RL, Mohr JP, et al. Thalamic stroke. Presentation and prognosis of infarcts and hemorrhages. Arch Neurol 1992; 49, 703–710.

202. Caplan LR. "Top of the basilar" syndrome. Neurology 1980; 30, 72–79.

203. Castaigne P, Lhermitte F, Buge A, et al. Paramedian thalamic and midbrain infarct: clinical and neuropathological study. Ann Neurol 1981; 10, 127–148.

204. Perren F, Clark S, Bogousslavsky J. The syndrome of combined polar and paramedian thalamic infarction. Arch Neurol 2005; 62, 1212–1216.

205. van Domburg PH, Ten Donkelaar HJ, Notermans SL. Akinetic mutism with bithalamic infarction. Neurophysiological correlates. J Neurol Sci 1996; 139, 58–65.

206. Krolak-Salmon P, Croisile B, Houzard C, et al. Total recovery after bilateral paramedian thalamic infarct. Eur Neurol 2000; 44, 216–218.

207. Weidauer S, Nichtweiss M, Zanella FE, et al. Assessment of paramedian thalamic infarcts: MR imaging, clinical features and prognosis. Eur Radiol 2004; 14, 1615–1626.

208. Stam J. Cerebral venous and sinus thrombosis: incidence and causes. Adv Neurol 2003; 92, 225–232.

209. Kimber J. Cerebral venous sinus thrombosis. QJM 2002; 95, 137–142.

210. Masuhr F, Mehraein S, Einhaupl K. Cerebral venous and sinus thrombosis. J Neurol 2004; 251, 11–23.

211. Urban PP, Muller-Forell W. Clinical and neuroradiological spectrum of isolated cortical vein thrombosis. J Neurol 2005; 252, 1476–1481.

212. Crawford SC, Digre KB, Palmer CA, et al. Thrombosis of the deep venous drainage of the brain in adults. Analysis of seven cases with review of the literature. Arch Neurol 1995; 52, 1101–1108.

213. Rahman NU, al Tahan AR. Computed tomographic evidence of an extensive thrombosis and infarction of the deep venous system. Stroke 1993; 24, 744–746.

214. Ciccone A, Canhao P, Falcao F, et al. Thrombolysis for cerebral vein and dural sinus thrombosis. Cochrane Database Syst Rev 2004; (1), CD003693.

215. Stam J. The treatment of cerebral venous sinus thrombosis. Adv Neurol 2003; 92, 233–240.

216. Nadeau SE. Neurologic manifestations of systemic vasculitis. Neurol Clin 2002; 20, 123–150.

217. Younger DS, Hays AP, Brust JC, et al. Granulomatous angiitis of the brain. An inflammatory reaction of diverse etiology. Arch Neurol 1988; 45, 514–518.

218. Moore PM. The vasculitides. Curr Opin Neurol 1999; 12, 383–388.

219. Kennedy PG. Viral encephalitis. J Neurol 2005; 252, 268–272.

220. Whitley RJ, Soong SJ, Linneman C Jr, et al. Herpes simplex encephalitis. Clinical assessment. JAMA 1982; 247, 317–320.

221. Tyler KL. Herpes simplex virus infections of the central nervous system: encephalitis and meningitis, including Mollaret's. Herpes 2004; 11 (Suppl 2), 57A–64A.

222. Wingerchuk DM. The clinical course of acute disseminated encephalomyelitis. Neurol Res 2006; 28, 341–347.

223. Menge T, Hemmer B, Nessler S, et al. Acute disseminated encephalomyelitis: an update. Arch Neurol 2005; 62, 1673–1680.

224. Gurdjian ES. Studies on experimental concussion. Clin Develop Med 1954; 40, 674–681.

225. Adams JH, Graham DI, Murray LS, et al. Diffuse axonal injury due to nonmissile head injury in humans: an analysis of 45 cases. Ann Neurol 1982; 12, 557–563.

226. Meythaler JM, Peduzzi JD, Eleftheriou E, et al. Current concepts: diffuse axonal injury-associated traumatic brain injury. Arch Phys Med Rehabil 2001; 82, 1461–1471.

227. Gennarelli TA, Thibault LE, Adams JH, et al. Diffuse axonal injury and traumatic coma in the primate. Ann Neurol 1982; 12, 564–574.

228. Adams JH, Graham DI, Gennarelli TA, et al. Diffuse axonal injury in non-missile head injury. J Neurol Neurosurg Psychiatry 1991; 54, 481–483.

229. Practice parameter: the management of concussion in sports (summary statement). Report of the Quality Standards Subcommittee. Neurology 1997; 48, 581–585.

230. Shaw NA. The neurophysiology of concussion. Prog Neurobiol 2002; 67, 281–344.

231. Giza CC, Hovda DA. The neurometabolic cascade of concussion. J Athl Train 2001; 36, 228–235.

232. Brooks WM, Friedman SD, Gasparovic C. Magnetic resonance spectroscopy in traumatic brain injury. J Head Trauma Rehabil 2001; 16, 149–164.

233. Shutter L, Tong KA, Holshouser BA. Proton MRS in acute traumatic brain injury: role for glutamate/glutamine and choline for outcome prediction. J Neurotrauma 2004; 21, 1693–1705.

234. Adams JH, Graham DI, Jennett B. The neuropathology of the vegetative state after an acute brain insult. Brain 2000; 123, 1327–1338.

235. Reilly PL, Graham DI, Adams JH, et al. Patients with head injury who talk and die. Lancet 1975; 2, 375–377.

236. Guskiewicz KM, McCrea M, Marshall SW, et al. Cumulative effects associated with recurrent concussion in collegiate football players: the NCAA Concussion Study. JAMA 2003; 290, 2549–2555.

237. McAllister TW, Arciniegas D. Evaluation and treatment of postconcussive symptoms. NeuroRehabilitation 2002; 17, 265–283.

238. Schwarz S, Egelhof T, Schwab S, et al. Basilar artery embolism. Clinical syndrome and neuroradiologic patterns in patients without permanent occlusion of the basilar artery. Neurology 1997; 49, 1346–1352.

239. Michotte A, de Keyser J, Dierckx R, et al. Brain stem infarction as a complication of giant-cell arteritis. Clin Neurol Neurosurg 1986; 88, 127–129.

240. Jentzen JM, Amatuzio J, Peterson GF. Complications of cervical manipulation: a case report of fatal brainstem infarct with review of the mechanisms and predisposing factors. J Forensic Sci 1987; 32, 1089–1094.

241. Hosoya T, Adachi M, Yamaguchi K, et al. Clinical and neuroradiological features of intracranial vertebrobasilar artery dissection. Stroke 1999; 30, 1083–1090.

242. Ferbert A, Bruckmann H, Drummen R. Clinical features of proven basilar artery occlusion. Stroke 1990; 21, 1135–1142.

243. Devuyst G, Bogousslavsky J, Meuli R, et al. Stroke or transient ischemic attacks with basilar artery stenosis or occlusion: clinical patterns and outcome. Arch Neurol 2002; 59, 567–573.

244. Moncayo J, Bogousslavsky J. Vertebro-basilar syndromes causing oculo-motor disorders. Curr Opin Neurol 2003; 16, 45–50.

245. Ehsan T, Hayat G, Malkoff MD, et al. Hyperdense basilar artery. An early computed tomography sign of thrombosis. J Neuroimaging 1994; 4, 200–205.

246. Ezaki Y, Tsutsumi K, Onizuka M, et al. Retrospective analysis of neurological outcome after intra-arterial thrombolysis in basilar artery occlusion. Surg Neurol 2003; 60, 423–429.

247. Levy EI, Hanel RA, Boulos AS, et al. Comparison of periprocedure complications resulting from direct stent placement compared with those due to conventional and staged stent placement in the basilar artery. J Neurosurg 2003; 99, 653–660.

248. Yu W, Binder D, Foster-Barber A, et al. Endovascular embolectomy of acute basilar artery occlusion. Neurology 2003; 61, 1421–1423.

249. Link MJ, Bartleson JD, Forbes G, et al. Spontaneous midbrain hemorrhage: report of seven new cases. Surg Neurol 1993; 39, 58–65.

250. Murata Y, Yamaguchi S, Kajikawa H, et al. Relationship between the clinical manifestations, computed tomographic findings and the outcome in 80 patients with primary pontine hemorrhage. J Neurol Sci 1999; 167, 107–111.

251. Barinagarrementeria F, Cantu C. Primary medullary hemorrhage. Report of four cases and review of the literature. Stroke 1994; 25, 1684–1687.

252. Posadas G, Vaquero J, Herrero J, et al. Brainstem haematomas: early and late prognosis. Acta Neurochir (Wien) 1994; 131, 189–195.

253. Sarkar A, Pollock BE, Brown PD, et al. Evaluation of gamma knife radiosurgery in the treatment of oligodendrogliomas and mixed oligodendroastrocytomas. J Neurosurg 2002; 97, 653–656.

254. Shuaib A. Benign brainstem hemorrhage. Can J Neurol Sci 1991; 18, 356–357.

255. Okudera T, Uemura K, Nakajima K, et al. Primary pontine hemorrhage: correlations of pathologic features with postmortem microangiographic, and

vertebralangiographic studies. Mt Sinai J Med 1978; 45, 305–321.

256. Shibata M. Hyperthermia in brain hemorrhage. Med Hypotheses 1998; 50, 185–190.

257. Morrison SF. Central pathways controlling brown adipose tissue thermogenesis. News Physiol Sci 2004; 19, 67–74.

258. Wijdicks EF, St Louis E. Clinical profiles predictive of outcome in pontine hemorrhage. Neurology 1997; 49, 1342–1346.

259. Wessels T, Moller-Hartmann W, Noth J, et al. CT findings and clinical features as markers for patient outcome in primary pontine hemorrhage. AJNR Am J Neuroradiol 2004; 25, 257–260.

260. Frequin ST, Linssen WH, Pasman JW, et al. Recurrent prolonged coma due to basilar artery migraine. A case report. Headache 1991; 31, 75–81.

261. Ducros A, Denier C, Joutel A, et al. The clinical spectrum of familial hemiplegic migraine associated with mutations in a neuronal calcium channel. N Engl J Med 2001; 345, 17–24.

262. Schon F, Martin RJ, Prevett M, et al. "CADASIL coma": an underdiagnosed acute encephalopathy. J Neurol Neurosurg Psychiatry 2003; 74, 249–252.

263. Kruit MC, van Buchem MA, Hofman PA, et al. Migraine as a risk factor for subclinical brain lesions. JAMA 2004; 291, 427–434.

264. Selby G, Lance JW. Observations on 500 cases of migraine and allied vascular headache. J Neurol Neurosurg Psychiatry 1960; 23, 23–32.

265. Thambisetty M, Biousse V, Newman NJ. Hypertensive brainstem encephalopathy: clinical and radiographic features. J Neurol Sci 2003; 208, 93–99.

266. Garg RK. Posterior leukoencephalopathy syndrome. Postgrad Med J 2001; 77, 24–28.

267. Hall WA. Infectious lesions of the brain stem. Neurosurg Clin N Am 1993; 4, 543–551.

268. Armstrong RW, Fung PC. Brainstem encephalitis (rhombencephalitis) due to Listeria monocytogenes: case report and review. Clin Infect Dis 1993; 16, 689–702.

269. Tyler KL, Tedder DG, Yamamoto LJ, et al. Recurrent brainstem encephalitis associated with herpes simplex virus type 1 DNA in cerebrospinal fluid. Neurology 1995; 45, 2246–2250.

270. Ho CL, Deruytter MJ. Manifestations of Neuro-Behcet's disease. Report of two cases and review of the literature. Clin Neurol Neurosurg 2005; 107, 310–314.

271. Fuentes S, Bouillot P, Regis J, et al. Management of brain stem abscess. Br J Neurosurg 2001; 15, 57–62.

272. Odaka M, Yuki N, Yamada M, et al. Bickerstaff's brainstem encephalitis: clinical features of 62 cases and a subgroup associated with Guillain-Barre syndrome. Brain 2003; 126, 2279–2290.

273. Weidauer S, Ziemann U, Thomalske C, et al. Vasogenic edema in Bickerstaff's brainstem encephalitis: a serial MRI study. Neurology 2003; 61, 836–838.

274. Lampl C, Yazdi K. Central pontine myelinolysis. Eur Neurol 2002; 47, 3–10.

Chapter 5

Multifocal, Diffuse, and Metabolic Brain Diseases Causing Delirium, Stupor, or Coma

DISORDERS OF GLUCOSE OR COFACTOR AVAILABILITY
Hypoglycemia
Hyperglycemia
Cofactor Deficiency

DISEASES OF ORGAN SYSTEMS OTHER THAN BRAIN
Liver Disease
Renal Disease
Pulmonary Disease
Pancreatic Encephalopathy
Diabetes Mellitus
Adrenal Disorders
Thyroid Disorders
Pituitary Disorders
Cancer

EXOGENOUS INTOXICATIONS
Sedative and Psychotropic Drugs
Intoxication With Other Common
    Medications
Ethanol Intoxication
Intoxication With Drugs of Abuse
Intoxication With Drugs Causing
    Metabolic Acidosis

ABNORMALITIES OF IONIC OR ACID-BASE ENVIRONMENT OF THE CENTRAL NERVOUS SYSTEM
Hypo-osmolar States
Hyperosmolar States
Calcium
Other Electrolytes
Disorders of Systemic Acid-Base Balance

DISORDERS OF THERMOREGULATION
Hypothermia
Hyperthermia

INFECTIOUS DISORDERS OF THE CENTRAL NERVOUS SYSTEM: BACTERIAL
Acute Bacterial Leptomeningitis
Chronic Bacterial Meningitis

INFECTIOUS DISORDERS OF THE CENTRAL NERVOUS SYSTEM: VIRAL
Overview of Viral Encephalitis
Acute Viral Encephalitis
Acute Toxic Encephalopathy During Viral
    Encephalitis
Parainfectious Encephalitis
    (Acute Disseminated Encephalomyelitis)
Cerebral Biopsy for Diagnosis of
    Encephalitis

CEREBRAL VASCULITIS AND OTHER VASCULOPATHIES
Granulomatous Central Nervous System
    Angiitis
Systemic Lupus Erythematosus
Subacute Diencephalic
    Angioencephalopathy
Varicella-Zoster Vasculitis
Behçet's Syndrome
Cerebral Autosomal Dominant
    Arteriopathy With Subcortical Infarcts
    and Leukoencephalopathy

MISCELLANEOUS NEURONAL AND GLIAL DISORDERS
Prion Diseases
Adrenoleukodystrophy (Schilder's
    Disease)
Marchiafava-Bignami Disease
Gliomatosis Cerebri
Progressive Multifocal
    Leukoencephalopathy
Epilepsy
Mixed Metabolic Encephalopathy

ACUTE DELIRIOUS STATES
Drug Withdrawal Delirium
    (Delirium Tremens)
Postoperative Delirium
Intensive Care Unit Delirium
Drug-Induced Delirium

This chapter describes the biochemical and physiologic mechanisms (where known) by which multifocal and diffuse disorders interfere with the metabolism of the brain to produce delirium, stupor, or coma. It also describes the signs and symptoms that characterize these disorders and differentiate them from localized intracranial mass lesions and unifocal destructive lesions.

Not all of the myriad disorders that cause delirium or coma can be included. Among the criteria for selection are (1) presentation to an emergency department with the acute or subacute onset of delirium or coma without a prior history that immediately explains the cause, (2) a condition that may be reversible if treated promptly but is potentially lethal otherwise, (3) an illness with characteristic clinical or laboratory findings that strongly suggest the diagnosis, or (4) a rare and unusual disorder that may be overlooked by physicians who are rushing to establish a diagnosis and start treatment.

A physician confronted by a stuporous or comatose patient must address the question, which of the major etiologic categories of dysfunction (i.e., supratentorial, subtentorial, metabolic, or psychologic) caused the coma? Chapters 3 and 4 discuss the signs that indicate whether a patient is suffering from a structural cause (supratentorial or subtentorial) of coma. This chapter describes some of the causes of diffuse and metabolic brain dysfunction. The next chapter describes psychologic dysfunction.

The initial section of this chapter describes the *clinical signs* of diffuse, multifocal, or metabolic disease of the brain. Once the physician has determined that the patient's signs and symptoms indicate such an illness, he or she must determine which of the large number of specific illnesses is responsible for this particular patient's stupor or coma. This question often requires a rapid answer because many metabolic disorders that cause coma are fully reversible if treated early and appropriately, but lethal if treatment is delayed or is inappropriate.

Table 5–1 lists some of the diffuse, multifocal, and metabolic causes of stupor and coma. It attempts to classify these causes in such a way that the table can be used as a checklist of the major causes to be considered when the physician is presented with an unconscious patient suspected of suffering from an illness in this category. Heading A concerns itself with deprivation of oxygen, substrates, or metabolic cofactors. Headings B through E are concerned with systemic diseases that cause abnormalities of cerebral metabolism (metabolic encephalopathy). Headings F and G are concerned with primary disorders of nervous system function, which, because of their diffuse involvement of brain, resemble the metabolic encephalopathies more than they do focal structural disease.

Heading H lists a variety of miscellaneous disorders whose cause is unknown. Although they represent a heterogeneous group of disorders, the diseases listed in Table 5–1, when they cause stupor and coma, can usually be distinguished by clinical signs alone from supratentorial and infratentorial focal lesions and from psychologic disorders.

One caveat: neither the neurologic examination nor the examiner is infallible, and some patients have more than one cause for coma. Hence, even when the diagnosis of metabolic disease is absolutely unequivocal, unless the response to treatment is rapid and equally robust, imaging is an essential part of a careful workup.

CLINICAL SIGNS OF METABOLIC ENCEPHALOPATHY

Each patient with metabolic coma has a distinctive clinical picture, depending on the particular causative illness, the depth of coma, and the complications provided by comorbid illnesses or their treatment. Despite these individualities, however, specific illnesses often produce certain clinical patterns that recur again and again, and once recognized, they betray the diagnosis. A careful evaluation of consciousness, respiration, pupillary reactions, ocular movements, motor function, and the electroencephalogram (EEG) may differentiate metabolic encephalopathy from psychiatric dysfunction (Chapter 6) on the one hand, and from supratentorial or infratentorial structural disease on the other (see Chapters 3 and 4). Because these general characteristics of metabolic coma are so important, they are discussed before the specific disease entities.

CONSCIOUSNESS: CLINICAL ASPECTS

In patients with metabolic encephalopathy, stupor or coma is usually preceded by delirium. Delirium is characterized by alterations of arousal (either increased or decreased),[1] disorientation, decreased short-term memory, reduced ability to maintain and shift attention, disorganized thinking, perceptual disturbances, delusions and/or hallucinations, and disorders of sleep-wake cycle.[2] Some workers believe that

Table 5–1 Some Diffuse, Multifocal, or Metabolic Causes of Delirium, Stupor, and Coma

A. Deprivation of oxygen, substrate, or metabolic cofactors
   1. Hypoxia° (interference with oxygen supply to the entire brain; cerebral blood flow [CBF] normal)
      a. Decreased blood PO_2 and O_2 content: pulmonary disease; alveolar hypoventilation; decreased atmospheric oxygen tension
      b. Decreased blood O_2 content, PO_2 normal: "anemic anoxia"; anemia; carbon monoxide poisoning; methemoglobinemia
   2. Ischemia° (diffuse or widespread multifocal interference with blood supply to brain)
      a. Decreased CBF resulting from decreased cardiac output: Stokes-Adams attack; cardiac arrest; cardiac arrhythmias; myocardial infarction; congestive heart failure; aortic stenosis; pulmonary embolism
      b. Decreased CBF resulting from decreased peripheral resistance in systemic circulation: syncope (see Table 5–8); carotid sinus hypersensitivity; low blood volume
      c. Decreased CBF associated with generalized or multifocal increased vascular resistance: hyperventilation syndrome; hyperviscosity (polycythemia, cryoglobulinemia or macroglobulinemia, sickle cell anemia); subarachnoid hemorrhage; bacterial meningitis; hypertensive encephalopathy
      d. Decreased CBF owing to widespread small-vessel occlusions: disseminated intravascular coagulation; systemic lupus erythematosus; subacute bacterial endocarditis; fat embolism; cerebral malaria; cardiopulmonary bypass
   3. Hypoglycemia° resulting from exogenous insulin: spontaneous (endogenous insulin, liver disease, etc.)
   4. Cofactor deficiency
      Thiamine (Wernicke's encephalopathy)
      Niacin
      Pyridoxine
      Cyanocobalamin
      Folic acid

B. Toxicity of endogenous products
   1. Due to organ failure
      Liver (hepatic coma)
      Kidney (uremic coma)
      Lung (CO_2 narcosis)
      Pancreas (exocrine pancreatic encephalopathy)
   2. Due to hyper- and/or hypofunction of endocrine organs: pituitary thyroid (myxedema-thyrotoxicosis); parathyroid (hypo- and hyperparathyroidism); adrenal (Addison's disease, Cushing's disease, pheochromocytoma); pancreas (diabetes, hypoglycemia)
   3. Due to other systemic diseases: diabetes; cancer; porphyria; sepsis

C. Toxicity of exogenous poisons
   1. Sedative drugs°: hypnotics, tranquilizers, ethanol, opiates
   2. Acid poisons or poisons with acidic breakdown products: paraldehyde; methyl alcohol; ethylene glycol; ammonium chloride
   3. Psychotropic drugs: tricyclic antidepressants and anticholinergic drugs; amphetamines; lithium; phencyclidine; phenothiazines; LSD and mescaline; ponoamine oxidase inhibitors
   4. Others: penicillin; anticonvulsants; steroids; cardiac glycosides; trace metals; organic phosphates; cyanide; salicylate

D. Abnormalities of ionic or acid-base environment of central nervous system (CNS)
   Water and sodium (hyper- and hyponatremia)
   Acidosis (metabolic and respiratory)
   Alkalosis (metabolic and respiratory)
   Magnesium (hyper- and hypomagnesemia)
   Calcium (hyper- and hypocalcemia)
   Phosphorus (hypophosphatemia)

Table 5–1 (cont.)

E. Disordered temperature regulation
   Hypothermia
   Heat stroke, fever

F. Infections or inflammation of CNS
   Leptomeningitis
   Encephalitis
   Acute "toxic" encephalopathy
   Parainfectious encephalomyelitis
   Cerebral vasculitis/vasculopathy
   Subarachnoid hemorrhage

G. Primary neuronal or glial disorders
   Creutzfeldt-Jakob disease
   Marchiafava-Bignami disease
   Adrenoleukodystrophy
   Gliomatosis, lymphomatosis cerebri
   Progressive multifocal leukoencephalopathy

H. Miscellaneous disorders of unknown cause
   Seizures and postictal states
   Concussion
   Acute delirious states°: sedative drugs and withdrawal; "postoperative" delirium; intensive care unit delirium; drug intoxications

°Alone or in combination, the most common causes of delirium seen on medical or surgical wards.

impairment of attention is the underlying abnormality in all acute confusional states; others emphasize clouding of consciousness as the core symptom.[3] The importance of these early behavioral warnings is so great that we will review briefly some of the mental symptoms that often precede metabolic coma and, by their presence, suggest the diagnosis. The mental changes are best looked for in terms of arousal, attention, alertness, orientation and grasp, cognition, memory, affect, and perception.

Tests of Mental Status

Assessing cognitive function in patients with impairment of attention and alertness is often difficult. However, careful quantitative assessment of these functions is exceedingly important, because changes in cognition often indicate whether the physician's therapeutic efforts are improving or worsening the patient's condition. Several validated bedside tests that can be given in a few minutes, even to confused patients, have been developed. These tests allow one to score cognitive functions and to follow the patient's course in quantitative fashion.[4–6] One test is specifically designed for patients in intensive care units, even those on respirators.[7] Table 5–2 illustrates one such scale.

Arousal can be defined as the degree of sensory stimulation required to keep the patient attending to the examiner's question. Patients with metabolic encephalopathy always have abnormalities of arousal. Some patients are hypervigilant, whereas in others arousal is decreased. In many delirious patients arousal alternates between hyper- and hypovigilance.[1] Hyperaroused patients are so distractible that they cannot maintain focus on relevant stimuli, whereas hypoaroused patients need constant sensory stimulation. In addition, most delirious patients have an altered sleep-wake cycle, often sleeping during the day but becoming more confused and hyperactive at night ("sundowning"). Abnormalities of arousal can also be reflected in motor activity, with hyperaroused patients demonstrating increased but purposeless motor activity and hypoaroused patients being relatively immobile. Although certain clinical states (i.e., drug withdrawal and fever) are more likely to produce a hyperaroused state than are other

Table 5–2 **The Confusion Assessment Method for the Intensive Care Unit (CAM-ICU)**

Delirium is diagnosed when both features 1 and 2 are positive, along with either feature 3 or feature 4.

Feature 1. Acute Onset of Mental Status Changes or Fluctuating Course
- Is there evidence of an acute change in mental status from the baseline?
- Did the (abnormal) behavior fluctuate during the past 24 hours, that is, tend to come and go or increase and decrease in severity?
  Sources of information: Serial Glasgow Coma Scale or sedation score ratings over 24 hours as well as readily available input from the patient's bedside critical care nurse or family

Feature 2: Inattention
- Did the patient have difficulty focusing attention?
- Is there a reduced ability to maintain and shift attention?
  Sources of information: Attention screening examinations by using either picture recognition or Vigilance A random letter test (see Methods and Appendix 2 for description of attention screening examinations). Neither of these tests requires verbal response, and thus they are ideally suited for mechanically ventilated patients.

Feature 3. Disorganized Thinking
- Was the patient's thinking disorganized or incoherent, such as rambling or irrelevant conversation, unclear or illogical flow of ideas, or unpredictable switching from subject to subject?
- Was the patient able to follow questions and commands throughout the assessment?
  1. "Are you having any unclear thinking?"
  2. "Hold up this many fingers." (Examiner holds two fingers in front of the patient.)
  3. "Now, do the same thing with the other hand." (Not repeating the number of fingers)

Feature 4. Altered Level of Consciousness
- Any level of consciousness other than "alert."
- Alert—normal, spontaneously fully aware of environment and interacts appropriately
- Vigilant—hyperalert
- Lethargic—drowsy but easily aroused, unaware of some elements in the environment, or not spontaneously interacting appropriately with the interview; becomes fully aware and appropriately interactive when prodded minimally
- Stupor—difficult to arouse, unaware of some or all elements in the environment, or not spontaneously interacting with the interviewer; becomes incompletely aware and inappropriately interactive when prodded strongly
- Coma—unarousable, unaware of all elements in the environment, with no spontaneous interaction or awareness of the interviewer, so that the interview is difficult or impossible even with maximum prodding

From Ely et al.,[6] with permission.

metabolic disorders such as drug intoxication and hypoxia/ischemia, in a given patient the state of arousal is not a reliable guide in diagnosis. In general, about one-quarter of patients with delirium are hyperaroused, one-quarter are hypoaroused, and one-half fluctuate between the two states. Although hyperaroused patients are often diagnosed earlier because of their florid behavior, their outcome appears no different from those patients who are hypoactive.[8,9]

ATTENTION AND ALERTNESS

Attention is a process whereby one focuses on relevant stimuli from the environment and is able to shift focus to other stimuli as they become relevant. Most observers believe that the core of delirium as an altered state of consciousness is failure of attention. Attention is assessed by the examiner during the course of the clinical examination by determining whether a patient continues to respond in an appropriate fashion to the questions posed by the examiner. Attention is tested formally by having a patient perform a repetitive task that requires multiple iterations, such as naming the days of the week or months of the year, or a random list of numbers or serial subtractions, backwards. Failure to complete the task and even inability to name what the task was indicate inattention.

Three different disorders of attention can be identified in delirious patients. The first disorder that usually occurs in patients who are hyperaroused is distractibility. Patients shift attention from the examiner to noises in the hallway or other extraneous stimuli. A second abnormality of attention is perseveration. Patients answer a new question or respond to a new stimulus with the same response they gave to the previous stimulus, failing to redirect behavior toward the new stimulus. The third abnormality is failure to focus on an ongoing stimulus. After being distracted by another stimulus, the patient will forget to return to the activity in which he or she was engaged before distraction.

Alterations of *alertness* preceding other changes are more characteristic of acute or subacutely developing metabolic encephalopathy than of more slowly developing dementia; demented patients tend to lose orientation and cognition before displaying an alteration in alertness. Severe metabolic encephalopathy eventually leads to stupor and finally coma, and of course, when this point is reached, mental testing no longer helps to distinguish metabolic from other causes of brain dysfunction.

ORIENTATION AND GRASP

Although attention and arousal are the first faculties to be impaired by metabolic encephalopathies, they are difficult to quantify. As a result, defects in orientation and immediate grasp of test situations often become the earliest

unequivocal symptoms of brain dysfunction. When examining patients suspected of metabolic or cerebral disorders, one must ask specifically the date, the time, the place, and how long it takes or the route one would take to reach home or some other well-defined place. Even uneducated patients or those with limited intellect should know the month and year, and most should know the day and date, particularly if there has been a recent holiday. Patients with early metabolic encephalopathy lose orientation for time and miss the year as frequently as the month or the day. Orientation for distance is usually impaired next, and finally, the identification of persons and places becomes confused. Disorientation for person and place but not time is unusual in structural disease but sometimes is a psychologic symptom. Disorientation for self is almost always a manifestation of psychologically induced amnesia.

COGNITION

The content and progression of thought are always disturbed in delirium and dementia, sometimes as the incipient symptoms. To detect these changes requires asking specific questions employing abstract definitions and problems. As attention and concentration are nearly always impaired, patients with metabolic brain disease usually make errors in serial subtractions, and rarely can they repeat more than three or four numbers in reverse. Thus, difficulty with mental arithmetic is not a sign necessarily of impaired calculation ability; writing the problem down, which eliminates the attentional component of the task, allows assessment of the underlying cognitive function. It is important to inventory language skills (including reading and writing), arithmetic skills, and visuospatial skills (including drawing), as well as to judge whether the patient is able to cooperate and to distinguish focal cognitive impairments (suggesting a focal lesion) from more global derangement that is seen in metabolic encephalopathy.

MEMORY

Loss of recent memory for recent events and inability to retain new memories for more than a few minutes is a hallmark of dementia and a frequent accompaniment of delirium. Most patients with metabolic brain disease have a memory loss that is proportional to other losses of cognitive functions. When the maximal pathologic changes involve the medial temporal lobe, however, recent memory loss outstrips other intellectual impairments. Thus, memory loss and an inability to form new associations can be a sign of either diffuse or bilateral focal brain disease.

AFFECT AND COMPORTMENT

Patients may appear apathetic and withdrawn, in which case they are often believed by their relatives to be depressed, or they may be ebullient and outgoing, particularly when hyperaroused. Inappropriate comments and behavior are common and often embarrassing to friends and relatives. Patients are usually unaware that their behavior is inappropriate.

PERCEPTION

Patients with metabolic brain disease frequently make perceptual errors, mistaking the members of the hospital staff for old friends and relatives and granting vitality to inanimate objects. Illusions are common and invariably involve stimuli from the immediate environment. Quiet and apathetic patients suffer illusory experiences, but these must be asked about since they are rarely volunteered. Anxious and fearful patients, on the other hand, frequently express concern about their illusions and misperceptions to the accompaniment of loud and violent behavior. Unlike patients with psychiatric disorders, visual or combined visual and auditory hallucinations are more common than pure auditory ones.[10,11]

Pathogenesis of the Mental Changes

Both global and focal cerebral functional abnormalities can cause the mental symptoms of metabolic brain disease. The global symptoms result from alterations of arousal that in turn interfere with attention, comprehension, and cognitive synthesis. Well-recognized focal cerebral abnormalities include specific abnormalities in language recognition and synthesis, in recent memory storage and recall, in gnosis (recognition of persons and/or objects [from

the Greek for *knowledge*]) and praxis (ability to preform an action [from the Greek for *action*]), and perhaps in the genesis of hallucinations. Focal lesions may mimic more diffuse causes of delirium. Perhaps the best example is the florid delirium that sometimes accompanies cerebral infarcts of the nondominant parietal lobe,[12] an area implicated in selective attention[13] that, as indicated above, may be the primary abnormality in delirium.

A combination of diffuse and focal dysfunction probably underlies the cerebral symptoms of most patients with metabolic encephalopathy. The extensive corticocortical physiologic connectivity of the human brain discussed in Chapter 1 implies that large focal abnormalities inevitably will cause functional effects that extend well beyond their immediate confines. Furthermore, the more rapidly the lesion develops, the more extensive will be the acute functional loss. Thus, the general loss of highest integrative functions in metabolic diseases is compatible with a diffuse dysfunction of neurons and, as judged by measurements of cerebral metabolism, the severity of the clinical signs is directly related to the mass of neurons affected. However, certain distinctive clinical signs in different patients and in different diseases probably reflect damage to more discrete areas having to do with memory and other selective aspects of integrative behavior. An example is the encephalopathy resulting from thiamine deficiency (Wernicke-Korsakoff syndrome; see page 223). In this illness, patients show acutely the clinical signs of delirium and, rarely, coma.[14] All neuronal areas are deprived of thiamine to the same extent, but certain cell groups such as the mamillary bodies, the mediodorsal nucleus of the thalamus, the periaqueductal gray matter, and the oculomotor nuclei are pathologically more sensitive to the deficiency and show the greatest anatomic evidence of injury. The final common pathway to neuronal destruction, as in many other disorders, is probably glutamate-induced excitotoxicity.[15,16] Thus, a diffuse disease may have a focal maximum. Clinically, eye movements, balance, and recent memory are impaired more severely than are other mental functions, and indeed, memory loss may persist to produce a permanent Wernicke-Korsakoff syndrome after other mental functions and overall cerebral metabolism have improved to a near-normal level.

RESPIRATION

Sooner or later, metabolic brain disease nearly always results in an abnormality of either the depth or rhythm of breathing. Most of the time, this is a nonspecific alteration and simply a part of a more widespread brainstem depression. Sometimes, however, the respiratory changes stand out separately from the rest of the neurologic defects and are more or less specific to the disease in question. Some of these specific respiratory responses are homeostatic adjustments to the metabolic process causing encephalopathy. The others occur in illnesses that particularly affect the respiratory mechanisms. Either way, proper evaluation and interpretation of the specific respiratory changes facilitate diagnosis and often suggest an urgent need for treatment.

As a first step in appraising the breathing of patients with metabolically caused coma, increased or decreased respiratory efforts must be confirmed as truly reflecting hyperventilation or hypoventilation. Increased chest efforts do not indicate hyperventilation if they merely overcome obstruction or pneumonitis, and conversely, seemingly shallow breathing can fulfill the reduced metabolic needs of subjects in deep coma. Although careful clinical evaluation usually avoids those potential deceptions, the bedside observations are most helpful when anchored by direct determinations of the arterial blood gases.

Neurologic Respiratory Changes Accompanying Metabolic Encephalopathy

Lethargic or slightly obtunded patients have posthyperventilation apnea, probably resulting from loss of the influence of the frontal lobes in causing continual if low-volume ventilation, even when there is no metabolic need to breathe.[17] Those in stupor or light coma commonly exhibit Cheyne-Stokes respiration. With more profound brainstem depression, transient neurogenic hyperventilation can ensue either from suppression of brainstem inhibitory regions or from development of neurogenic pulmonary edema.[18,19] As an illustration, poisoning with short- or intermediate-acting barbiturate preparations often induces brief episodes of hyperventilation and motor hypertonus, either during the stage of deepening coma or as patients reawaken. Hypoglycemia and anoxic damage are even more frequent causes of transient hyperpnea. Diabetic ketoacidosis and other causes of coma that cause a metabolic acidosis may produce slow, deep (Kussmaul) respirations. Both hepatic encephalopathy and systemic inflammatory states cause persistent hyperventilation, resulting in a primary respiratory alkalosis. In these instances, the increased breathing sometimes outlasts the immediate metabolic perturbation, and if the subject also has extensor rigidity, the clinical picture may superficially resemble structural disease or severe metabolic acidosis. However, attention to other neurologic details usually leads to the proper diagnosis, as the following case illustrates.

Patient 5–1

A 28-year-old man was brought unconscious to the emergency department. Fifteen minutes earlier, with slurred speech, he had instructed a taxi driver to take him to the hospital, then "passed out." His pulse was 100 per minute, and his blood pressure was 130/90 mm Hg. His respirations were 40 per minute and deep. The pupils were small (2 mm), but the light and ciliospinal reflexes were preserved. Oculocephalic reflexes were present. Deep tendon reflexes were hyperactive; there were bilateral extensor plantar responses, and he periodically had bilateral extensor spasms of the arms and legs. His blood glucose was 20 mg/dL. After 25 g of glucose was given intravenously, respirations quieted, the extensor spasms ceased, and he withdrew appropriately from noxious stimuli. After 75 g of glucose, he awoke and disclosed that he was diabetic, taking insulin, and had neglected to eat that day.

Comment: This man's hyperpnea and decerebrate rigidity initially suggested structural brainstem disease to the emergency department physicians. Normal oculocephalic responses, normal pupillary reactions, and the absence of other focal signs made metabolic coma more likely, and the diagnosis was confirmed by the subsequent findings.

The effectiveness of respiration must be evaluated repeatedly when metabolic disease depresses the brain, because the brainstem reticular formation is especially vulnerable to chemical depression. Anoxia, hypoglycemia, and drugs all are capable of selectively inducing hypoventilation or apnea while concurrently sparing other brainstem functions such as pupillary responses and blood pressure control.

Acid-Base Changes Accompanying Hyperventilation During Metabolic Encephalopathy

Respiration is the first and most rapid defense against systemic acid-base imbalance. Chemoreceptors located in the carotid body and aortic arterial wall, as well as in the lower brainstem, quickly respond to alterations in the blood of either hydrogen ion concentration or PCO_2. Hypoxia sensitizes peripheral chemoreceptors and activates central chemoreceptors, but under most circumstances carbon dioxide levels, which are linked to blood pH, are more important in determining respiration (see Chapter 2). Table 5–3 lists some causes of abnormal ventilation in unresponsive patients.

HYPERVENTILATION

In a stuporous or comatose patient, hyperventilation is a danger sign meaning one of two things: either compensation for metabolic acidosis or a response to primary respiratory stimulation (respiratory alkalosis). Metabolic acidosis and respiratory alkalosis are differentiated by blood biochemical analyses. In the first instance, the arterial blood pH is low (less than 7.30 if hyperpnea is to be attributed to acidosis) and the serum bicarbonate is also low (usually below 10 mEq/L). In the second case, the arterial pH is high (over 7.45) and the serum bicarbonate is normal or reduced. In both primary respiratory alkalosis and metabolic acidosis with respiratory compensation, the arterial carbon dioxide tension ($PaCO_2$) is reduced, usually below 30 mm Hg. Respiratory compensation for metabolic acidosis is a normal brainstem reflex response and, hence, occurs in most cases of metabolic acidosis. Mixed primary metabolic acidosis and primary respiratory alkalosis (which persists after the acidotic load is removed) also occurs in several conditions, particularly salicylate toxicity and hepatic coma. A diagnosis of mixed metabolic abnormality can be made when the degree of

Table 5–3 Some Causes of Abnormal Ventilation in Unresponsive Patients

I. Hyperventilation
  A. Metabolic acidosis
    1. Anion gap
      Diabetic ketoacidosis°
      Diabetic hyperosmolar coma°
      Lactic acidosis
      Uremia°
      Alcoholic ketoacidosis
      Acidic poisons°
        Ethylene glycol
        Propylene glycol
        Methyl alcohol
        Paraldehyde
        Salicylism (primarily in children)
    2. No anion gap
      Diarrhea
      Pancreatic drainage
      Carbonic anhydrase inhibitors
      NH_4Cl ingestion
      Renal tubular acidosis
      Ureteroenterostomy
  B. Respiratory alkalosis
    Hepatic failure°
    Sepsis°
    Pneumonia
    Anxiety (hyperventilation syndrome)
  C. Mixed acid-base disorders (metabolic acidosis and respiratory alkalosis)
    Salicylism
    Sepsis°
    Hepatic failure°
II. Hypoventilation
  A. Respiratory acidosis
    1. Acute (uncompensated)
      Sedative drugs°
      Brainstem injury
      Neuromuscular disorders
      Chest injury
      Acute pulmonary disease
    2. Chronic pulmonary disease°
  B. Metabolic alkalosis
    Vomiting or gastric drainage
    Diuretic therapy
    Adrenal steroid excess (Cushing's syndrome)
    Primary aldosteronism
    Bartter's syndrome

°Common causes of stupor or coma.

respiratory or metabolic compensation is excessive. Table 5–4 lists some of the causes of hyperventilation in patients with metabolic encephalopathy.

Table 5–4 **Pathophysiology of Metabolic Acidosis**

Cause	Rate of Acid Accumulation
Failure of renal acid excretion	2–4 mEq/hour
Decreased H^+ secretion	
Distal renal tubular acidosis	
Decreased NH_4^+ production	
Generalized renal failure	
Adrenal insufficiency/ hypoaldosteronism	
Loss of bicarbonate and alkaline equivalents	1–20 mEq/hour
Gastrointestinal	
Diarrhea	
Pancreatic, biliary, and enteric drainage	
Urinary diversion	
Renal	
Carbonic anhydrase inhibitors	
Proximal renal tubular acidosis	
Posthypocapnic state	
Dilutional acidosis	
Addition and/or overproduction of acid	2–500 mEq/hour
Endogenous	
Lactic acidosis	
Ketoacidosis	
Alcoholic	
Starvation	
Diabetes	
Hereditary metabolic enzyme disorders	
Exogenous	
Acid administration	
Hydrochloric acid	
Ammonium chloride	
Cationic amino acids in total parenteral nutrition	
Toxins converted to acid	
Methanol	
Ethylene glycol, propylene glycol	
Paraldehyde	
Salicylate	

From Swenson,[20] with permission.

Metabolic acidosis sufficient to produce coma and hyperpnea has four important causes: uremia, diabetes, lactic acidosis (anoxic or spontaneous), and the ingestion of poisons that are acidic or have acidic breakdown products (Table 5–4).

In any given patient, a quick and accurate selection can and must be made from among these disorders. Diabetes and uremia are diagnosed by appropriate laboratory tests, and diabetic acidosis is confirmed by identifying serum ketonemia. It is important to remember that severe alcoholics without diabetes occasionally can develop ketoacidosis after prolonged drinking bouts.[21] An important observation is that diabetics, especially those who have been treated with the oral hypoglycemic agent metformin, are subject to lactic acidosis as well as to diabetic ketoacidosis, but in the former condition ketonemia is lacking.[22] If diabetes and uremia are eliminated in a patient as causes of acidosis, it can be inferred either that he or she has spontaneous lactic acidosis or has been poisoned with an exogenous toxin such as ethylene glycol, propylene glycol (which is metabolized to a racemic mixture of lactate), methyl alcohol, or decomposed paraldehyde. Anoxic lactic acidosis would be suspected only if anoxia or shock was present, and even then severe anoxic acidosis is relatively uncommon. Although laboratory tests can identify and quantify the ingested agents, these tests are not usually immediately available (see Chapter 7). However, the toxins are osmotically active and measurement of serum osmolality can detect the presence of an osmotically active substance, indicating exposure to a toxic agent.[23] Severe toxic alcohol poisonings can be treated with fomepizole and, if necessary in patients with renal failure, hemodialysis.[24] One report suggests that diethylene glycol poisoning can cause delayed neurologic sequelae including cranial neuropathies and bulbar palsy.[25]

The treatment of metabolic acidosis depends first on treating the inciting factor. Intravenous bicarbonate is indicated to treat hyperkalemia and to help clear acidic toxins from cells. Bicarbonate does not appear helpful in treating diabetic ketoacidosis.[20]

Sustained *respiratory alkalosis* has five important causes among disorders producing the picture of metabolic stupor or coma: salicylism, hepatic coma, pulmonary disease, sepsis, and psychogenic hyperventilation (Table 5–5).

Table 5–5 **Pathophysiology of Respiratory Alkalosis**

Hypoxia
Parenchymal lung disease
   Pneumonia
   Bronchial asthma
   Diffuse interstitial fibrosis
   Pulmonary embolism
   Pulmonary edema
Medications and mechanical ventilation
   Medications
     Salicylate
     Nicotine
     Xanthine
     Catecholamines
     Analeptics
   Mechanical ventilation
Central nervous system disorders
   Meningitis, encephalitis
   Cerebrovascular disease
   Head trauma
   Space-occupying lesion
   Anxiety
Metabolic
   Sepsis
   Hormonal
   Pyrexia
   Hepatic disease
Hyperventilation syndrome

From Foster et al.,[26] with permission.

Neurogenic pulmonary edema and central neurogenic hyperventilation may also cause respiratory alkalosis in patients with metabolic stupor or coma. As is true with metabolic acidosis, these usually can be at least partially separated by clinical examination and simple laboratory measures.

Salicylate poisoning causes a combined respiratory alkalosis and metabolic acidosis that lowers the serum bicarbonate disproportionately to the degree of serum pH elevation. Salicylism should be suspected in a stuporous hyperpneic adult if the serum pH is normal or alkaline, there is an anion gap, and the serum bicarbonate is between 10 and 14 mEq/L. Salicylism in children lowers serum bicarbonate still more and produces serum acidosis. A bedside laboratory test can rapidly establish a diagnosis of salicylate intoxication,[27] although usually in an awake patient the positive history and the presence of respiratory alkalosis are sufficient. A single serum salicylate measurement may be somewhat misleading, particularly if the patient has taken enteric-coated tablets that may delay absorption. Therefore, in a patient with a suspected salicylate overdose, careful measurements should be done every 3 hours until levels have peaked. The ingestion of sedative drugs in addition to salicylates may blunt the hyperpnea and lead to metabolic acidosis, a picture that may mislead the examiner.

Salicylates directly activate the respiratory centers of the brainstem, although the mechanism is not known. Acetaminophen poisoning, more common than salicylate poisoning, may cause either metabolic acidosis (lactic acidosis) or respiratory alkalosis resulting from its hepatic toxicity (see below).[28,29]

The treatment includes, where appropriate, gastric lavage and activated charcoal. Urinary alkalization helps promote excretion of the drug; hemodialysis may be necessary if there is renal failure.[30] Acetylcysteine may limit the degree of hepatic toxicity by acetaminophen (see Chapter 7).

Hepatic coma, producing respiratory alkalosis, rarely depresses the serum bicarbonate below 16 mEq/L, and the diagnosis usually is betrayed by other signs of liver dysfunction. The associated clinical abnormalities of liver disease are sometimes minimal, particularly with fulminating acute liver failure or when gastrointestinal hemorrhage precipitates coma in a chronic cirrhotic patient. Liver function tests and measurement of arterial ammonia must be relied upon in such instances.

Sepsis is always associated with hyperventilation, probably a direct central effect of the cascade of cytokines and prostaglandins initiated by endotoxinemia. In fact, a respiratory rate of more than 20 breaths per minute, or a PCO_2 of less than 30 torr, is part of the definition of sepsis.[31] Early in the course of the illness the acid-base defect is that of a pure respiratory alkalosis (HCO_3 greater than 15 mEq/L), but in critically ill patients, lactic acid later accumulates in the blood and the stuporous patient usually presents a combined acid-base defect of respiratory alkalosis and metabolic acidosis (HCO_3 less than 15 mEq/L). Fever, or in severe cases hypothermia and hypotension, may accompany the neurologic signs and suggest the diagnosis.

Respiratory alkalosis caused by *pulmonary congestion, fibrosis, or pneumonia* rarely depresses the serum bicarbonate significantly. This diagnosis should be considered in hypoxic, hyperpneic comatose patients who have normal or slightly lowered serum bicarbonate levels and no evidence of liver disease.

Psychogenic hyperventilation does not cause coma, but may cause delirium, and may be present as an additional symptom in a patient with psychogenic "coma." Severe alkalosis, by itself, has been reported to cause seizures and coma. The decreased ionizable calcium complicating alkalosis may lead to muscle twitching, muscle spasms, and tetany, as well as positive Chvostek and Trousseau's signs.[32]

Acid-Base Changes Accompanying Hypoventilation During Metabolic Encephalopathy

In an unconscious patient, hypoventilation means either respiratory compensation for metabolic alkalosis or respiratory depression with consequent acidosis. The differential diagnosis is outlined in Table 5–3. In metabolic alkalosis the arterial blood pH is elevated (greater than 7.45), as is the serum bicarbonate (greater than 35 mEq/L). In untreated respiratory acidosis with coma, the serum pH is low (less than 7.35) and the serum bicarbonate is either normal or

high, depending on prior treatment and how rapidly the respiratory failure has developed. The $PaCO_2$ is always elevated in respiratory acidosis (usually greater than 55 mm Hg) and is often elevated in metabolic alkalosis as well because of respiratory compensation in metabolic alkalosis. In respiratory acidosis, the pH of the cerebrospinal fluid (CSF) is always low if artificial ventilation has not been used.[33,34] The PCO_2 is elevated in respiratory acidosis, and in metabolic alkalosis with respiratory compensation, but is usually less than 50 mm Hg in primary metabolic alkalosis and almost invariably rises considerably higher than this when primary respiratory acidosis causes stupor or coma. In both disorders, the oxygen tension is reduced due to hypoventilation. A normal serum bicarbonate level is consistent with untreated respiratory acidosis of short duration but not with metabolic alkalosis.

Metabolic alkalosis results from (1) excessive loss of acid via gastrointestinal or renal routes, (2) excessive bicarbonate load, or (3) failure to fully correct the posthypocapnic state (Table 5–6).[32]

To find the specific cause often requires exhaustive laboratory analyses, but delirium and obtundation owing to metabolic alkalosis are rarely severe and never life threatening, so that

Table 5–6 **Pathophysiology of Metabolic Alkalosis**

Generation	Examples
1. Loss of acid from extracellular space A. Loss of gastric fluid (HCl)	Vomiting Primary aldosteronism and diuretic administration
B. Acid loss in the urine: increased distal Na^+ delivery in presence of hyperaldosteronism	
C. Acid shifts into cells	Potassium deficiency
D. Loss of acid into stool	Congenital chloride-losing diarrhea
2. Excessive HCO_3 loads A. Absolute 1. Oral or parenteral HCO_3	Milk alkali syndrome
2. Metabolic conversion of the salts of organic acids in HCO_3^1	Lactate, acetate, or citrate administration (especially in conditions with underlying liver disease)
B. Relative	$NaHCO_3$ dialysis
3. Posthypercapnic states	Correction of chronic hypercapnia in presence of low-salt diet or in a patient with congestive heart failure

From Khanna and Kurtzman,[32] with permission

Table 5–7 **Pathophysiology of Respiratory Acidosis**

Acute	Chronic
Acute central nervous system depression	Central sleep apnea
Drug overdose (benzodiazepines,	Primary alveolar
narcotics, barbiturates,	hypoventilation
propofol, major tranquilizers)	Obesity hypoventilation
Head trauma	syndrome
Cerebrovascular accident	Spinal cord injury
Central nervous system infection	Diaphragmatic paralysis
(encephalitis)	Amyotrophic lateral sclerosis
Acute neuromuscular disease	Myasthenia gravis
Guillain-Barré syndrome	Muscular dystrophy
Spinal cord injury	Multiple sclerosis
Myasthenic crisis	Poliomyelitis
Botulism	Hypothyroidism
Organophosphate poisoning	Kyphoscoliosis
Acute airways disease	Thoracic cage disease
Status asthmaticus	Chronic obstructive
Upper airway obstruction (laryngospasm,	pulmonary disease
angioedema, foreign body aspiration	Severe chronic interstitial lung
Exacerbation of chronic obstructive	disease
pulmonary disease	
Acute parenchymal and vascular disease	
Cardiogenic pulmonary edema	
Acute lung injury	
Multilobular pneumonia	
Massive pulmonary embolism	
Acute pleural or chest wall disease	
Pneumothorax	
Hemothorax	
Flail chest	

From Epstein and Singh,[36] with permission.

time exists for careful diagnostic considerations. Respiratory compensation from metabolic alkalosis leads to hypocapnia, but the PCO_2 rarely is higher than 50 torr. Higher levels suggest coexistent pulmonary disease.[35]

Respiratory acidosis is a more pressing problem,[36] caused by either severe pulmonary or neuromuscular disease (peripheral respiratory failure) or by depression of the respiratory center (central respiratory failure) (Table 5–7).

Both causes induce hypoxia as well as CO_2 retention. Chest examinations almost always can differentiate neuromuscular from pulmonary disease, and the presence of tachypnea distinguishes pulmonary or peripheral neuromuscular failure from central failure with its irregular or slow respiratory patterns. Severe respiratory acidosis of any origin is best treated by artificial ventilation. Acute respiratory acidosis causes encephalopathy, sometimes associated with headache, which may reflect intracranial vasodilation. If the PCO_2 exceeds 70 torr, the patient may become stuporous or comatose. If awake, there may be asterixis, myoclonus, and sometimes papilledema, the last resulting from increased intracranial pressure (ICP) due to the carbon dioxide-induced cerebral vasodilation.

PUPILS

Among patients in deep coma, the state of the pupils becomes the single most important criterion that clinically distinguishes between metabolic and structural disease. The presence of preserved pupillary light reflexes, despite concomitant respiratory depression, vestibulo-ocular caloric unresponsiveness, decerebrate rigidity, or motor flaccidity, suggests metabolic coma. Conversely, if asphyxia, anticholinergic or glutethimide ingestion, or pre-existing pupillary disease can be ruled out, the absence of pupillary light reflexes strongly implies that the disease is structural rather than metabolic.

Pupils cannot be considered conclusively nonreactive to a light stimulus unless care has been taken to examine them with magnification using a very bright light and maintaining the stimulus for several seconds. Infrared pupillometry is more reliable than the flashlight.[38] Ciliospinal reflexes are less reliable than light reflexes but, like them, are usually preserved in metabolic coma even when motor and respiratory signs signify lower brainstem dysfunction.[37]

OCULAR MOTILITY

The eyes usually rove randomly with mild metabolic coma and come to rest in the forward position as coma deepens. Although almost any eye position or random movement can be observed transiently when brainstem function is changing rapidly, a maintained conjugate lateral deviation or dysconjugate positioning of the eyes at rest suggests structural disease. Conjugate downward gaze, or occasionally upward gaze, can occur in metabolic as well as in structural disease and by itself is not helpful in the differential diagnosis.[39]

HISTORICAL VIGNETTE

Patient 5–2

A 63-year-old woman with severe hepatic cirrhosis and a portacaval shunt was found in coma. She groaned spontaneously but otherwise was unresponsive. Her respirations were 18 per minute and deep. The pupillary diameters were 4 mm on the right and 3 mm on the left, and both reacted to light. Her eyes were deviated conjugately downward and slightly to the right. Oculocephalic responses were conjugate in all directions. Her muscles were flaccid, but her stretch reflexes were brisk

and more active on the right with bilateral extensor plantar responses. No decorticate or decerebrate responses could be elicited. Her arterial blood pH was 7.58, and her $PaCO_2$ was 21 mm Hg. Two days later she awoke, at which time her eye movements were normal. Four days later she again drifted into coma, this time with the eyes in the physiologic position and with sluggish but full oculocephalic responses. She died on the sixth hospital day with severe hepatic cirrhosis. No structural central nervous system (CNS) lesion was found at autopsy.

Comment: This patient was seen prior to the availability of computed tomography (CT) scanning, but the later autopsy confirmed the clinical impression that these focal abnormalities were due to her liver failure, not a structural lesion. The initial conjugate deviation of the eyes downward and slightly to the right had suggested a deep, right-sided cerebral hemispheric mass lesion. But the return of gaze to normal with awakening within 24 hours and nonrepetition of the downward deviation when coma recurred ruled out a structural lesion. At autopsy, no intrinsic cerebral pathologic lesion was found to explain the abnormal eye movements. We have observed transient downward as well as transient upward deviation of the eyes in other patients in metabolic coma.

Because reflex eye movements are particularly sensitive to depressant drugs, cold caloric stimulation often provides valuable information about the depth of coma in patients with metabolic disease. The ocular response to passive head movement is less reliable than the caloric test, as absence of oculocephalic responses may imply purposeful inhibition of the reflex and does not dependably distinguish psychogenic unresponsiveness from brainstem depression. Cold caloric stimulation produces tonic conjugate deviation toward the irrigated ear in patients in light coma and little or no response in those in deep coma. If caloric stimulation evokes nystagmus, cerebral regulation of eye movements is intact and the impairment of consciousness is either very mild or the "coma" is psychogenic. If the eyes spontaneously deviate downward following lateral deviation, one should suspect drug-induced coma.[39] Finally, if caloric stimulation repeatedly produces dysconjugate eye movements, structural brainstem disease should be suspected (but see Chapter 2).

Patient 5–3

A 20-year-old woman became unresponsive while riding in the back seat of her parents' car. There was no history of previous illness, but her parents stated that she had severe emotional problems. On examination, her vital signs and general physical examination were normal. She appeared to be asleep when left alone, with quiet shallow respiration and no spontaneous movements. Her pupils were 3 mm and reactive. Oculocephalic responses were absent. She lay motionless to noxious stimuli but appeared to resist passive elevation of her eyelids. Cold caloric testing elicited tonic deviation of the eyes with no nystagmus. Blood and urine toxicology screens were positive for barbiturates, and she awoke the next morning and admitted ingesting a mixture of sedative drugs to frighten her mother.

Comment: The coma in this patient initially appeared light or even simulated. However, tonic deviation of the eyes in response to cold caloric irrigation signified that normal cerebral control of eye movements was impaired and indicated that her unresponsiveness was the result of organic, but probably toxic or metabolic, and not structural brain dysfunction. Toxicology screening discovered at least one cause, but drug overdosages are often mixed, and not all of the components may be picked up on screening.

MOTOR ACTIVITY

Patients with metabolic brain disease generally present two types of motor abnormalities: (1) nonspecific disorders of strength, tone, and reflexes, as well as focal or generalized seizures, and (2) certain characteristic adventitious movements that are almost diagnostic of metabolic brain disease.

"Nonspecific" Motor Abnormalities

Diffuse motor abnormalities are frequent in metabolic coma and reflect the degree and distribution of CNS depression (Chapter 1). Paratonia and snout, suck, or grasp reflexes may be seen in dementia, as well as in patients in light coma. With increasing brainstem depression, flexor and extensor rigidity and sometimes flaccidity appear. The rigid states are sometimes asymmetric.

Patient 5–4

A 60-year-old man was found in the street, stuporous, with an odor of wine on his breath. No other history was obtainable. His blood pressure was 120/80 mm Hg, pulse rate 100 per minute, and respirations 26 per minute and deep. After assessing radiographically for cervical spine injury, his neck was found to be supple. There was fetor hepaticus and the skin was jaundiced. The liver was palpably enlarged. He responded to noxious stimuli only by groaning. There was no response to visual threat. His left pupil was 5 mm, the right pupil was 3 mm, and both reacted to light. The eyes diverged at rest, but passive head movement elicited full conjugate ocular movements. The corneal reflexes were decreased but present bilaterally. There was a left facial droop. The gag reflex was present. He did not move spontaneously, but grimaced and demonstrated extensor responses to noxious stimuli. The limb muscles were symmetrically rigid and stretch reflexes were hyperactive. The plantar responses were extensor. An emergency CT scan was normal. The lumbar spinal fluid pressure was 120 mm/CSF and the CSF contained 30 mg/dL protein and one white blood cell. The serum bicarbonate was 16 mEq/L, chloride 104 mEq/L, sodium 147 mEq/L, and potassium 3.9 mEq/L. Liver function studies were grossly abnormal.

The following morning he responded appropriately to noxious stimulation. Hyperventilation had decreased, and the extensor posturing had disappeared. Diffuse rigidity, increased deep tendon reflexes, and bilateral extensor plantar responses remained. Improvement was rapid, and by the fourth hospital day he was awake and had normal findings on neurologic examination. However, on the seventh hospital day his blood pressure declined and his jaundice increased. He became hypotensive on the ninth hospital day and died. The general autopsy disclosed severe hepatic cirrhosis. An examination of the brain revealed old infarcts in the frontal lobes and the left inferior cerebellum. There were no other lesions.

Comment: In this patient, the signs of liver disease suggested the diagnosis of hepatic coma. At first, however, anisocoria and decerebrate rigidity hinted at a supratentorial mass lesion such as a subdural hematoma. The normal pupillary and oculocephalic reactions favored metabolic disease and the subsequent CT scan and absence of signs of rostral-caudal deterioration supported that diagnosis.

Focal weakness is surprisingly common with metabolic brain disease. Several of our patients with hypoglycemia or hepatic coma were transiently hemiplegic, and several patients with uremia or hyponatremia had focal weakness of upper motor neuron origin. Others have reported similar findings.[40,41]

HISTORICAL VIGNETTE

Patient 5–5

A 37-year-old man had been diabetic for 8 years. He received 35 units of protamine zinc insulin each morning in addition to 5 units of regular insulin when he believed he needed it. One week before admission he lost consciousness transiently upon arising, and when he awoke, he had a left hemiparesis, which disappeared within seconds. The evening before admission the patient had received 35 units of protamine zinc and 5 units of regular insulin. He awoke at 6 a.m. on the floor and was soiled with feces. His entire left side was numb and paralyzed. His pulse was 80 per minute, respirations 12, and blood pressure 130/80 mm Hg. The general physical examination was unremarkable. He was lethargic but oriented. His speech was slurred. There was supranuclear left facial paralysis and left flaccid hemiplegia with weakness of the tongue and the trapezius muscles. There was a left extensor plantar response but no sensory impairment. The blood sugar was 31 mg/dL. EEG was normal with no slow-wave focus. He was given 25 g of glucose intravenously and recovered fully in 3 minutes.

Comment: This patient, who was seen prior to the availability of CT scanning, provides a closer look at the range of physical signs and EEG phenomena that may occur in hypoglycemia. Today, fingerstick glucose testing would have occurred much earlier, often before reaching the hospital, and the physician rarely gets to see such cases. In this man, the occurrence of a similar brief attack of left hemiparesis a week previously suggested right

carotid distribution infarction initially.[41] However, the patient was a little drowsier than expected with an uncomplicated unilateral carotid stroke in which the damage was apparently rather limited. The fact that his attack might have begun with unconsciousness and the fecal staining made his physicians suspect a seizure. However, hypoglycemia also can cause unconsciousness as well as focal signs in conscious patients. After treatment of the low glucose, the hemiplegia cleared rapidly.

Patients with metabolic brain disease may have either focal or generalized seizures that can be indistinguishable from the seizures of structural brain disease. However, when metabolic encephalopathy causes focal seizures, the focus tends to shift from attack to attack, something that rarely happens with structural seizures. Such migratory seizures are especially common and hard to control in uremia.

Motor Abnormalities Characteristic of Metabolic Coma

Tremor, asterixis, and multifocal myoclonus are prominent manifestations of metabolic brain disease; they are less commonly seen with focal structural lesions unless these latter have a toxic or infectious component.

The *tremor* of metabolic encephalopathy is coarse and irregular and has a rate of 8 to 10 per second. Usually these tremors are absent at rest and, when present, are most evident in the fingers of the outstretched hands. Severe tremors may spread to the face, tongue, and lower extremities, and frequently interfere with purposeful movements in agitated patients such as those with delirium tremens. The physiologic mechanism responsible for this type of tremor is unknown. It is not seen in patients with unilateral hemispheric or focal brainstem lesions.

First described by Adams and Foley[42] in patients with hepatic coma, *asterixis* is now known to accompany a wide variety of metabolic brain diseases and even some structural lesions.[43] Asterixis was originally described as a sudden palmar flapping movement of the outstretched hands at the wrists.[44] It is most easily elicited in lethargic but awake patients by directing them to hold their arms outstretched with hands dorsiflexed at the wrist and fingers extended and abducted (i.e., "stopping traffic"). Incipient asterixis comprises a slight irregular tremor of the fingers, beginning after a latent period of 2 to 30 seconds that is difficult to distinguish from the tremor of metabolic encephalopathy. Leavitt and Tyler[45] have described the two separate components of this tremulousness. One is an irregular oscillation of the fingers, usually in the anterior-posterior direction but with a rotary component at the wrist. The second consists of random movements of the fingers at the metacarpal-phalangeal joints. This second pattern becomes more and more marked as the patient holds his or her wrist dorsiflexed until finally the fingers lead the hand into a sudden downward jerk followed by a slower return to the original dorsiflexed position. Both hands are affected, but asynchronously, and as the abnormal movement intensifies, it spreads to the feet, tongue, and face (dorsiflexion of the feet is often an easier posture for obtunded patients to maintain). Indeed, with severe metabolic tremors it sometimes becomes difficult to distinguish between intense asterixis and myoclonus, and there is some evidence that the two types of movements represent the same underlying phenomenon (sudden and transient loss of muscle tone followed by sudden compensation). Asterixis is generally seen in awake but lethargic patients and generally disappears with the advent of stupor or coma, although occasionally one can evoke the arrhythmic contraction in such subjects by passively dorsiflexing the wrist. Asterixis can also be elicited in stuporous patients by passively flexing and abducting the hips.[46] Flapping abduction-adduction movements occurring either synchronously or asynchronously suggest metabolic brain disease (Figure 5–1).

Unilateral, or less commonly bilateral, asterixis has been described in patients with focal brain lesions.[43] Electromyograms recorded during asterixis show a brief absence of muscular activity during the downward jerk followed by

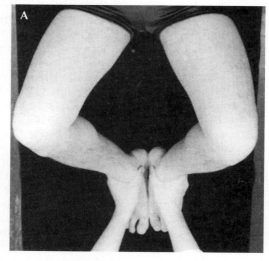

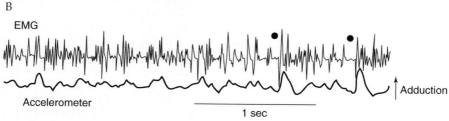

Figure 5–1. (A) Technique of hip flexion-abduction. (B) Electromyographic (EMG) recording from the hip adductors (upper trace) and accelerometric recording from the patella (lower trace). Brief periods of EMG silence (black dots) are followed by a burst of high-voltage electrical activity and a striking change in acceleration. (From Noda et al.,[46] with permission.)

a sudden muscular compensatory contraction, much like the sudden bobbing of the head that normally accompanies drowsiness. The sudden electrical silence is unexplained and not accompanied by EEG changes.[42,45,47]

Multifocal myoclonus consists of sudden, nonrhythmic, nonpatterned gross twitching involving parts of muscles or groups of muscles first in one part of the body, then another, and particularly affecting the face and proximal limb musculature. Multifocal myoclonus most commonly accompanies uremic encephalopathy, a large dose of intravenous penicillin, CO_2 narcosis, and hyperosmotic-hyperglycemic encephalopathy. Multifocal myoclonus, in a patient who is stuporous or in coma, is indicative of severe metabolic disturbance. However, it may be seen in some waking patients with neurodegenerative disorders (e.g., Lewy body dementia or Alzheimer's disease) or prion disorders (Creutzfeldt-Jakob disease and related disorders). Its physiology is unknown; the motor twitchings are not always reflected by a specific EEG abnormality and have, in fact, been reported in a patient with electrocerebral silence.[48]

DIFFERENTIAL DIAGNOSIS

Distinction Between Metabolic and Psychogenic Unresponsiveness

In awake patients, differences in the mental state, the EEG, the motor signs, and, occasionally, the breathing pattern distinguish metabolic from psychiatric disease. Most conscious patients with metabolic brain disease are confused and many are disoriented, especially for time. Their abstract thinking is defective; they cannot concentrate well and cannot easily retain new information. Early during the illness, the outstretched dorsiflexed hands show irregular tremulousness and, frequently, asterixis. Snout, suck, and grasp reflexes are seen. The EEG is generally slow. Posthyperventilation apnea may be elicited and there may be hypoventilation or hyperventilation, depending on the specific metabolic illness. By contrast, awake patients with psychogenic illness, if they will cooperate, are not disoriented and can retain new information. If they seem disoriented, they are disoriented to self (i.e., they report

that they don't know who they are) as well as to time and place; disorientation to self almost never occurs in delirious patients. They also lack abnormal reflexes or adventitious movements, although they may have irregular tremor, and they have normal EEG frequencies. Ventilatory patterns, with the exception of psychogenic hyperventilation, are normal.

Unresponsive patients with metabolic disease have even slower activity in their EEGs than responsive patients with metabolic disease, and caloric vestibulo-ocular stimulation elicits either tonic deviation of the eyes or, if the patient is deeply comatose, no response. Psychogenically unresponsive patients have normal EEGs and a normal response to caloric irrigation, with nystagmus having a quick phase away from the side of ice water irrigation; there is little or no tonic deviation of the eyes (see page 65). In some patients with psychogenic coma, the eyes deviate toward the ground when the patient is placed on his or her side.[49] Forced downward deviation of the eyes has been described in patients with psychogenic seizures.[50]

Distinction Between Coma of Metabolic and Structural Origin

As discussed in Chapter 2, the key to distinguishing coma of metabolic versus structural origin is to identify focal neurologic signs that distinguish structural coma. On the other hand, certain characteristic motor and EEG findings can help confirm the diagnosis of a metabolic encephalopathy when patients are merely obtunded or lethargic. Most patients with metabolic brain disease have diffusely abnormal motor signs including tremor, myoclonus, and, especially, bilateral asterixis. The EEG is diffusely, but not focally, slow. The patient with gross structural disease, on the other hand, generally has abnormal focal motor signs and if asterixis is present, it is unilateral. The EEG may be slow, but in addition with supratentorial lesions, a focal abnormality will usually be present.

Finally, metabolic and structural brain diseases are distinguished from each other by a combination of signs and their evolution. Comatose patients with metabolic brain disease usually suffer from partial dysfunction affecting many levels of the neuraxis simultaneously, yet concurrently retain the integrity of other functions originating at the same levels. The orderly rostral-caudal deterioration that is characteristic of supratentorial mass lesions does not occur in metabolic brain disease, nor is the anatomic defect regionally restricted as it is with subtentorial damage.

ASPECTS OF CEREBRAL METABOLISM PERTINENT TO COMA

Earlier chapters of this book have described the physiologic relationships among the brainstem, the diencephalon, and the cerebral hemispheres that underlie the wakeful state and normally generate the psychologic activities that constitute full consciousness. The brain's sensorimotor and mental activities are closely coupled to cerebral metabolism so that neurochemical impairment or failure from any cause is likely to produce rapidly evolving neurologic abnormalities.

Neurons and glial cells undergo many chemical processes in fulfilling their specialized functions. The nerve cells must continuously maintain their membrane potentials, synthesize and store transmitters, manufacture axoplasm, and replace their always decaying structural components (Figure 5–2). Glia, which constitute 90% of the brain's cells, have several functions, some of which have been recently recognized.[51,52] The oligodendroglial cells have as their major role the generation and maintenance of myelin. Microglia (macrophages) are the brain's immune cells. Astrocytes regulate much of the ion homeostasis of the brain's extracellular fluid. In addition, they may aid neuronal function by supplying substrate (lactate)[51] (although the degree, if any, to which neurons metabolize lactate in vivo is controversial[53]). Astrocytes also participate in controlling blood flow[52] and in maintaining the blood-brain barrier.[54] All of these complex activities require energy, in fact, more of it per kilogram weight of cells than in any other organ in the body. Furthermore, many of the enzymatic reactions of both neurons and glial cells, as well as of the specialized cerebral capillary endothelium, must be catalyzed at some point by the energy-yielding hydrolysis of adenosine triphosphate (ATP) to adenosine diphosphate (ADP) and inorganic phosphate. Without a constant and generous supply of

ATP, cellular synthesis slows or halts, neuronal functions decline or cease, and cell structures quickly crumble.

Oxygen, glucose, and cerebral blood flow (CBF) operate interdependently to supply the brain with the substrate and cofactors it requires to carry out the chemical reactions that generate its energy and synthesize its structural components. Awake or asleep, the brain metabolizes at one of the highest rates of any organ in the body. However, although the overall metabolism of the brain is relatively constant, different areas of the brain metabolize at different rates, depending on how active an area is.[55] For example, during exercise, the activity of the motor cortex increases dramatically, compensated for by decreased metabolism elsewhere in the brain.[56] Changes in regional metabolism are best demonstrated by functional magnetic resonance imaging (MRI) or positron emission tomography (PET) imaging (Figure 5–3). The brain suffers a special vulnerability in that it possesses almost no reserves of its critical nutrients, so that even a brief interruption of blood flow or oxygen supply threatens the tissue's vitality. These considerations are central to an understanding of many of the metabolic encephalopathies, and the following paragraphs discuss them in some detail.

CEREBRAL BLOOD FLOW

Under normal resting conditions, the total CBF in man is about 55 mL/100 g/minute, an amount that equals 15% to 20% of the resting cardiac output. A number of studies have found that the overall CBF remains relatively constant during the states of wakefulness or slow-wave sleep as well as in the course of various mental and physical activities. PET and functional MRI scanning reveal that this apparent uniformity masks a regionally varying and dynamically fluctuating CBF, which is closely adjusted to meet the metabolic requirements posed by local physiologic changes in the brain. Overall flow in gray matter, for example, is normally three to four times higher than in white matter.[55]

When neural activity increases within a region, cerebral metabolism increases to meet the increased demand.[57] Cerebral metabolic rate for glucose and CBF each increase about 50% in the active area, whereas the metabolic rate for oxygen increases only about 5%.[57]

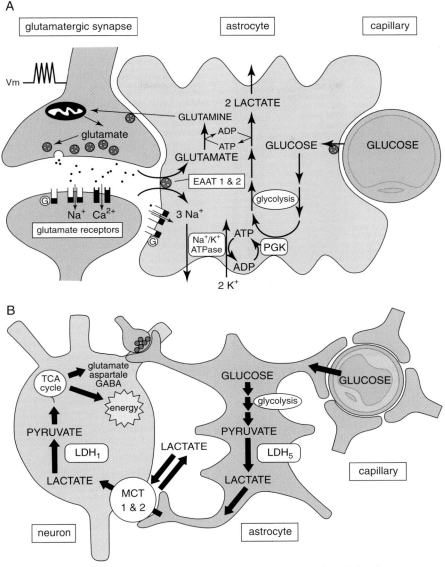

Figure 5–2. (A) Schematic representation of the mechanism for glutamate-induced glycolysis in astrocytes during physiologic activation. At glutamatergic synapses, presynaptically released glutamate depolarizes postsynaptic neurons by acting at specific receptor subtypes. The action of glutamate is terminated by an efficient glutamate uptake system located primarily in astrocytes. Glutamate is cotransported with Na^+, resulting in an increase in the intra-astrocytic concentration of Na^+, leading to an activation of the astrocyte Na^+/K^+-ATPase. Activation of the Na^+/K^+-ATPase stimulates glycolysis (i.e., glucose use and lactate production). Lactate, once released by astrocytes, can be taken up by neurons and serves them as an adequate energy substrate. (For graphic clarity, only lactate uptake into presynaptic terminals is indicated. However, this process could also occur at the postsynaptic neuron.) This model, which summarizes in vitro experimental evidence indicating glutamate-induced glycolysis, is taken to reflect cellular and molecular events occurring during activation of a given cortical area. (B) Schematic representation of the proposed astrocyte-neuron lactate shuttle. Following neuronal activation and synaptic glutamate release, glutamate reuptake into astrocytes triggers increased glucose uptake from capillaries via activation of an isoform of the Na^+/K^+-ATPase, which is highly sensitive to ouabain, possibly the alpha-2 isoform (Pellerin and Magistretti 1994, 1997). Glucose is then processed glycolytically to lactate by astrocytes that are enriched in the muscle form of lactate dehydrogenase (LDH_5). The exchange of lactate between astrocytes and neurons is operated by monocarboxylate transporters (MCTs). Lactate is then converted to pyruvate since neurons contain the heart form of LDH (LDH_1). Pyruvate, via the formation of acetyl-CoA by pyruvate dehydrogenase (PDH), enters the tricarboxylic acid (TCA) cycle, thus generating 17 adenosine triphosphate (ATP) molecules per lactate molecule. ADP, adenosine diphosphate. (From Magistretti and Pellerin,[58] with permission.)

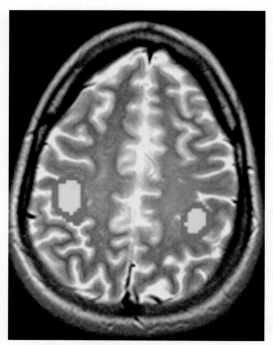

Figure 5–3. A functional magnetic resonance imaging scan of the normal individual flexing and extending his fingers. Blood flow increases to a greater degree than oxygen consumption in the motor areas, leading to an increase in oxyhemoglobin. The paramagnetic oxyhemoglobin causes an increased blood oxygen level-dependent signal in the motor cortex bilaterally. (Image courtesy Dr. Andrei Holodny.)

Thus, the oxygen extraction falls, increasing the concentration of oxyhemoglobin in venous blood. This is the basis for the blood oxygenation level dependent (BOLD) signal obtained using functional MRI. The increase in glucose metabolism over oxygen metabolism results in increased lactate production, possibly the substrate for the increased demand of neurons[58] (Figure 5–4). The stimulus for the increase in regional CBF is complex.[59] A number of vasoactive substances are released by neurons and glia during increased neural activity. Important among these are adenosine, nitric oxide, dopamine, acetylcholine, vasoactive intestinal polypeptide, and arachidonic acid metabolites.[59] Several pathologic states of brain are marked by a disproportionately high rate of local blood flow in relation to metabolism. Examples of such reactive hyperemia or "uncoupling" of flow and metabolism occur in areas of traumatic or postischemic tissue injury, as well as in regions of inflammation or in the regions surrounding certain brain tumors. So far, the nature of the local stimulus to such pathologic vasodilation also has eluded investigators. The effects of the process, however, can act to increase the bulk of the involved tissue and thereby accentuate the pathologic effects of compartmental swelling in the brain, as discussed in Chapter 2.

Reduced CBF has several causes. As described in Chapter 3, the cerebral vasculature's capacity for autoregulation protects the CBF against all but the most profound drops in systemic blood pressure. The process of autoregulation also means that conditions causing a lowered cerebral metabolism are usually accompanied by a secondary fall in CBF, although in many such cases the initial decline in CBF is less than the metabolic reduction.[60] This delayed response may reflect the relatively slow adaptation of the tonic contractile state of vascular smooth muscle rather than a true uncoupling of flow and metabolism. Intrinsic arterial spasm in cerebral vessels, which reduces tissue flow below metabolic needs, is an uncommon phenomenon limited largely to arteries at the base of the brain (e.g., with local surgical trauma as well as with subarachnoid bleeding and sometimes with meningitis [see Chapter 4]). Multifocal cerebral arteriolar spasm had been invoked to explain the regional cerebral vascular injury of malignant hypertension; recent work, however, offers a different interpretation of the pathogenesis of that disorder (see page 168).

Primary reductions in CBF can be regional or general (global). *Regional impairments of CBF* results from intrinsic diseases of the cervical and cerebral arteries (atherosclerosis, thrombosis, and, rarely, inflammation), from arterial embolism, and from the extrinsic pressure on individual cerebral arteries produced by compartmental herniation. *General or global reductions in CBF* result from systemic hypotension, complete or functional cardiac arrest (e.g., ventricular arrhythmias in which output falls below requirements of brain perfusion), and increased ICP. As noted earlier in this volume, however, unless some primary abnormality of brain tissue acts to increase regional vascular resistance, an increase in the ICP must approach the systemic systolic pressure before the CBF declines sufficiently to cause recognizable changes in neurologic functions.

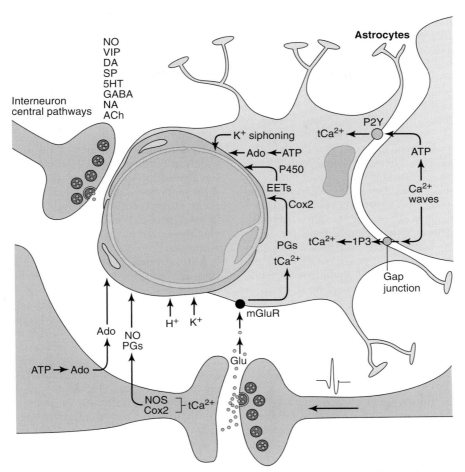

Figure 5–4. Vasoactive mediators released from neurons and glia by neural activity. Ions (H$^+$ and K$^+$) contribute to the extracellular currents that are associated with synaptic transmission. Adenosine (Ado) is produced through adenosine triphosphate (ATP) catabolism. Glutamate (Glu)-induced increases in the intracellular concentration of Ca^{2+} in neurons and glia activate the synthesis of nitric oxide (NO), of the cyclooxygenase-2 (Cox2) products prostaglandins (PGs), and of the cytochrome P450 epoxygenase products epoxyeicosatrienoic acids (EETs). In astrocytes, the [Ca^{2+}] increase is produced by activation of metabotropic glutamate receptors (mGluRs) and by propagation of Ca^{2+} waves from neighboring astrocytes through activation of purinergic receptors (P2Y) or entry of IP3 (inositol (1,4,5)-triphosphate) through gap junctions. Astrocytic lipoxygenase products could also produce vasodilation by inducing NO release from endothelial cells. Spatial buffering currents in astrocytes release K$^+$ from perivascular end-feet, where K$^+$ conductance is greatest (K$^+$ siphoning). Interneurons and projecting neurons with perivascular contacts release vasoactive neurotransmitters and neuropeptides, including NO, vasoactive intestinal polypeptide (VIP), dopamine (DA), substance P (SP), serotonin (5HT), gamma-aminobutyric acid (GABA), noradrenaline (NA), and acetylcholine (ACh). (From Iadecola,[59] with permission.)

Cessation of blood flow to the brain (*ischemia*), as discussed in subsequent paragraphs, appears to cause a greater risk of irreversible tissue damage than does even a profound reduction in the arterial oxygen tension (*anoxemia*). The precise lower level of arterial perfusion required to maintain the vitality of the tissue in man is not known. Extrapolations based on animal experiments suggest that the CBF of 20 mL/100 g of brain per minute causes loss of consciousness but not permanent damage. If the flow falls to 10 mL/100 g/minute, membrane integrity is lost and calcium influx into the cells leads to irreversible damage. Time is also an important factor. Flows of 18 mL can be tolerated for several hours without leading to infarction, whereas flows of 5 mL lasting for more than 30 minutes will cause infarction.[61]

Several factors may explain why ischemia so severely threatens tissue structure. A change in pH or lactic acid concentration is one factor. Anaerobic metabolism produces large amounts of lactic acid and lowers the pH. The increased concentration of hydrogen ions leads to cell death[62] by increasing brain edema, interfering with mitochondrial ATP generation, increasing calcium levels, and the formation of free radicals, all of which can cause cellular death.[63] Hypoglycemia (see below), by increasing lactate production, contributes to the brain damage.

Several other factors play a role in helping regulate CBF, the most important of which is PCO_2 or, more accurately, cerebral pH. Cerebral acidosis is a potent vasodilator, as is potassium, which leaks into the brain extracellular space during hypoxia. Other factors that serve to increase CBF include nitric oxide (which in older literature was referred to as endothelial-derived relaxing factor), adenosine (probably working through nitric oxide), and prostaglandins (for a review see [59,64]).

GLUCOSE METABOLISM

Glucose is the overwhelmingly predominant blood-borne substrate for brain metabolism. One might question why this is so since it is known that slices of cerebral cortex in vitro can utilize a variety of substrates, including fatty acids and other compounds, to synthesize acetoacetate for entry into the citric acid cycle. The answer appears to lie in the specialized properties of the blood-brain barrier, which, by rigorously limiting or facilitating the entry or egress of substances to and from the brain, guards the narrow homeostasis of that organ. Glucose is transported across the blood-brain barrier by a carrier-mediated glucose transporter (Glut-1). The uptake of glucose into neurons is also facilitated by a glucose transporter (Glut-3), and glucose uptake into astrocytes by Glut-1. Under normal circumstances, brain glucose concentration is approximately 30% of that of plasma. Insulin is not required for the entry of glucose into brain or for its metabolism by brain cells. Nevertheless, the brain is rich in insulin receptors with substantial regional variation, the richest area being the olfactory bulb.[65] Insulin itself reaches the brain using a transporter that is partially saturated at euglycemic levels. The exact function of insulin and its receptor in the brain is not known.

In net metabolic terms, each 100 g of brain in a normal human being utilizes about 0.31 mol (5.5 mg) of glucose per minute so that in the basal, prolonged fasting state, the brain's consumption of glucose almost equals the total amount that the liver produces. This net figure, however, hides the fact that glucose consumption in local regions of the brain varies widely according to local functional changes. Because of its rapid transfer into brain, glucose represents essentially the organ's only substrate under normal physiologic conditions. However, neurons probably utilize lactate produced from glucose by astrocytes when stimulated with glutamate.[66]

Ketone bodies can diffuse into brain and also are transported across the blood-brain barrier. These substances provide increased fuel to the brain when beta-hydroxybutyrate, acetoacetate, and other ketones increase in the blood during states such as starvation, the ingestion of high-fat diets, or ketoacidosis. During starvation, in fact, liver gluconeogenesis may fall below the level required to meet cerebral substrate needs; at such times ketone utilization can contribute as much as 30% of the brain's fuel for oxidative metabolism. For unknown reasons, however, the brain does not appear able to subsist entirely on ketone bodies, and as mentioned below, some investigators believe that ketones contribute to the neurologic toxicity of diabetic ketoacidosis.

Under normal circumstances, all but about 15% of glucose uptake in the brain is accounted for by combustion with O_2 to produce H_2O and energy, the remainder going to lactate production. The brain contains about 1 mmol/kg of free glucose in reserve and a considerable amount of glycogen, perhaps as high as 10 mg/L, which is present in astrocytes.[67,68] With the addition of either increased metabolic demand or decreased metabolic supply, glycogen in astrocytes can break down to lactate to support neuronal function. Despite this, deprivation of glucose and oxygen to the brain rapidly results in loss of consciousness, normal cerebral function being maintained for only a matter of seconds.

The energy balance of the brain is influenced both by its supply of energy precursors (i.e., its input) and by the work the organ does (i.e., its output). Just as intrinsic mechanisms appropriately increase or decrease the rate of metabolism in different regions of the brain during periods of locally increased or decreased functional activity, intrinsic mechanisms appear able to "turn down" general cerebral metabolic activity and produce stupor or coma when circumstances threaten to deplete blood-borne substrate.

Several metabolic disorders are known to cause a decrease in the brain's rate of metabolism and physiologic function without initially resulting in any encroachment on the energy reserves of the tissue. The reversible hypometabolism of anesthesia is discussed in a following section. Mechanistically less well understood than anesthesia is a reversible hypometabolism that accompanies the early stages of hypoglycemia, severe hypoxemia, reduced states of CBF, and hyperammonemia. The response appears to be important in protecting the brain against irreversible damage, however, and is well illustrated by describing the neurochemical changes that accompany hypoglycemia. Both hyperglycemia and hypoglycemia can damage the brain.

Hyperglycemia

Brain damage from chronic hyperglycemia (i.e., either type 1 or type 2 diabetes) is well established.[69] Sustained hyperglycemia causes hyperosmolality, which in turn induces compensatory vasopressin secretion. Although adaptive in the short term, in the long term sustained hyperglycemia damages vasopressin-secreting neurons in the hypothalamus and supraoptic nucleus. In addition, some evidence suggests that sustained hyperglycemia damages hippocampal neurons as well,[70] leading to cognitive defects in both humans[71] and experimental animals. These effects appear to be independent of diabetes-induced damage to brain vasculature leading to stroke, a common complication of chronic poorly controlled diabetes.

The effect of hyperglycemia on patients with damaged brains is less clear cut. Clinical evidence demonstrates that patients who are hyperglycemic after brain injury, either due to global or focal ischemia[72] or to brain trauma, do less well than patients who are euglycemic. The same may well be true for critically ill patients, even those without direct brain damage. These findings have led investigators to recom-

mend careful control of blood glucose in critically ill patients and those with brain injury of various types.[73]

The mechanism by which hyperglycemia worsens the prognosis in such patients is not clear. Some believe that the increased production of lactate and lowering of the pH leads to the cellular damage. However, lactate is probably a good substrate for neurons, and the increased blood glucose should be protective. In fact, in experimental animals, a glucose load given 2 to 3 hours before an ischemic insult is protective, but the same glucose load administered 15 to 60 minutes before ischemia aggravates the ischemic outcome,[74] although these findings have been challenged.[75] Another possible mechanism by which hyperglycemia may damage the brain is that a glucose load leads to release of glucocorticoids that in turn can cause cellular damage.[70] Whatever the mechanism, careful control of blood glucose allowing neither hyper- nor hypoglycemia appears essential for the best care of critically ill and brain-injured patients.

Hypoglycemia

Hypoglycemia deprives the brain of its major substrate and can be expected to interfere with cerebral metabolism by reducing the brain's energy supply in a manner similar to that caused by hypoxia. With very severe or prolonged hypoglycemia this turns out to be true, but with less severe or transient reductions of glucose availability, one finds that brain function and metabolism decline before one can detect a decline in ATP levels in the tissue.

Soon after insulin came into clinical use, it was realized that hypoglycemic coma could last for up to an hour or so without necessarily leaving any residual neurologic effects or structural brain damage. (This capacity to induce transient but fully reversible coma was important in developing the ineffective[76] use of insulin coma in attempts to treat psychiatric disorders.) Since equally long periods of hypoxemic coma always leave neurologic damage in their wake, the difference between the effects of a deficiency of oxygen and a deficiency of substrate has engendered considerable interest. Accordingly, the mechanism of hypoglycemic coma has received repeated attention by biochemists with results important to the understanding of many aspects of human cerebral metabolism.

Hypoglycemia affects CBF, glucose consumption, and oxygen consumption in different ways. Clinical studies of CBF and metabolism during hypoglycemia in humans indicate that at all levels of blood sugar thus far studied, CBF remains the same or may occasionally rise,[77] perhaps from nitric acid release,[78] or fall slightly.[79] Overall changes in CBF do not reflect regional changes. At modest levels of hypoglycemia (3.0 mmol/L), CBF increases in several areas including the medial prefrontal cortex, whereas it falls in others, such as the hippocampus.[79] In an experimental study, a sharp rise in CBF (57%) occurred when blood glucose concentrations fell below 2 mmol/L, at which point brain glucose concentrations approached zero.[80] With a relatively mild reduction of blood glucose in humans down to levels of 1.7 to 2.6 mmol/dL (31 to 46 mg/dL), consciousness is preserved, and cerebral glucose consumption (CMRglu) declines moderately but cerebral oxygen consumption remains normal. Despite the preservation of consciousness, at levels of approximately 2.5 mmol/L the latency of the P300 readiness potential increases as does reaction time, suggesting an altered ability to make decisions.[81] In patients with hypoglycemic coma, cerebral metabolic rate for oxygen ($CMRO_2$) declines only to an insignificant degree, but CMRglu falls disproportionately by more than half.[77] These changes imply that during hypoglycemia the brain is utilizing substrates other than glucose for oxidative metabolism, such as endogenous glycogen[82] and lactate.[83] Furthermore, despite a normal oxygen consumption, the qualitative change in substrate results in profound functional changes in the neural systems that normally subserve consciousness.

Studies in animals extend the above studies in man and indicate that even with degrees of hypoglycemia sufficient to produce convulsions or deep coma, whole brain energy reserves are at least briefly maintained. Levels of phosphocreatine and ATP remain normal in the brains of mice or rats so long as EEG activity remained. Energy reserves fail only after prolonged convulsive activity or after the EEG becomes isoelectric ($\sim$1 mmol/L[84]).

Cerebral metabolic studies imply that hypoglycemic confusion, stupor, and even coma in its early stages cannot be attributed simply to a failure of overall cerebral energy supply. The mechanism by which hypoglycemia causes irreversible neurologic dysfunction is not known, but experimental evidence suggests that impaired acetylcholine metabolism[85] or a rise in aspartic acid levels leading to excessive excitation of neurons[86] may be involved. Profound hypoglycemia causes pathologic changes in the brain, probably due in part to the massive release of aspartate into the brain extracellular space, flooding excitatory amino acid receptors and causing an influx of calcium, leading to neuronal necrosis.[84] Evidence also implicates apoptosis, probably resulting from release of cytochrome C, causing an increase in caspase-like activity.[87]

Other mechanisms may add to the neurologic dysfunction caused by hypoglycemia. Neurogenic pulmonary edema resulting from a massive sympathetic discharge adds hypoxia to the hypoglycemic insult.[88] Transient cerebral edema, either vasogenic[89] from increased blood-brain barrier permeability or cytotoxic,[90] may also complicate the development of hypoglycemia. A single case report describes the development of central pontine myelolysis (see page 171) associated with hypoglycemic coma, but without electrolyte disturbance, in a patient with anorexia nervosa[91]; the cause is unknown.

The above discussion on hypoglycemia indicates that the presence or absence of energy failure in the tissue may be the major factor that determines whether cells die or recover. The following section extends the point and compares some of the cerebral metabolic effects of reversible anesthesia with those of anoxic-ischemic and other metabolic conditions producing stupor or coma.

Many directly applied physical and chemical agents can injure the brain. For example, trauma can shear axons and displace tissue sufficiently to cause neuronal death. However, in addition to direct injury, many lethal injuries of the brain exert their effects by producing tissue anoxia. As discussed above, the body normally maintains its nervous tissue in a constant "high-energy" state in which the oxidative metabolism of glucose generates a constant supply of ATP and phosphocreatine to maintain membrane potentials, transmit neuronal impulses, and synthesize protoplasm. When the mechanisms that sustain these energy reserves go awry, ATP and phosphocreatine levels decline, membranes lose their pumping mechanisms, the cells swell, and, at some point, the neuron loses its capacity to recover. Histologic evidence, discussed below, indicates that the mitochondria bear the initial brunt of irreversible damage, while histochemical evidence suggests that oxidative enzymes themselves are destroyed.[92] As the precise lethal point of no return is unknown in cellular-molecular terms, one generally must turn to physiologic models when trying to find out just when and why the nervous system dies. Evidence from such models indicates that the brain can harmlessly suspend its activities almost indefinitely when metabolically depressed or cooled, but quickly succumbs when it loses its functional activities in the absence of oxygen or substrate.

ANESTHESIA

General anesthesia and slow-wave sleep are states comparable to pathologic coma, but which maintain normal levels of energy metabolites and are easily reversible. Both may affect the same structures[93] in the brain, but the mechanisms of neither are fully understood. In both sleep and anesthesia, there is inhibition of the neuronal pathways making up the ascending arousal system. During sleep, gamma-aminobutyric acid (GABA)-ergic neurons in the ventrolateral preoptic nucleus inhibit the components of the ascending arousal system via $GABA_A$ receptors (see Chapter 1). Most general anesthetics are potential $GABA_A$ receptor agonists that inhibit the activity of the arousal system by activating the same $GABA_A$ receptors used by the ventrolateral preoptic nucleus during sleep. The result is slowing of thalamocortical activity in both sleep and general anesthesia.[94,95]

General anesthetic agents produce immobility and block pain, largely the effect of the anesthetics on the descending brainstem modulatory systems and directly on the spinal cord, and cause amnesia and loss of consciousness when given in high doses.[95,96] These actions for most anesthetic agents (benzodiazepines, barbiturates, propofol, ethanol, gas anesthetics) are due to activation of different classes of $GABA_A$ receptors that contain alpha-1 subunits (most important in sedative and amnestic effects) and alpha-2, -3, and -5 subunits (most important for anxiolytic and muscle relaxant effects).[97] Other anesthetic agents, such as nitrous oxide

and ketamine, act mainly as N-methyl-D-aspartate (NMDA) antagonists. These agents distort, rather than depress, thalamocortical activity, and hence are sometimes called dissociative agents rather than anesthetics. Thus, whereas $GABA_A$ agonist general anesthetics decrease cerebral metabolism, ketamine increases CBF and maintains oxygen and glucose metabolism at a waking level.[98] The depth of anesthesia and the degree of diminution of cerebral metabolism with $GABA_A$ agonist anesthetics can be roughly measured by the EEG. As anesthesia deepens, electroencephalographic activity is suppressed; the degree of suppression from none to a completely isoelectric EEG correlates roughly with the cerebral metabolic rate.[99] Some general anesthetics actually increase CBF, but they still diminish cerebral metabolism. Thus, clinically, anesthesia depresses the function of the brain but keeps that organ in a high-energy state poised for the resumption of normal function. Well-ventilated animals subject to various concentrations of general anesthetics maintain normal concentrations of ATP and phosphocreatine and normal lactate pyruvate ratios, indicating that no tissue hypoxia has occurred.[100] *The brain can be depressed to essentially functionless levels by anesthetic depressant drugs, yet lose none of its capacity for total recovery when the anesthetic disappears.* Several investigators have demonstrated that experimental animals and humans can be resuscitated to full functional activity after periods of deep anesthesia producing hours to days of isoelectric EEG flattening.[101] This tolerability is used clinically in cases of status epilepticus to prevent continuous seizure activity from damaging the brain. A corollary is that in cases of coma due to sedative overdose, the depth and duration of coma are not indicative of the potential for recovery of function.

In animal experiments, general anesthesia, either before or within a few hours of an ischemic insult to the brain, protects against brain damage when measured a few days after the insult. However, at 3 weeks there is no difference in the degree of neuronal damage between the anesthetized animals and those treated without anesthesia,[102,103] indicating no protection against the delayed effects of anoxia (see page 219).

Clinical experience with barbiturate anesthesia and drug poisoning indicates that given good medical care, most patients usually survive anesthesia, even profound suppression of neu-ral activity resulting from self-administered bar-biturates or other sedative drugs. Even when coma is so deep that artificial respiration must be provided for several days and the blood pressure supported by vasopressor agents for a week or more, patients can awaken with no apparent or measurable impairment of brain function. Hence, it is critical to determine the presence of sedative overdose when evaluating the prognosis of a patient in coma, even those with other causes of coma.

The complete reversibility of anesthetic coma, plus the low metabolic rate that accom-panies deep anesthesia, has inspired efforts to determine whether barbiturate anesthesia can minimize the expected extent of postanoxic is-chemic brain damage. Barbiturates also scav-enge free radicals from reoxygenated tissue, but it remains to be proved that this represents an important biologic function in resuscitation. On the other hand, phenobarbital also induces cytochrome P450, which serves as a source of reactive oxygen species. Whether these oppo-site effects help, hurt, or have no effect on the brain is unclear.[104,105] Of some interest, a ran-domized trial of neonates with hypoxic-ischemic encephalopathy indicates that phe-nobarbital in a dose of 20 mg/kg given intra-venously within 6 hours of birth in term and near-term neonates was associated with a de-crease in lipid peroxides. There was also a de-crease in antioxidant enzymes and antioxidant vitamins in the CSF. A trend suggested that lower levels of lipid peroxides in the CSF were associated with a better outcome.[106] Barbitu-rate coma is effective in controlling intractable status epilepticus, but its role in any other brain injury is, at this writing, uncertain.[101] Barbitu-rate anesthesia has been applied to patients in coma from head trauma. It lowers ICP, but it is unclear if it affects outcome.[107]

MECHANISMS OF IRREVERSIBLE ANOXIC-ISCHEMIC BRAIN DAMAGE

Anoxia, ischemia, and hypoglycemia, although biologically different,[108] can combine under several circumstances to damage the brain. Somewhat different but overlapping patho-logic changes characterize the irreversible brain injury caused by each of these three conditions. Systemic and local circulatory dif-ferences among them influence the exact ge-ography and type of cellular response. Similar changes in the brain mark the postmortem findings of several conditions, including pa-tients dying in coma after fatal status epi-lepticus, carbon monoxide poisoning, or several of the systemic metabolic encephalopathies.

Global Ischemia

Complete cerebral ischemia, as in cardiac ar-rest in man, causes loss of consciousness in less than 20 seconds. Within 5 minutes, glucose and high-energy phosphate stores are depleted. Following that the patient, even if successfully resuscitated, may be left severely brain dam-aged. This is especially true in elderly pa-tients who most frequently suffer cardiac ar-rest because their brains are more vulnerable to ischemic damage. By definition, during car-diac arrest the CBF falls to zero. Resuscita-tion results in transient hyperemia with in-creased blood flow and oxygen metabolism; subsequently, both decrease in a heteroge-neous fashion.[109] In most patients, when blood flow is re-established, cerebral autoregulation is either absent or the curve is shifted to the right, such that CBF begins to fall at a higher mean arterial pressure than it did before the cardiac arrest. As a result, it is important to maintain normal and perhaps slightly elevated blood pressure after cardiac arrest.

Both vascular and neuronal factors play a role in the seemingly brief periods of global ischemia that can damage the brain in clinical circum-stances. Changes to vascular endothelium dur-ing the course of ischemia, as well as additional changes to glial cells (swelling to compress en-dothelial vessels, viscosity changes in blood), may lead to poor perfusion once cardiac func-tion is restored. This so-called "no-reflow phe-nomenon"[110] increases with prolonged duration of ischemia.[110–112] Loss of autoregulation can aggravate edema formation, lead to hemor-rhage, and cause additional neuronal damage, so-called "reperfusion injury."[113] The combi-nation of the ischemia and its aftermath results in neuronal necrosis,[114] particularly in the hip-pocampus, but if the ischemia is prolonged, elsewhere in the hemispheres as well.

Although the exact mechanisms are not un-derstood, it is likely that during the ischemia the loss of high-energy phosphates causes cellular depolarization that induces the release of glutamate, which in turn causes entry of toxic levels of calcium into neurons. In the reperfusion phase, the restoration of oxidative metabolism probably produces a burst of excess free radicals that are also cytotoxic.[113]

Cardiac arrest can either cause death of neurons, particularly in vulnerable areas associated with reactive astrocytes, or microinfarcts and areas of pancellular necrosis associated with perivascular diffuse tissue spongiosis. The latter lesions appear in a laminar distribution and are more profound in watershed zones between the major territories of arterial supply. Both types of lesions are more intense and heterogeneous in patients dying after a period of prolonged coma.[115]

Particularly vulnerable areas include the occipital cortex, the frontoparietal cortex, the hippocampus, the basal ganglia, the thalamic reticular nucleus, Purkinje cells of the cerebellum, and the spinal cord (Figure 5–5). Laminar necrosis of the cortex generally involves layers III and V, which contain the greatest numbers of large pyramidal cells. The most vulnerable area is the CA1 region of the hippocampus. Some patients with lesions restricted to the CA1 region who recover from cardiac arrest can develop a residual severe anterograde amnesia (see Patient 5–6).[116]

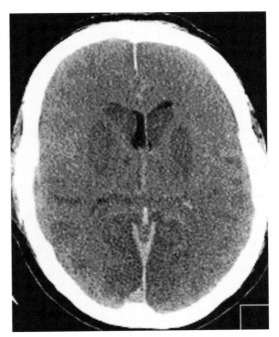

Figure 5–5. Computed tomography scan of a comatose patient after prolonged cardiopulmonary resuscitation. The scan was taken at a time when the patient was deeply comatose but breathing. The brain is swollen, with cortical sulci virtually obliterated. No signal differentiation can be seen between gray and white matter. The lentiform nuclei are hypointense, suggesting basal ganglia infarction. (Scan courtesy Dr. Sasan Karimi.)

Focal Ischemia

Focal ischemia differs from global ischemia in that it allows for collateral circulation to deliver at least some blood to the areas surrounding the area of no perfusion induced by the vascular occlusion. The surrounding area, called the penumbra,[117] suffers low flow but not cellular death. It is the goal of the physician treating the patient to try to preserve that area and return its metabolism to normal. Like global ischemia, damage can occur either during the ischemic period or during reperfusion.[118] Schaller and Graf[118] have diagramed a three-peaked curve presenting times at which the penumbra is susceptible to tissue damage. The first occurs during ischemia with damage resulting from oxygen depletion, energy failure, depolarization of neurons and synapses, and homeostasis failure. The second occurs after reperfusion with damage caused by excitotoxicity as well as disturbed homeostasis. The third occurs several weeks later with late damage to neurons and glial cells via both necrosis and apoptosis. As indicated above, interventions that appear to ameliorate the first two peaks, such as the use of anesthetic agents at the time of ischemia, do not appear to have any effect on the delayed necrosis.[103]

Focal ischemia also differs from global ischemia in its therapeutic window. The physician has minutes to restore circulation in a patient with cardiac arrest before irreversible brain damage with a significant neurologic deficit occurs. With focal ischemia there is, by definition, collateral blood flow to the surrounding tissue and often an area of partial ischemia, the penumbra that surrounds the area of most intense ischemia. The tissue constituting the penumbra may have blood flow below the level at which it functions normally, but yet not so low as to cause immediate infarction. Hence, there is often a window of time that may persist for several hours, during which the tissue in the penumbra can be saved; in some cases this will reduce the area of what would otherwise be infarcted tissue to the point where there may be little or no neurologic deficit. The exact time window undoubtedly varies depending on the individual vascular anatomy and the nature of the vascular obstruction, but evidence from trials of thrombolytic therapy indicates that it often persists for as long as 3 hours. The time window may, in fact, be longer, but by 3 hours the risk of a hemorrhage into the infarcted tissue becomes greater than the benefit from salvaging partially ischemic tissue.[118]

Hyperglycemia during reperfusion increases infarct volume and may cause hemorrhage. It also reduces the CBF. The mechanism for this effect is not clear, but it could result from damage to endothelium, increased expression of adhesion molecules, or glycosylation of critical proteins that lead to vasodilation.

Patient 5–6

A 44-year-old woman was found unconscious in her room when her husband returned home. He called for paramedics and she was transported to the hospital, where a diagnosis of carbon monoxide poisoning was made. She had a brief period of cardiac arrest from which she was resuscitated. She remained first unconscious and then poorly responsive for about 10 days before recovering. When she recovered she appeared a little euphoric but was able to relate to her husband and family in perfectly logical fashion. She returned home and tried to go back to work as a college teacher of Spanish. Unfortunately, she rapidly discovered that she could not remember where she had parked her car and could not remember what she was to teach that day, although once she was involved in teaching, she was able to do relatively well. With careful preparation of lesson plans in advance and arrangements for her car to be in the same place and described to her in writing, she was able to continue to function at the community college.

Hypoxia

Unlike ischemia and hypoglycemia, hypoxia alone is rarely responsible for brain necrosis.[114]

In fact, hypoxic preconditioning of experimental animals by exposure to moderate hypoxia of 8% to 10% oxygen for 3 hours protects against cerebral ischemia delivered 1 or 2 days later.[119] Miyamoto and Auer exposed rats to an arterial PO_2 of 25 torr for 15 minutes and failed to find necrotic neurons.[114] Unilateral carotid ligation (ischemia) caused necrosis even in animals exposed to an arterial O_2 of 100 torr. In these experiments, hypoxia exacerbated the effects of ischemia. In most situations in humans, hypoxia leads to either hypotension or cardiac arrest so that hypoxic insults are for the most part a mixture of hypoxic and ischemic injury.

Pure hypoxia, such as occurs in carbon monoxide poisoning, is more likely to lead to delayed injury to the subcortical structures of the hemispheres. Typically the damage will occur 1 to several days after the patient awakens from the hypoxic episode and involves a characteristic distribution, including the posterior hemispheric white matter and basal ganglia, often leaving the patient blind and with a choreic movement disorder. A similar pattern of brain injury is seen with a variety of mitochondrial encephalopathies and deficits in carbohydrate metabolism, suggesting that the injury is due to failure of oxidative metabolism. The reason that the injury has a predilection for these sites is unknown, although the neurons in the globus pallidus have a particularly high constitutive firing rate, and this may predispose them to hypoxic injury.

EVALUATION OF NEUROTRANSMITTER CHANGES IN METABOLIC COMA

Several neurotransmitters control arousal, sleep-wake cycles, and consciousness. They are probably also involved in metabolic encephalopathies and their role, where known, is discussed in the sections below on specific encephalopathies.[120]

Acetylcholine

The cholinergic system described in Chapter 1 plays an important role in consciousness.[121] The nicotinic alpha-4-beta-2 receptor is inhibited by clinically relevant doses of volatile anesthetics and ketamine, although whether the inhibition is clinically relevant is not clear.[122] However, anticholinergic agents that cross the blood-brain barrier can cause memory loss and florid delirium, and anticholinergic medications are an independent risk factor for delirium in older medical inpatients.[123]

Dopamine

Dopamine plays a key role in arousal. A wide range of stimulant drugs (amphetamine, methylphenidate, modafinil) are antagonists of the dopamine reuptake pump, and if mice lack this dopamine transporter, the drugs do not have a stimulatory effect. Patients with Parkinson's disease have increased sleepiness, as do patients treated with dopamine antagonists. Paradoxically, D2 agonist drugs can also cause sleepiness. The reason for this puzzling response appears to be due to the fact that the D2 receptor can be either pre- or postsynaptic. Dopamine has its major stimulatory effects via postsynaptic receptors, but the D2 receptor is also found presynaptically on dopamine terminals, where it down-regulates dopamine release. Thus, D2 agonist drugs reduce endogenous dopamine release. Interestingly, dopamine agonists can cause delirium, whereas dopamine blockers are often used to treat delirium. Dopamine antagonists also cause EEG slowing.[124] Dopamine release is increased in hypoxia at a time when acetylcholine release is decreased.[120]

Gamma-Aminobutyric Acid

As indicated above, the $GABA_A$ receptor is a major target of many general anesthetic agents. Benzodiazepines, which are $GABA_A$ potentiators, can cause memory loss, delirium,[125] and, rarely, coma.[126] Increased concentrations of endogenous GABA agonists, both benzodiazepine-like and non-benzodiazepine-like, have been found in patients with hepatic encephalopathy.[127] A variety of $GABA_B$ receptor agonists, such as baclofen, are also sedating. Gamma-hydroxybutyrate (GHB), which has recently been approved for use in narcolepsy, binds both to $GABA_B$ receptors and probably to specific GHB receptors. This drug causes profound impairment of consciousness

and high-voltage delta-wave EEG activity. It has achieved a reputation as a "date rape" drug because in lower doses it causes memory loss and sometimes delirium.

Serotonin

Several investigators have implicated the evolutionary very old serotonin in the pathogenesis of delirium. Both high and low levels of serotonin have been associated with delirium.[128–130] Serotonin levels are dependent on the transport of tryptophan, a large neutral aromatic amino acid that crosses the blood-brain barrier. Because several other large amino acids, including isoleucine, leucine, methionine, phenylalanine, and tyrosine, use the same saturable carrier, they compete with one another. Thus, changes in the amino acid levels in the plasma affect serotonin metabolism in the brain. For example, recent studies suggest that ingestion of tryptophane-rich alpha-lactalbumin at bedtime improves morning alertness and brain measures of attention in normal individuals.[131] The effect of serotonin withdrawal is a little less clear. Increased tryptophan uptake results in increased brain serotonin activity in patients with hepatic encephalopathy.[120]

Histamine

Histamine is now known to play a key role in maintaining a waking state. Histamine neurons in the tuberomammillary nucleus in the hypothalamus comprise a major component of the ascending arousal system. Inhibition of the histamine neurons with a GABA agonist in cats causes sleepiness, and disinhibition with bicuculline causes wakefulness and prevents the sedating effects of anesthetics. Animals with knockouts either of the gene for histidine decarboxylase, which synthesizes histamine, or the H_1 receptor, which is found in the cerebral cortex, are more sleepy and do not respond to other arousing neurotransmitters such as orexin. Those H_1 antagonists that are used to treat allergies and also cross the blood-brain barrier cause considerable sleepiness in humans. H_2 antagonists, such as cimetidine, ranitidine, and famotidine, have, on rare occasions, been associated with delirium, particularly in the elderly.[132,133] This response may be due to nonspecific interaction with other histamine receptor subtypes.

Glutamate

The most common excitatory neurotransmitter in the brain, glutamate is used by almost all neurons involved in thalamocortical and long-range corticocortical transmission. Drugs that block NMDA receptors, which are required for memory phenomena such as long-term potentiation (LTP), including ketamine, nitrous oxide, and phencyclidine, cause intense delirium. However, these drugs do not reduce activity in the arousal system, and may in fact heighten it. As a result, subjects who have had ketamine often report bizarre and distorted experiences, but may be aware even when they appear not to be. Up-regulation of glutamate neurotransmission has been associated with alcohol withdrawal delirium (delirium tremens).[134]

Norepinephrine

Norepinephrine is used by neurons of the locus coeruleus, which also is a major component of the ascending arousal system. Although ablation of the locus coeruleus has minimal effects on consciousness, due to redundant pathways from other monoaminergic systems, its neurons fire in association with novel stimuli in the environment and are most active during wakefulness. Beta blockers can cause depression, but not impairment of consciousness. Alpha blockers mainly impair consciousness when they cause peripheral vasodilation and orthostatic hypotension. CSF norepinephrine is elevated during alcohol withdrawal[135] and may be involved in opiate withdrawal as well; treatment with the alpha-2 agonist clonidine can relieve the withdrawal symptoms. Cocaine, which blocks reuptake of norepinephrine as well as dopamine, has convulsive, respiratory, and circulatory toxicity, but it is not clear what part of this syndrome can be attributed to norepinephrine.[135]

SPECIFIC CAUSES OF METABOLIC COMA

The diagnosis of specific causes of metabolic coma is not always easy. The history often is unobtainable and the neurologic examination in many instances suggests only that the cause of coma is metabolic without identifying the specific etiology. Thus, laboratory examinations are usually required to make a final diagnosis. But when the patient is acutely and severely ill and time is short, the major treatable causes of acute metabolic coma (which are comparatively few) must be considered systematically. In obscure cases, it is remarkable how often an accurate clue is derived from careful observation of the respiratory pattern accompanied, when indicated, by analysis of blood gases, determination of blood sugar, and lumbar puncture.

Because hypoglycemic coma is frequent, dangerous, and often clinically obscure, one should check a fingerstick glucose on any patient in whom the cause of delirium, stupor, or coma is not immediately known. Because hyperglycemia can worsen the prognosis in patients with cerebral infarction or head trauma, glucose should not be given unless the patient is known to be hypoglycemic. In potentially malnourished patients, thiamine should be given along with glucose to minimize the risk of acute Wernicke's encephalopathy (see page 313).[136]

Brain oxygen tension can be measured directly by inserting a sensor[137,138] into the brain or indirectly by measuring cerebral venous oxygen into the jugular bulb.[139] However, jugular venous oxygen tension gives no hint as to oxygen tension in specific regions of the brain.

ISCHEMIA AND HYPOXIA

Hypoxia of the brain almost always arises as part of a larger problem in oxygen supply, either because the ambient pressure of the gas falls or systemic abnormalities in the organism interrupt its delivery to the tissues. Although there are many causes of tissue hypoxia,[140] disturbances in oxygen supply to the brain in most instances can be divided into hypoxic hypoxia, anemic hypoxia, histotoxic hypoxia, and ischemic hypoxia. Though caused by different conditions and diseases, all four categories share equally the potential for depriving brain tissue of its critical oxygen supply. The main differences between the hypoxic, anemic, and ischemic forms are on the arterial side. All three forms of anoxia share the common effect of producing *cerebral venous hypoxia*, which, save for oxygen sensors inserted into brain,[138] is the best guide in vivo to estimate the partial pressure of the gas in the tissue.[141] However, with histotoxic hypoxia, blood oxygen levels may be normal.

In *hypoxic hypoxia*, insufficient oxygen reaches the blood so that both the arterial oxygen content and tension are low. This situation results either from a low oxygen tension in the environment (e.g., high altitude or displacement of oxygen by an inert gas such as nitrogen[142] or methane) or from an inability of oxygen to reach and cross the alveolar capillary membrane (pulmonary disease, hypoventilation). With mild or moderate hypoxia, the CBF increases to maintain the cerebral oxygen delivery and no symptoms occur. However, clinical evidence suggests that even in chronic hypoxic conditions, the CBF can only increase to about twice normal. When the increase is insufficient to compensate for the degree of hypoxia, the $CMRO_2$ begins to fall and symptoms of cerebral hypoxia occur. Because hypoxic hypoxia affects the entire organism, all energy-intensive tissues are affected, and eventually, if the oxygen delivery is sufficiently impaired, the myocardium fails, the blood pressure drops, and the brain becomes ischemic. Most of the pathologic changes in patients who die after an episode of hypoxic hypoxia are related to ischemia[114]; therefore, it is difficult to define the actual damage done by hypoxic hypoxia alone.[143] For example, glutamate release causing excitocytotoxicity occurs in vitro with ischemia but not anoxia.[144] Loss of consciousness due to hypoxic hypoxia before blood pressure drops may be a result of enhanced spontaneous transmitter release, which probably disrupts normal neural circuitry.[145]

In *anemic hypoxia*, sufficient oxygen reaches the blood, but the amount of hemoglobin available to bind and transport it is decreased. Under such circumstances, the blood oxygen content is decreased even though oxygen tension in the arterial blood is normal. Either low hemoglobin content (anemia) or chemical changes in hemoglobin that interfere with oxygen binding (e.g., carbon monoxyhemoglobin, methemoglobin) can be responsible. Coma occurs if the oxygen content drops so low that the brain's metabolic needs are not met even by an increased CBF. The lowered blood viscosity that occurs in anemia makes it somewhat easier for the CBF to increase than in carbon monoxide poisoning. Most of the toxicity from carbon monoxide poisoning is not due to hemoglobin binding but is histotoxic, a result of its binding to cytochromes.[146]

In *ischemic hypoxia*, the blood may or may not carry sufficient oxygen, but the CBF is insufficient to supply cerebral tissues. The usual causes are diseases that greatly reduce the cardiac output, such as myocardial infarction, arrhythmia, shock, and vasovagal syncope, or diseases that increase the cerebral vascular resistance by arterial occlusion (e.g., stroke) or spasm (e.g., migraine).

Histotoxic hypoxia results from agents that poison the electron transport chain. Such agents include cyanide and carbon monoxide. Carbon monoxide intoxication is by far the most common; smoke from house fires can cause both carbon monoxide and cyanide poisoning (see page 240). Because the electron transport chain is impaired, glycolysis is increased leading to increased lactic acid; thus, high levels of lactic acid (greater than 7 mmol/L) in the blood are encountered in patients with severe cyanide poisoning. Some cyanide antidotes increase methemoglobin, which may add to the anemic hypoxic burden of patients who have also been poisoned with carbon monoxide[147]; hydroxycobalamine treatment does not help under such conditions.

The development of neurologic signs in most patients with ischemia or hypoxia depends more on the severity and duration of the process than on its specific cause. Ischemia (vascular failure) is generally more dangerous than hypoxia alone, in part because potentially toxic products of cerebral metabolism such as lactic acid are not removed. The clinical categories of hypoxic and ischemic brain damage can be subdivided into acute, chronic, and multifocal.

Acute, Diffuse (or Global) Hypoxia or Ischemia

This circumstance occurs with conditions that rapidly reduce the oxygen content of the blood or cause a sudden reduction in the brain's overall blood flow. The major causes include obstruction of the airways, such as occurs with drowning, choking, or suffocation; massive obstruction to the cerebral arteries, such as occurs with hanging or strangulation; and conditions causing a sudden decrease in cardiac output, such as asystole, severe arrhythmias, vasodepressor syncope, pulmonary embolism, or massive systemic hemorrhage. Embolic or thrombotic disorders, including thrombotic thrombocytopenic purpura, disseminated intravascular coagulation, acute bacterial endocarditis, falciparum malaria, and fat embolism, can all cause such widespread multifocal ischemia that they can give the clinical appearance of acute diffuse cerebral ischemia. If the cerebral circulation stops completely, consciousness is lost rapidly, within 6 to 8 seconds. It takes a few seconds longer if blood flow continues but oxygen is no longer supplied. Fleeting lightheadedness and blindness sometimes precede unconsciousness. Generalized convulsions, pupillary dilation (due to massive adrenal and sympathetic release of catecholamines as part of the emergency stress response), and bilateral extensor plantar responses quickly follow if anoxia is complete or lasts longer than a few seconds. If tissue oxygenation is restored immediately, consciousness returns in seconds or minutes without sequelae. If, however, the oxygen deprivation lasts longer than 1 or 2 minutes, or if it is superimposed upon pre-existing cerebral vascular disease, then stupor, confusion, and signs of motor dysfunction may persist for several hours or even permanently. Under clinical circumstances, total ischemic anoxia lasting longer than 4 minutes starts to kill brain cells, with the neurons of the cerebral cortex (especially the hippocampus) and cerebellum (the Purkinje cells) dying first. In humans, severe diffuse ischemic anoxia lasting 10 minutes or more begins to destroy the brain. In rare instances, particularly drowning, in which cold water rapidly lowers brain temperature, recovery of brain function has been noted despite more prolonged periods of anoxia, although such instances are more common in children than adults. Thus, resuscitation efforts after drowning (particularly in children) should not be abandoned just because the patient has been immersed for more than 10 minutes.

As noted above, much experimental evidence indicates that the initial mechanism of anoxia's rapidly lethal effect on the brain may, to some degree, lie in the inability of the heart and the cerebral vascular bed to recover from severe ischemia or oxygen deprivation. It has

been reported that if one makes meticulous efforts to maintain the circulation, the brains of experimental animals can recover from as long as 30 minutes of very severe hypoxemia with arterial PO_2 tensions of 20 mm Hg or less. Equally low arterial blood oxygen tensions have been reported in conscious humans who recovered without sequelae. These laboratory findings suggest that guaranteeing the integrity of the systemic circulation offers the strongest chance of effectively treating or preventing hypoxic brain damage. Interestingly, previous episodes of hypoxia may protect against ischemic brain injury by inducing hypoxia inducible factor (HIF-1) that in turn induces vascular endothelial growth factor, erythropoietin, glucose transporters, glycolytic enzymes, heat shock proteins, and other genes that may protect against ischemia.[119]

Vigorous and prolonged attempts at cardiac resuscitation are justified, particularly in young and previously healthy individuals in whom recovery of cardiac function is more likely to occur.

Acute, short-lived hypoxic-ischemic attacks causing unconsciousness are most often the result of transient global ischemia caused by syncope (Table 5–8). Much less frequently, transient attacks of vertebrobasilar ischemia can cause unconsciousness. Such attacks may be accompanied by brief seizures, which often present problems in differential diagnosis as seizures themselves cause loss of consciousness.

Syncope or fainting results when cerebral perfusion falls below the level required to supply sufficient oxygen and substrate to maintain tissue metabolism. If the CBF falls below about 20 mL/100 g/minute, there is a rapid failure of cerebral function. Syncope has many causes, the most frequent being listed in Table 5–8. Among young persons, most syncope results from dysfunction of autonomic reflexes producing vasodepressor hypotension, so-called neurocardiogenic, vasovagal, or reflex syncope.[148] These events are typically driven by a beta-adrenergic vasodilation in response to increased blood norepinephrine, often during an episode of pain involving tissue invasion (e.g., having blood drawn) or even witnessing such an event in another person. Vasodepressor responses remain the predominant cause of syncope in older persons as well, but with advancing age, syncopal attacks are more likely to

Table 5–8 **Principal Causes of Brief Episodic Unconsciousness***

1. SYNCOPE
Primarily vascular
A. Decreased peripheral resistance
   1. Vasodepressor
      a. Psychophysiologic
      b. Reflex from visceral sensory stimulation (deep pain, gastric distention, postmicturition, etc.)
      c. Carotid sinus syncope, type 2 (vasodepressor)
      d. Cough syncope (impaired right heart return)
   2. Blood volume depletion
   3. Neurogenic autonomic insufficiency

Primarily cardiac
A. Cardiodecelerator attacks (transient sinus arrest)
      a. Psychophysiologic
      b. Visceral sensory stimulation (tracheal stimulation, glossopharyngeal neuralgia, swallow syncope, etc.)
      c. Carotid sinus syncope, type 1 (cardiodecelerator)
B. Cardiac arrhythmia or asystole
C. Aortic stenosis
D. Carotid origin emboli in the presence of severe vascular disease of other cervical cranial arteries
2. AKINETIC OR ABSENCE SEIZURES
3. DROP ATTACKS
4. VERTEBROBASILAR TRANSIENT ISCHEMIC ATTACKS
5. HYPOGLYCEMIA
6. CONVERSION REACTION

*In conditions 1 and 2, the altered consciousness is apparent to the observer. Condition 3 often is so brief (especially if the head falls below the level of the heart, resulting in improved cerebral blood flow) that neither subject nor observer can be sure whether full consciousness was retained. In conditions 4 and 5, the patient may appear awake and "conscious" to observers, but has no exact memory of the episode and often recalls it simply as an unconscious attack.

occur as a result of cardiac arrhythmia or hyperactive baroreceptor reflexes due to peripheral, CNS, or cardiac disease.

Vasodepressor syncope is usually heralded by a brief sensation of giddiness, weakness, and sweating before consciousness is lost. This is an important diagnostic point if present, but about 30% of patients with true syncope may be amnesic from the loss of consciousness and

thus report the episode as a "drop attack"[149] (see below).

Reflex syncopal attacks almost always occur when the victim is in the standing position, rarely when sitting, and almost never when prone or supine. Asystole, on the other hand, characteristically produces unheralded, abrupt unconsciousness regardless of position. If upright, the subject suddenly sinks or falls to the ground. The brevity of the unconsciousness, the rapid restoration of wakefulness when the head is at position equal to or lower than the heart, and the appearance of pallor prior to and during the loss of consciousness differentiate asystolic syncope from transient vertebrobasilar insufficiency.

Drop attacks, defined as sudden collapse of the legs in someone who is standing resulting in a fall, generally occur in middle-aged[150] and older adults.[151] Some are caused by syncope, the patient having amnesia for the loss of consciousness. Others are otologic in origin,[152] although the patient is sometimes unaware of vertigo. Occasionally drop attacks occur as a result of bilateral ischemia of the base of the pons or the medullary pyramids, or as a result of transient, positional compression of the upper cervical spinal cord due to atlantoaxial subluxation or fracture of the dens.[153] In such cases, there is no loss of consciousness.

Vertebrobasilar transient ischemic attacks produce short-lived neurologic episodes characterized by symptoms of neurologic dysfunction arising from subtentorial structures, especially vertigo, nausea, and headache[154] (Table 5–9). As a result, *vertebrobasilar ischemic attacks rarely cause isolated syncope.* Brief confusion or amnesic episodes sometimes occur, but stupor and coma are rare, perhaps because ischemia sufficient to affect such a large part of the brainstem bilaterally generally causes additional signs of brainstem ischemia. Basilar ischemia involving the descending motor pathways in the basis pontis or the medullary pyramids sometimes results in drop attacks, which may superficially resemble asystolic syncope. The absence of either unconsciousness or the physical appearance of circulatory failure differentiates the condition from true syncope.

Epileptic seizures may occasionally be difficult to distinguish from syncope as a cause of unconsciousness. Tonic seizures and a few clonic jerks are not rare in patients with syncopal

Table 5–9 **Prodromal Symptoms in 53 of 85 Patients With Basilar Artery Occlusion**

Symptom	No. of Patients
Vertigo, nausea	26*
Headache, neckache	18
Hemiparesis	9
Double vision	9
Dysarthria	9
Hemianopia	5
Hemihypesthesia	5
Tinnitus, hearing loss	5
Drop attack	4
Confusion	3
Other	6

*Only four of these patients did not experience other prodromal symptoms.

attacks, but unless the patient is kept in an upright position they are generally quite brief, whereas grand mal epileptic attacks usually last 2 to 4 minutes and tend to recur independently of body position. Some patients suffer from akinetic seizures that can cause sudden loss of consciousness without motor activity, resembling cardiac syncope or drop attacks.[155–157] Other patients with subclinical or partial complex seizures may suddenly enter a twilight state in which there is loss of contact with the outside world, but usually no loss of posture.

Pulmonary embolism presents as syncope in about 10% of patients.[158] Seizures may also be a presenting symptom of a pulmonary embolus.[159] Focal signs without cerebral infarction are occasionally present.[160] Factors causing symptoms include cerebral ischemia, hypoxia, and hypocapnia resulting from the fall in cardiac output, blood oxygenation, compensatory respiratory alkalosis that accompanies sudden occlusion of a major pulmonary artery, or vasovagal reflex syncope.[158] An occasional patient suffers cerebral infarction as well, probably from a paradoxic embolus. A pulmonary embolus raises right atrial pressure, opening a potentially patent foramen ovale, thus allowing a subsequent venous embolus to reach the brain. One clue to the presence of a pulmonary embolus in a patient who has suffered syncope or is confused is the presence of unexpected tachypnea or tachycardia in a patient recovering from a syncopal episode or a seizure, as Patient 5–7 illustrates.

Patient 5–7

A 39-year-old woman with a primary brain tumor was doing well after radiation and chemotherapy when, without warning, she had a generalized convulsion. She was taken to the emergency department where she was slightly confused and disoriented but otherwise had a nonfocal neurologic examination. Her pulse was 120 and respirations were 20. A CT scan of the brain revealed no acute changes. The emergency department physician called the treating neurologist, thinking that the patient must have suffered a seizure as a result of the brain tumor. The patient had had seizures before, but the tachypnea and tachycardia led the neurologist to suspect the possibility of a pulmonary embolus. A CT of the chest was performed, which revealed the pulmonary embolus. The patient was anticoagulated and made a full recovery.

Comment: The treating neurologist (not one of us) was very astute in considering possibilities in addition to the presence of a brain tumor as the cause of seizures. There was no reason that the patient, having recovered consciousness, would be tachycardic and tachypneic, but because many patients with primary brain tumors suffer thromboembolic disease, he requested the chest examination, which led to the correct diagnosis and appropriate treatment. However, one can be led astray. Focal seizures can cause dyspnea, leading one to incorrectly suspect pulmonary disease[161]; generalized seizures can cause pulmonary edema, which also leads to tachypnea. In addition, after a prolonged grand mal seizure, there is often an elevated serum lactate level (presumably due to poor oxygenation during the seizure) and thus it may take 10 to 15 minutes for the breathing and heart rate to return to normal. On the other hand, prolonged tachypnea should be evaluated by arterial blood gases. Respiratory alkalosis, hypoxia, and hypocapnia indicate pulmonary embolus (the sum of PaO_2 and $PaCO_2$ is usually less than 100), whereas metabolic acidosis with respiratory compensation suggests postseizure lactic acidosis.

Intermittent or Sustained Hypoxia

Intermittent hypoxia is exemplified by diminished cognitive functions and sometimes acute delirium in patients suffering from obstructive sleep apnea.[162] Sustained hypoxia is illustrated by delirium and sometimes focal neurologic signs that occur in young people at altitudes above 10,000 feet (3,000 meters).[163,164] These disorders are fully reversible. In addition, extreme degrees of anemia or low arterial oxygenation due to myocardial infarction, congestive heart failure, and pulmonary disease can, under appropriate circumstances, produce delirium, stupor, or coma. This is particularly true when more than one cause of hypoxia is present. For example, a myocardial infarct may cause encephalopathy in moderately anemic elderly subjects who also have chronic pulmonary disease. Happily, often correcting only one of the problems may ameliorate the encephalopathy.

Multifocal cerebral ischemia occurs in a number of conditions affecting the arterial bed or its contents. Hypertensive encephalopathy,[165] also referred to as hyperperfusion encephalopathy[166] or posterior reversible leukoencephalopathy (PRES),[167] is relatively rare, but often misdiagnosed. Its importance lies in the fact that if the disorder is appropriately identified and treated, it is usually (but not always) reversible. Formerly associated only with acute hypertensive emergencies, particularly eclampsia, the illness is now seen in a variety of settings including after the administration of cyclosporin or tacrolimus, as well as after several cancer chemotherapeutic agents.[168,169] It is also seen in a slightly different form after carotid endarterectomy and in a variety of small vessel diseases including systemic lupus erythematosus, scleroderma, and cryoglobulinemia. In one series of 110 patients, 30 suffered from pre-eclampsia or eclampsia and 24 from cyclosporin or tacrolimus neurotoxicity.[166] Most but not all of the patients in whom the disorder is induced by chemotherapy are also hypertensive, although the hypertension may be quite transitory and missed unless the patient's blood pressure is being monitored. Typically the patient, previously neurologically normal, complains of severe headache and may become agitated, leading to progressive confusion, delirium, stupor, or coma. Many patients suffer from focal or generalized seizures and multifocal neurologic signs, especially cortical blindness, but also hemiplegia or other focal signs. On neurologic examination, one clue is retinal artery spasm and papilloretinal edema; retinal exudates may also be present.

The imaging findings are characteristic and best seen on MRI[168] (CT scans may be normal or may show hypodensity in the parietal-occipital areas bilaterally). The MRI shows increased intensity on T2 and fluid-attenuated inversion recovery (FLAIR) images bilaterally and often symmetrically involving the posterior hemispheres and, less commonly, the cerebellum, thalamus, brainstem, and splenium of the corpus callosum. Rarely, more frontal areas may be involved as well. T1 images may show hypointensity in the same areas and occasionally contrast enhancement. Diffusion-weighted images are usually normal, but in its more severe form, may indicate restricted diffusion. Perfusion studies demonstrate hyperperfusion in the areas of abnormal signal. These MR findings are characteristic of vasogenic cerebral edema. Abnormal diffusion images indicate cerebral ischemia or infarction and suggest a poorer prognosis.

The pathogenesis of the disorder is believed to be a breakdown of the blood-brain barrier resulting from damage to endothelial cells when hypertension exceeds the boundaries of autoregulation and small vessels dilate, opening the blood-brain barrier. Other factors that also play a role include up-regulation of aquaporin-4 (a water channel in cerebral blood vessels that is also up-regulated in normal pregnancy),[170] interleukin-6 (an inflammatory cytokine that opens the blood-brain barrier), and nitric oxide, which induces vasodilation, particularly when intravascular flow rates are high, overcoming autoregulation.[165] The posterior distribution of the changes is not understood, but may be a result of the tendency for swelling of the medial temporal lobes to compress the posterior cerebral arteries, which may further diminish blood flow to this territory.

In less severe cases neuropathologic findings only reveal edema of white matter,[171] and if treated (e.g., for pre-eclampsia), the MRI changes and functional impairment may be entirely reversible. In more severe cases, microangiopathy with endothelial swelling and fibrinoid necrosis of small vessels and sometimes frank infarction occurs.[172]

The treatment consists first of recognizing the syndrome and lowering the blood pressure. Blood pressure lowering should be done judiciously, preferably in an intensive care unit with an arterial line in place. Most authorities recommend reduction of mean arterial pressure by no more than 20% to 25% within a period of minutes to a couple of hours; more rapid reduction may lead to cerebral infarction.[173] In patients with eclampsia or preeclampsia, intravenous magnesium sulfate has been shown in controlled trials to improve outcome, perhaps by its action as a vascular calcium channel blocker.[174]

The blood pressure may not be very high, particularly in children in whom resting blood pressure is usually quite low, or in pregnant women in whom the resting blood pressure is usually considerably lower than other adults. In fact, in a pregnant woman, an increase in blood pressure to a level that is still in the high normal range (e.g., 140/90) may be sufficient to cause the symptoms. Often, these patients present with a migrainous syndrome in the predelivery period or up to 2 weeks after delivery. It is the sudden rise from baseline level that causes the problem. In many patients, at the time the illness is recognized the blood pressure has already returned toward normal and these patients need only be treated with careful observation.

Patient 5–8

A 63-year-old man with a history of hypertension who had been complaining of headache for approximately 2 months was brought to an emergency department having been found unconscious in his home. When he arrived at the emergency department he was poorly responsive and had a right hemiplegia. His blood pressure was 200/130 mm Hg. An MR scan revealed large T2 and FLAIR hyperintense lesions in both posterior hemispheres with a rim of contrast enhancement surrounding the larger left-sided lesion (Figure 5–6). His physicians, concerned about the enhancing lesions representing a tumor, undertook an extensive workup, which included two lumbar punctures, which were unrevealing; a PET image of the

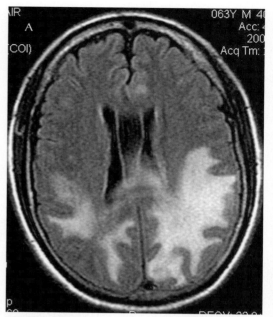
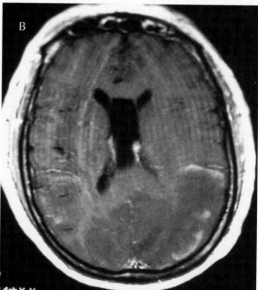

Figure 5–6. Posterior reversible leukoencephalopathy. Fluid-attenuated inversion recovery (FLAIR) image (A) and contrast-enhanced T1 (B). This was the magnetic resonance imaging (MRI) scan that led to the brain biopsy in Patient 5–8. The area of enhancement at the margin was interpreted as compatible with a glioma. (MRI courtesy Dr. Alexis Demopoulos.)

brain, showing decreased activity in the involved regions; and a body PET, which was negative. The family was informed that he probably had a brain tumor and a brain biopsy was performed that revealed only edematous tissue. Finally, attempts were made to control his blood pressure. He remained confused for 7 days and then began to improve. An MR scan done a week later continued to reveal hyperintensity on the FLAIR image with the added changes in the cerebellum and brainstem. The patient continued to improve and his neurologic signs eventually returned to normal with complete resolution on the MR scan. He was discharged on antihypertensive agents.

Disseminated intravascular coagulation is characterized by the intravascular activation of coagulation leading to occlusion of multiple small vessels. It has several different causes,[175] including sepsis,[176] trauma (particularly head injury),[177] malignancy,[178] hepatic failure, and several severe toxic and immunologic reactions.[179] The disorder may cause either small cerebral infarcts or cerebral hemorrhages including subdural hematomas. On the other hand, diffuse vascular plugging, particularly on the venous side, may reduce CBF so that the neurologic symptoms are nonspecific and include fluctuating focal neurologic signs, delirium, and sometimes stupor or coma. The diagnosis is established by examination of coagulation factors in the blood.[180] The presence of disseminated intravascular coagulation in an illness such as sepsis or head trauma confers a poor prognosis.

Cerebral malaria is a common and feared complication of infection with *Plasmodium falciparum*. In adults it is generally part of multiorgan failure and is characterized by delirium, stupor, or coma usually following a generalized seizure. Patients often have disconjugate eye movements and may have flexor or extensor rigidity. Mortality in adults is about 20% and most deaths occur within 24 hours of the onset of the illness. Because the encephalopathy follows systemic manifestations of malaria (i.e., chills and fever), the diagnosis is not difficult. About 15% of patients have retinal hemorrhages, which aid in the diagnosis. The pathogenesis of the disorder includes obstruction of the cerebral microvasculature. There may be raised ICP with edema, both vasogenic and cytotoxic. The disorder may

be complicated by hypoglycemia and the sequelae of generalized convulsions.[181]

Fat embolism, frequently a complication of skeletal trauma particularly involving fracture of the large, long bones that contain substantial amounts of marrow, is characterized by the release of fat droplets that plug small vessels from the marrow into the venous circulation. These may be sufficiently compliant to squeeze through lung capillaries, reaching the arterial circulation and causing diffuse plugging of small arterioles and capillaries. Two clinical syndromes arise from fat embolus. The first, or pulmonary syndrome, is a result of the initial multiple pulmonary microemboli that lead to progressive hypoxia with resulting tachypnea and hypocarbia (similar to other forms of pulmonary embolus). The hypoxia can be initially corrected by oxygen, but if the emboli occlude enough alveolar capillaries, the patient eventually develops respiratory failure. The second, or cerebral syndrome, is characterized by confusion, lethargy, stupor, or coma.[182] Characteristically, the symptoms are not present immediately following the traumatic injury, but rather after a period of several hours to as long as 2 or 3 days during which the fat emboli pass from the pulmonary to the arterial circulation. The patient becomes lethargic and, in fulminant instances, comatose. Accompanying the diffuse neurologic signs of stupor and coma can be a variety of focal signs including focal seizures, hemiparesis, or conjugate deviation of the eyes. The diagnosis can be difficult to establish in mild to moderately severe cases. In severe or fulminating instances, a characteristic petechial rash usually develops over the neck, shoulders, and upper part of the anterior thorax on the second or third day after injury. Biopsy of the petechiae reveals lipid emboli in small vessels. However, because standard tissue processing involves delipidation, it is necessary to alert the pathologist to the possibility of fat emboli so that frozen tissue sections can be stained for fat. Similar petechiae may be seen in the conjunctivae and eye grounds. Magnetic resonance spectroscopy (MRS) suggests the presence of lipid in the brain before there is evidence of cerebral hypoxic ischemia due to small vessel occlusions.[183] Later, the MRI gives evidence of multiple high-intensity lesions on diffusion-weighted image presenting as bright spots on a dark background (star field patterns).[184] The prognosis with supportive care is good, and patients who survive an acute episode usually recover without significant neurologic residua. An occasional patient may suffer prolonged coma usually with diffuse cerebral edema.[185] Silicone emboli injected for cosmetic purposes may mimic the fat embolism syndrome.[186]

HISTORICAL VIGNETTE

Patient 5–9

A previously healthy 27-year-old woman was examined through the courtesy of Dr. Philip Swanson of the University of Washington, Seattle. While skiing, she suffered a noncompound fracture of the left tibia and fibula. Except for pain, her condition was uncomplicated until 36 hours later when nurses recorded that she was not making verbal responses. Shortly thereafter, she received pentothal sodium and nitrous oxide-oxygen anesthesia for closed reduction of the fracture and failed to awaken postoperatively. Examination revealed intact pupillary responses and intermittent abnormal extensor posturing of the extremities, more on the left than the right. Blood gases showed a PaO_2 of 60 mm Hg and $PaCO_2$ of 20 mm Hg. Fat droplets were found in the urine and the CSF, and successive small numbers of petechial hemorrhages appeared in the optic fundi and the conjunctivae. No episode of hypotension or cardiac arrhythmia was ever recorded.

Seven days after the onset of coma, the woman lay in an eyes-open state with roving eye movements and gave no sign of psychologic awareness. Constant posturing of the head and extremities was present. She perspired heavily and chewed briskly during times that the eyes were open. There was hypertonus in all four extremities with the postures as noted. The left leg remained in a cast.

The patient remained in a vegetative state for another 48 hours, then began to talk and follow commands. Her somatic neurologic defects gradually subsided. Successive psychologic tests reflected gradual intellectual improvement. Four months following the accident, the neurologic examination showed that she had returned to normal. She scored 100 on the Wechsler Adult Intelligence Scale and 110 on the Memory Scale. She returned to full employment.

Comment: This patient had a characteristic course for fat embolism, so that despite the lack of scanning available at the time, the diagnosis is clear and the natural history of the disorder is apparent.

Cardiopulmonary bypass surgery results in virtually continuous bombardment of the brain with emboli. These may be recorded during surgery with intracranial Doppler monitoring. The embolic barrage results in four different patterns of neurologic complications[187]: cerebral infarction, postoperative delirium, transient cognitive dysfunction, and long-term cognitive dysfunction. Infarction occurs in 1% to 5% of patients; a postoperative delirium complicates 10% to 30% of patients. The delirium is often hyperactive and florid, usually beginning 1 or 2 days after the operation and persisting for several days (see page 283). Short-term cognitive dysfunction has been reported in 30% to 80% of patients, with long-term cognitive changes in 20% to 60% of patients. In addition to the multiple emboli, hypotension during anesthesia with hypoxia during extracorporal circulation may contribute to this outcome. Early reports suggested that there was permanent cognitive dysfunction after pulmonary bypass surgery. On the other hand, recent reports[188] conclude that control groups with similar levels of coronary artery disease also have worse cognitive scores than healthy controls.

Emboli to the brain from the heart originate from cardiac valves infected with bacteria,[189] from cardiac valves encrusted with fibrin-platelet vegetations in patients with nonbacterial thrombotic endocarditis,[190] from prosthetic cardiac valves,[191] and from cardiac thrombus or cardiac myxoma.[192] Depending on the size and number of the emboli, the vessels in which they lodge, and the rapidity of their resolution, patients can present with either focal signs due to fairly large cerebral infarcts or more diffuse neurologic signs including delirium and stupor, either accompanied or unaccompanied by focal neurologic signs. Patients with nonbacterial thrombotic endocarditis are more likely to exhibit a pattern of numerous small infarcts in multiple territories than are patients with infective endocarditis, who are more likely to have lesions restricted to a single territory.[193] An MRI showing multiple areas of abnormality, only some of which are positive on diffusion-weighted image, indicates multiple infarcts of different ages. If the abnormalities are in several different vascular territories, it is likely that the emboli come from a central source, such as the heart or aorta. Echocardiography helps establish the diagnosis. If transthoracic echocardiography is negative, a transesophageal echocardiogram may establish the diagnosis.[194]

vegetations may be difficult to visualize even with transesophageal echocardiogram, possibly because the vegetations are very friable and may embolize shortly after they form. However, cerebral infarcts or a fluctuating level of consciousness, with or without focal signs, should prompt a diligent search for a coagulopathy in a cancer patient.

Patient 5–10

A 58-year-old man was admitted to the hospital for left-sided weakness. He had lost about 30 pounds over the previous 2 months, and on general examination he had a distended liver. On examination he was slightly lethargic, but other cognitive functions were intact. There was weakness of adduction of the left eye on looking to the right, with nystagmus in the abducting eye. He showed left upper motor neuron facial paresis and weakness of his left arm and leg. In addition, there was loss of appreciation of the position of his left limbs in space. CT scan disclosed both a right middle cerebral artery distribution infarct as well as a small infarct in the paramedian portion of the upper pons. Because these infarcts were apparently in two different vascular distributions, a central cause of emboli was suspected.

CT of the abdomen disclosed a mass in the head of the pancreas, diagnosed as pancreatic carcinoma, as well as multiple liver metastases. Transthoracic and transesophageal echocardiogram was negative, as was heart rhythm monitoring. Blood coagulation testing showed a mild elevation of the prothrombin time and elevated fibrin degradation products. He subsequently had fluctuating drowsiness and passed into a coma, and a decision was made by the family to provide only comfort care. He died several days later.

At autopsy, the diagnosis of metastatic pancreatic carcinoma was confirmed. Examination of the heart disclosed vegetations on the mitral valve consisting of fibrin-platelet thrombi. There was diffuse thrombosis in both arteries and veins within the brain and the kidneys, but limited evidence of disseminated coagulation in other organs.

Comment: Coagulopathies, including disseminated intravascular coagulation, venous thrombosis (which may cause paradoxic emboli), nonbacterial thrombotic endocarditis, or some combination of these syndromes, are a common cause of stroke in patients with cancer. Hematologic signs and involvement of other organ systems may be minimal, as in this case. Fibrin-platelet

Sequelae of Hypoxia

Following apparent recovery from an acute hypoxic insult, about 3%[195] of patients relapse into a severe *delayed postanoxic encephalopathy.* Our own experience with this disorder now extends to well over 20 cases (Patient 1–1). The onset in our patients has been as early as 4 days and as late as 14 days after the initial hypoxia; reports from other authors give an even longer interval.[196] The clinical picture includes an initial hypoxic insult that usually is sufficiently severe that patients are in deep coma when first found but awaken within 24 to 48 hours. Occasionally, however, relapse has been reported after a mild hypoxic insult that was sufficient only to daze the patient and not to cause full unconsciousness.[196] In either event, nearly all patients resume full activity within 4 or 5 days after the initial insult and then enjoy a clear and seemingly normal interval of 2 to 40 days. Then, abruptly, affected subjects become irritable, apathetic, and confused. Some are agitated or develop mania. Walking changes to a halting shuffle, and diffuse spasticity or rigidity appears. The deterioration may progress to coma or death or may arrest itself at any point. Most patients have a second recovery period that leads to full health within a year,[195] although some remain permanently impaired. Hyperbaric oxygen given at the initial insult does not appear to prevent the development of this neurologic problem.[197]

The MRI reveals a low apparent diffusion coefficient, which recovers over several months to a year. The typical distribution of lesions includes the deep white matter, particularly in the posterior part of the hemisphere, and the basal ganglia. This pattern is similar to the distribution of infarcts seen in patients with mitochondrial encephalopathies and may be due to the impairment of cellular oxidative metabolism in both cases. The serial changes are consistent with cytotoxic edema, perhaps from apoptosis triggered by the hypoxia.[198] The pathogenesis of the delay to neurologic deterioration is not known.

Patient 5–11

A 35-year-old electrical engineer was diagnosed with hypokalemic periodic paralysis. Attacks were often precipitated by eating foods rich in sugar, which caused a sudden drop in potassium. One day, after eating a jelly doughnut he went to exercise in the gym. He became gradually weaker and called for help, but soon was so weak that he became apneic. Despite the eventual participation of bystanders in artificial ventilation, he suffered an estimated period of about 5 minutes of severe hypoxia. He was resuscitated by paramedics and brought to the hospital, where he awoke quickly and resumed normal activity. On the fourth day after his hypoxic event he became drowsy, then lapsed into a stuporous state and then a coma. After about a week he again woke up but was blind, and soon developed athetotic limb movements. When he was seen 3 months later he was of normal intelligence, had normal pupillary light responses, but did not have conscious light perception. There was facial grimacing and constant chorea and athetosis in all four limbs. MRI scan of the brain demonstrated white matter injury in both the posterior parts of both cerebral hemispheres as well as the basal ganglia bilaterally.

Delayed coma after hypoxia has been reported most often after carbon monoxide or asphyxial gas poisoning, but as shown in Patient 5–11, cases are known in which other injuries, including hypoglycemia, cardiac arrest, strangulation, or a complication of surgical anesthesia, have provided the antecedent insult. Often, the neurologic changes are at first mistaken for a psychiatric disorder or even a subdural hematoma because of the lucid interval. Mental status examination clarifies the first of these errors, and the diffuse distribution of the neurologic changes, the lack of headache, and the absence of signs of rostral caudal deterioration as well as MRI eliminate the second.

Pathologically, the brains of patients dying of delayed postanoxic deterioration contain diffuse, severe, and bilateral leukoencephalopathy of the cerebral hemispheres with sparing of the immediate subcortical connecting fibers and, usually, of the brainstem.[199] Demyelination is prominent and axis cylinders appear reduced in number. The basal ganglia are sometimes infarcted,[200] but the nerve cells of the cerebral hemispheres and the brainstem remain mostly intact. The mechanism of the unusual white matter response is unknown. A few patients have been reported to have had aryl-sulfatase-A pseudodeficiency. This genetic defect is not known to cause cerebral disease and its relationship to the demyelination is unclear.[201] The diagnosis of coma caused by postanoxic encephalopathy is made from the history of the initial insult and by recognizing the characteristic signs and symptoms of metabolic coma. There is no specific treatment, but bedrest for patients with acute hypoxia may prevent the complication.

Another sequela of severe diffuse hypoxia is the syndrome of *intention or action myoclonus.*[202] Patients suffering from this syndrome generally have had an episode of severe hypoxia caused by cardiac arrest or airway obstruction and have usually had generalized convulsions during the hypoxic episode. About 40% of patients who do not regain consciousness after cardiac resuscitation develop myoclonic status epilepticus.[203] The development of myoclonic status epilepticus in the comatose patient portends a poor prognosis, although we have seen an occasional patient recover. Affected patients who awaken from posthypoxic coma usually are dysarthric, and attempted voluntary movements are marked by myoclonic jerks of trunk and limb muscles. The pathophysiologic basis of this disorder has not been established. Electrophysiologically, the myoclonus can be either cortical or subcortical.[204] The cortical form may respond to levetiracetam; the subcortical may respond to 5-hydroxytryptophan.[204]

DISORDERS OF GLUCOSE OR COFACTOR AVAILABILITY

Hypoglycemia

Hypoglycemia is a common and serious cause of metabolic coma and one capable of remarkably varied combinations of signs and symptoms.[205] Among patients with severe hypoglycemic coma, most have been caused by excessive doses of insulin or oral hypoglycemic agents for the treatment of diabetes. In one series of 51 patients admitted to the hospital for hypoglycemia, 41 were diabetics, 36 being treated with insulin and five with sulfonylurea drugs. In nondiabetic patients, the hypoglycemia had been induced by excessive alcohol and one patient had injected herself with insulin in a suicide attempt.[206] Less frequent causes of hypoglycemic coma were insulin-secreting pancreatic adenomas, retroperitoneal sarcomas, and hemochromatosis with liver disease. In patients taking either insulin or oral hypoglycemics, the addition of fluoroquinolones, mostly gatifloxacin or ciprofloxacin, may induce severe hypoglycemia[207] (gatifloxacin can also cause hyperglycemia[208]). The intake of alcohol and perhaps psychoactive drugs in insulin-treated diabetics with severe hypoglycemia is relatively common. In fact, alcohol alone is responsible for a significant percentage of patients with severe hypoglycemia.[209] It is therefore important to check blood glucose even in patients in whom cognitive impairment can be attributed to alcohol ingestion. Fortunately, in most emergency departments a blood glucose from a fingerstick is done as a matter of course in any patient with altered mental status.

Pathologically, hypoglycemia directs its main damage at the cerebral hemispheres, producing laminar or pseudolaminar necrosis in fatal cases, but largely sparing the brainstem. Clinically, the picture of acute metabolic encephalopathy caused by hypoglycemia usually presents in one of four forms: (1) as a delirium manifested primarily by mental changes with either quiet and sleepy confusion or wild mania; (2) coma accompanied by signs of multifocal brainstem dysfunction including neurogenic hyperventilation and decerebrate spasms. In this form pupillary light reactions, as well as oculocephalic and oculovestibular responses, are usually preserved to suggest that the underlying disorder is metabolic. The patients sometimes have shiver-like diffuse muscle activity and many are hypothermic (33°C to 35°C); (3) as a stroke-like illness characterized by focal neurologic signs with or without accompanying coma. In one series of patients requiring hospital admission, 5% suffered transient focal neurologic abnormalities.[206] In patients with focal motor signs, permanent motor paralysis is uncommon and the weakness tends to shift from side to side during different episodes of metabolic worsening. This kind of shifting deficit, as well as the fact that focal neurologic signs also occur in children in coma with severe hypoglycemia, stands against explaining the localized neurologic deficits as being caused by cerebral vascular disease; (4) as an epileptic attack with single or multiple generalized convulsions and postictal coma. In one series, 20% had generalized seizures.[206] Many hypoglycemic patients convulse as the blood sugar level drops, and some have seizures as their only manifestation of hypoglycemia leading to an erroneous diagnosis of epilepsy. The varying clinical picture of hypoglycemia often leads to mistaken clinical diagnoses, particularly when in a given patient the clinical picture varies from episode to episode, as in Patient 5–12.

Patient 5–12

A 45-year-old woman was hospitalized for treatment of a large pelvic sarcoma. She had liver metastases and was malnourished. On morning rounds she was found to be unresponsive. Her eyes were open, but she did not respond to questioning, although she moved all four extremities in response to noxious stimuli. She was sweating profusely. The blood glucose was 40 mg/dL. Her symptoms cleared immediately after an intravenous glucose infusion. The next day her roommate called for help when the patient did not respond to her questions. This time she was awake and alert but globally aphasic with a right hemiparesis. Again she was hypoglycemic, and the symptoms resolved after the infusion of glucose.

Comment: The variability and neurologic findings from episode to episode make hypoglycemia a great imitator, particularly of structural disease of the nervous system, raising the question of whether prehospital blood glucose measurement should be done in all patients suspected by emergency medical services of having had a stroke. In one such series of 185 patients suspected of "cerebral vascular accident," five were found to be hypoglycemic and all were medication-controlled diabetics. All of these patients improved after receiving glucose.[210]

Neither the history nor the physical examination reliably distinguishes hypoglycemia from other causes of metabolic coma, although (as is true in hepatic coma) an important clinical point is that the pupillary and vestibulo-ocular reflex pathways are almost always spared. The great danger of delayed diagnosis is that the longer hypoglycemia lasts, the more likely it is to produce irreversible neuronal loss. This may be the reason that more diabetics treated with insulin have EEG abnormalities than those treated with diet alone.[211] Insidious and progressive dementia is not rare among zealously controlled diabetics who often suffer recurrent minor hypoglycemia. Hypoglycemic seizures cause permanent cognitive deficits in children with diabetes,[212] but even repetitive episodes of hypoglycemia without seizures can lead to cognitive dysfunction.[213] Patients with severe hypoglycemia often have changes on MRI suggesting cerebral infarction (hyperintensity on diffusion-weighted images).[90] These abnormalities may reverse after treatment with glucose and thus do not imply permanent damage.[214] Subtle hypoglycemia can go unrecognized, as Patient 5–13 illustrates.

Patient 5–13

A 77-year-old man with unresectable mesothelioma who had lost his appetite and was losing weight awoke one morning feeling "unusually good" and for the first time in weeks having an appetite. He got dressed and while descending the stairs from his bedroom slipped and fell but did not injure himself. He seated himself at the breakfast table, but despite indicating an appetite did not attempt to eat. His wife noticed that his speech was slurred, his balance was poor, and he did not respond appropriately to questions. She finally coaxed him to eat and after breakfast he returned entirely to normal. The following morning the same thing happened and his wife brought him to the emergency department, where his blood sugar was determined to be 40 mg/dL. He responded immediately to glucose.

Comment: What appeared to be hunger should have been a clue that he was hypoglycemic, but because the patient was not a diabetic, neither he nor his family had any suspicion of the nature of the problem. His wife dismissed the first episode because he recovered after breakfast. Alert emergency department physicians recognized the nature of the second episode and treated him appropriately.

Once recognized, the treatment is simple. Ten percent glucose given intravenously in 50-mL (5g) aliquots to restore blood glucose to normal levels prevents the possible deleterious overshoot of giving 50% glucose.[215] Restoring blood glucose will almost always return neurologic function to normal, although sometimes not immediately. However, prolonged coma and irreversible diffuse cortical injury can occasionally result from severe hypoglycemia. Relapses, particularly in patients taking sulfonylureas, are common. The sulfonylurea agents cause hypoglycemia by binding to a receptor on pancreatic beta cells, the inactive ATP-dependent potassium channels causing depolarization of the beta cell and opening voltage-gated calcium channels to release insulin. Octreotide binds to a second receptor of the pancreatic beta cell and inhibits calcium influx, reducing the secretion of insulin after depolarization. This drug has been used to treat those patients with sulfonylurea overdose who are resistant to IV glucose.[147]

Hyperglycemia

The diabetic patient must walk a tight line between hypoglycemia and hyperglycemia, as both can damage the brain. As indicated on page 203, increasing evidence suggests that hyperglycemia deleteriously affects the prognosis in patients with brain injury whether due to trauma or stroke. Increasing efforts are being made to control blood glucose in intensive care units, although it is not yet clear how that affects prognosis.[73] Hyperglycemia is associated with cognitive defects and an increased risk of dementia, particularly in the elderly.[216] Diabetic encephalopathy can be caused at least in part by toxic effects of hyperglycemia on the brain that include increased polyol pathway flux, sorbitol accumulation, myoinositol depletion, increased oxidative stress, nonenzymatic protein glycation, and disturbed calcium homeostasis.[216] Hyperglycemia also has acute effects on the brain, as in the syndrome of diabetic nonketotic hyperosmolar states, as discussed in the section on hyperosmolality (page 255), and can result in delirium, stupor, or coma.

Cofactor Deficiency

Deficiency of one or more of the B vitamins can cause delirium, stupor, and ultimately dementia, but only thiamine deficiency seriously contends for a place in the differential diagnosis of coma.[136,217,218]

Thiamine deficiency produces Wernicke's encephalopathy, a symptom complex caused by neuronal dysfunction that, if not reversed, promptly leads to damage of the gray matter and blood vessels surrounding the third ventricle, cerebral aqueduct, and fourth ventricle.[217] Why the lesions have such a focal distribution is not altogether understood since, when thiamine is not ingested, it disappears from all brain areas at about the same rate. One investigator has proposed that with severe thiamine deficiency, glutamate and glutamic acid decarboxylase accumulate in peripheral tissues. The elevated levels of glutamate in the blood pass through circumventricular organs (brain areas without a blood-brain barrier) into the cerebral ventricles and contiguous brain, finally diffusing into the extracellular space of diencephalic and brainstem tissues. The damage to cells in this area is then produced by glutamate excitotoxicity.[16] Because alpha-ketoglutarate dehydrogenase is thiamine dependent and rate limiting in the tricarboxylic acid cycle, focal lactic acidosis, decreases in cerebral energy, and resultant depolarization have also been postulated as causes of the focal defect.[15] In addition, a thiamine-dependent enzyme, transketolase, loses its activity in the pontine tegmentum more rapidly than in other areas, and it is presumed that a focal effect such as this is related to the restricted pathologic changes. Thiamine reverses at least some of the neurologic defects in Wernicke's encephalopathy so rapidly that for years physicians have speculated that the vitamin is involved in synaptic transmission. Thiamine-deficient animals have a marked impairment of serotonergic neurotransmitter pathways in the cerebellum, diencephalon, and brainstem.[219] The areas of diencephalic and brainstem involvement in animals correspond closely to the known distribution of pathologic lesions in humans with Wernicke's encephalopathy. Thiamine affects active ion transport at nerve terminals and is necessary for regeneration and maintenance of the membrane potential.[220]

The ultimate cause of thiamine deficiency is absence of the vitamin from the diet, and the most frequent reason is that patients have substituted alcohol for vitamin-containing foods. A danger is that the disease can be precipitated by giving vitamin-free glucose infusions to chronically malnourished subjects. A significant number of elderly hospitalized patients have evidence of moderate to severe thiamine deficiency. Before it was routine to add thiamine to intravenous infusions in hospitalized patients, we encountered on the wards in a cancer hospital one or two very sick patients a year who were not eating and developed Wernicke's disease when being nourished by IV infusions[221] without vitamins. We still encounter occasional such patients on the wards in a general hospital. In some cases that we have seen, thiamine had been prescribed orally. However, its absorption orally is unreliable, particularly in patients who are malnourished; hence, it must be supplied by IV or IM injection for at least the first few days in any patient with suspected Wernicke's encephalopathy.

As would be expected with lesions involving the diencephalic and periaqueductal structures, patients are initially obtunded and confused, and often have striking memory failure. Deep stupor or coma is unusual, dangerous, and often a preterminal development. However, such behavioral symptoms are common to many disorders. They can be attributed to Wernicke's disease only when accompanied by nystagmus, oculomotor paralysis, and impaired vestibulo-ocular responses that are subsequently reversed by thiamine treatment. In advanced cases, involvement of oculomotor muscles may be sufficient to cause complete external ophthalmoplegia; fixed, dilated pupils are a rarity. Most patients also suffer from ataxia, dysarthria, and a mild peripheral neuropathy in addition to the eye signs. Many affected patients show a curious indifference to noxious stimulation and some are hypothermic and hypophagic. Autonomic insufficiency is so common that orthostatic hypotension and shock are constant threats. The hypotension of Wernicke's disease appears to result from a combination of neural lesions and depleted blood volume and is probably the most common cause of death.

The MRI is characteristic. T2 and FLAIR images are symmetrically hyperintense in the mammillary bodies, dorsal medial thalami, periventricular areas of the hypothalamus, periaqueductal gray matter, and tectum of the midbrain. On rare occasions, hemorrhage can be demonstrated in the mammillary bodies by hyperintensity on T1-weighted image. Lesions do not usually contrast enhance.[136,222] Diffusion-weighted images may show restricted diffusion within the areas, a finding that may be more sensitive than standard sequences.[222,223] Restricted diffusion has also been reported in the splenium of the corpus callosum in acute Wernicke's encephalopathy.[223] Corpus callosum atrophy has been demonstrated in patients with Wernicke's disease related to alcohol, but not those with Wernicke's disease related to intestinal surgery, anorexia, or hyperemeses gravidarum.[224]

DISEASES OF ORGAN SYSTEMS OTHER THAN BRAIN

Liver Disease

Liver disease can damage the brain in several ways. Acute liver failure causes brain edema with resultant intracranial hypertension.[225] About 30% of patients with acute liver failure succumb when ICPs increase to levels that impair CBF causing brain infarction, increased edema, and eventual transtentorial herniation. Chronic liver failure, usually from cirrhosis or after portocaval shunting, is usually characterized only by defects in memory and attention with increased reaction time and poor concentration. One striking and frustrating problem in liver failure is that the encephalopathy may fluctuate widely without obvious cause. More severe forms can lead to delirium, stupor, and coma. The most severe forms often occur in a cirrhotic patient with mild, chronic hepatic encephalopathy who develops an infection, has gastrointestinal bleeding, or takes in an excessive amount of protein (so-called meat intoxication).[226] Cerebral dysfunction occurs either when liver function fails or when the liver is bypassed so that the portal circulation shunts intestinal venous drainage directly into the systemic circulation.

The major site of pathology appears to reside in astrocytes. In chronic liver disease, morphologic changes include an increase in large Alzheimer type-2 astrocytes.[227] The astrocytes exhibit an alteration in the expression of benzodiazepine receptors, glutamate transporters, and glial acidic fibrillary protein. In the more acute encephalopathy, or with deterioration of chronic encephalopathy, permeability of the blood-brain barrier increases without loss of tight junctions. The resultant cerebral edema, along with an increase in CBF, leads to intracranial hypertension.[228] All these pathologic processes are believed to be initiated by an elevated blood ammonia level with increased ammonia uptake into the brain. The ammonia is metabolized by astrocytes to glutamine. The glutamine may be retained within the cell, leading to swelling. There is no consistent correlation between the level of ammonia and the patient's clinical symptoms, suggesting that there are other factors; sepsis is certainly one. Cytokines, particularly tumor necrosis factor (TNF)-alpha, may play a role. Oxidative stress may be another.[227]

The clinical picture of hepatic encephalopathy is fairly consistent, but its onset often is difficult to define. The incipient mental symptoms usually consist of a quiet, apathetic delirium, which either persists for several days or rapidly evolves into profound coma. Less often, in perhaps 10% to 20% of cases, the earliest symptoms are of a boisterous delirium verging on mania, an onset suggesting rapidly progressive liver disease. One of our patients with chronic cirrhosis suffered two episodes of hepatic coma spaced 2 weeks apart. The first began with an agitated delirium; the second, with quiet obtundation. It was impossible to distinguish between the two attacks by biochemical changes or rate of evolution. Respiratory changes are a hallmark of severe liver disease. Hyperventilation, as judged by low arterial PCO_2 and high pH levels, occurs at all depths of coma and usually becomes clinically obvious as patients become deeply comatose. This almost invariable hyperventilation is well confirmed by our own series of 83 patients; all had plasma alkalosis and all but three had low PCO_2 values. These three exceptions had concomitant metabolic alkalosis, correction of which was followed by hyperventilation and respiratory alkalosis. Although some authors have reported instances of metabolic acidosis, particularly in terminal patients, in our experience it is likely that encephalopathy unaccompanied by either respiratory or metabolic alkalosis is not hepatic. Moderately obtunded patients with hepatic encephalopathy sometimes have nystagmus on lateral gaze. Tonic conjugate downward or downward and lateral ocular deviation has marked the onset of coma in several of our patients; we have once observed reversible, vertical skew deviation during an episode of hepatic coma. Focal neurologic signs are not rare. In one series of 34 cirrhotic patients with 38 episodes of hepatic encephalopathy, eight demonstrated focal signs, two hemiplegia and four hemiparesis, two had agnosia, and one developed a lower limb monoplegia.[40] Other signs that have been described include disconjugate eye movements[229] and ocular bobbing.[230] Only one of our patients convulsed. Others have reported the seizure incidence to be between 2% and 33%. When seizures occur they may be related to alcohol withdrawal, cerebral edema, or hypoglycemia accompanying the liver failure.[231] Peripheral oculomotor paralyses are rare in hepatic coma unless patients have concomitant Wernicke's disease, and, in fact, easily elicited brisk and conjugate oculocephalic and oculovestibular responses are generally a striking finding in unresponsive patients with hepatic encephalopathy. The pupils are usually small but react to light. Asterixis[44] or miniasterixis[232] (see page 195) is characteristic and frequently involves the muscles of the feet, tongue, and jaw, as well as the hands. Patients with mild to moderate encephalopathy are usually found to have bilateral gegenhalten. Decorticate and decerebrate posturing responses, muscle spasticity, and bilateral extensor plantar responses frequently accompany deeper coma.

Hepatic coma is rarely a difficult diagnosis to make in patients who suffer from severe chronic liver disease and gradually lose consciousness displaying the obvious stigmata of jaundice, spider angiomata, fetor hepaticus, and enlarged livers and spleens. The diagnosis can be more difficult in patients whose coma is precipitated by an exogenous factor and who have either mild unsuspected liver disease or portal-systemic shunts. In this situation, hepatic coma can be suspected by finding clinical evidence of metabolic encephalopathy combined with respiratory alkalosis and brisk oculocephalic reflexes. The diagnosis is strengthened by identifying a portal-systemic shunt, plus an elevated serum ammonia level. The blood sugar should be measured in patients with severe liver disease since diminished liver glycogen stores may induce hypoglycemia and complicate hepatic coma. When the diagnosis remains doubtful, analysis of spinal fluid may reveal markedly elevated levels of either glutamine or alpha-ketoglutaramate (α-KGM). Of the two, α-KGM levels give almost no false positives as well as the strongest discrimination between patients with and without brain involvement.[233] The spinal fluid in hepatic encephalopathy is usually clear and free of cells, and has a normal protein content. In severe cases, the opening pressure may be elevated, sometimes to very high levels. It is rare to detect bilirubin in the CSF unless patients have serum bilirubin levels of at least 4 to 6 mg/dL and chronic parenchymal liver failure as well. The EEG undergoes progressive slowing in hepatic coma, with slow activity beginning symmetrically in the frontal leads and spreading posteriorly as unconsciousness deepens. The changes are characteristic but not specific; they thus help in identifying a diffuse abnormality but do not necessarily diagnose hepatic failure.

CT or MRI is usually only helpful in ruling out structural disease such as cerebral hematomas, although in advanced stages there may be substantial cerebral edema. In cases of severely elevated ICP, compromise of CBF may even result in global cerebral infarction. MRS identifies a lowered myoinositol and choline with increased glutamine levels in the basal ganglia of patients in early stages of hepatic encephalopathy when compared with cirrhotic controls[234] (Figure 5–7). The basal ganglia may be hyperintense on the T1-weighted image, believed to be a result of manganese deposits. Mild cerebral atrophy is frequently present. PET scanning demonstrates hypometabolism in frontal and parietal lobes, sometimes with increased uptake in the infra- and medial temporal regions, cerebellum, and posterior thalamus.[226] Fluorodeoxy PET studies of the brain in cirrhotics shows a relative decrease of glucose utilization in the cingulate gyrus, the medial and lateral frontal regions, and the

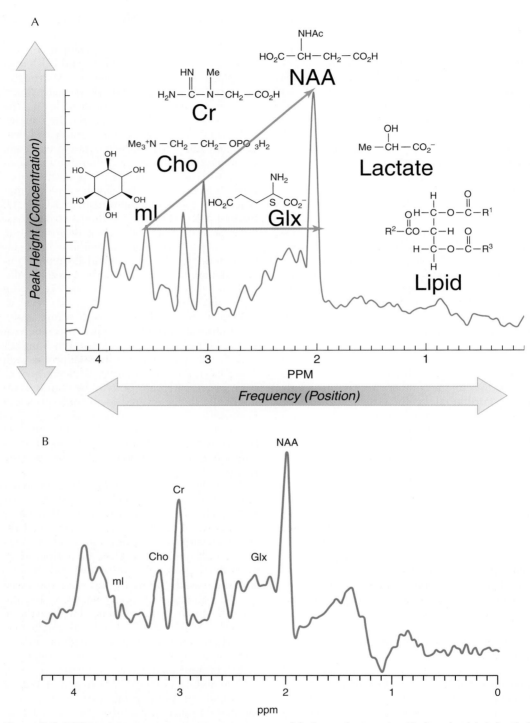

Figure 5–7. (A) Representative magnetic resonance spectrum of the human brain in vivo. Each peek is labeled with the molecule and its structure. The absorption spectra of lipid and lactate are not observed in a normal brain. The diagonal arrow represents Hunter's angle, which is drawn starting from myoinositol to N-acetylaspartate. In a normal spectrum, Hunter's angle is 45 degrees and is formed by the peaks of myoinositol, creatinine, choline, and N-acetylaspartate. (B) MRS in a patient with chronic hepatic encephalopathy, demonstrating the three changes characteristic of hepatic encephalopathy: decreased myoinositol, increased glutamate-glutamine, and decreased choline. After transplant and metabolic changes, the patient returned to normal. (From Lin et al. Neuro Rx 2005, 2, 197–214, with permission.)

Multifocal, Diffuse, and Metabolic Brain Diseases Causing Delirium, Stupor, or Coma   227

parieto-occipital cortex, with a relative increase in the basal ganglia, hippocampus, and cerebellum.[235]

Mild hepatic encephalopathy may fluctuate markedly in severity, and it is sometimes confused with psychiatric disturbances or acute alcoholism. Comatose patients in whom hepatic coma has developed rapidly often have motor signs (but not neuro-ophthalmologic changes) that may suggest structural disease of the brainstem. They are sometimes mistakenly believed to have subdural hematoma or basilar artery thrombosis. In anything short of preterminal hepatic coma, however, pupillary and caloric responses are normal, patients hyperventilate, and signs of rostral-caudal deterioration are absent, all of which rule out subdural hematoma. Subtentorial structural disease is ruled out by the normal pupillary and caloric responses as well as the fluctuating and inconstant quality of motor signs.

Renal Disease

Renal failure causes uremic encephalopathy. The treatment of uremia, in turn, potentially causes two additional disorders of cerebral function: the dialysis dysequilibrium syndrome and progressive dialysis encephalopathy. Confusion, delirium, stupor, and sometimes coma can occur with each of these conditions.

UREMIC ENCEPHALOPATHY

Before the widespread use of dialysis and renal transplantation, the uremic syndrome was common in North America and Western Europe. Today, the early correction of biochemical abnormalities in patients with known acute or chronic renal disease often prevents the development of cerebral symptoms. As a result, the physician more often encounters uremic encephalopathy as a problem of differential diagnosis in patients with a systemic disease causing multiorgan failure such as a collagen vascular disorder, malignant hypertension, the ingestion of a toxin, bacteremia, or disseminated anoxia-ischemia. Most of these primary disorders themselves produce abnormalities of brain function, adding to the complexities of diagnosis.

Despite extensive investigations, the precise cause of the brain dysfunction in uremia eludes identification. However, certain notable associations exist. Once azotemia develops, the uremic syndrome correlates only in a general way with biochemical changes in the blood. As with other metabolic encephalopathies, the more rapid the development of the toxic state, the less disturbed is the systemic chemical equilibrium. The level of the blood urea nitrogen (BUN) associated with uremic encephalopathy can vary widely. Urea itself cannot be the toxin, as urea infusions do not reproduce uremic symptoms and hemodialysis reverses the syndrome, even when urea is added to the dialyzing bath so as not to lower the blood level. Although it is rare to see uremic encephalopathy with a creatine lower than 7.0, levels of creatinine and other serum biochemical or electrolyte abnormalities do not correlate with the neurologic state. Serum sodium or potassium levels can be abnormally low or high in uremia, depending on its duration and treatment, but symptoms associated with these electrolyte changes are distinct from the typical panorama of uremic encephalopathy. Systemic acidosis is not the cause; the systemic acidosis does not involve the CNS, and treatment of the reduced blood pH has no effect on uremic cerebral symptoms.

Morphologically, the brains of patients dying of uremia show no consistent abnormality. Uremia uncomplicated by hypertensive encephalopathy does not cause cerebral edema. The cerebral oxygen consumption declines in uremic stupor, just as it does in most other metabolic encephalopathies, although perhaps not as much as might be expected from the degree of impaired alertness. Levels of cerebral high-energy phosphates remain high during experimental uremia, while rates of glycolysis and energy utilization are reduced below normal. Uremic brains show a decrease in sodium and potassium flux along with depressed sodium-stimulated, potassium-dependent ATPase activity. However, all the above changes appear to be effects rather than causes of the disorder.

Calcium concentration in the brain is elevated,[236] and in humans with uremia both cognitive function and the EEG may be improved by parathyroidectomy,[237] suggesting that calcium plays a role. In addition, 1-guanidino compounds are elevated in uremia, and this may affect the release of gamma-aminobutyric acid.[238] In uremic experimental animals, tryptophan is diminished both in plasma and brain, but levels of its metabolic product, 3-hydroxykinurine, a known neurotoxin, are elevated in the brain, particularly in the striatum and the medulla.[239] Also in uremic animals, up-regulation of the superoxide-producing enzyme nicotinamide adenine dinucleotide phosphate oxidase and down-regulation of supraoxide dismutase cause oxidative stress in the brain via the nitration of brain proteins and the oxidation of myelin. Oxidative stress is also caused during dialysis treatment by interaction of the patient's blood with both the dialysis membrane and dialysate impurities.[240] Turnover of dopamine in the striatum, mesencephalon, and hypothalamus is decreased in uremic animals, whereas turnover of norepinephrine and 5-hydroxytriptomine is unchanged. Whether suppression of central dopamine turnover contributes to motor impairment in uremic animals is not clear.[241]

The clinical picture of uremic encephalopathy is nonspecific in most instances, although the characteristic combination of dulled consciousness, hyperpnea, and motor hyperactivity should immediately give high suspicion to the diagnosis. Untreated patients with uremic encephalopathy have metabolic acidosis, generally with respiratory compensation. Like many other metabolic encephalopathies, uremia, particularly when it develops rapidly, can produce a florid delirium marked by noisy agitation, delusions, and hallucinations. More often, however, progressive apathetic, dull, quiet confusion with inappropriate behavior blends slowly into stupor or coma accompanied by characteristic respiratory changes, focal neurologic signs, tremor, asterixis, muscle paratonia, and convulsions or, more rarely, nonconvulsive status epilepticus.[242] In uremic patients, both generalized convulsions and nonconvulsive status epilepticus may be caused by antibiotics, particularly cephalosporins.[243] Untreated patients with uremic encephalopathy all have serum acidosis. Pupillary and oculomotor functions are seldom disturbed in uremia, certainly not in any diagnostic way. On the other hand, motor changes are rarely absent. Patients with chronic renal disease are weak and unsteady in their movements. As uremia evolves, many of them develop diffuse tremulousness, intense asterixis, and, often, so much multifocal myoclonus that the muscles can appear to fasciculate. Action myoclonus (see page 195) has also been reported.[244,245] Tetany is frequent. Stretch reflex asymmetries are common, as are focal neurologic weaknesses; 10 of our 45 patients with

uremia had a hemiparesis that cleared rapidly after hemodialysis or shifted from side to side during the course of the illness.

Laboratory determinations tell one only that patients have uremia, but do not delineate this as the cause of coma. Renal failure is accompanied by complex biochemical, osmotic, and vascular abnormalities, and the degree of azotemia varies widely in patients with equally serious symptoms. One of our patients, a child with nephritis, had severe delirium proceeding to stupor despite a BUN of only 48 mg/dL. Other patients were free of cerebral symptoms with BUN values over 200 mg/dL. Uremia also causes aseptic meningitis accompanied by stiff neck with as many as 250 lymphocytes and polymorphonuclear leukocytes/mm^3 in the CSF. The spinal fluid protein often rises as high as 100 mg/dL and the CSF pressure can be abnormally elevated to over 160 to 180 mm in some patients. EEG slowing correlates with increasing degrees of azotemia, but many patients with slow records have little or no accompanying mental changes.[246] The electrophysiologic changes are nonspecific and of no help in establishing the diagnosis.

In differential diagnosis, uremia must be distinguished from other causes of acute metabolic acidosis, from acute water intoxication, and from hypertensive encephalopathy. Penicillin and its analogs can be a diagnostic problem when given to uremic patients, as these drugs can cause delirium, asterixis, myoclonus, convulsions, and nonconvulsive status epilepticus.[243] Laboratory studies distinguish uremia from other causes of metabolic acidosis causing the triad of clouded consciousness, hyperpnea, and a low serum bicarbonate (uremia, diabetes, lactic acidosis, ingestion of exogenous poisons), but only uremia is likely to cause multifocal myoclonus, tetany, and generalized convulsions, and the others do not cause azotemia during their early stages.

Hyponatremia is common in uremia and can be difficult to dissociate from the underlying uremia as a cause of symptoms. Patients with azotemia are nearly always thirsty, and they have multiple electrolyte abnormalities. Excessive water ingestion, inappropriate fluid therapy, and hemodialysis all potentially reduce the serum osmolarity in uremia and thereby risk inducing or accentuating delirium and convulsions. The presence of water intoxication is confirmed by measuring a low serum osmolarity (less than 260 mOsm/L), but the disorder can be suspected when the serum sodium concentration falls below 120 mEq/L (see page 253). Interestingly, rapid correction of hyponatremia does not seem to be associated with pontine myelinolysis (see page 171) when it occurs in uremic patients. The osmotic pressure of urea in the brain that is eliminated more slowly than in the blood appears to protect the brain against the sudden shifts in brain osmolality, although such shifts may emerge during treatment unless special precautions are taken (see below).[247] Patients with uremia are often deficient in thiamine, which may cause neurologic manifestations that mimic uremia.[248]

It may be difficult to separate the symptoms of uremia from those of hypertensive encephalopathy if both azotemia and advanced hypertension plague the same patient. Each condition can cause seizures, focal neurologic signs, increased ICP, and delirium or stupor. The MRI of typical posterior leukoencephalopathy (see page 215) establishes the diagnosis of hypertensive encephalopathy.

The treatment of uremia by hemodialysis sometimes adds to the neurologic complexity of the syndrome. Neurologic recovery does not always immediately follow effective dialysis, and patients often continue temporarily in coma or stupor. One of our own patients remained comatose for 5 days after his blood nitrogen and electrolytes returned to normal. Such a delayed recovery did not imply permanent brain damage, as this man, like others with similar but less protracted delays, enjoyed normal neurologic function on chronic hemodialysis.

DIALYSIS DYSEQUILIBRIUM SYNDROME

Some patients undergoing dialysis, particularly during the first treatment, develop headache, nausea, muscle weakness, cramps, and fatigue. At one time, occasional patients had more serious symptoms caused by a sudden osmolar gradient shifting of water into the brain, including asterixis, myoclonus, delirium, convulsions, stupor, coma, and very rarely death,[249] but these are now prevented by slower dialysis and the addition of osmotically reactive solutes such as urea, glycerol, mannitol, or sodium to the dialysate.[238] An occasional patient will de-velop a subdural hematoma, probably resulting from a combination of anticoagulants used for dialysis and the coagulopathy that often accompanies uremia. Wernicke's encephalopathy with its attendant confusional state (page 223) has developed in patients receiving chronic dialysis who were not being given vitamin supplements.[248]

All agree on the general mechanism of the dialysis dysequilibrium syndrome, although not on the details.[250] The blood-brain barrier is only slowly permeable to urea as well as to a number of other biologic molecules, including electrolytes and idiogenic osmols[251] (molecules, e.g., organic acids, amino acids, that form during pathologic processes and increase tissue osmolality), that form in brain during serum hyperosmolarity. The brain and blood are in osmotic equilibrium in steady states such as uremia; electrolytes and other osmols are adjusted so that brain concentrations of many biologically active substances (e.g., H^+, Na^+, Cl^-) remain more normal than those in blood. A rapid lowering of the blood urea by hemodialysis is not paralleled by equally rapid reductions in brain osmols. As a result, during dialysis the brain becomes hyperosmolar relative to blood and probably loses sodium, the result being that water shifts from plasma to brain, potentially resulting in water intoxication. Concurrently, rapid correction of blood metabolic acidosis can induce brain tissue acidosis because the increased PCO_2 in the blood rapidly diffuses into the brain, whereas the bicarbonate moves much more slowly because of the slow movement of bicarbonate into the brain. Symptoms of water intoxication can be prevented by slower dialysis and by adding agents to maintain blood osmolarity.

RENAL TRANSPLANT

Immunosuppression accompanying renal transplant can lead to a variety of neurologic disorders.[246,252] As indicated on page 215, cyclosporin and taxolimus can cause posterior leukoencephalopathy and the anti-CD3 murine monoclonal antibody, muromonab-CD3, can be neurotoxic, causing aseptic meningitis with headache and blurred vision and sometimes encephalopathy and seizures.[252,253] MRI shows patchy enhancement in the corticomedullary junction, indicating blood-brain barrier dysfunction. The pathogenesis of the encephalopathy is believed to be cerebral edema from a capillary leak syndrome.[254]

Renal transplant patients also are at risk for a variety of opportunistic infections and tumors similar to other immune-suppressed patients, such as those with HIV infection. These include lymphomas, which may occur primarily in the CNS, as the patient description indicates on page 362, and lead to stupor or coma. Opportunistic infections include fungi, such as *Aspergillus, Cryptococcus,* or *Candida,* and viruses, including cytomegalovirus, varicella-zoster, papova virus (JC virus), or progressive multifocal leukoencephalopathy. On rare occasions, the transplanted kidney carries a virus and may cause encephalitis within a few days of the transplant.[252]

Pulmonary Disease

Hypoventilation owing to advanced lung failure or neurologic causes can lead to a severe encephalopathy or coma.[255] The mechanistic basis for the neurologic changes has not been fully explained, and in most instances the encephalopathy probably depends on a variable interaction of hypoxemia, hypercapnia, congestive heart failure, and other factors such as systemic infection and the fatigue of prolonged, ineffective respiratory efforts. Airway obstruction due to obstructive sleep apnea may awaken patients at night, adding to their daytime lethargy.[256] However, unless some complication such as respiratory arrest occurs leading to prolonged hypoxia, permanent changes in the brain are lacking and the encephalopathy is fully reversible. Serum acidosis per se is probably not an important factor, as alkali infusions unaccompanied by ventilatory therapy fail to improve the neurologic status of these patients. Also, although hypoxia may potentiate the illness, it is unlikely that it is the sole cause of the cerebral symptoms, as patients with congestive heart failure commonly tolerate equal degrees of hypoxia with no encephalopathy. Of all the variables, the degree of carbon dioxide retention correlates most closely with the neurologic symptoms. The development of cerebral symptoms also depends in part on the duration of the condition. For example, some subjects with chronic hypercarbia have no cerebral symptoms despite

$PaCO_2$ levels of 55 to 60 mm Hg, whereas patients with previously compensated, but marginal, pulmonary function suddenly become hypoxic and hypercapnic because of an infection or excess sedation. Such patients may be erroneously suspected of having sedative poisoning or other causes of coma, but as in the following example, blood gas measurements make the diagnosis.

Patient 5–14

A 60-year-old woman with severe chronic pulmonary disease went to a physician complaining of nervousness and insomnia. An examination disclosed no change in her pulmonary function, and she was given a sedative to help her sleep. Her daughter found her unconscious the following morning and brought her to the hospital. She was comatose but withdrew appropriately from noxious stimuli. She was cyanotic, and her respirations were labored at 40 per minute. Her pupils were 3 mm in diameter and reacted to light. There was a full range of extraocular movements on passive head turning. No evidence of asterixis or multifocal myoclonus was encountered, and her extremities were flaccid with slightly depressed tendon reflexes and bilateral extensor plantar responses. The arterial blood pH was 7.17, the $PaCO_2$ was 70 mm Hg, the serum bicarbonate was 25 mEq/L, and the PaO_2 was 40 mm Hg. She was intubated and received artificial ventilation with a respirator for several days before she awakened and was able by her own efforts to maintain her arterial $PaCO_2$ at its normal level of 45 mm Hg.

Comment: This is not an unusual history. It is possible that the increased nervousness and insomnia were symptoms of increasing respiratory difficulty. The sedative hastened the impending decompensation and induced severe respiratory insufficiency as sleep stilled voluntary respiratory efforts. The rapidity with which her $PaCO_2$ rose from 45 to 70 mm Hg is indicated by her normal serum bicarbonate, there having been no time for the development of the renal compensation that usually accompanies respiratory acidosis.

When CO_2 accumulates slowly, the complaints of insidiously appearing headache, somnolence, and confusion may occasionally attract more attention than the more direct signs of respiratory failure. The headache, like other headaches associated with increased ICP, may be maximal when the patient first awakens from sleep and disappears when activity increases respiration, lowering the PCO_2 and, thus, the ICP.

In its most severe form, pulmonary encephalopathy may cause increased ICP, papilledema,[257] and bilateral extensor plantar responses, symptoms that may at first raise the question of a brain tumor or some other expanding mass. The important differential features are that in CO_2 retention focal signs are rare, blood gases are always abnormal, and the encephalopathy usually improves promptly if artificial ventilation is effectively administered.

Two associated conditions are closely related to CO_2 narcosis and often accentuate its neurologic effects. One is hypoxemia and the other is metabolic alkalosis, which often emerges as the result of treatment. Hypoxia accompanying CO_2 retention must be treated, because lack of oxygen is immediately dangerous both to the heart and brain. Traditional teaching has been that oxygen therapy for hypercapnic patients with an acute exacerbation of chronic obstructive pulmonary disease may be dangerous, as it may reduce respiratory drive and further worsen hypercapnia. Recent evidence suggests that most patients tolerate oxygen replacement well,[258] and for those who are not comatose but require artificial ventilation, noninvasive ventilation with a face mask appears to suffice.[259] Renal bicarbonate excretion is a relatively slow process. As a result, correction of CO_2 narcosis by artificial respiration sometimes induces severe metabolic alkalosis if the carbon dioxide tension is returned quickly to normal in the face of a high serum bicarbonate level. Although metabolic alkalosis is usually asymptomatic, Rotheram and colleagues[260] reported five patients with pulmonary emphysema treated vigorously by artificial ventilation in whom metabolic alkalosis was associated with serious neurologic symptoms. These patients, after initially recovering from CO_2 narcosis, developed severe alkalosis with arterial blood pH values above 7.55 to 7.60 and again became obtunded. They developed multifocal myoclonus, had severe convulsions, and three died. Two patients regained consciousness after blood CO_2 levels were raised again by deliberately reducing the level of

ventilation. We have observed a similar sequence of events in deeply comatose patients treated vigorously with artificial ventilation, but have found it difficult to conclude that alkalosis and not hypoxia, possibly from hypotension,[261] was at fault. What seems likely is that too sudden hypocapnia induces cerebral vasoconstriction, which more than counterbalances the beneficial effects to the brain of raising the blood oxygen tension. Rotheram and his colleagues believe that the PCO_2 should be lowered gradually during treatment of respiratory acidosis to allow renal compensation to take place and prevent severe metabolic alkalosis. This is a reasonable approach so long as hypoxemia is prevented.

Pancreatic Encephalopathy

Failure of either the exocrine or endocrine pancreas can cause stupor or coma. Failure of the endocrine pancreas (diabetes) is discussed in the next section. Failure of the exocrine pancreas causes pancreatic encephalopathy, a rare complication of acute or chronic pancreatitis. Chronic relapsing pancreatitis may cause episodic stupor or coma.[262] Estrada and associates reported that six of 17 nonalcoholic patients with acute pancreatitis, whom they followed prospectively, developed encephalopathy.[263] The pathogenesis of pancreatic encephalopathy is not known. Postmortem evidence of patchy demyelination of white matter in the brain has led to the suggestion that enzymes liberated from the damaged pancreas are responsible for the encephalopathy.[263] Other hypotheses include coexistent viral pancreatitis and encephalitis, disseminated intravascular coagulation complicating pancreatitis, and fat embolism. In one patient with relapsing pancreatitis and episodic coma, there were marked increases in CSF, plasma citrulline, and arginine levels, and moderate increases of other amino acids.[262] Acute pancreatitis raises dopamine levels in brains of rats.[264] Pathologically, autopsies have revealed cerebral edema, patchy demyelination, occasional perivascular hemorrhages, and, at times, plugging of small vessels with fat or fibrin thrombi.[265] Biochemical complications of acute pancreatitis also may cause encephalopathy. These include cerebral ischemia secondary to hypotension, hyperosmolality, hypocalcemia,[266] and diabetic acidosis.

Pancreatic encephalopathy usually begins between the second and fifth day after the onset of pancreatitis. The clinical features include an acute agitated delirium with hallucinations, focal or generalized convulsions, and often signs of bilateral corticospinal tract dysfunction. The mental status may wax and wane, and patients often become stuporous or comatose. The CSF is usually normal or occasionally has a slightly elevated protein concentration. The CSF lipase level is elevated.[263] The EEG is always abnormal with diffuse or multifocal slow activity. The diagnosis usually suggests itself when, after several days of abdominal pain, the patient develops acute encephalopathy. The MRI may be normal[267] or show diffuse white matter lesions.[265] The differential diagnosis should include other factors complicating pancreatitis listed above, including, of course, mumps that can cause both pancreatitis and encephalopathy. CSF lipase is elevated in pancreatic encephalopathy.

Patient 5–15

A 72-year-old male with no significant past medical history presented to the hospital with abdominal pain and was diagnosed with acute pancreatitis. The next day the patient was noted to be confused with waxing and waning mental status changes, which became an acute agitated delirium on the fifth day requiring four-point restraints. EEG done at the time showed a diffuse theta rhythm. Initial CT and MRI studies were unrevealing and the patient remained mute in an awake state for several days, following which he recovered to a confused state with occasional lucid periods. Neurologic examination was notable for preserved arousal and confabulation, decreased spontaneous movements of the lower extremities, and increased muscle tone. Diffuse hyperreflexia and bilateral extensor plantar response were noted. Repeat MRI reveal diffuse white matter abnormalities consistent with demyelination.

Diabetes Mellitus

Diabetes is the most common endocrine disease presenting as undiagnosed stupor or coma.

Pituitary, adrenal, or thyroid failure may occasionally present similarly, and these disorders are the subject of this section. Hyper- and hypoparathyroidism are discussed with abnormalities of electrolyte metabolism (page 256).

Diabetes, an illness increasing alarmingly in incidence,[268] is an endocrine disease with protean systemic manifestations. The clinical effects of diabetes may appear in virtually any organ of the body, either alone or in combination with other organs. The brain is both directly and indirectly affected by diabetes; delirium, stupor, and coma are common symptoms of certain stages of the disease.[269–271] The potential causes of stupor or coma in patients with diabetes are many; some are listed in Table 5–10. When a diabetic patient develops stupor or coma, more than one of the defects listed in Table 5–10 may be present, and all must be dealt with if one is to bring about an adequate recovery.

Hyperosmolality is the single most common cause of coma in the diabetic patient.[270] This disorder, which is discussed in detail on page 255, can be an isolated cause of coma in a nonketotic hyperglycemic state or a contributing cause in patients with diabetic ketoacidosis or lactic acidosis.

Diabetic ketoacidosis[269,272] causes impairment of consciousness in about 20% of affected patients and coma in about 10%. In general, patients with alteration of consciousness generally have arterial pHs below 7.0,[271] but neither the arterial nor the CSF pH (which

Table 5–10 Some Causes of Stupor or Coma in Diabetic Patients

Nonketotic hyperglycemic hyperosmolar coma
Ketoacidosis
Lactic acidosis
Central nervous system acidosis complicating treatment
Cerebral edema complicating treatment
Hyponatremia (inappropriate secretion of antidiuretic hormone)
Disseminated intravascular coagulation
Hypophosphatemia
Hypoglycemia
Uremia-hypertensive encephalopathy
Cerebral infarction
Hypotension
Sepsis

is typically normal) correlates well with level of consciousness.[273] There is poor correlation between the plasma glucose level and the severity of diabetic ketoacidosis, but patients who are comatose from severe diabetic ketoacidosis almost always have some degree of hyperosmolality as well. The hyperglycemia is caused both by glucose underuse (usually from insulin deficiency) and from overproduction of glucose, a result of glucagon stimulating hepatic glycogenolysis and gluconeogenesis. Spillage of glucose into the urine causes an osmotic diuresis and leads to dehydration, which in turn leads to hyperosmolarity (see page 255). Ketogenesis is caused by the breakdown of triglycerides and release of free fatty acids into the blood. In the absence of insulin, fatty acids are unable to enter the citric acid cycle, but instead enter the mitochondria, where they are oxidized to ketone bodies, mostly acetoacetate and beta-hydroxybutyrate. Although ketone bodies are weak acids, as they accumulate they overcome the body's buffering capacity and produce acidosis.[269]

Diabetic ketoacidosis usually develops in the insulin-dependent (type 1) diabetic but also occurs, albeit at lesser incidence, in patients with non-insulin-dependent (type 2) diabetes. The most common precipitating factor is infection; other precipitating causes include failure to take hypoglycemic medications, alcohol abuse, pancreatitis, cerebral or cardiovascular events, and drugs.[269] Corticosteroids may precipitate diabetic complications and represent a significant problem among neuro-oncology patients with diabetes who require steroids to reduce brain edema from tumors. The catabolic effect of corticosteroids provides increased amino acid precursors for gluconeogenesis.

Most affected patients are awake when they come to the hospital and have a history of thirst, polyuria, anorexia, and fatigue. They are obviously dehydrated, and deep regular (Kussmaul) respirations mark the hyperventilation, which partially compensates for the metabolic acidosis. The breath generally has the hallmark fruity smell of ketosis. There is often some degree of hypotension and tachycardia because the hyperglycemic-induced osmotic diuresis has reduced the blood volume. Such patients are rarely febrile, and if stuporous or comatose, are likely to be mildly hypothermic even when an acute infection has precipitated the ketoacidosis. The lack of fever, coupled with the fact that ketoacidosis itself can produce a leukocytosis, makes the diagnosis of a concomitant infection difficult. Nausea, vomiting, and acute abdominal pain also may complicate the early course of patients with diabetic ketoacidosis; some patients develop hemorrhagic gastritis.

Although it may be difficult to identify the precipitating factors, the diagnosis of ketoacidosis is rarely difficult; the obvious hyperventilation in all but terminal patients should lead the physician to suspect metabolic acidosis and diabetic ketoacidosis as one of its common causes (see Table 5–4, page 189).

Diabetic lactic acidosis usually occurs in patients receiving oral hypoglycemic agents, particularly metformin,[274] but has also been reported in patients not being treated for diabetes. The mechanism of excess lactate production is unknown. Clinical signs and symptoms are the same as those of diabetic ketoacidosis or any other severe metabolic acidosis, with the exception that patients with lactic acidosis are more likely to be hypotensive or in shock. Lactic acidosis in diabetics is distinguished from diabetic ketoacidosis by the absence of high levels of ketone bodies in the serum.[271]

The *treatment* of diabetic ketoacidosis or lactic acidosis, although usually lifesaving, can itself sometimes have serious or even fatal consequences. The CSF, which is usually normal in the untreated patient with diabetic acidosis, may become transiently acidotic if the serum acidosis is treated by intravenous bicarbonate infusion, and this may be associated with some short-lived worsening of the patient's state of consciousness.[273,275] Potentially more dangerous is the sudden lowering of serum osmolality that occurs as insulin lowers the serum glucose and intravenous fluids correct the dehydrated state. This lowering of serum osmolality causes a shift of water into the brain, leading to cerebral edema, which is sometimes fatal.[269,276] The condition should be suspected clinically when patients recovering from diabetic ketoacidosis or lactic acidosis complain of headache and become lethargic and difficult to arouse. Assuming that no evidence of meningitis is present, patients affected with cerebral edema may then develop hyperpyrexia, hypotension, tachycardia, and signs of transtentorial herniation, which, if not promptly and effectively treated with hyperosmolar agents, can culminate in death. At autopsy, the brain shows edema with transtentorial herniation. In a study of eight children and adolescents after treatment for a diabetic ketoacidosis who were scanned for headache and confusion, hyperintensity was found in the medial frontal cortex on FLAIR and diffusion-weighted images, suggesting edema. However, apparent diffusion coefficient values were normal, indicating vasogenic edema rather than cytotoxic edema from infarction. Spectroscopy demonstrated increased levels of myo-inositol and glucose with decreased levels of taurine. The abnormalities were more marked in the frontal than in the occipital region. Changes gradually resolved over time.[277] Cerebral edema in adults is much rarer.

Also complicating the treatment of diabetic ketoacidosis and lactic acidosis is the fact that some patients who suffer from the syndrome of inappropriate release of antidiuretic hormone may become more easily hypo-osmolar during rehydration. Other factors that may complicate the course of diabetic ketoacidosis and add to stupor or coma include disseminated intravascular coagulation (see page 217), hypokalemia, and hypophosphatemia. Profound hypophosphatemia can cause generalized convulsions, stupor, and coma.[278] Fluid overload, acute respiratory distress syndrome, thromboembolism including cerebral infarction, and acute gastric dilation[269] can also cause problems.

Increasing evidence suggests that hyperglycemia may worsen symptoms in patients with brain injury from either head trauma[279,280] or acute stroke[281] (see page 203)[72] or even acutely ill patients in intensive care units.[73] Hyperglycemia is an independent risk factor for stroke, both in people with and without diabetes.[282] The cause of worsening brain injury from hyperglycemia is not clear. Some evidence suggests that preischemic hyperglycemia enhances the accumulation of extracellular glutamate, perhaps causing excitotoxic nerve damage.[283] Other evidence suggests that hyperglycemia affects protein kinase and protein phosphorylation in the brain.[284] Furthermore, hyperglycemia in and of itself appears to deleteriously affect cognition. In adult diabetics, when the blood glucose is greater than 15 mmol/L (270 mg/dL), cognition was deleteriously affected.[71] Chronic diabetes may lead to permanent changes in cognition (diabetic

encephalopathy)[216] that are not believed to be solely related to vascular changes. Diabetes both facilitates long-term depression and inhibits long-term potentiation in the hippocampus.[285] This effect on synaptic plasticity could impair memory. In animals, hyperglycemia during brain ischemia causes cytochrome C release, activates caspase 3, and exacerbates DNA fragmentation induced by ischemia, mechanisms by which hyperglycemia may cause neuronal apoptosis.[286]

Hypoglycemia (see page 203) is a common and serious cause of stupor or coma in diabetic patients[269,287,288] and usually occurs in those taking hypoglycemic agents or during the correction of severe diabetic ketoacidosis. However, spontaneous hypoglycemia, particularly reactive hypoglycemia,[289] can be an early manifestation of diabetes in patients not known to be diabetic,[290,291] presumably a result of insulin dysregulation, or in those known to be diabetic and suffering from renal insufficiency. We have also seen hypoglycemia as a cause of sudden loss of consciousness in rare patients with insulin-secreting tumors of the pancreas.

Diabetes can lead to severe *renal insufficiency*, producing uremic coma or hypertensive encephalopathy. Severe *cerebral arteriosclerosis* associated with diabetes is a cause of cerebral infarction that can produce coma if in the posterior fossa distribution.

Finally, *autonomic neuropathy* caused by diabetes can be a cause of syncope or coma, resulting from cardiac arrhythmia, orthostatic hypotension, cardiac arrest, or painless myocardial infarction. Hypoglycemic unawareness[292] is the failure of the patient to recognize the prodromal symptoms of hypoglycemia, often leading to stupor or coma without warning. This is particularly common in patients who take a combination of hypoglycemic drugs as well as beta blockers, which eliminate most of the warning signs of hypoglycemia (sweating, tachycardia) that are due to catecholamine release. However, hypoglycemic unawareness may also be a result of autonomic neuropathy[293] or impaired epinephrine secretion of unknown cause.[292]

Adrenal Disorders

Both hyper- and hypoadrenal corticosteroid states are occasional causes of altered consciousness,[294] but the exact mechanisms responsible for those alterations are not fully understood. Adrenal corticosteroids have profound effects on the brain, influencing genes that control enzymes and receptors for biogenic amines and neuropeptides, growth factors, and cell adhesion factors.[294]

ADDISON'S DISEASE[295,296]

The pathogenesis of the encephalopathy of adrenal cortical failure in Addison's disease probably involves several factors in addition to the removal of the effect of cortisol on brain tissue. The untreated disease also produces hypoglycemia as well as hyponatremia and hyperkalemia due to hypoaldosteronism. Hypotension is the rule and, if severe, this alone can cause cerebral symptoms from orthostatic hypotension. Symptoms do not entirely clear until both mineralocorticosteroids and glucocorticosteroids are replaced. Some untreated and undertreated patients with Addison's disease are mildly delirious. In a series of 86 patients with adrenal insufficiency associated with the antiphospholipid syndrome, altered mental status was present in only 16 (19%). The major symptoms were abdominal pain (55%), hypotension (54%), and nausea or vomiting (31%). Weakness, fatigue, malaise, or asthenia was present in 31%.[297] Stupor and coma usually appear, if at all, only during addisonian crises. Changes in consciousness, respiration, pupils, and ocular movements are not different from those of several other types of metabolic coma. The presence of certain motor signs, however, may be helpful in suggesting the diagnosis. Patients in addisonian crises have flaccid weakness and either hypoactive or absent deep tendon reflexes, probably resulting from hyperkalemia; a few suffer from generalized convulsions, which have been attributed to hyponatremia and water intoxication. Papilledema is occasionally present and presumably results from brain swelling caused by fluid shifts perhaps exacerbated by increased capillary permeability, which is normally limited by corticosteroids. The EEG is diffusely slow and not different from the pattern in other causes of metabolic encephalopathy.[298]

The neurologic signs of addisonian coma are only rarely sufficiently distinctive to be diagnostic, although the combination of metabolic coma, absence of deep tendon reflexes, and papilledema may suggest adrenal insufficiency.

A pigmented skin and hypotension are helpful supplementary signs and, when combined with a low serum sodium and a high serum potassium level, strongly suggest the diagnosis. The definitive diagnosis of adrenal insufficiency is made by the direct measurement of low blood or urine cortisol levels.

Surgical procedures and other acute illnesses put severe stress on the adrenal glands. A patient whose adrenal function has been marginal prior to an acute illness or surgical procedure may suddenly develop adrenal failure with its attendant delirium. The symptoms may be attributed inappropriately to the acute illness or to a "postoperative delirium" (see page 283) unless adrenal function studies are carried out. Some patients without known pre-existing adrenal insufficiency develop acute adrenal failure following surgical procedures, particularly cardiac surgery. Acute pituitary failure, as in pituitary apoplexy, may also cause an addisonian state.

The main error in differential diagnosis of Addison's disease is with regard to the hyponatremia, hyperkalemia, or hypoglycemia as the primary cause of the metabolic coma, rather than recognizing the combination as caused by underlying adrenal insufficiency. This error can be avoided only by considering Addison's disease as a potential cause of metabolic coma and by heeding the other general physical signs and laboratory values. Hypotension and hyperkalemia, for example, rarely combine together in other diseases causing hyponatremia or hypoglycemia. Patients with Addison's disease are exceedingly sensitive to sedative drugs, including barbiturates and narcotics; ingestion of standard doses of these drugs may produce coma.

CUSHING'S SYNDROME

Cushing's syndrome,[299] whether naturally occurring or iatrogenic in origin, causes increased levels of blood corticosteroids, which frequently leads to an encephalopathy characterized primarily by behavioral changes (either elation or depression) and only rarely by stupor or coma. The changes in behavior associated with glucocorticoid excess are almost always a direct result of that agent on the brain. In a pilot study assessing the psychologic effects of high-dose steroids, we gave 100 mg of dexamethasone daily for 3 days to 10 patients suffering from epidural spinal cord compression and compared psychologic changes in those patients with 10 other patients suffering from vertebral body lesions, but not cord compression, who did not receive steroids. Four of the 10 steroid-treated patients developed behavioral changes, which included hallucinations. None displayed abnormalities of alertness or state of consciousness. The control patients did not develop similar symptoms.

Depression is a more common complication in Cushing's disease (excess pituitary adrenocorticotropic hormone [ACTH] secretion), and elation is more common after ingestion of glucocorticoids. This finding has led some investigators to hypothesize that the depressive effect of Cushing's disease is caused by ACTH rather than cortisol. This hypothesis would be consistent with the observation that patients who have been treated with corticosteroids often become depressed as the dose is tapered and endogenous ACTH is again generated. Similar behavioral changes may be the presenting complaint in patients with paraneoplastic Cushing's syndrome in which there is ectopic production of ACTH by a tumor (usually occult).[300]

Occasionally, patients with Cushing's syndrome, particularly with adrenocorticotropin-secreting tumors, develop delirium or stupor that is not a direct result of glucocorticoid excess. Profound hypokalemic metabolic alkalosis may occur after a long period of steroid excess, and the respiratory compensation for the alkalosis may raise $PaCO_2$ and lower PaO_2, resulting in deleterious effects on the state of consciousness. Diabetes and hypertension with their attendant neurologic manifestations often complicate Cushing's syndrome.

Thyroid Disorders

Both hyperthyroidism and hypothyroidism interfere with normal cerebral function,[301,302] but exactly how the symptoms are produced is unclear. Thyroid hormone (or more strictly triiodothyronine) binds to nuclear receptors that function as ligand-dependent transcription factors. The hormone is absolutely essential for development of the brain, such that in infantile hypothyroidism the neurologic abnormality is rarely reversed unless the defect is almost immediately recognized and corrected.[303] One reason may be that thyroid hormone regulates hippocampal neurogenesis in both the juvenile and adult brain.[304] Thyroid hormone also has effects on cerebral metabolism[305]; hypothyroidism causes a generalized decrease in regional CBF by over 20% and a 12% decrease in cerebral glucose metabolism without specific regional changes. On the other hand, hyperthyroidism appears to have little effect on cerebral metabolism.

HYPOTHYROIDISM

Coma is a rare complication of myxedema[306–308] but one that is often associated with a fatal outcome. In a series of 11 patients either stuporous or comatose from hypothyroidism, three of four patients who were in a coma on admission died, whereas only one of seven patients with less severe changes of consciousness died.[308] Many authors have commented on the appearance of "suspended animation" in these profoundly hypometabolic patients. Characteristically, the patients are hypothermic with body temperatures between 87°F and 91°F. They appear to hypoventilate and, indeed, usually have elevated blood PCO_2 values and mild hypoxia. The EEG is slow and the voltage may be either depressed or increased.[309] Triphasic waves have been reported.[310] The onset of myxedema coma is usually acute or subacute and precipitated by stresses such as infection, congestive heart failure, trauma, exposure to cold, or sedative or anesthetic drug administration in an untreated hypothyroid patient.

The diagnosis of myxedema in a patient in coma is suggested by cutaneous or subcutaneous stigmata of hypothyroidism, plus a low body temperature and the finding of pseudomyotonic stretch reflexes (i.e., normal jerk, but slow relaxation phase). The diagnosis is also often suggested by the presence of elevated muscle enzyme levels in the serum but can be confirmed definitively only by thyroid function tests. As myxedema coma frequently results in death, however, treatment with intravenous administration of triiodothyronine or thyroxine as well as treatment of the precipitating cause should begin once the clinical diagnosis has been made and blood for laboratory tests has been drawn; treatment should not be delayed while awaiting laboratory confirmation.

The greatest diagnostic challenge in myxedema coma is to regard one or more of its complications as the whole cause of the encephalopathy. Carbon dioxide narcosis may be suspected if hypoventilation and CO_2 retention are present, but $PaCO_2$ values are rarely above 50 to 55 mm Hg in hypothyroidism, and hypothermia is not part of CO_2 narcosis. Some authors have attributed the cause of coma and profound hypothyroidism to respiratory failure with carbon dioxide retention, but this is unlikely as not all patients with myxedema hypoventilate. Hyponatremia is often present in severe myxedema, probably the result of inappropriate antidiuretic hormone (ADH) secretion, and sometimes is severe enough to cause seizures. Gastrointestinal bleeding and shock also can complicate severe myxedema and divert attention from hypothyroidism as a cause of coma. Hypothermia, which is probably the most dramatic sign, should always suggest hypothyroidism, but may also occur in other metabolic encephalopathies, especially hypoglycemia, depressant drug poisoning, primary hypothermia due to exposure, and brainstem infarcts.

Hashimoto's encephalopathy is an encephalopathy associated with autoimmune thyroiditis characterized by high titers of antithyroid antibodies in the serum.[311,312] Patients may be hypothyroid, but also may be euthyroid or even hyperthyroid. The disorder is a relapsing and remitting encephalopathy, and may be characterized by seizures, either focal or generalized; myoclonus; confusion; and in some instances stupor and coma. There may be associated pyramidal tract and cerebellar signs. MRI is generally uninformative; in the few cases that have come to autopsy, there is no evidence of vasculitis.[313] The EEG shows generalized slowing with frontal intermittent rhythmic delta activity and often triphasic waves.[314] Antithyroid antibodies are found in serum and spinal fluid, and antineuronal antibodies have also been reported in some cases, although the pathophysiologic significance of either type of antibody for the encephalopathy is not clear.[313] The importance of the syndrome is that it is steroid responsive and should be suspected when a hypothyroid patient does not show an improved level of consciousness in response to thyroxin. The diagnosis is established by elevated thyroid antibodies and responsiveness to steroids.

HYPERTHYROIDISM

Thyrotoxicosis usually presents with signs of increased CNS activity (i.e., anxiety, tremor, or hyperkinetic behavior).[302,306] Subtle changes in cognitive function accompany the more obvious emotional disturbances. Rarely, in "thyroid storm," these symptoms can progress to confusion, stupor, or coma.[306] Thyroid storm usually develops in a patient with pre-existing thyrotoxicosis, often partially treated, who encounters precipitating factors such as an infection or a surgical procedure. The early clinical picture is dominated by signs of hypermetabolism. Fever is invariably present, profuse sweating occurs, there is marked tachycardia, and there may be signs of pulmonary edema and congestive heart failure. A more difficult problem is so-called *apathetic* thyrotoxicosis.[315,316] Such patients are usually elderly and present with neurologic signs of depression and apathy. If untreated, the clinical symptoms progress to delirium and finally to stupor and coma. Nothing distinctive marks the neurologic picture. Hypermetabolism is not clinically prominent, nor can one observe the eye signs generally associated with thyrotoxicosis. However, almost all patients show evidence of severe weight loss and have cardiovascular symptoms, particularly atrial fibrillation and congestive heart failure. Many have signs of a moderately severe proximal myopathy. The diagnosis is established by obtaining tests that reflect thyroid hyperfunction and the neurologic signs are reversed by antithyroid treatment.

Pituitary Disorders

Pituitary failure can be associated with stupor or coma under two circumstances: (1) Pituitary apoplexy (Figure 5–8) is the term applied to hemorrhage or infarction usually of a pituitary tumor, but less commonly of the normal pituitary gland. Encephalopathy is caused by an acutely expanding mass lesion compressing the diencephalon or by inflammation due to ejection of noxious substances (blood or necrotic tissue) into the subarachnoid space. Patients generally present with headache, vomiting, photophobia, fever, visual loss, and ocular palsies. About 10% of patients are stuporous or comatose, in part due to the subarachnoid inflammation, and in part due to pituitary failure resulting from the hemorrhagic infarct.[306,317] Sheehan's syndrome, also called postpartum pituitary necrosis, is another form of pituitary

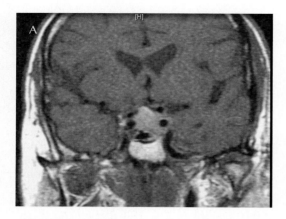

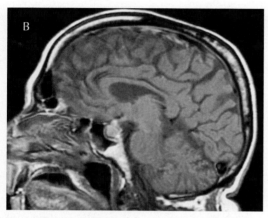

Figure 5–8. Coronal (A) and sagittal (B) unenhanced T1 magnetic resonance imaging (MRI) scans of a patient with pituitary apoplexy. This 76-year-old male had been hospitalized for treatment of rectal carcinoma when he suddenly complained of headache, visual blurring, diplopia, and confusion. The MRI revealed a sellar and suprasellar mass compressing the optic chiasm and the cavernous sinuses. Surgery revealed a necrotic lesion with a few cells that probably represented a pituitary adenoma.

apoplexy. The acute form begins hours to days after delivery with signs of acute adrenal insufficiency (see above). In the past, symptoms began in the hospital before the patient went home, but because of the advent of short obstetric stays, most patients return home and then present to an emergency department with hypotension, tachycardia, hypoglycemia, fatigue, nausea, and vomiting; unrecognized, the disease is fatal.[318] (2) Patients with panhypopituitarism, if the levels of corticosteroids or thyroid hormone fall low enough or if there is a disturbance of water balance, may become stuporous or comatose. In addition, similar to pa-

tients with primary adrenal or thyroid failure, patients with pain are sensitive to narcotic and sedative drugs.

Pituitary excess causes encephalopathy by hyperfunction of the pituitary-adrenal axis (i.e., during Cushing's syndrome; see previous section).

Cancer

Diffuse encephalopathy leading to delirium, stupor, or coma is frequently seen in patients with disseminated cancer.[319] About 20% of the neurologic consultations in a cancer hospital are requested for the evaluation of confused or stuporous patients.[320] The causes of the mental changes are many (Table 5–11) and may

Table 5–11 **Some Neurologic Complications of Cancer Causing Stupor or Coma**

Lesion	Example
Primary brain tumor	Hypothalamic glioma
	Gliomatosis cerebri
Brain metastasis	Carcinomatous encephalitis
Leptomeningeal	
metastasis	Hydrocephalus
Vascular disease	
Large stroke	Nonbacterial
	thromboendocarditis
	Cerebral venous
	occlusion
Multiple small	Disseminating intravascular
strokes	coagulation
	Intravascular lymphoma
Infections	
Viral	Progressive multifocal
	encephalopathy
	Herpes simplex/zoster
Fungi	*Aspergillus*
Bacteria	*Listeria*
Side effects of	
therapy	
Radiation	Radiation dementia
Chemotherapy	MTX leukoencephalopathy
Metabolic	Hypoglycemia
	Liver, renal failure
Nutritional	Wernicke's
	Pellagra
	B_{12} deficiency
	encephalopathy

include all those discussed in this book.[321] In a series of 140 patients with encephalopathy and cancer, two-thirds had multiple causes of their encephalopathy. However, when a single cause was identified, multiple brain metastases were the most common. In some cases, the metastases are leptomeningeal and may be discovered only by lumbar puncture. Other single causes included drugs, sepsis, multiorgan failure, and hypoxia.[321] As with other patients suffering from metabolic encephalopathy, the cancer patient can often be restored to a fully sentient state if the underlying metabolic cause is corrected.

Patient 5–16

A 60-year-old man with multiple myeloma became obtunded while in the hospital. Treatment with chemotherapy had produced a severe pancytopenia, which had led to pneumonia. In addition, he suffered from renal failure and required intermittent hemodialysis. At 6:50 a.m. he was given 4 mg of levorphanol because of low back pain. Early in the afternoon he began hemodialysis, but he became hypotensive and hemodialysis was stopped. He was noted early in the evening to be markedly obtunded, with the right eye slightly deviated outward and upward. His respirations "appeared agonal." On neurologic examination the patient was stuporous. With vigorous stimuli, however, he could be aroused to say his name and to identify Memorial Hospital. No other verbal responses could be secured. His pupils were 1.5 mm and reactive. In the resting position, the left eye was straight ahead and the right eye was slightly externally and superiorly deviated. Ice water calorics yielded a few beats of nystagmus in the appropriate direction. His respirations were 8 per minute, irregular, and shallow. Bilateral asterixis and extensor plantar responses were present. Laboratory abnormalities that morning had included a white blood cell count of 1,100/mm³, a hemoglobin of 9.3 g/dL, and platelets of 21,000/mm³, and D-dimer concentrations (fibrin degradation products suggesting mild disseminated intravascular coagulation) were elevated. The serum sodium was 130 mEq/L, BUN 82 mg/dL, creatinine 5.7 mg/dL, total protein 8.1 g/L with an albumin of 3.0 g, and alkaline phosphatase of 106. Because of the small pupils and slow and shallow respiration, despite the pneumonia, the patient

was given 0.4 mg of naloxone intravenously. The pupils dilated to 6 mm, respirations went from 8 to 24 per minute, and he became awake and alert, complaining of the low back pain for which he had been given the drug that morning. The following morning he again became obtunded but less than the evening before. Pupils were 3 mm, and respirations were 20 and relatively deep. Another 0.4 mg of naloxone was given, the pupils dilated to 7 mm, respirations accelerated to 30 and deeper, and again he became alert and oriented.

Comment: The clues to opioid overdosage in this patient were the small pupils and the shallow, irregular respirations despite pneumonia. The patient's other metabolic defects made him particularly sensitive to small doses of opioids, as did the fact that he had not received the drug in the past for pain and thus had not developed tolerance to it. Furthermore, the long action of levorphanol induced a relapse the next morning after the effects of the naloxone had worn off.

Patient 5–17

A 42-year-old woman with breast cancer known to be metastatic to bone was admitted to the hospital because of stupor. When stimulated vigorously she would answer with her name, but could not answer other questions or follow commands. On examination there was bilateral papilledema. Pupils were 2 mm bilaterally, with roving eye movements and full responses to oculocephalic maneuvers. There were diminished tendon reflexes in the left triceps and right knee jerk. Toes were upgoing. A CT scan with contrast disclosed several small enhancing lesions along the surface of the cerebral cortex. Lumbar puncture showed increased opening pressure of 300 mm/CSF, protein of 228, 14 WBCs, no RBCs, and multiple large atypical cells, which, on cytologic examination, were similar to the adenocarcinoma cells of her breast cancer. She was treated with dexamethasone and whole brain radiation therapy, resulting in rapid clearing of her cognitive function. Intraventricular chemotherapy with methotrexate and cytosine arabinoside was initiated. When she died of a pulmonary embolus 18 months later, autopsy revealed no evidence of residual cancer in the brain.

Comment: Leptomeningeal metastasis from cancer generally presents with multilevel dysfunction of the CNS, spinal cord, and spinal nerve roots. The loss of several tendon reflexes in this setting is a critical clue to the diagnosis. Radiologic evaluation may show nothing, or it may reveal superficial tumor implants along the surface of the brain, the meninges, or the spinal roots. Although often a sign of far advanced cancer, in occasional patients, particularly with breast cancer or lymphoma, vigorous treatment may clear the tumor cells and dramatically improve and extend the patient's life.

EXOGENOUS INTOXICATIONS

Sedative and Psychotropic Drugs

Many drugs in common use can cause delirium, stupor, or coma when taken in large amounts (Table 5–12).

Table 5–12 Drugs Causing Delirium, Stupor, or Coma

Medicinal agents
  Amphetamines
  Anticholinergics
  Psychotropic
    Tricyclics
    Selective serotonin reuptake inhibitors
    Lithium
    Phenothiazine
  Sedatives
    Benzodiazepines
    Barbiturates
    Glutethimide
    Methaqualone
  Opioids
  Acetaminophen
  Anticonvulsants
Nonmedical agents
  Alcohols
    Alcohol
    Ethylene glycol/propylene glycol
    Methanol
Illicit drugs
  Cocaine
  Methamphetamine
  Gamma-hydroxybutyrate
  Methylenedioxymethamphetamine (MDMA)
  Phencyclidine
  Ketamine
  Rohypnol

The list of such drugs is legion; also, the agents favored by drug abusers change from time to time and differ in different geographic areas. Agents causing delirium or coma may include (1) medicinal agents prescribed but taken in overdose, (2) medicinal agents procured illicitly (e.g., opioids), (3) agents substituted for alcohol such as ethylene glycol and methanol, and (4) illicit drugs (e.g., "party" or "club" drugs).[322] If it is known what agents the patient has taken, there is not much of a diagnostic problem. However, patients who are stuporous but arousable may deny drug ingestion and, if comatose, no history may be available at all.

A few drugs such as salicylates and acetaminophen can be tested at the bedside.[27] Combined HPLC-immunoenzymatic screening is available in some emergency departments to detect amphetamines, barbiturates, benzodiazepines, cocaine, opioids, and phencyclidine and other drugs in 20 to 45 minutes.[323] Others can be inferred from the physical examination (e.g., pupil size and response to antidotes) or rapidly procured laboratory tests. Examples include an anion gap, unidentifiable osmoles, or an oxygen saturation gap[324] (Table 5–13). Measurement of the anion gap helps in establishing a diagnosis. An increased anion gap is found in toxic ingestion of drugs such as ethylene glycol, propylene glycol, methanol, paraldehyde, and salicylates. A decreased anion gap may be found after ingestion of lithium, bromides, or iodides.[324] An increased osmol gap (see page 241) can be found with ethanol and ethylene ingestion. The so-called oxygen saturation gap exists when there is more than a 5% difference between calculated saturation, as measured from arterial blood, and that as measured by an oximeter. If the oximeter reading is too high after carbon monoxide intoxication, there may be severe methemoglobinemia. In addition, if the venous blood has a high oxygen content with the appearance of arterial blood, one should consider cyanide or hydrogen sulfide poisoning.[324]

However, in many instances, an accurate immediate diagnosis leans heavily upon the physical findings and clinical deduction. Laboratory confirmation of the clinical diagnosis is desirable, but the delay in conducting the tests often means that the information becomes available too late to be useful in guiding treatment. Furthermore, blood levels of sedatives

Table 5–13 Laboratory Clues to Specific Toxins

Anion gap
  Increased
    Ethylene glycol
    Methanol
    Paraldehyde
    Salicylate
    Acetaminophen
    Cocaine
  Decreased
    Bromides
    Lithium
    Iodide

Osmolal gap
  Increased
    Ethanol
    Ethylene glycol
    . Propylene glycol

O_2 saturated gap
  Increased
    Carbon monoxide
    Methemoglobin
    Cyanide
    Hydrogen sulfate

Modified from Fabbri et al.[323] and Mokhlesi and or-bridge,[324] with permission.

or alcohol sometimes provide a poor guide to the depth or anticipated duration of coma. Several reasons account for the potential discrepancy. Persons who chronically take these drugs develop a tolerance to their effects and require larger doses with resulting higher blood levels to produce coma. Pharmacologic interaction between drug mixtures and the inability to anticipate the effects of still unabsorbed material in the gut further interfere with making a correlation.

Sedatives such as benzodiazepines, neuroleptics, antihistamines, alcohol, and sedating antidepressants, as well as older drugs such as meprobamate and bromides, can all produce coma if enough is taken. The mechanism of action of each drug depends partly on its structure and partly on the dose. Many of the sedative drugs cause delirium or coma by increasing GABAergic input to the ascending arousal system, thus extinguishing wakefulness.[324,326] Antidepressant drugs interfere with the reuptake of neurotransmitters, including serotonin and norepinephrine, and neuroleptics block dopamine receptors, but the more sedating ones also have antihistamine and anticholinergic effects. These effects may produce autonomic dysfunction, and in fact, the most dangerous effect of overdose with tricyclic antidepressants is their cardiotoxicity.

Overdoses with most depressant drugs produce fairly consistent clinical findings; individual drugs usually cause relatively minor clinical differences. Almost all of these agents depress vestibular and cerebellar function as readily as cerebral cortical function so that nystagmus, ataxia, and dysarthria accompany or even precede the first signs of impaired consciousness. Larger amounts of drug produce coma, and at this quantity all the agents depress brainstem autonomic responses. With few exceptions, such as the benzodiazepines or neuroleptics, respiration tends to be depressed at least as much as and sometimes more than somatic motor function. The pupils are usually small and reactive and ciliospinal reflexes are preserved. The oculocephalic responses are depressed or absent, and the oculovestibular responses to cold caloric testing are depressed and may be lost altogether in deep coma. Patients with depressant drug poisoning are usually flaccid with stretch reflexes that are diminished or absent. This typical picture is not always immediately seen, especially if coma develops rapidly after the ingestion of a fast-acting barbiturate such as secobarbital or pentobarbital. In such cases, respiratory depression may ensue almost as rapidly as does unconsciousness; signs in the motor system may initially evolve as if function was being depressed in a rostral-caudal fashion, with a brief appearance of hyperreflexia and even clonus and extensor plantar responses. Failure to recognize this short-lived phase (it rarely lasts more than 30 to 45 minutes) as being due to depressant drugs can be fatal if one leaves the patient temporarily unattended or delays needed ventilatory assistance. The identifying clue to the toxic-metabolic basis of the changes in such cases is that the pupillary reflexes are preserved and the motor signs are symmetric. Treatment is discussed in Chapter 7.

Supportive care involves prevention of further absorption of the poison, elimination of the toxin that has already been absorbed, and, when necessary, supportive respiration, blood pressure, and cardiac rhythm. Some toxins have specific antidotes that have been recently reviewed.[324,327]

Table 5–14 Clues to Specific Drugs Frequently Causing Delirium, Stupor, or Coma

Drug	Chemical Diagnosis	Behavior	Physical Signs
Amphetamine	Blood or urine	Hypertension; aggressive, sometimes paranoid, repetitive behavior progressing into agitated paranoid delirium; auditory and visual hallucinations	Hyperthermia, hypertension, tachycardia, arrhythmia; pupils dilated; tremor, dystonia, occasionally convulsions
Cocaine	None available	Similar to above but more euphoric, less paranoid	Variable
Club drugs such as Methylenedioxy-methamphetamine (MDMA), phenocyclidine	Blood or urine	Confused, disoriented, perceptual distortions, distractible, withdrawn or eruptive; can lead to accidents or violence	See text
Atropine-scopolamine	None available	Delirium; often agitated; responding to visual hallucinations; drowsiness; rarely coma	Fever, flushed face; dilated pupils; sinus or supraventricular tachycardia; hot dry skin
Tricyclic antidepressants	Blood or urine	Drowsiness; delirium; agitation; rarely coma	Fever; supraventricular tachycardia; conduction defects; ventricular tachycardia or fibrillation; hypotension; dystonia
Phenothiazines	Blood	Somnolence; coma rare	Arrhythmias, hypotension, dystonia (see text page 261)
Lithium	Blood	Lethargic confusion, mute state, eventually coma. Multifocal seizures can occur. Onset can be delayed by hours or days after overdose	Appearance of distraction; roving conjugate eye movement; pupils intact; paratonic resistance; tremors, akathisia
Benzodiazepines	Blood or urine	Stupor, rarely unarousable	Essentially no cardiovascular or respiratory depression
Methaqualone	Blood or urine	Hallucinations and agitation blend into depressant drug coma	Mild: resembles barbiturate intoxication. Severe: increased tendon reflexes, myoclonus, dystonia, convulsions. Tachycardia and heart failure
Barbiturates	Blood or urine	Stupor or coma	Hypothermia; skin cool and dry; pupils reactive; doll's eyes absent; hyporeflexia; flaccid hypotension; apnea
Alcohol	Blood or breath	Dysarthria, ataxia, stupor. Rapidly changing level of alertness with stimulation	With stupor: hypothermia, skin cold and moist; pupils reactive, midposition to wide; tachycardia
Opioids/opiates	Blood or urine	Stupor or coma	Hypothermia; skin cool and moist; pupils symmetrically pinpoint reactive; bradycardia, hypotension; hypoventilation; pulmonary edema

Alcoholic stupor can be a difficult diagnosis because so many patients who are unconscious for other reasons (e.g., head trauma or drug ingestion) will have the odor of "alcohol" (actually caused by impurities in the liquor) on their breath. Measurement of breath ethanol is not as accurate as measurement of blood ethanol and often underestimates the degree of toxicity.[328] However, in a stuporous or comatose patient with a breath ethanol level of less than 50 mg/dL, alcohol intoxication is probably not the culprit and other causes need to be searched for.

The patient in an alcoholic stupor (blood level 250 to 300 mg/dL, although highly tolerant alcoholics may be awake at these levels) usually has a flushed face, a rapid pulse, a low blood pressure, and mild hypothermia, all resulting from the vasodilatory effects of alcohol. As the coma deepens (blood levels of 300 to 400 mg/dL), such patients become pale and quiet, and the pupils may dilate and become sluggishly reactive. With deeper depression respiration fails. The depth of alcoholic stupor or coma may be deceptive when judged clinically. Repetitive stimulation during medical examinations often arouses such patients to the point where they awaken and require little further stimulation to remain awake, only to lapse into a deep coma with respiratory failure when left alone in bed. Alcohol is frequently taken in conjunction with psychotropic or sedative drugs in suicide attempts. Because ethanol is also a GABA$_A$ agonist, it synergizes with the other depressant drugs. Under such circumstances of double ingestion, blood levels are no longer reliable in predicting the course, and sudden episodes of respiratory failure or cardiac arrhythmias are more frequent than in patients who have taken only a barbiturate.

HEROIN-OPIATE OVERDOSAGE

These drugs can be taken either by injection or sniffing. Overdosage with narcotics may occur from suicide attempts or, more commonly, when an addict or neophyte misjudges the amount or the quality of the heroin he or she is injecting or sniffing. Characteristic signs of opioid coma include pinpoint pupils that generally contract to a bright light and dilate rapidly if a narcotic antagonist is given. Respiratory slowing, irregularity, and cessation are prominent features and result either from di-

rect narcotic depression of the brainstem or from pulmonary edema, which is a frequent complication of heroin overdosage,[329] although the pathogenesis is not understood. Opiates can cause hypothermia, but by the time such patients reach the hospital, they frequently have pneumonitis due to aspiration, so that body temperatures may be normal or elevated. Some opioids such as propoxyphene and meperidine can cause seizures. Intravenous naloxone at an initial dose of 0.2 to 0.4 mg usually reverses the effects of opioids. In patients who are physically dependent, the drug may also cause acute withdrawal. Repeated boluses at intervals of 1 to 2 hours may be needed, as naloxone is a short-acting agent and the patient may have taken a long-acting opioid.[327]

SEDATIVE DRUGS

The neurologic examination itself cannot categorically separate drug poisoning from other causes of metabolic brain disease. The most common diagnostic error is to mistake deep coma from sedative poisoning for the coma of brainstem infarction. The initial distinction between these two conditions may be difficult, but small, reactive pupils, absence of caloric responses, failure to respond to noxious stimuli, absence of stretch reflexes, and muscular flaccidity suggest a profound metabolic disorder. Persistent extensor responses, hyperactive stretch reflexes, spasticity, dysconjugate eye movements to caloric tests, and unreactive pupils more likely occur with brainstem destruction. If both the pupillary light reflexes and ciliospinal responses are present, deep coma is metabolic in origin. However, even if both the pupillary reactions and the ciliospinal reflexes are lost, deep coma can still be due to severe sedative intoxication. Thus, demonstration of brain death requires eliminating the possibility of a sedative overdose (see Chapter 7).

Patient 5–18

A 48-year-old woman ingested 50 g of chloral hydrate, 1.5 g of chlordiazepoxide (150 tablets of Librium), and 2.4 g of flurazepam (80 capsules of Dalmane) in a suicide attempt. Shortly afterward, her family found her in a lethargic condition and by the time they brought her to the emergency department she was deeply comatose, hypotensive, and apneic. Examination following endotracheal intubation and the initiation of artificial ventilation showed a blood pressure of 60/40 mm Hg, pupils that were 2 mm in diameter and light fixed, absent corneal and oculovestibular responses, and total muscle flaccidity accompanied by areflexia. Arterial and Schwann-Ganz catheters were placed to assist in physiologic monitoring in view of the overwhelmingly large depressant drug dose. There was already evidence of aspiration pneumonia by the time she reached the hospital. A broad-spectrum antibiotic was given and a dopamine infusion was started, which initially succeeded in raising the blood pressure to 80/60 mm Hg. By 12 hours following admission, progressively increasing amounts of dopamine to a level of 40 pg/kg/minute were unable to keep the blood pressure above 60/40 mm Hg and urine flow ceased. Treatment with L-norepinephrine was initiated at an intravenous dose that reached 12 pg/minute. This induced a prompt rise in blood pressure to 80/40 mm Hg accompanied by a brisk urine flow. Toxicologic analysis of an admission blood sample showed the qualitative presence of chloral hydrate (quantitative assay was not available). Chlordiazepoxide level was 59.4 μg/mL and flurazepam was 6.6 μg/mL.

Early management was complicated by the effects of radiographically demonstrated aspiration pneumonia and by pulmonary edema, as well as by atrial, junctional, and ventricular premature cardiac contractions. Hypotension hovering between 80/60 and 60/40 mm Hg was a serious problem for the first 48 hours, and declines in blood pressure were repeatedly accompanied by a marginal urinary flow. The woman remained unresponsive, but by day 4 it was possible to maintain mean blood pressures above 80/60 mm Hg using dopamine; the L-norepinephrine was discontinued. Isosthenuria and polyuria developed, reflecting the probable complication of renal tubular necrosis, but meticulous attention to electrolyte balance, pulmonary toilet, and the avoidance of overhydration managed to prevent the various complications from worsening. Ice water caloric stimulation first elicited a reaction of ocular movement on day 4 and the pupillary light reflexes reappeared on the same day. On day 8 spontaneous breathing began and one could detect stretch reflexes in the extremities. She first responded to noxious stimuli by opening her eyes and withdrawing her limbs on day 10 and she

mumbled words 1 day later. Not until day 13 did she fully awaken to follow commands and answer questions. The quick phase of nystagmus to caloric stimulation did not return until day 15. She subsequently made a complete physical and intellectual recovery and received psychiatric treatment.

Comment: This woman's course emphasizes the maxim that if patients with depressant drug poisoning survive to reach the hospital, they are potentially salvageable no matter what the blood levels of the ingested agent. The toxicologic analyses in this instance showed an amount of drug in the body that is generally regarded as a fatal dose. Whether hemodialysis would have shortened this patient's course can be questioned, since none of the ingested agents was dialyzable. Generally speaking, among younger patients seen with drug intoxication, only those who have ingested large amounts of barbiturates have periods of unconsciousness that approach the length of this woman's coma. However, patients put into pentobarbital coma therapeutically to treat status epilepticus may have a very similar course, and prolonged drug-induced coma does not appear to injure the brain. Her case illustrates that any sedative taken in sufficiently large amounts is capable of producing many days of coma that require meticulous systemic care to accomplish survival. Her outcome further emphasizes that even very long periods of unresponsive coma need not produce any measure of brain injury so long as blood gases and arterial perfusion pressures are maintained at levels close to the physiologic norm.

In diagnosing coma caused by depressant drug poisoning, one must not only identify the cause, but also judge the depth of coma, for the latter influences the choice of treatment. Several years ago, Reed and colleagues[330] suggested a grading scheme for patients with depressant drug poisoning, as outlined in Table 5–15. The practical aspect of the classification is that only patients with grade 3 or 4 depression are at risk of losing their lives. By the same token, comparisons of the potential value of one treatment over another can only be judged by comparing them on patients in grade 3 or 4 coma, where essentially all deaths occur.

Benzodiazepines and nonbenzodiazepine agonists of the same receptors (e.g., drugs like zolpidem and eszopiclone) have replaced barbiturates as hypnotic agents. They cause much

Table 5–15 **Severity of Depressant Drug Coma***

Grade: 0 Asleep but arousable
   1 Unarousable to talk but withdraws
      appropriately
   2 Comatose; most reflexes intact;
      no cardiorespiratory depression
   3 Comatose; no tendon reflexes;
      no cardiorespiratory depression
   4 Respiratory failure, hypotension,
      pulmonary edema or arrhythmia present.
      Comatose for more than 36 hours

*Adapted from Reed et al.[330]

less respiratory depression, but at very high dosages may still cause respiratory arrest, particularly if the patient has underlying chronic pulmonary disease. An overdose can be reversed by the specific antagonist flumazenil.[331] Flumazenil is useful in assessing multiagent poisoning because it reverses the side effects of the benzodiazepine; however, in some circumstances it may cause acute withdrawal seizures.[332] Flumazenil does not affect coma due to alcohol, barbiturates, tricyclic antidepressants, or opioids.

INTOXICATION WITH ENDOGENOUSLY PRODUCED "BENZODIAZEPINES"

Over the years there have been scattered case reports of patients with recurrent episodes of stupor resembling drug overdose,[333] but no drug ingestion could be identified. Lugaresi and colleagues suggested the possibility that such attacks might be due to elevated levels of an endogenous benzodiazepine-like agent called "endozepine."[334,335] Patients clinically resemble those who have taken benzodiazepines in overdose and, in fact, some have called into question whether the disorder is really due to surreptitious ingestion of benzodiazepines[336]; at least one of Lugaresi's cases turned out to be due to surreptitious lorazepam ingestion.[337] Stupor in such patients may last hours or days; it has an unpredictable onset and frequency. Patients are entirely normal between attacks. Like patients with benzodiazepine intoxication, these patients respond to flumazenil, which both wakes the patient and normalizes the EEG. Measures of endogenous benzodiazepine-like levels are increased during the stupor. Patients can be treated with oral flumazenil to reduce the frequency of attacks. The first reports of the disorder may have been by Haimovic and Beresford in 1992.[333]

Intoxication With Other Common Medications

Acetaminophen overdose is the most common poisoning reported to poison information centers. The drug's metabolite (NAPQI)[338] can cause acute liver necrosis, and doses above 5 g can lead to liver failure and hepatic coma. Alkalosis and grossly elevated liver function studies are a clue to its presence; prompt treatment with *N*-acetylcysteine often prevents fatality.[339]

ANTIDEPRESSANTS

These drugs include the tricyclic agents such as amitriptyline, selective serotonin reuptake inhibitors such as paroxetine and fluoxetine, and monoamine oxidase (MAO) inhibitors. All can produce delirium, and the tricyclic antidepressants can cause stupor or coma. The major toxicity of the tricyclic antidepressants is on the cardiovascular system, causing cardiac arrhythmias and hypotension. The CNS is affected by the change in blood pressure as well as the anticholinergic effects of the drugs that can lead to anhydrosis, fever, and multifocal monoclonus.[327] Selective serotonin reuptake inhibitors and MAO inhibitors taken alone generally are not neurotoxic. When taken together, however, they may result in the serotonin syndrome characterized by delirium, myoclonus, hyperreflexia, diaphoresis, flushing, fever, nausea, and diarrhea. Disseminated intravascular coagulation may be a side effect and add to the CNS difficulties. Methysergide and cyproheptadine have been reported to be effective in reversing this disorder.[327]

Lithium intoxication is characterized by tremor, ataxia and nystagmus, choreoathetosis, photophobia, and lethargy. It may also induce nephrogenic diabetes insipidus, resulting in volume depletion and hyperosmolarity. Delirium, seizures, coma, and cardiovascular instability may occur with severe intoxication.[339] Cerebellar toxicity occurs at levels higher than 3.5 mEq/L and may be nonreversible.[340] With a decreased serum anion gap, hemodialysis may be required for severe intoxication.[339]

Many other drugs are proconvulsive and may produce seizures, as indicated in Table 5–17.

Ethanol Intoxication

One would hardly think that it takes a medical education to diagnose a drunk, but the appraisal of ethanol intoxication sometimes turns out to be deceptively difficult. In Belfast, for example, where events should provide no lack of experience, the diagnosis of alcohol or non-alcohol ingestion in patients with head injury was incorrectly made a full 12% of the time. Of even greater potential consequence, six of 42 subjects with blood levels over 100 mg/dL were clinically unrecognized as being intoxicated.[341]

Alcohol exerts its main sedative effect by potentiating the $GABA_A$ receptor. However, it also affects other neurotransmitters, including causing increases in dopaminergic transmission, which is a critical component of the reward system to the brain. It also promotes the release of noradrenaline, blocks the NMDA glutamate receptor, and stimulates the $5HT_3$ receptor.[342]

Moderately large doses of ethanol represent a frequent cause of stupor, most examples of which recover spontaneously without medical attention. Large doses produce a coma that at greater than 400 mg/dL can be fatal, primarily due to respiratory depression. A major problem with alcohol ingestion is that the ensuing uninhibited behavior leads to the impulsive ingestion of other sedative, hypnotic, or anti-depressant drugs or to careless, headstrong, and uncoordinated activity (e.g., fighting, driving while intoxicated) that invites head trauma. As a result, the major diagnostic problem in altered states of consciousness associated with acute alcoholic intoxication lies in separating the potentially benign and spontaneously reversible signs of alcoholic depression from evidence of more serious injury from other drugs or head trauma.

As noted above, in pure alcohol intoxication, blood levels correlate fairly well with clinical signs of intoxication. Dose levels correlate less well because the rate of absorption from the stomach and intestine depends heavily on the presence or absence of other stomach contents. Chronic ingestion induces moderate tolerance, but in general, the associations in Table 5–16 represent dependable guidelines. When estimating dosage, the physician should recall that in the United States the alcoholic content of distilled spirits equals 50% of the stated proof on the label.

Clinical signs of acute drunkenness can closely resemble those caused by several other metabolic encephalopathies, especially including other depressant drug intoxication, diabetic ketoacidosis, and hypoglycemia. Innate psychologic traits influence the behavior of many drunks, adding to the complexities of diagnosis. As mentioned above, the odor of the breath depends on impurities and is an unreliable sign. Patients with alcohol intoxication are ataxic, clumsy, and dysarthric. They are easily confused, are often uninhibited and boisterous (or, more severely, stuporous), and commonly vomit. The conjunctivae are often hyperemic and with severe poisoning the pupils react sluggishly to light. Severe intoxication or stupor produces a remarkable degree of analgesia ("feeling no pain") to noxious stimuli such that prior to the discovery of modern anesthetics, alcohol was often used for this purpose.

Table 5–16 Clinical Effects and Blood Levels in Acute Alcoholism

Symptoms	Blood Level (mg/dL)
Euphoria, giddiness, verbosity	25–100
Long reaction time, impaired mental status examination	
Mild incoordination, nystagmus	
Hypalgesia to noxious stimuli	
Boisterousness, withdrawal, easily confused	100–200
Conjunctival hyperemia	
Ataxia, nystagmus, dysarthria	
Pronounced hypalgesia	
Nausea, vomiting, drowsiness	200–300
Diplopia, wide sluggish pupils	
Marked ataxia and clumsiness	
Hypothermia, cold sweat, amnesic stupor	>300
Severe dysarthria or anarthria	
Anesthesia	
Stertor, hypoventilation	
Coma	

Table 5–17 Proconvulsant Agents: Classification by Source and Use

	Pharmaceuticals		Nonpharmaceuticals	
Class	**Class**	**Example(s)**	**Class**	**Example(s)**
Analgesics		Meperidine/normeperidine, propoxyphene, pentazocine, salicylate, tramadol	Alcohols	Methanol, ethanol (withdrawal)
Anesthetics		Local anesthetics (lidocaine, benzocaine)	Antiseptics/preservatives	Ethylene oxide, phenol
Anticonvulsants		Carbamazepine	Biologic toxins	
Antidepressants		Tricyclics (amitriptyline/nortriptyline), amoxapine, bupropion, selective serotonin reuptake inhibitors (citalopram), venlafaxine	Marine animals	Domoic acid (shellfish [blue mussels])
			Mushrooms	Monomethylhydrazine (*Gyromitra* spp.)
			Plants	Coniine (poison hemlock), viral A (water hemlock) camphor
Antihistamines		Diphenhydramine, doxylamine, tripelennamine	Gases (naturally and/or anthropogenically occurring)	Carbon monoxide, hydrogen sulfide, hydrogen cyanide
Antimicrobials			Metals/organometallics	Alkyl mercurials (dimethylmercury), arsenic, lead, thallium, tetraethyl lead, organotins (trimethyltin)
Antineoplastics		Alkylating agents (chlorambucil, busulfan)	Metal hydrides	Pentaborane, phosphine
Antipsychotics		Clozapine, loxapine	Pesticides	
Asthma medications			Fungicides/herbicides	Dinitrophenol, diquat, glufosinate
Cardiovascular drugs		Propranolol, quinidine	Insecticides	Organochlorines (lindane, DDT, organophosphates (parathion), pyrethroids (type II), sulfuryl fluoride, alkyl halides (methyl bromide)
Cholinergics		Pilocarpine, bethanechol	Molluscacides	Metaldehyde
Muscle relaxants		Baclofen, orphenadrine	Rodenticides	Strychnine, zinc or aluminum phosphide
Nonsteroidal anti-inflammatory drugs		Mefenamic acid, phenylbutazone		
Psychostimulants/anorectics		Amphetamine, caffeine, cocaine, methamphetamine, methylenedioxymethamphetamine (MDMA)		
Vitamins/supplements		Vitamin A, iron salts (ferrous sulfate)		

A secure diagnosis of alcoholic intoxication and its severity requires blood level determinations. When these are unavailable, determining serum osmolality helps.[324] Alcohol adds osmols to blood in a degree proportional to its blood level. A blood level over 150 mg/dL produces a serum osmolality of less than 320 mOsm/kg, and patients with blood alcohol levels of 200 mg/dL had a serum osmolality of greater than 340 mOsm/kg. Because alcohol is uniformly distributed in body water, the hyperosmolality does not lead to fluid shifts out of the brain, and thus, the hyperosmolality produced by alcohol is not in itself a cause of symptoms.

Intoxication With Drugs of Abuse

Party or club drugs include GHB, ketamine, Rohypnol (flunitrazepam), methamphetamine, lysergic acid diethylamide (LSD), and 3,4-methylenedioxymethamphetamine (MDMA; Ecstasy).[322,343] Other drugs include cocaine, opioids (see above), and phencyclidine. These drugs may be taken alone or in combination and can cause critical illness.[327]

Cocaine may be taken nasally, orally, or intravenously. The drug inhibits neuronal uptake of catecholamines and causes CNS stimulation. Patients are often euphoric and may be anxious, agitated, and delirious, and sometimes have seizures. Agitation can be controlled with benzodiazepines. Some patients are febrile and require cooling. There is no specific antidote. Some patients develop a CNS vasculitis that can result in cerebral infarction, myocardial infarction, and sometimes cerebral hemorrhage. This is currently one of the most common causes of stroke in young adults without the usual risk factors for atherosclerotic disease.

GHB causes a state of deep sleep with high-voltage delta EEG. It has been released in the United States to treat narcolepsy, in which fragmented sleep at night contributes to daytime symptoms such as cataplexy. Because it induces such deep unresponsiveness, it has achieved a reputation as a date rape drug[344] and, at high doses, can cause coma and respiratory insufficiency. It has a rather short half-life, so that recovery usually occurs within several hours. Some uncontrolled studies have suggested physostigmine as an antidote, but the evidence for this is poor and experimental studies have failed to find an effect.[345,346]

Phencyclidine, or "angel dust," is a glutamate NMDA receptor antagonist.[347] It results in bizarre behavior and agitation and, at higher doses, can produce delirium and coma. Both vertical and horizontal nystagmus are common. Seizures and dystonic reactions are less common. Many patients have pinpoint pupils when they are awake and agitated, and this can be a clue to the diagnosis. Patients may develop hypertensive encephalopathy; intracranial and subarachnoid hemorrhages have been reported. Ketamine, another NMDA antagonist, has been used as an anesthetic agent and is still used in the veterinary setting.[348] As a club drug it can either be ingested or smoked. It causes delirium, often with hallucinations. Side effects may include hypothermia and respiratory depression.[349] With either drug, a benzodiazepine may help control violent behavior.[327]

MDMA has its major effect on the serotonin system. It is an indirect serotonin agonist that inhibits tryptophan hydroxylase and thus decreases serotonin production. It also induces the release of serotonin and blocks serotonin reuptake. The drug also increases the release of dopamine and norepinephrine from presynaptic neurons and prevents their metabolism by inhibiting monamine oxidase. The usual adverse effects include anxiety, ataxia, and difficulty concentrating; seizures can occur and pupillary dilation is common. Hyperthermia may lead to death.[349] Agitation and seizures can be treated with benzodiazepines.

Flunitrazepam (Rohypnol) is a benzodiazepine and like other drugs in this class potentiates $GABA_A$ receptors. Its effects are similar to other drugs in this class, such as benzodiazepines or alcohol intoxication, except that it is more likely to produce respiratory depression, so that overdose can be life threatening. Flumazenil, a benzodiazepine antagonist, can reverse the toxicity.[349]

Intoxication With Drugs Causing Metabolic Acidosis

The metabolism and mechanisms of neurologic changes in acid-base disorders are discussed on pages 188–192. This section considers specific exogenous poisons causing metabolic acidosis.[325] These include methyl alcohol, ethylene glycol, and paraldehyde. Salicylate poisoning also produces a metabolic acidosis in the tissues, but in adults this aspect of the disorder often is overshadowed in the blood by evidence of respiratory alkalosis.

The metabolic acidosis and neurotoxicity of methyl alcohol, ethylene glycol, and paraldehyde all result from their metabolic breakdown products rather than the original agent. Poisoning from all three drugs is most common in chronic alcoholics who ingest the agents either by mistake or in ignorance of their risks as a substitute for ethanol. All three agents initially cause symptoms of alcohol intoxication, progressing to confusion and stupor, by which point symptoms and signs of severe acidosis and systemic organ complications usually emerge as well.

Methanol is degraded by alcohol dehydrogenase into formic acid.[327] The presence of ethanol in the system slows its metabolic breakdown, thereby influencing the clinical course. The earliest and most frequent neurologic damage of methyl alcohol poisoning affects retinal ganglion cells. The symptoms of methanol poisoning can evolve over several days or appear abruptly. Stupor, coma, or seizures occur only in severely poisoned patients. Most subjects at first give the appearance of advanced inebriation and develop visual loss ("blind drunk"). Hyperpnea (respiratory compensation for metabolic acidosis) is the rule. Effective early intervention depends on recognizing the presence of an organic acidosis and treating it vigorously by using an inhibitor of alcohol dehydrogenase, such as fomepizole.[24] Because ethanol competes with methanol for alcohol dehydrogenase and thus slows its metabolism, it may be used to minimize the damage from methanol if a specific inhibitor is not readily available. If these drugs fail, hemodialysis may be indicated.[327] The following patient illustrates the point.

Patient 5–19

A 39-year-old man had been intermittently drinking denatured alcohol for 10 days. He was admitted complaining that for several hours his vision was blurred and he was short of breath. He was alert, oriented, and coherent, but restless. His blood pressure was 130/100 mm Hg, his pulse was 130 per minute, and his respirations were 40 per minute, regular and deep. The only other abnormal physical findings were 20/40 vision, engorged left retinal veins with pink optic disks, and sluggishly reactive pupils, 5 mm in diameter. His serum bicarbonate level was 5 mEq/L, and his arterial pH was 7.16. An intravenous infusion was begun immediately; 540 mEq of sodium bicarbonate was infused during the next 4 hours. By that time his arterial pH had risen to 7.47 and his serum bicarbonate to 13.9 mEq/L. He was still hyperventilating but less restless. The infusion was continued at a slower rate for 20 hours to a total of 740 mEq of bicarbonate. He recovered completely.

Comment: Denatured alcohol, usually sold as a solvent, contains about 83% ethanol and 16% methanol. Hence, it is not unusual for alcoholics to ingest denatured alcohol, despite the required warnings on the label, and this source should be sought in the emergency department when a patient who appears intoxicated with ethanol complains of visual symptoms and is hyperventilating. It is likely that the presence of ethanol sufficiently slowed the metabolism of methanol in this patient so that he was able to recover. This patient had profound acidosis, as was reflected by the requirement of 540 mEq of parenteral sodium bicarbonate to raise his serum bicarbonate from 5 to 13 mEq/L. However, it is not clear that bicarbonate therapy improves outcome.[325] Some patients suffer from hypercalcemia and hypoglycemia, and these need to be corrected. Patients may be chronically malnourished and treatment with vitamins, particularly thiamine but also folate and pyridoxine, should be administered. These same general guidelines apply to ingestion of other alcohols as indicated below. The acidosis of methyl alcohol poisoning can be lethal with alarming rapidity. One of our patients walked into the hospital complaining of blurred vision. He admitted drinking "a lot" of methyl alcohol and was hyperventilating. During the 10 minutes that it took to transfer him to a treatment unit he lost consciousness. By the time an intravenous infusion could be started, his breathing and heart had stopped and resuscitation was unsuccessful. No bicarbonate could be detected in a serum sample drawn simultaneously with death.

Paraldehyde is no longer available in the United States, as it has been replaced by other drugs for treating status epilepticus, although it may still be available in other countries.[350]

Paraldehyde is metabolized to acetic acid, which may cause acidosis, but the degree of acidosis in these patients exceeds the amount of detectable acetic acid in the serum, implying the presence of other acid products as well. Distinctive clinical features, in addition to the manifestations of metabolic acidosis, include the odor of paraldehyde on the breath, abdominal pain, a marked leucocytosis, and obtunded, lethargic behavior. All patients reported to date have recovered.

Ethylene glycol (antifreeze) is metabolized by alcohol dehydrogenase, the end products being formic, glyoxylic, and oxalic acids.[327] A relatively severe metabolic acidosis occurs during the early hours of toxicity. The initial clinical signs are similar to alcohol intoxication but without ethanol's characteristic odor. Patients with severe poisoning go on to disorientation, stupor, coma, convulsions, and death. Neuro-ophthalmologic abnormalities including papilledema, nystagmus, and ocular bobbing can be prominent. Metabolic abnormalities, if uncorrected, can lead to cardiopulmonary failure. A late complication of ethylene glycol poisoning is renal damage caused by oxalate crystalluria. Diagnosis should be suspected by a history of ingestion of antifreeze in an alcoholic or after a suicide attempt, the identification of an anion gap metabolic acidosis, and the detection of characteristic oxalic acid crystals in the urine. The treatment is the same as that of methanol poisoning (see above).[339]

Propylene glycol is a widely available organic solvent used in a variety of oral and injectable pharmaceutical agents, food preparations, and cosmetic materials. Because of its typically pharmacologically inert nature, propylene glycol overdose is not considered in the differential diagnosis of acute large anion gap acidosis and is not included in standard toxicologic studies (or may be used as an internal standard masking overdose). However, propylene glycol overdose may produce profound CNS compromise including stupor and coma, cardiovascular collapse, and marked hematologic changes including leukocytosis, thrombocytosis, microcytic anemia, and bone marrow abnormalities. Animal studies indicate reduction in arousal following repeated intoxication, suggesting that long-term CNS depression results from chronic propylene glycol exposure.[351] Commercial preparations of propylene glycol contain a racemic mixture and are metabolized in vivo to both D- an L-lactic acid isomers. Cats that developed CNS depression were noted to accumulate D-lactate on a dose-dependent basis that was positively correlated with an elevated anion gap. Preferential accumulation in the brain is thought to occur because of the low level of catabolizing enzyme in this site. D-lactic acidosis is known to produce a toxic encephalopathy in humans, usually in the setting of short bowel syndrome.[352]

Lactic acidosis has emerged increasingly in recent years as a metabolic disorder sometimes associated with neurologic symptoms and a poor prognosis.[353] Mild and asymptomatic elevations of serum lactate up to 6 mEq/L accompany a number of conditions including alkalosis, carbohydrate infusions, anxiety, and other conditions that elevate blood epinephrinemia, diabetic ketoacidosis, and alcohol intoxication. More intense, but still systemically benign, lactic acidosis with arterial blood levels of 20 mEq/L or more and blood pH levels below 7.00 can follow vigorous muscular exercise. We have observed similar degrees of acidosis and acidemia following major motor convulsions, but in neither exercise nor epilepsy was there evidence that the lactacidemia affected brain function. Lactic acid crosses the blood-brain barrier via a carrier mechanism that saturates at about three to four times the normal plasma concentration of 1 mEq/L. Thus, although high concentrations of lactate in the brain are believed to be neurotoxic, possibly by promoting excitotoxicity,[354] these probably only occur when produced by local brain ischemia or in conditions in which systemic hypoxia, circulatory failure, or drug poisoning also affect directly the oxidative metabolism of the CNS.

In adults, *salicylate intoxication* appears in two principal forms. Relatively younger persons sometimes take aspirin or similar agents in suicide attempts. Although many become severely ill and a few die with terminal coma or convulsions, most of these younger patients lack prominent neurologic complaints except for tinnitus and dyspnea. Older persons, by contrast, often ingest salicylates in excessive amounts more or less accidentally in proprietary analgesics; in these patients, neurologic symptoms can dominate the early illness, producing an encephalopathy that initially obscures the etiologic diagnosis. Salicylates act as a "metabolic uncoupler" in oxidative phosphorylation and stimulate net organic acid production. Aspirin (acetylsalicylic acid) also contains 1.7 mEq of acid per 300-mg tablet. In experimental animals, death from salicylate poisoning comes from convulsions and relates directly to the concentration of the drug in the brain; clinical evidence suggests that similar principles apply in humans.

Salicylates in adults stimulate respiration neurogenically to a degree that nearly always produces a respiratory alkalosis in the blood unless simultaneous ingestion of a sedative drug suppresses the respiratory response.[327] The metabolic acidosis of the tissues is reflected usually by a disproportionately lowered serum bicarbonate and always by an acid urine. Depending on age, associated illness, and the rapidity of accumulation, the first symptoms of salicylate intoxication usually appear at a blood level of about 40 to 50 mg/dL. Blood levels over 60 mg/dL usually produce symptoms of severe toxicity. Initial complaints are of tinnitus and, less often, deafness. As many as one-half of older persons with severe salicylate intoxication develop confusion, agitation, slurred speech, hallucinations, convulsions, stupor, or coma. Hyperpnea, intact pupillary responses, intact oculocephalic responses, diffuse paratonia, and, in many instances, extensor plantar responses are present. In a patient with metabolic encephalopathy, a respiratory alkalosis and mildly abnormal anion gap in the blood combined with aciduria are almost

always diagnostic of salicylism and can be quickly confirmed by determination of salicylate blood levels. Salicylate intoxication may be complicated by gastrointestinal bleeding, pulmonary edema, and multiorgan failure. Hemodialysis may be necessary to treat the disorder. The following patient illustrates the problem.

Patient 5–20

A 74-year-old woman with osteoarthritis, self-treated with aspirin, developed peptic ulcer disease. She was admitted to the hospital, where she was noted to be lethargic and confused after she fell out of bed. With a dysarthric, deepened voice, she complained of a recent loss of hearing. The examination showed fluctuating lethargy, asterixis, and bilateral extensor plantar responses, but little else. A CT scan was unremarkable and the changes were at first ascribed to the nonfocal effects of trauma. The next day, however, she was barely arousable, severely dysarthric, and disoriented when she did respond. The pupils were 2 mm and equal, the oculocephalic responses full and conjugate, and prominent bilateral asterixis involved the upper extremities. Both plantar responses were extensor and the respiratory rate was 32 per minute. Arterial blood gases were pH 7.48, PCO_2 24 mm Hg, PO_2 81 mm Hg, and HCO_3 19 mEq/L. Serum sodium was 134, potassium 3.5, and chloride 96 mEq/L, giving an anion gap of approximately 19. Serum salicylate level was 54 mg/dL. She was treated cautiously with alkaline diuresis and became alert without abnormal neurologic symptoms or signs within 48 hours. Her aspirin was found in the bedside table.

Many poisons have specific antidotes, and some of the most common are indicated in Table 5–18.

Table 5–18 Selected Drugs and Poisons With Specific Antidotes

Drug/Poison	Antidotes
Acetaminophen	N-acetylcysteine
Anticholinergics	Physostigmine
Anticholinesterases	Atropine
Benzodiazepines	Flumazenil
Carbon monoxide	Oxygen
Cyanide	Amyl nitrite, sodium nitrite, sodium thiosulfate, hydroxocobalamin
Ethylene glycol	Ethanol/fomepizole, thiamine, and pyridoxine
Hypoglycemic agents	Dextrose, glucagon, octreotide
Methanol	Ethanol or fomepizole, folic acid
Methemoglobinemia	Methylene blue
Opioids	Naloxone
Organophosphate	Atropine, pralidoxamine

Modified from Fabbri et al.,[323] with permission.

ABNORMALITIES OF IONIC OR ACID-BASE ENVIRONMENT OF THE CENTRAL NERVOUS SYSTEM

The term *osmolality* refers to the number of solute particles dissolved in a solvent. Osmolality is usually expressed as milliosmoles per liter

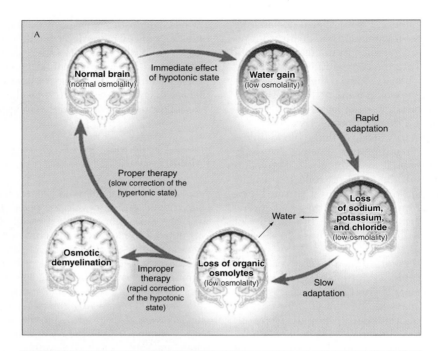

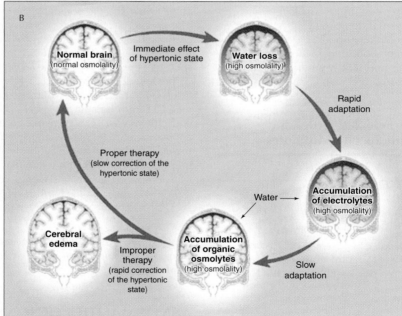

Figure 5–9. (A) Effects of hyponatremia on the brain and adaptive responses. Within minutes after the development of hypotonicity, water gain causes swelling of the brain and a decrease in osmolality of the brain. Partial restoration of brain volume occurs within a few hours as a result of cellular loss of electrolytes (rapid adaptation). The normalization of brain volume is completed within several days through loss of organic osmolytes from brain cells (slow adaptation). Low osmolality in the brain persists despite the normalization of brain volume. Proper correction of hypotonicity re-establishes normal osmolality without risking damage to the brain. Overly aggressive correction of hyponatremia can lead to irreversible brain damage. (B) Effects of hypernatremia on the brain and adaptive responses. Within minutes after the development of hypertonicity, loss of water from brain cells causes shrinkage of the brain and an increase in osmolality.

of water (mOsm/L). It can either be measured directly in the serum by the freezing point depression method or, for clinical purposes, calculated from the concentrations of sodium, potassium, glucose, and urea (the predominant solutes) in the serum (assuming that there is no intoxication). The formula below gives a rough but clinically useful approximation of the serum osmolality:

$$mOsm/kg = 2(Na + K) + \frac{glucose}{18} + \frac{BUN}{2.8}$$

Sodium and potassium are expressed in mEq/L, and the divisors convert glucose and BUN expressed in mg/dL to mEq/L. If the glucose and BUN are normal, the serum osmolality can be approximated by doubling the serum Na^+ and adding 10.

Normal serum osmolality is 290 ± 5 mOsm/kg. As indicated on page 248, a measured osmolality higher than the calculated osmolality indicates a substantial concentration of an unmeasured osmolar substance, usually a toxin. Hypo-osmolality leads to an increased cellular water content and tissue swelling. Only a few agents are equally and rapidly distributed throughout the body water (e.g., alcohol); therefore, hyperosmolality due to excess ethanol does not affect water distribution within the brain. However, the blood-brain barrier prevents most agents from entering the CNS. As a result, hyperosmolality due to these agents results in redistribution of water from within the CNS to the circulation. This property is used clinically when mannitol (a nonmetabolizable sugar) is injected intravenously to draw fluid out of the brain and temporarily decrease cerebral edema. However, the brain has protective mechanisms against osmolar shifts,[355] including slow redistribution of solutes, so that rapid changes in serum osmolality produce more prominent neurologic symptoms than slow changes. Direct measurement of osmolar substances using MRS demonstrates decreases

in myelinositol, choline, creatine, phosphocreatine, and probably glutamate/glutamine. Interestingly, in the patients studied who had chronic hyponatremia (mean serum sodium 120 mEq/L), there was no increase in water content.[356] Accordingly, it is not possible to give exact values above or below normal at which symptoms will develop. However, subacute changes in serum osmolalities below about 260 mEq/L, or above about 330 mEq/L over hours or a few days, are likely to produce cerebral symptoms. In addition, cerebral symptoms can be produced by sudden restorations of osmolality toward normal when an illness has produced a sustained osmolar shift away from normal. In extreme cases, this can cause central pontine myelinolysis (page 171).

Hypo-osmolar States

Sodium is the most abundant serum cation, and for practical purposes, systemic hypo-osmolarity occurs only in hyponatremic states. On the other hand, not all hyponatremic states are necessarily hypo-osmolar. For example, hyponatremia may be hyperosmolar, as with severe hyperglycemia (see page 171), or iso-osmolar, as, for example, during transurethral prostatic resection when large volumes of sodium-free irrigants are systemically absorbed.

Hyponatremia or *"water intoxication"* can cause delirium, obtundation, and coma, examples being encountered annually in almost all large hospitals. Symptoms result from water excess in the brain, hence the name water intoxication (Figure 5–9A). The pathogenesis of the symptoms caused by hyponatremia is probably multifactorial.[357,358] Water entering both neurons and glia causes brain edema and thus increased ICP. Brain herniation is probably the event leading to death. In an attempt to compensate, sodium and potassium are excreted from cells via a sodium-potassium

---

Partial restitution of brain volume occurs within a few hours as electrolytes enter the brain cells (rapid adaptation). The normalization of brain volume is completed within several days as a result of the intracellular accumulation of organic osmolytes (slow adaptation). The high osmolality persists despite the normalization of brain volume. Slow correction of the hypertonic state re-establishes normal brain osmolality without inducing cerebral edema, as the dissipation of accumulated electrolytes and organic osmolytes keeps pace with water repletion. In contrast, rapid correction may result in cerebral edema as water uptake by brain cells outpaces the dissipation of accumulated electrolytes and organic osmolytes. Such overly aggressive therapy carries the risk of serious neurologic impairment due to cerebral edema. (From Adrogue and Madias,[367] with permission.)

ATPase pump, altering membrane excitability[359] and perhaps causing the seizures that are common in severe hyponatremia. Seizures may lead to hypoxia, but whether hypoxia plays a significant role in the development of the clinical symptoms is unclear.[357]

Although acute hyponatremia can be fatal, chronic hyponatremia is usually only mildly symptomatic. The reason appears to be that the brain adapts to the hyponatremia by decreasing organic osmols within the cell, especially amino acids.[359,360] Acute hyponatremia is rarely a cause of emergency department visits. In a total of 44,826 emergency department visits, only 2.9% were hyponatremic, and of those only 11 (0.8%) of the hyponatremic patients presented with acute neurologic symptoms. The cause of the symptomatic hyponatremia was variable, but included increased water intake either from polydipsia or the use of herbal teas for weight reduction, drug abuse with MDMA, and use of diuretic agents. Women appear more susceptible than men. Of the 11 patients in this series, nine were women.[361] We have also encountered this problem in Shapiro's syndrome, in which there is paroxysmal hypothermia and sometimes hyponatremia in association with agenesis of the corpus callosum.[362]

The entry of water into the brain is promoted by aquaporin, a water channel protein present in both brain and choroid plexus.[363] In experimental animals, hyponatremia increases aquaporin-1 expression in the choroid plexus, allowing more water to enter the CSF and leading to apoptosis of cells surrounding the ventricular system.[363] There is also increased immunoreactivity of aquaporin-4, a channel that allows entry of water into glia.[364]

Most patients with slowly developing or only moderately severe hyponatremia are confused or delirious (Table 5–19).

With more severe or more rapidly developing hyponatremia, asterixis and multifocal myoclonus often appear. Coma is a late and life-threatening phase of water intoxication, and both coma and convulsions are more common with acute than chronic hyponatremia. Neurologic symptoms are rare with serum sodium above 120 mg/L and convulsions or coma generally do not occur until the serum sodium values reach 95 to 110 mEq/L (again, the more rapidly the serum sodium falls, the more likely the symptoms are to occur at a higher level). Permanent brain damage may follow hypona-

Table 5–19 Clinical Manifestations of Hyponatremic Encephalopathy

Early°	Anorexia
	Headache
	Nausea
	Emesis
	Muscular cramps
	Weakness
Advanced°	Impaired response to verbal stimuli
	Impaired response to painful stimuli
	Bizarre (inappropriate) behavior
	Hallucinations (auditory or visual)
	Asterixis
	Obtundation
	Incontinence (urinary or fecal)
	Respiratory insufficiency
Far advanced°	Decorticate and/or decerebrate posturing
	Bradycardia
	Hyper- or hypotension
	Altered temperature regulation (hypo- or hyperthermia)
	Dilated pupils
	Seizure activity (usually grand mal)
	Respiratory arrest
	Coma
	Polyuria (secondary to central diabetes insipidus)

°Any manifestation may be observed at any stage, and some patients will have only minimal symptoms.

From Videen et al.,[356] with permission.

tremic convulsions, and treatment with antiepileptic drugs is generally useless. The primary treatment must be directed at reversing the hyponatremia. Fraser and Arieff measured plasma sodium in 136 patients with hyponatremic encephalopathy. Premenopausal women developed severe symptoms at higher sodium levels than either postmenopausal women or men.[357]

Patient 5–21

A 33-year-old schoolteacher was admitted to the hospital in a coma. She had been working regularly until 2 days prior to admission when she stayed home with nausea and vomiting. Two hours before admission she was noted to be dysarthric when speaking on the telephone. Later she was found by friends on the floor, unconscious and cyanotic. She had three generalized convulsions and was brought to the hospital. Her blood pressure was 130/180 mm Hg, her pulse 140 per minute, her respirations 24 per minute and regular, and her body temperature 38.7°C. She did not respond to noxious stimulation. Her eyes deviated conjugately to the left at rest but turned conjugately to the right with passive head turning. Her pupils were 6 mm on the right and 5 mm on the left, and they briskly constricted to light stimulation. Both corneal reflexes were present. Her arms, hands, and fingers were flexed with spastic rigidity and irregular athetoid movements. Her legs and feet were rigidly extended. There were bilateral extensor plantar responses. She had three more convulsions that began in the right hand and then rapidly became generalized.

Despite extensive investigations and tests for metabolic aberrations or poisons, the only abnormalities found in this woman were of acute water intoxication. Her serum values were as follows: sodium 98 mEq/L, potassium 3.4 mEq/L, and osmolality 214 mOsm/L (normal = 290 ± 5). The BUN was 10 mg/dL. Water restriction and infusion of 5% NaCl returned the electrolyte values to normal. After several days she opened her eyes, grimaced when pinched, and moved all extremities. Her muscles remained rigid, however, especially on the right side, and she continued to have bilateral extensor plantar responses. She had no further seizures. Six months later she remained severely demented and unable to care for herself.

Comment: The cause of this patient's hyponatremia was never discovered. Excessive water intake in patients with no underlying metabolic problem, such as psychogenic polydipsia, is sometimes the cause. Hyponatremia has no pathognomonic signs or symptoms to suggest it in preference to other metabolic abnormalities, but should be suspected in patients who suddenly develop an unexplained encephalopathy or seizures, particularly if they are receiving diuretics, have carcinoma of the lung, or have neurologic disease. The diagnosis is possible if the serum sodium level falls below 120 mEq/L and highly likely when the sodium is below 115 mEq/L. The treatment of hyponatremia is to restore serum sodium to normal levels. This is usually done using hypertonic saline.[355,357,365] However, if the hyponatremia is corrected rapidly (greater than 25 mEq/L in the first

24 to 48 hours), patients, particularly those with liver disease or other severe illnesses, are at risk for developing demyelinating lesions in the brain.[357] Although called central pontine myelinolysis (see page 171), the disorder actually can affect the corpus callosum and other myelinated areas as well. Clinical symptoms include dysarthria, vertigo, quadriparesis, pseudobulbar palsy, confusion, and coma. The disorder can lead to death.[339] Hence, rapid reversal of hyponatremia is generally limited to patients with severe and acute symptoms and is controlled at about 15 mEq/L/day, although there is no absolute cutoff below which central pontine myelinolysis does not occur.

Hyperosmolar States

Physicians sometimes induce transient hyperosmolality by therapeutically using hypertonic solutions containing sodium chloride or mannitol to treat cerebral edema. Complications of hyperosmolarity only occasionally arise during such efforts. Much more frequent are hyperosmolarity problems arising with hypernatremia or with severe hyperglycemia. *Hypernatremia*[355] (Figure 5–9B) can be chronic or acute, the latter type being more prone to produce neurologic symptoms. Mild chronic hypernatremia occasionally occurs in chronic untreated diabetes insipidus caused by uncompensated water loss, but severe chronic hypernatremia with serum sodium levels in excess of 155 to 160 mEq/L is practically confined to the syndrome of essential hypernatremia. Essential hypernatremia usually is caused by a diencephalic abnormality and is characterized by a lack of thirst and a failure of ADH secretion to respond to osmoreceptor stimulation. In essential hypernatremia, serum sodium concentrations sometimes rise in excess of 170 mEq/L.[366] We have seen this disorder mainly in patients with lesions of the preoptic area along the lamina terminalis, but patients have been reported without macroscopic lesions. Most patients with significant hypernatremia complain of fatigue and weakness. They usually become lethargic when sodium levels exceed 160 mEq/L; with elevations above 180 mEq/L, most become confused or stuporous and some die. A danger is that too rapid rehydration of such chronically hypernatremic subjects can produce symptoms of water intoxication in the presence of serum sodium levels as high as 155 mEq/L (i.e., about 25 to 30 mEq below the level at which hydrating efforts began). The problem is especially frequent in children.[367,368]

Severe water depletion, producing acute hypernatremia, occurs in children with intense diarrhea and, occasionally, in adults with diabetes insipidus during circumstances that impair their thirst or access to adequate water replacement. Acute hypernatremia also occurs in obtunded patients receiving excessively concentrated solutions by tube feeding. As with other hyperosmolar states, blood volumes tend to be low because of excess free water losses (solute diuresis). Elevated levels of urea nitrogen, and sometimes glucose, contribute to the hyperosmolality. Symptoms of encephalopathy usually accompany serum sodium levels in excess of about 160 mEq/L or total osmolalities of 340 or more mOsm/kg, the earliest symptoms being delirium or a confusional state. Hypernatremic osmolality also should be considered when patients in coma receiving tube feedings show unexplained signs of worsening, especially if their treatment has included oral or systemic dehydrating agents. In the hypernatremic patient, sodium enters muscle cells, displacing potassium, and the eventual result is hypokalemia and a hypopolarized muscle cell that can be electrically inexcitable. Rhabdomyolysis may be the eventual result. Clinically patients have weak, flaccid muscles and absent deep tendon reflexes, and the muscles are electrically inexcitable.[366]

Nonketotic hyperglycemic hyperosmolality is a relatively common cause of acute or subacute stupor and coma, especially in elderly subjects.[369] The condition occurs principally in patients with mild or non-insulin-requiring diabetes, but has occasionally been encountered in nondiabetics with a hyperglycemic response after severe burns. Most, but not all, of the affected subjects are middle-aged or older, and a large percentage have an associated acute illness precipitating the hyperglycemic attack. In patients with symptoms, blood sugars may range from 800 to 1,200 mg/dL or more with total serum mOsm/kg in excess of 350.[270] An absence of or very low levels of ketonemia differentiates the condition from diabetic ketoacidosis with coma. In addition, one finds substantially more evidence of dehydration and hemoconcentration than in most

examples of early diabetic ketoacidosis. The pathogenesis of nonketotic hyperglycemia is believed to relate to a partial insulin deficiency, severe enough to interfere with glucose entry into cells, but not intense enough so that activation of the hepatic ketogenic sequence occurs. Certain drugs, including phenytoin, corticosteroids, and immunosuppressive agents, enhance the tendency to hyperglycemia. Dehydrating agents such as mannitol given unthinkingly to such patients can greatly intensify the hyperosmolality. In addition to its spontaneous occurrences, nonketotic hyperglycemia represents a prominent risk in neurologic patients, already obtunded from other illnesses, who receive corticosteroid drugs that have mineralocorticoid effects (e.g., hydrocortisone, prednisone) and whose fluids are restricted.

The clinical presentation of hyperglycemic hyperosmolar coma consists of signs of systemic dehydration accompanied by lethargic confusion progressing into deep stupor or coma. Generalized, focal, or partial continuous seizures occur in about one-fifth of the cases, and focal, stroke-like motor deficits affect about one-quarter. Laboratory studies disclose severe hyperglycemia combined with evidence of severe dehydration of body fluids. Perhaps one-quarter of the patients have a mild to moderate lactic acidosis, and many have signs of at least mild renal insufficiency. Untreated, all patients die, and even the best efforts at therapy fail in some, largely because of the seriousness of associated illnesses. Hyperglycemia in and of itself can affect cognitive function. In a study of adults with either type 1 or type 2 diabetes, blood glucose levels greater than 270 mg/dL were associated with slow cognitive performance tests, impacting around 50% of the 105 subjects investigated.[71] A rare complication of the diabetic hyperosmolar nonketotic state is acute nontraumatic rhabdomyolysis that may lead to renal failure.[370]

Calcium

Both high and low serum calcium values can be associated with neurologic abnormalities.[371]

HYPERCALCEMIA

An elevated serum calcium level may be due to the effects of primary hyperparathyroidism, immobilization, or cancer. Hypercalcemia is a common and important complication of cancer, resulting from either metastatic lesions that demineralize the bones or as a remote effect of parathyroid hormone-secreting tumors. Hyperparathyroidism due to a benign parathyroid adenoma is also a common cause.[372] The systemic clinical symptoms of hypercalcemia include anorexia, nausea and frequently vomiting, intense thirst, polyuria, and polydipsia. Muscle weakness can be prominent and neurogenic atrophy has been reported. Some patients with hypercalcemia have as their first symptom a mild diffuse encephalopathy with headache. Delusions and changes in affect can be prominent, so that many such patients have been initially treated for a psychiatric disorder until the blood calcium level was measured. With severe hypercalcemia, stupor and finally coma occur. Generalized or focal seizures are rare. The posterior leukoencephalopathy syndrome (see page 215) has been reported in association with severe hypercalcemia.

Hypercalcemia should be suspected in a delirious patient who has a history of renal calculi, recent immobilization, cancer, or evidence of any other systemic disease known to cause the condition.[373] A serum calcium determination is therefore a routine part of the evaluation in patients with unexplained delirium or confusional states.

HYPOCALCEMIA

Hypocalcemia is usually caused by hypoparathyroidism (often occurring late and unsuspected after thyroidectomy), pancreatitis, or, rarely, an idiopathic disorder of calcium metabolism. The cardinal peripheral manifestations of hypocalcemia are neuromuscular irritability and tetany, but these may be absent when hypocalcemia develops insidiously. Accordingly, patients with hypoparathyroid hypocalcemia can sometimes present with a mild diffuse encephalopathy as their only symptom. Seizures, either focal or generalized, are common, especially in children. With more severe cases, excitement, delirium, hallucinations, and stupor have been reported. Except postictally, however, coma is rare. Papilledema has been reported, associated with an increased ICP. This hypocalcemic pseudotumor cerebri apparently is a direct effect of the metabolic abnormality, but the precise mechanism remains unexplained.[371]

Hypocalcemia is commonly misdiagnosed as mental retardation, dementia, or epilepsy, and occasionally a brain tumor is suspected. Hypocalcemia should be suspected if the patient has cataracts, and the correct diagnosis sometimes can be inferred from observing calcification in the basal ganglia on CT scan. Normally, serum calcium levels run from 8.5 to 10.5 mg/dL. About half of this is bound to albumin and half represents free ions. For each 1.0 g/dL drop in serum albumin below about 5, the serum calcium falls by about 0.8 mg/dL. Thus, with an albumin of 2.0 g/dL, a normal serum calcium may be as low as 7.0 mg/dL. To avoid making this extrapolation, if there is any question about the calcium level, the free serum calcium should be measured. A free calcium level below 4.0 mg/dL is diagnostic of hypocalcemia.

Chronic hypocalcemia may cause chorea and parkinsonism, along with calcifications in the basal ganglia. Tetany caused by spontaneous, irregular repetitive nerve action potentials is a common complication of hypocalcemia, as Patient 5–22 demonstrates.

Patient 5–22

An 18-year-old woman had been treated for an osteogenic sarcoma. Surgery was followed by cisplatin-based chemotherapy. Five years later following reconstructive surgery on her leg, she complained of numbness and tingling of both hands and arms spreading into the face and followed by spasms of her arms, which lasted several hours. A diagnosis of panic attack was made and after sedation the symptoms cleared. Other attacks followed but were milder until 2001; while the patient was in bed with a viral illness, the symptoms were so severe that she was taken to an emergency department where sedation was again applied. She was referred for evaluation of anxiety and panic attacks. The general neurologic examination was entirely normal. However, a Trousseau's sign elicited by raising the pressure in a blood pressure cuff above systolic pressure for 3 minutes demonstrated carpal spasms bilaterally. Voluntary hyperventilation for 2 minutes reproduced the carpal spasms and paresthesias in both hands. Chvostek's sign elicited by tapping over the facial nerve in front of the ear also elicited contraction of the facial muscles, particularly the orbicularis oculi. Serum calcium was 7.5 mEq/L (normal = 8.5 to 10.5); serum albumin was normal, but ionized calcium was 3.8 mEq/L (normal = 4.8 to 5.3). Serum magnesium and potassium were also low. The patient responded to electrolyte replacement.

Comment: Cisplatin and ifosfamide are drugs that can cause calcium- and magnesium-losing nephropathy. Both low magnesium (see below) and low ionized calcium that result from a magnesium loss can cause hyperventilation that further lowers ionized calcium, presumably by increasing the binding of calcium to albumin, thus causing tetany. The patient's two severe attacks probably resulted from anxiety-induced hyperventilation.

Other Electrolytes

Hypo- and hypermagnesemia are rare causes of neurologic symptomatology.[371] Hypomagnesemia, like hypercalcemia, causes irritability and tetany as described in the case above, sometimes with seizures and confusion. Focal neurologic signs sometimes occur. Because hypomagnesemia and hypocalcemia often occur together, it is sometimes difficult to determine which is the culprit. Both should be corrected.

Hypermagnesemia is even rarer than hypomagnesemia. It is mainly seen in the obstetric suite when eclampsia is treated with intravenous infusion of magnesium sulfate. Magnesium blocks calcium channels, so there is failure of neurotransmission. Muscles are flaccid and deep tendon reflexes disappear early. The muscle weakness may involve respiratory muscles, causing hypoxia. If high levels persist, they may equilibrate across the blood-brain barrier, resulting in lethargy and confusion and rarely coma.

Hypophosphatemia can occur during nutritional repletion, with gastrointestinal malabsorption, use of phosphate binders, starvation, diabetes mellitus, and renal tubular dysfunction. Delirium, stupor, and coma have been reported, as have generalized convulsions.[374] Phosphate repletion reverses the symptoms. Hyperphosphatemia can occur with rhabdomyolysis or during the tumor lysis syndrome, but does not appear to cause neurologic symptoms.[278]

Disorders of Systemic Acid-Base Balance

Systemic acidosis and alkalosis accompany several diseases that cause metabolic coma, and the attendant respiratory and acid-base changes can give important clues about the cause of coma (see page 188 and Table 5–3). However, of the four disorders of systemic acid-base balance (respiratory and metabolic acidosis and respiratory and metabolic alkalosis), only respiratory acidosis acts as a direct cause of stupor and coma with any regularity.[255] Even then, the associated hypoxia may be as important as is the acidosis in producing the neurologic abnormality. Metabolic acidosis, the most immediately medically dangerous of the acid-base disorders, by itself only rarely produces coma. Usually, metabolic acidosis is associated with delirium or, at most, confused obtundation. Respiratory alkalosis under most circumstances causes no more than light-headedness and confusion, which is believed to be due to decreased CBF in the face of low PCO_2. However, when respiratory alkalosis[26] is caused by overcorrection of chronic pulmonary failure, the resulting large drop in PCO_2, while serum bicarbonate corrects more slowly, can cause stupor or coma associated with multifocal myoclonus due to cerebral ischemia resulting from the large decrease of CBF.[375] Severe metabolic alkalosis has occasionally been reported to cause encephalopathy and rarely seizures. Tetany may occur, probably related to decreased ionizable calcium.[32] Compensation for metabolic alkalosis with hypoventilation and a rising PCO_2 may play a role in decreasing consciousness, and in adult patients with cystic fibrosis may contribute to respiratory failure.[35] If patients with acid-base disorders other than respiratory acidosis or severe and protracted metabolic acidosis are in stupor or coma, it is unlikely that the acid-base disturbance by itself is responsible. Instead, it is more likely is that the metabolic defect responsible for the acid-base disturbance (e.g., uremia, hepatic encephalopathy, or circulatory depression leading to lactic acidosis) also is directly interfering with brain function.

A useful clinical clue to the presence and possible cause of metabolic acidosis or certain other electrolyte disorders comes from estimating the anion gap from the measured blood electrolytes. The calculation is based on the known electroneutrality of the serum, which requires the presence of an equal number of anions (negative charges) and cations (positive charges). For practical purposes, sodium and potassium (or sodium alone) represent 95% of the cations, whereas the most abundant and conveniently measured anions, chloride and bicarbonate, add up to only 85% of the normal total. The result is an anion gap in unmeasured electrolytes that amounts normally to about 12 ± 4 mEq/L:

$$(Na + K) - (Cl^- + HCO_3)$$
$$= 8 \text{ to } 16 \text{ mEq/L}$$

An increase in the anion gap ordinarily implies the presence of an undetected electrolyte (either an endogenous or exogenous toxin) causing a metabolic acidosis, and should prompt an immediate search by deduction and specific test for the "missing anion."

DISORDERS OF THERMOREGULATION

Both hyperthermia and hypothermia can interfere with cerebral metabolism, causing diffuse neurologic signs including delirium, stupor, or coma. Brain temperature is affected both by body temperature and the intrinsic metabolic activity of the brain. Under normal circumstances, the brain is about 0.4°C warmer than arterial blood with considerable variability from area to area.[376] Brain temperature can fluctuate 3°C to 4°C during normal behavioral activity and more so when exposed to certain drugs (see below). Current evidence suggests that brain cells can tolerate temperatures of no more than 41°C.[376] After that, cellular death of neurons such as Purkinje cells of the cerebellum begins; as a result, patients recovering from heat stroke may suffer severe and permanent ataxia.[377] When brain temperature rises, either because of its own activity or an increase in body temperature, there is an increase in blood flow, which is usually greater than that required by the increase in metabolism. Vasodilation from the increased blood flow reduces brain temperature toward that of blood but increases blood volume and, therefore, ICP. This can harm the brain, particularly when ICP is already elevated from the brain injury or tumor. Thus, hyperthermia is more damaging to injured brain, for example, after traumatic brain injury, than it is to normal brain, for example, after heat stroke. Hyperthermia also can be devastating in patients who have suffered a cerebral infarct, because the CBF cannot increase to meet metabolic demands in the ischemic area, but the increase in flow to other brain areas may be at the expense of perfusion of the ischemic penumbra.

Hypothermia

Hypothermia results from a variety of illnesses including disorders of the hypothalamus, myxedema, hypopituitarism, and bodily exposure.[378,379] A low body temperature may accompany metabolic coma, particularly hypoglycemia and drug-induced coma, especially that resulting from barbiturate overdose, phenothiazine overdose, or alcoholism. With decreasing body temperature, cerebral metabolic needs decrease and, thus, CBF and oxygen consumption fall. In the absence of any underlying disease that may be causing both coma and hypothermia, there is a rough correlation among the body temperature, cerebral oxygen uptake, and state of consciousness. Unless there is some other metabolic reason for stupor or coma, patients with body temperatures above 32.2°C are usually conscious. Initially, patients are tachypneic, tachycardic, and shivering with intense peripheral vasoconstriction and sometimes elevated blood pressure. As time passes, patients may become apathetic, uncoordinated, and hypobulic.[378] At temperatures between 28°C and 32.2°C, patients become stuporous or comatose with slowed respiration and bradycardia. Hypotension and atrial dysrhythmias may occur. Below 28°C respirations may cease, pupils become nonreactive, and the EEG may become flat. Patients may develop pulmonary edema or ventricular dysrhythmias.

Clinically, accidental hypothermia (i.e., hypothermia in the absence of any predisposing cause) is a disease mainly of elderly people exposed to a moderately cold environment (i.e., mainly during the winter months). It is also seen with ethanol intoxication, and may be an important component of suppression of cerebral function in many drownings. Hypothermic patients are often found unconscious in a cold environment, although fully one-third are found in their beds rather than out in the street. The patients who are unconscious are strikingly pale, have a pliable consistency of subcutaneous tissue, and may have the appearance of myxedema even though that disease is not present. Shivering is absent if the temperature falls below 30°C, but there may be occasional fascicular twitching over the shoulders and trunk, and there is usually a diffuse increase in muscle tone leading almost to the appearance of rigor mortis. The body feels cold to the touch even in protected areas such as the perineum. Respirations are slow and shallow and there can be CO_2 retention. The blood pressure may be immeasurable and the pulse very slow or absent. Some patients are thought to be dead when first encountered. At times the deep tendon reflexes are absent, but usually they are present and may be hyperactive; they may, however, have a delayed relaxation phase resembling that of myxedema. The pupils may be constricted or dilated and reportedly may not respond to light. The EEG is diffusely slow without reduction in amplitude. One makes the diagnosis by recording the body temperature and ruling out precipitating causes other than exposure. Standard clinical thermometers do not register below 34.4°C (94°F); thus, simple perusal of the chart of temperatures taken by the nursing staff may not reveal the true severity of the hypothermia. Furthermore, it is not clear how accurate tympanic thermometers are in patients with severe hypothermia. The perceptive physician must procure a thermometer that records sufficiently low readings to verify his or her clinical impression. Hypothermia carries a high mortality rate (40% to 60%). However, those who do recover rarely suffer residual neurologic changes. In fact, hypothermia is neuroprotective and is routinely used by cardiothoracic surgeons to extend the amount of time they can suspend cerebral circulation during surgery on the heart or the aortic arch. Therapeutic hypothermia is also being increasingly used for the treatment of a variety of neurologic disorders, particularly head injuries and cardiac arrest.[380] Similarly, hypothermic drowning victims, particularly children, may be successfully resuscitated after much longer periods of respiratory arrest than normothermic individuals. Brain injuries

in patients who die include perivascular hemorrhages in the region of the third ventricle with chromatolysis of ganglion cells. Multifocal infarcts have been described in several viscera, including the brain, and probably reflect the cardiovascular collapse that complicates severe hypothermia. Hypothermia may be complicated by rhabdomyolysis leading to renal failure.

A rare cause of hypothermia is paroxysmal hypothermia, a condition in which patients with developmental defects in the anterior hypothalamus have intermittent episodes of hypothermia, down to a body temperature of 30°C or even lower, lasting several days at a time, accompanied by ataxia, stupor, and sometimes coma. Shapiro and colleagues pointed out an association with agenesis of the corpus callosum, which is sometimes accompanied by episodic hyponatremia (see above).[381] Although spontaneous and complete recovery is the rule with supportive care, we have treated these patients with non-steroidal anti-inflammatory drugs and this, anecdotally, has increased body temperature.

Hyperthermia

Fever, the most common cause of hyperthermia in humans, is a regulated increase in body temperature in response to an inflammatory stimulus. Fever is caused by the action of prostaglandin E2, which is made in response to inflammatory stimuli, on neurons in the preoptic area. The preoptic neurons then activate thermogenic pathways in the brain that increase body temperature. It is rare for fever to produce a body temperature above 40°C to 41°C, which has only limited effects on cognitive function. Hence, changes in consciousness in patients with fever are mainly due to neuronal effects of the underlying inflammatory condition itself, not the change in body temperature (see section on infectious and inflammatory disorders of the CNS, page 262).

On the other hand, hyperthermia of 42°C or higher, which is sufficient to produce stupor or coma, can occur with *heatstroke*.[382] Heat stroke, caused by failure of the brain's physiologic mechanisms for heat dissipation, occurs most commonly in young people who exercise unduly in heat to which they are not acclimatized, and in older people (who presumably possess less plastic adaptive mechanisms), particularly during the summer's first hot spell.[382] It is a particular threat in patients taking anticholinergic drugs, which interfere with heat dissipation by inhibiting sweating, and is also seen in rare patients with hypothalamic lesions who lack appropriate thirst and vasopressin responses to conserve fluid.

Clinically, heat stroke typically begins with headache and nausea, although some patients may first come to attention due to a period of agitated and violent delirium, sometimes punctuated by generalized convulsions, or they may just lapse into stupor or coma. The patient's skin is usually hot and dry, although sweating occasionally persists during the course of heat stroke. The patient is tachycardic, may be normotensive or hypotensive, and may have a serum pH that is normal or slightly acidotic. The pupils are usually small and reactive, caloric responses are present except terminally, and the skeletal muscles are usually diffusely hypotonic in contradistinction to malignant hyperthermia (see below). The diagnosis is made by recording an elevated body temperature, generally in excess of 42°C.[383] As with hypothermia, clinical thermometers usually reach a maximum at 108°F or 42°C, but a temperature of this level does not mean that the patient cannot be warmer.

Heatstroke is easily distinguished from fever because fever of all types is governed by neural mechanisms and does not reach 42°C. It is produced by peripheral vasoconstriction and increased muscle tone and shivering (i.e., the opposite pattern to hyperthermia). The main danger of heatstroke is vascular collapse due to hypovolemia often accompanied by ventricular arrhythmias. Patients with heat stroke must be treated emergently with rapid intravenous volume expansion and vigorous cooling by immersion in ice water, or ice, or evaporative cooling (a cooling blanket is far too slow). If cardiac arrest is avoided, permanent neurologic sequelae are rare. However, some patients exposed to very high temperatures for a prolonged time are left with permanent neurologic residua including cerebellar ataxia, dementia, and hemiparesis.

Hyperthermia may also occur in patients after severe traumatic brain injury.[384] In most cases this is a fever response due to the presence of inflammatory cytokines within the blood-brain barrier. However, in some cases (e.g., preoptic lesions or pontine hemorrhages) it may be due to damage to descending neural pathways that inhibit thermogenesis. Risk factors in patients with traumatic brain injury include diffuse axonal injury and frontal lobe injury of any type, but hyperthermia is common when there is subarachnoid hemorrhage as well. Characteristically the patient is tachycardic, the skin is dry, and the temperature rises to a plateau that does not change for days to a week. The fever is resistant to antipyretic agents and usually occurs several days after the injury. The prognosis in patients with fever due to brain injury is worse than those without it, but whether that is related to the extent of the injury or the hyperthermia is unclear.[384]

Three related syndromes related to intake of drugs may cause severe hyperthermia. These syndromes are the neuroleptic malignant syndrome, malignant hyperthermia, and the serotonin syndrome. The syndromes, although clinically similar, can be distinguished both by the setting in which they occur and by some differences in their physical sign. The *neuroleptic malignant syndrome* is an idiosyncratic reaction either to the intake of neuroleptic drugs or to the withdrawal of dopamine agonists. The disorder is rare and generally begins shortly after the patient has begun the drug (typical drugs include high-potency neuroleptics such as haloperidol, and atypical neuroleptics such as risperidone or prochlorperazine, but phenothiazines and metoclopramide have also been reported). The onset is usually acute with hyperthermia greater than 38°C and delirium, which may lead to coma. Patients are tachycardic and diaphoretic with rigid muscles and may have dystonic or choreiform movements.[385] There is usually leukocytosis and there may be a dramatically elevated creatine kinase level. Rhabdomyolysis leading to renal failure may occur.[386] The diagnosis can be made by recognizing that the patient has been on a neuroleptic agent (usually for a short time) or has withdrawn from dopamine agonists. Hyperreflexia, clonus, and myoclonus, which characterize the serotonin syndrome (see below), are usually not present. The neuroleptic malignant syndrome does not typically occur on first exposure to the drug, or if the patient is rechallenged, and may be due to the coincident occurrence of a febrile illness and increased muscle tone in a patient with limited dopaminergic tone.

Malignant hyperthermia occurs in about one in 50,000 adults during induction of general anesthesia.[387] As the name indicates, the patients become hyperthermic and develop tachycardia and muscle rigidity with lactic acidosis. Serum creatine kinase is elevated and patients may develop rhabdomyolysis. Pulmonary and cerebral edema can develop late and be potentially fatal.[387] The syndrome occurs with a variety of anesthetics and muscle relaxants in patients who have genetic defects of one of several receptors controlling the release of sarcoplasmic calcium in skeletal muscle. When exposed to the agent, sudden increases in intracellular calcium result in the clinical findings. Dantrolene sodium is an effective antidote.

The *serotonin syndrome* results when patients take agents that either increase the release of serotonin or inhibit its uptake. Common causes include cocaine and methamphetamine as well as serotonin reuptake inhibitors. Less common causes include dextromethorphan, meperidine, L-dopa, bromocriptine, tramadol, and lithium.[387] Patients become delirious or stuporous. They are febrile, diaphoretic, and tachycardic and demonstrate mydriasis. Reflexes are hyperactive with clonus. Spontaneous myoclonus as well as muscular rigidity may be present. More serious intoxication may lead to rhabdomyolysis, metabolic acidosis, and hyperkalemia. The disorder usually begins within 24 hours of having taken the medication. It is rather abrupt in onset; patients usually recover.

INFECTIOUS DISORDERS OF THE CENTRAL NERVOUS SYSTEM: BACTERIAL

This section describes a group of disorders in which an accurate diagnosis of stupor or coma carries the highest priority. The conditions are relatively common and many of them perturb or depress the state of consciousness as a first symptom. Symptoms of CNS infection can easily mimic those of other illnesses. Quick and accurate action is nowhere more necessary, because proper treatment often is brain saving or even lifesaving, whereas delays or errors often result in irreversible neurologic deficits or death.

CNS infections in immunocompromised patients are particularly difficult to diagnose and treat for two reasons: (1) symptoms and signs, save for delirium or stupor, may be absent and the patient may have other reasons for being encephalopathic. Furthermore, the immunosuppression may prevent the patient from mounting an inflammatory response and thus the spinal fluid may not suggest infection. In addition, imaging may either be normal or nonspecific. (2) The organisms infecting the CNS in an immunocompromised patient are different from those encountered in the general population. However, being aware of the nature of the immunocompromise, and the variety of organisms that tend to affect such patients, can often lead to an effective early diagnosis and treatment.[388,389]

Acute Bacterial Leptomeningitis

Acute leptomeningeal infections frequently cause alterations in consciousness. In one series of 696 episodes of community-acquired acute bacterial meningitis, 69% of patients had some alteration of consciousness and 14% were comatose. Seizures had occurred in 5%.[390] In a review of 317 patients with CNS *Listeria*, 59 (19%) were stuporous and 76 (24%) were comatose.[391] Leptomeningeal infections produce stupor and coma in one of several ways, as follows.

TOXIC ENCEPHALOPATHY

Both the bacterial invaders and the inflammatory response to them can have profound effects on cerebral metabolism, causing neuronal injury or death. The injury is mediated by a release of reactive oxygen species, proteases, cytokines, and excitatory amino acids. Both apoptosis and necrosis can occur.[392]

BACTERIAL ENCEPHALITIS AND VASCULITIS

The bacteria that cause acute leptomeningitis often invade the cerebrum, penetrating via the Virchow-Robin perivascular spaces and causing inflammation of both penetrating meningeal vessels and the brain itself.[393] The effects on the brain are both vascular and metabolic. Vasculitis induces diffuse or focal ischemia of the underlying brain and can lead to focal areas of necrosis. Diffuse necrosis of the subcortical white matter has also been reported as a complication of such bacterial vasculitis. Cerebral veins may be occluded, as well as arteries.[393]

INAPPROPRIATE THERAPY

The fluid therapy employed for patients with acute leptomeningitis carries a potential risk of inducing acute water intoxication unless carefully regulated. Many patients with bacterial meningitis suffer from inappropriate ADH secretion, which leads to hyponatremia and cerebral edema when excessive amounts of water are infused.

CEREBRAL HERNIATION

As a result of the above mechanisms, severe leptomeningeal infection is often accompanied by considerable cerebral edema, especially in young persons. Cerebral edema is an almost invariable finding in fatal leptomeningitis, and the degree may be so great that it causes both transtentorial and cerebellar tonsillar herniation. In a series of 87 adults with pneumococcal meningitis, diffuse brain edema was encountered in 29%.[393] In addition, leptomeningeal infections occlude CSF absorptive pathways and, depending on the site of occlusion, cause either communicating or noncommunicating hydrocephalus in about 15% of patients.[393] Shunting of the ventricles may be required to relieve the pressure. The enlargement of the ventricles by nonreabsorbed CSF adds to increased ICP and increases the risk of cerebral herniation.

All of these mechanisms lead to a form of stupor and coma that closely resembles that produced by other metabolic diseases, leading us to include acute leptomeningitis in this section. However, it is important not to lose sight of the possibility that as the patient's condition worsens, a structural component may also supervene.

The meningeal infections that produce coma are principally those caused by acute bacterial organisms. The major causes of community-acquired bacterial meningitis include *Streptococcus pneumoniae* (51%) and *Neisseria meninigitis* (37%).[390] In immunocompromised patients, *Listeria monocytogenes* meningitis accounts for about 4% of cases.[391,394,395] *Listeria* meningitis may be noticeably slower in its course, but has a tendency to cause brainstem abscesses. *Staphylococcus aureus* and, since a vaccine became available, *Haemophilus influ-*

enzae are uncommon causes of community-acquired meningitis.[390]

CLINICAL FEATURES

The clinical appearance of acute meningitis is one of an acute metabolic encephalopathy with drowsiness or stupor accompanied by the toxic symptoms of chills, fever, tachycardia, and tachypnea. Most patients have either a headache or a history of it. However, the classic triad of fever, nuchal rigidity, and alteration of mental status was present in only 44% of patients in a large series of community-acquired meningitis.[390] Focal neurologic signs were present in one-third and included cranial nerve palsies, aphasia, and hemiparesis; papilledema was found in only 3%. CT or MRI may show enhancement in cerebral sulci (Figure 5–10).

Meningitis, particularly in children, can cause acute brain edema with transtentorial herniation as the initial sign. Clinically, such children rapidly lose consciousness and develop hyperpnea disproportionate to the degree of fever. The pupils dilate, at first moderately and then widely, then fix, and the child develops decerebrate motor signs. Urea, mannitol, or other hyperosmotic agents, if used properly, can prevent or reverse the full development of the ominous changes that are otherwise rapidly fatal. In this situation, some believe that a diagnostic lumbar puncture may lead to transtentorial herniation and death. On the other hand, delaying lumbar puncture to procure a CT scan places the patient at major risk, and if the edema is diffuse, the scan does not indicate the risk of herniation.[396–398] Hence, it is now standard practice to draw blood cultures, start empiric antibiotic therapy, procure a CT scan, and then do a lumbar puncture if there does not appear to be evidence of marked cerebral edema or shift.[399]

In elderly patients, bacterial meningitis sometimes presents as insidiously developing stupor or coma in which there may be focal neurologic signs but little evidence of severe systemic illness or stiff neck. In older patients, a stiff neck may result from cervical osteoarthritis. However, the neck is usually also stiff in the lateral direction as well as in the anterior-posterior direction, a finding not present in meningitis. Furthermore, a positive Kernig sign (resistance to extension of the knee when the hip is flexed) or Brudzinski sign (flexion

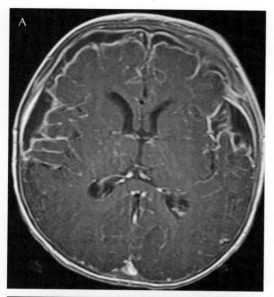

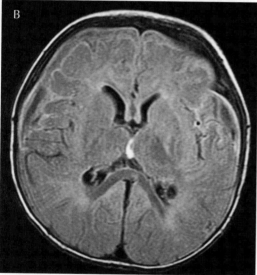

Figure 5–10. (A) A contrast-enhanced T1 image of a patient with acute bacterial meningitis. There is marked enhancement in several of the cerebral sulci. The cortex and the underlying brain appear normal. Hyperintensity in cerebral sulci is apparent on the FLAIR (B) image. (Magnetic resonance image courtesy Dr. Linda Hier.)

of the hips when the neck is flexed) is pathognomonic of meningeal irritation.

In one series, 50% of patients with meningitis were admitted to the hospital with an incorrect diagnosis.[397,398] Such patients can be regarded incorrectly as having suffered a stroke, but this error is readily avoided by accurate spinal fluid

examinations. Another pitfall is the difficulty of assessing the CSF when blood due to a traumatic lumbar puncture obscures the elevated spinal fluid white cell count. With acute subarachnoid bleeding, there is approximately one white cell to each 1,000 red cells in the CSF. When there are more than two or three white cells beyond this ratio, the patient should be treated as if there were meningitis until proven otherwise by a repeat tap or negative cultures.

Patients are occasionally observed who develop the encephalopathy of meningitis before white cells appear in the lumbar spinal fluid. The series of Carpenter and Petersdorf[400] includes several such cases, and the following is an example from our own series.

Patient 5–23

A 28-year-old man complained of mild diurnal temperature elevation for several days with intermittent sore throat, chills, and malaise. He had no muscle or joint complaints or cough, but his chest felt tight. He saw his physician, who found him to be warm and appear acutely ill, but he lacked significant abnormalities on examination, except that his pharynx and ear canals were reddened. A diagnosis of influenza was made, but the next afternoon he had difficulty thinking clearly and was admitted to the hospital.

His blood pressure was 90/70 mm Hg, pulse 120 per minute, respirations 20 per minute, and body temperature 38.6°C. He was acutely ill, restless, and unable to sustain his attention to cooperate fully in the examination. No rash or petechiae were seen. There was slight nuchal rigidity and some mild spasm of the back and hamstring muscles. The remainder of the physical and the neurologic examination was normal. The white blood count was 18,000/mm³ with a left shift. Urinalysis was normal. A lumbar puncture was performed with the patient in the lateral recumbent position; the opening pressure was 210 mm, the closing pressure was 170 mm, and the clear CSF contained one red cell and no white cells. The next morning the protein was reported as 80 mg/dL, the glucose content as 0.

The first evening at 9 p.m. his temperature had declined to 38°C and he was seemingly improved. Two hours later he had a chill followed by severe headache and he became slightly irrational. The body temperature was 37.6°C. There was an increase in the nuchal rigidity with increased hamstring and back muscle spasm. The white blood count had increased to 23,000/mm³. Shortly before 1:30 a.m., he became delirious and then comatose with irregular respiration. The pupils were equal and reactive; the optic fundi were normal; the deep tendon reflexes were equal and active throughout. The left plantar response was extensor, the right was equivocal. Because of the high white cell count, fever, and coma, administration of large doses of antibiotics was started, but the diagnosis was uncertain.

The next morning the spinal fluid and throat cultures that had been obtained the evening before were found to contain *Neisseria meningitides* and a lumbar puncture now revealed purulent spinal fluid containing 6,000 white cells/mm³ under a high pressure, with high protein and low glucose contents.

Comment: The error in diagnosis in this patient was in failing to ensure that a CSF Gram stain, protein, and glucose were done and checked immediately by the physicians, who were lured into a false sense of security by the absence of white blood cells in the CSF. In addition, if meningitis or other CNS infection is suspected, even if no cells are found in the initial examination, the lumbar puncture should be repeated in about 6 hours. Patients with overwhelming meningococcal septicemia, and few or no polymorphonuclear leukocytes in their spinal fluid, represent the worst prognostic group of patients with acute bacterial meningitis. Although a high concentration of polymorphonuclear leukocytes and a decreased spinal fluid glucose strongly suggest the diagnosis of bacterial meningitis, viral infections including mumps and herpes simplex can also occasionally cause hypoglycorrhachia.

Chronic Bacterial Meningitis

Although there are many bacterial causes of chronic meningitis, including syphilis, Lyme disease, nocardia, and actinomycosis, only two commonly come into the differential diagnosis of impairment of consciousness.

TUBERCULOUS MENINGITIS

Although tuberculosis is usually considered a subacute or chronic disease, tuberculous men-

ingoencephalitis may have a fulminant course. Fewer than 50% of adults with meningoencephalitis have a history of pulmonary tuberculosis.[401] On examination patients are lethargic, stuporous, or comatose with nuchal rigidity. The CSF is characterized by an elevated opening pressure with one to 500 white blood cells, which are mainly lymphocytes or monocytes, resembling more an aseptic than an infective meningitis. The protein concentration is elevated (above 100 mg/dL) and the glucose concentration is usually decreased, but rarely below 20 mg/dL. Organisms are seen on smear in a minority of patients. Cultures of the CSF may be negative, but even if positive, take several weeks to develop. Polymerase chain reaction (PCR) techniques are rapid and specific; however, sensitivity has been reported to range from 25% to 80%.[401] Neuroimaging is nonspecific, demonstrating contrast enhancement of the meninges and often hydrocephalus.

Because the cell count in the spinal fluid is often low or even absent, the disorder may be confused with other causes of so-called aseptic meningitis including sarcoidosis, leptomeningeal metastases, Wegener's granulomatosis, and Behçet's disease. The severity of the illness should lead one to suspect the possibility of tuberculosis. Untreated, patients usually die within a few weeks.

WHIPPLE'S DISEASE

Whipple's disease is a systemic inflammatory disorder caused by a bacterium, *Trophermyma whippleii*.[402] It most commonly affects middle-aged men. There may be systemic symptoms including weight loss, abdominal pain, diarrhea, arthralgias, and uveitis. However, in some cases the symptoms are restricted to the CNS and often are characterized by encephalopathy or even coma.[403] Brainstem signs, especially ataxia and focal or generalized seizures, are common, as is dementia. The characteristic neurologic abnormality in these patients is oculomasticatory myorhythmia, a slow convergence nystagmus accompanied by synchronous contraction of the jaw. The myorhythmias are present in only about 20% of patients and are always associated with a supranuclear vertical gaze palsy. The spinal fluid may demonstrate a pleocytosis but may be entirely benign. MRI is nonspecific showing hyperintense signal in the hypothalamus and brainstem sometimes with abnormal enhancement, but without mass effect. Lesions are frequently multiple.

The diagnosis, if suspected, can often be made by intestinal biopsy or sometimes by PCR of the spinal fluid, but may require meningeal biopsy.[404] The disease is curable with antibiotics but lethal if not treated.

INFECTIOUS DISORDERS OF THE CENTRAL NERVOUS SYSTEM: VIRAL

Overview of Viral Encephalitis

Viruses, bacteria, rickettsia, protozoa, and nematodes can all invade brain parenchyma. However, only viruses, bacteria, and the rickettsial infection Rocky Mountain spotted fever[405] invade the brain acutely and diffusely enough to cause altered states of consciousness and to demand immediate attention in the diagnosis of stupor or coma. Bacterial encephalitis has been considered above as a part of meningitis. Viral encephalitis is discussed in this section.

Viral encephalitis can be divided into four pathologic syndromes. These syndromes are sometimes clinically distinct as well, but the clinical signs of the first three are often so similar as to preclude specific diagnosis without biopsy, CSF PCR,[406] or, sometimes, autopsy. (1) *Acute viral encephalitis* results from invasion of the brain by a virus that produces primarily or exclusively a CNS infection.[407] (2) *Parainfectious encephalomyelitis* also occurs during or after viral infections, particularly the childhood infections of measles, mumps, and varicella.[407] (3) *Acute toxic encephalopathy* usually occurs during the course of a systemic infection with a common virus. (4) *Progressive viral infections* are encephalitides caused by conventional viral agents but occurring in susceptible patients, usually those who are immunosuppressed, or who develop the infection in utero or during early childhood. Such infections lead to slow or progressive destruction of the nervous system. During intrauterine development these disorders include cytomegalovirus, rubella, and herpes infections, although nonviral causes such as toxoplasma or syphilis can have a similar result. During

childhood, progressive brain damage may occur with subacute sclerosing panencephalitis, subacute measles encephalitis, or progressive rubella panencephalitis, but all of these are now rarely seen in vaccinated populations. Progressive multifocal leukoencephalopathy, a slow infection with JC virus, may occur at any time of life in an immune-compromised host. These latter disorders are subacute or gradual in onset, producing stupor or coma in their terminal stages. Hence, they do not cause problems in the differential diagnosis of stupor or coma, and are not dealt with here in detail. Progressive multifocal leukoencephalopathy is considered along with the primary neuronal and glial disorders of brain (Table 5–1, heading G). *Prion infections,*[408,409] including Creutzfeldt-Jakob disease, Gerstmann-Sträussler disease, and fatal familial insomnia,[410] were at one time also thought to be "slow viral" illnesses, but they are now known to be due to a misfolded protein. With the occasional exception of Creutzfeldt-Jakob disease, these disorders likewise are gradual in onset; they do not represent problems in differential diagnosis and are not discussed here.

In each of the pathologically defined viral encephalitides, the viruses produce neurologic signs in one of three ways: (1) they invade, reproduce in, and destroy neurons and glial cells (acute viral encephalitis). Cell dysfunction or death may occur even in the absence of any inflammatory or immune response. (2) They evoke an immune response that can cause hemorrhage, inflammation, and necrosis, or demyelination (parainfectious encephalomyelitis). (3) They provoke cerebral edema and sometimes vascular damage (toxic encephalopathy), both of which increase the ICP and, like a supratentorial mass lesion, lead to transtentorial herniation

The clinical findings in each of the viral encephalitides are sometimes sufficiently different to allow clinical diagnosis even when the illness has progressed to the stage of stupor or coma. Furthermore, within each of these categories, specific viral illnesses may have individual clinical features that strongly suggest the diagnosis. Unfortunately, all too often the first three categories, which cause acute brain dysfunction, cannot be distinguished on a clinical basis, and the generic term acute encephalitis must be used unless PCR, biopsy, or autopsy material establishes the exact pathologic change. To compound the complexity, certain viruses can cause different pathologic changes in the brain depending on the setting. For example, acute toxic encephalopathy, parainfectious encephalomyelitis, subacute sclerosing panencephalitis, and subacute measles encephalitis were all reported to be caused by the measles virus (although now this is rarely seen). Despite these difficulties in diagnosis, an attempt should be made to separate the acute encephalitides into pathologic categories and to establish the causal agent, since the treatment and prognosis are different in the different categories. Brain biopsy is only rarely necessary, as discussed in detail on page 273.

Acute Viral Encephalitis

Although a number of viruses cause human encephalitis, only two major types are both common and produce coma in the United States: arboviruses (Eastern equine, Western equine, and St. Louis encephalitis) and herpes viruses.

Uncommon causes of stupor and coma include West Nile virus (especially between August and October),[411,412] severe acute respiratory syndrome (SARS), and other emerging neurotropic viruses that may become more common causes of encephalitis-induced coma in the future.[413] (The varicella-zoster virus, a rare cause of stupor in the normal adult population, may produce cerebral vasculitis [page 275]).

HERPES SIMPLEX ENCEPHALITIS (FIGURE 5–11)

This disease is pathologically characterized by extensive neuronal damage in the cerebral hemispheres with a remarkable predilection by the virus for the gray matter of the medial temporal lobe as well as other limbic structures, especially the insula, cingulate gyrus, and inferior frontal lobe. Neuronal destruction is accompanied by perivascular invasion with inflammatory cells and proliferation of microglia with frequent formation of glial nodules. The vascular endothelium often swells and proliferates. Areas of focal cortical necrosis are

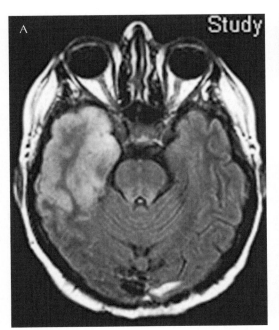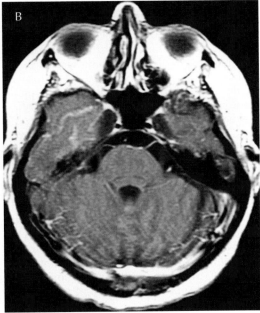

Figure 5–11. Magnetic resonance images of herpes simplex encephalitis. (A) and (B) are, respectively, the FLAIR and contrast-enhanced images of a patient with acute herpes simplex encephalitis. She also suffered from non-small cell lung cancer, and a left occipital metastasis had been previously resected (scar obvious on FLAIR image).

common. Local hemorrhage into brain tissue may occur. Cowdry type A inclusion bodies in neurons and glial cells are a distinctive feature.

Clinically, herpes simplex encephalitis begins with the acute onset of a confusional state, aphasia, or behavioral changes, often accompanied by headache, fever, and seizures. The illness progresses acutely or subacutely to produce stupor or coma. In one series of 45 patients, 28 had Glasgow Coma Score of less than 10 and 13 were deeply comatose.[414] This early stage may be fulminating, and in some instances may transition from full health to stupor in only a few hours. Often, behavioral disturbances or agitated delirium, particularly with olfactory or gustatory hallucinations, precedes coma by hours or days, a pattern so characteristic as to suggest the diagnosis. Focal motor signs frequently accompany the onset of coma, and tremors of the extremities, face, and even trunk commonly complement the agitated delirium of herpes encephalitis. Occasionally the neurologic signs of herpes simplex encephalitis, either type 1[415] or type 2,[416] are limited to the brainstem, with cranial nerve palsies predominating.

The CSF pressure is usually increased (180 to 400 mm CSF) and the white cell count is usually elevated (10 to 1000/mm^3, mostly mononuclear). Both may be normal, particularly early in the course of the illness. Up to 500 red cells/mm^3 are common and the CSF protein content usually is elevated (values up 870 mg/dL having been reported). The CSF sugar is usually normal but occasionally depressed. Identification of viral DNA by PCR establishes the diagnosis and obviates the need for a biopsy.[417,418] The EEG is always abnormal. Distinctive, periodic, high-voltage, 1-Hz sharp waves from one or both temporal lobes are highly characteristic of herpes simplex encephalitis and suggest a poor prognosis. Imaging with MRI typically identifies the lesions much earlier than CT. Abnormalities in the temporal lobes, and sometimes the frontal lobe as well, suggest the diagnosis. Functional imaging identifies hyperperfusion in the temporal lobe.[417] Extratemporal involvement on MRI is found in a significant minority of patients.[419] Early diagnosis of herpes simplex encephalitis is vital as treatment with acyclovir or an equivalent antiviral drug yields the best results when administered before patients become comatose.

Sometimes, as in the following cases, severe hemispheral brain swelling produces transtentorial herniation and may lead to death.

Patient 5–24

A 71-year-old woman was brought into the emergency department for a headache and confusion. Her temperature was 98°F and she complained of a diffuse headache, but could not answer questions coherently. Neurologic examination showed a mild left hemiparesis and some left-sided inattention. A right hemisphere ischemic event was suspected, but the CT did not disclose any abnormality. She was admitted to the stroke service. The following day her temperature spiked to 102°F, and a lumbar puncture was done showing seven white blood cells, 19 red blood cells, a protein of 48, and a glucose of 103 with a normal opening pressure. An MRI showed T2 signal involving the medial and lateral temporal lobe, as well as the insular and cingulate cortex on the right, with less intense but similar involvement of the right cingulate cortex. By this time she had lapsed into a stuporous state, with small but reactive pupils, full roving eye movements, and symmetric increase in motor tone. She was started on acyclovir. Despite treatment she developed edema of the right temporal lobe with uncal herniation.

Comment: Because the initial presentation suggested a right hemisphere ischemic event, the patient was treated according to standard stroke protocols, which do not require lumbar puncture. By the time the MRI scan was done, revealing the typical pattern of herpes simplex encephalitis, the patient had progressed to a stuporous state and acyclovir was not able to prevent the swelling and herniation of her right temporal lobe.

The following case was seen in the era prior to CT and antiviral therapy. It is presented because it illustrates the natural history of herpes encephalitis and included a pathologic examination.

HISTORICAL VIGNETTE

Patient 5–25

A 32-year-old children's nurse was admitted to the hospital in coma. She had felt vaguely unwell 5 days before admission and then developed occipital headache and vomiting. Two days before admission, a physician carefully examined her but found only a temperature of 39°C and a normal blood count. She remained alone for the next 48 hours and was found unconscious in her room and brought to the emergency department.

Examination showed an unresponsive woman with her head and eyes deviated to the right. She had small ecchymoses over the left eye, left hip, and knee. Her neck was moderately stiff. The right pupil was slightly larger than the left, both reacted to light, and the oculocephalic reflex was intact. The corneal reflex was bilaterally sluggish and the gag reflex was intact. Her extremities were flaccid, the stretch reflexes were 3+, and the plantar responses were flexor. In the emergency department she had a generalized convulsion associated with deviation of the head and the eyes to the left. The opening pressure on lumbar puncture was 130 mm of CSF. There were 550 mononuclear cells and 643 red blood cells/mm^3. The CSF glucose was 65 and the protein was 54 mg/dL. Skull x-ray findings were normal. A right carotid arteriogram showed marked elevation of the sylvian vessels with only minimal deviation of the midline structures. Burr holes were placed; no subdural blood was found. A ventriculogram showed the third ventricle curved to the right. The EEG contained 1- to 2-Hz high-amplitude slow waves appearing regularly every 3 to 5 seconds from a background of almost complete electrical silence. Low-amplitude 10- to 12-Hz sharp-wave bursts of gradually increasing voltage began over either frontal area and occurred every 1 to 2 minutes; they lasted 20 to 40 seconds and were associated with seizure activity.

Her seizures were partially controlled with anticonvulsants and she received 20 million units of penicillin and chloramphenicol for possible bacterial meningitis. Her condition gradually deteriorated, and on the eighth hospital day she developed midposition fixed pupils with absence of oculovestibular responses, and diabetes insipidus with a serum osmolality of 313 mOsm/L and urine specific gravity of 1.005. Eight days after admission, lumbar puncture yielded a serosanguineous fluid with 26,000 red blood cells and 2,200 mononuclear cells. The protein was 210 mg/dL. CSF antibody titers for herpes simplex virus were 1:4 at admission but 1:32 by day 8. She died 10 days after admission, having been maintained with artificial ventilation and pressor agents for 48 hours.

At autopsy, herpes simplex virus was cultured from the cerebral cortex. The leptomeninges were congested, and the brain was swollen and soft with bilateral deep tentorial grooving along the hippocampal gyrus. The diencephalon was displaced an estimated 8 to 10 mm caudally through the tentorial notch. On cut section, the medial and anterior temporal lobes as well as the insula were bilaterally necrotic, hemorrhagic, and soft. Linear and oval hemorrhages were found in the thalamus bilaterally and extended down the central portion of the brainstem as far as the pons. Hemorrhages were also found in the cerebellum, and there was a small, intact arteriovenous malformation in the right sylvian fissure. There were meningeal infiltrations predominantly of lymphocytes, some plasma cells, and polymorphonuclear leukocytes. The perivascular spaces were also infiltrated in places extending to the subcortical white matter. In some areas the entire cortex was necrotic with shrunken and eosinophilic nerve cells. Numerous areas of extravasated red blood cells were present in the cortex, basal ganglia, and upper brainstem. Marked microglial proliferation and astrocytic hyperplasia were present. Cowdry type A intranuclear inclusion bodies were present primarily in the oligodendroglia, but were also seen in astroglia, small neurons, and occasional capillary endothelial cells.

Comment: This patient's history, findings, and course in the days before imaging, PCR, or antiviral agents were available were characteristic of herpes simplex encephalitis. The pathologic examination of the brain complements the imaging available in modern cases, and was able to demonstrate the presence of viral inclusions.

Many noninfectious illnesses may mimic infections. Some present as acute meningeal reactions, others as more chronic reactions. Table 5–20 lists some of these.

Acute Toxic Encephalopathy During Viral Encephalitis

Acute toxic encephalopathy is the term applied to a nervous system disorder, seen predominantly in children under the age of 5, which usually occurs during or after a systemic viral infection and is characterized clinically by the acute onset of increased ICP, with or without focal neurologic signs, and without CSF pleocytosis. The disorder is distinguished pathologically from acute viral encephalitis by the

Table 5–20 Disorders That Imitate Central Nervous System Infections and the Types of Infection That They Most Commonly Mimic

Acute Meningitis	Chronic Meningitis	Encephalitis/ Meningoencephalitis
Behçet's disease	Chemical meningitis	Acute disseminated encephalomyelitis
Chemical meningitis	Granulomatous angiitis	
Cyst rupture	Lymphomatoid granulomatosi	Acute hemorrhagic leukoencephalitis
Drug-induced meningitis		Acute toxic encephalopathy
Meningism	Meningeal malignancy	Behçet's disease
Parameningeal infection	Systemic lupus erythematosus	Serum sickness
Sarcoidosis	Sarcoidosis	Systemic lupus erythematosus
Systemic lupus erythematosus		
Vogt-Koyanagi-Harada syndrome		Vogt-Koyanagi-Harada syndrome

Modified from Wasay et al.,[419] with permission.

absence of inflammatory change or other pathologic abnormalities of acute viral encephalitis, save for cerebral edema and its consequences. Edema is induced by inflammatory cytokines, inducible nitric oxide synthase, adhesion molecules, and miniplasmin.[421] The cause of acute toxic encephalopathy is unknown and may represent several different illnesses. The best characterized of these was Reye's syndrome (see below), which rarely is seen anymore, after the use of aspirin was abandoned in children with febrile illnesses. It often accompanies viral infection, particularly influenza,[422] but also the common exanthems such as measles and mumps; it also appears without evidence of preceding systemic viral infection. In some instances, viruses have been identified in the brain at autopsy. There may be accompanying evidence of an acute systemic illness, such as liver and kidney damage in Reye's syndrome, or the patient may be free of symptoms other than those of CNS dysfunction. Death is caused by cerebral edema with transtentorial herniation. At autopsy neither inflammation nor demyelination are encountered in the brain, only evidence of severe and widespread cerebral edema.

Clinically, the disease is characterized by an acute or subacute febrile onset associated with headache, sometimes nausea and vomiting, and often delirium or drowsiness followed by stupor or coma. Focal neurologic signs usually are absent but may be prominent and include hemiparesis or hemiplegia, aphasia, or visual field defects. In its most fulminant form, the untreated illness progresses rapidly, with signs of transtentorial herniation leading to coma with impaired ocular movements, abnormal pupillary reflexes, abnormal posturing, and, eventually, respiratory failure and death. Status epilepticus marks the early course of a small proportion of the patients. Patient 5–26 illustrates such a case.

Patient 5–26

A 46-year-old man was in hospital 10 days following a negative inguinal lymph node dissection for the treatment of urethral cancer. He was well and ready for discharge when he complained of a sudden left temporal headache and was noted by his roommate to be confused. Neurologic examination revealed a modest temperature elevation to 38.1°C in an awake but confused individual who was disoriented to time and had difficulty carrying out three-step commands. The neurologic examination was entirely intact, and laboratory evaluation for infection or metabolic abnormalities was entirely normal. The EEG was bilaterally slow, more so on the right side than the left. The lumbar puncture pressure was 160 mm CSF. There were two red cells, one white cell, and a protein of 41 mg/dL. The glucose was 75 mg/dL. Within 48 hours he became agitated and mildly aphasic, with a right homonymous visual field defect. He then had a generalized convulsion. The day following the seizure, the lumbar puncture pressure was 230 mm CSF; there was one white cell, a protein of 90 mg/dL, and glucose of 85 mg/dL. A CT scan was normal, as were bilateral carotid arteriograms. Cultures of blood and CSF for bacteria, viruses, and viral titers were all negative, as was a coagulation profile. Within 48 hours after the convulsion, the patient lapsed into coma with evidence of transtentorial herniation leading to respiratory arrest and death despite treatment with mannitol and steroids. At autopsy, the general examination was normal except for evidence of his previous surgery. There was no evidence of residual cancer. The brain weighed 1,500 g and was grossly swollen, with evidence of both temporal lobe and tonsillar herniation and a Duret hemorrhage in the pons. Microscopic examination was consistent with severe cerebral edema and herniation, but there was no inflammation, nor were there inclusion bodies.

Comment: Except for his age and a somewhat protracted course, this patient is typical of patients with acute toxic encephalopathy.

A clinical distinction between acute, sporadic viral encephalitis and acute, toxic encephalopathy often cannot be made. Certain clues, when present, help to differentiate the two entities: acute encephalopathy appears with or shortly after a banal viral infection, usually occurs in children under 5 years of age, may be associated with hypoglycemia and liver function abnormalities, and usually produces only a modest degree of fever. Rapidly developing increased ICP in the absence of focal signs or neck stiffness also suggests acute toxic encephalopathy. Conversely, prominent focal signs, particularly those of temporal lobe dysfunction accompanied by an abnormal CT or MRI, indicate an acute viral encephalitis such as herpes simplex. The presence of pleocytosis (with or without additional red cells) in the CSF suggests acute viral encephalitis, whereas a spinal fluid under very high pressure, but with

a normal cellular content, suggests acute toxic encephalopathy. In many instances, however, neither a clinical nor laboratory diagnosis can be made immediately.

REYE'S SYNDROME

A variant of acute toxic encephalopathy is Reye's syndrome. This disorder seemed to appear out of nowhere in the 1950s and then, except for rare reports, disappeared before 1990. In children it was believed to be precipitated by the use of aspirin to treat viral infections. Whether this is true has been questioned.[423] This disorder, like other acute toxic encephalopathies, was characterized by progressive encephalopathy with persistent vomiting often following a viral illness (particularly influenza B and varicella). It differs from other forms of acute toxic encephalopathy in that it occurred in epidemics and there was usually evidence of hepatic dysfunction and often hypoglycemia. The illness was pathologically characterized by fatty degeneration of the viscera, particularly the liver but also the kidney, heart, lungs, pancreas, and skeletal muscle. The cause of death in most cases, as in acute toxic encephalopathy, was cerebral edema with transtentorial and cerebellar herniation.

Parainfectious Encephalitis (Acute Disseminated Encephalomyelitis)

Parainfectious disseminated encephalomyelitis and acute hemorrhagic leukoencephalopathy are terms applied to distinct but related clinical and pathologic disorders, both of which are probably caused by an immunologic reaction either to the virus itself or to antigens exposed due to viral injury. Another term for this disorder is acute disseminated encephalomyelitis (ADEM). The same reaction can also be triggered by vaccination and rarely by bacterial or parasitic infection.[424,425] Two pathogenetic mechanisms have been advanced. In the first, the invading organism or vaccine is molecularly similar to a brain protein (molecular mimicry), but sufficiently different for the immune system to recognize it as nonself and mount an immune attack against the brain or spinal cord. In the second, the virus invades the brain causing tissue damage and leakage of antigens into the systemic circulation. Because the brain is a relatively immune protected site, the immune system may not have been exposed to the brain protein before and it mounts an immune attack.[424] Similar clinical and pathologic disorders can be produced in experimental animals by the injection of brain extracts of myelin basic protein mixed with appropriate adjuvants (experimental allergic encephalomyelitis [EAE]) and by Theiler virus.[424] Hemorrhagic changes appear to signify a hyperacute form of allergic encephalomyelitis (see *encephalomyelitis*, below). The disorder largely affects children, but adults and even the elderly are sometimes affected. The estimated incidence is 0.8 per 100,000 population per year.[424] Fifty to 75% of patients have a febrile illness within the 30 days preceding the onset of neurologic symptomatology.

In parainfectious disseminated encephalomyelitis, the brain and spinal cord contain multiple perivascular zones of demyelination in which axis cylinders may be either spared or destroyed. There is usually striking perivascular cuffing by inflammatory cells. Clinically, the illness occasionally arises spontaneously, but usually it follows by several days a known or presumed viral infection, frequently an exanthem (e.g., rubella, varicella), but occasionally a banal upper respiratory infection or another common viral infection (e.g., mumps or herpes). The onset is usually rapid, with headache and a return of fever. In most cases, there is early evidence of behavioral impairment, and as the disorder progresses, the patient may lapse into delirium, stupor, or coma. In one series of 26 patients, five (19%) were comatose.[426] Nuchal rigidity may be present. Both focal and generalized convulsions are common, as are focal motor signs such as hemiplegia or paraplegia.

Careful examination often discloses evidence for disseminated focal CNS dysfunction in the form of optic neuritis, conjugate and dysconjugate eye movement abnormalities, and sensory losses or motor impairment. In 80% of cases, the CSF white cell count is elevated, usually to less than 500 lymphocytes/mm^3, but in the remainder there may be no elevation of CSF white blood count. The CSF protein may be slightly increased, but the glucose is normal. Oligoclonal bands may be present, but are commonly absent. In about one out of five patients, the CSF is normal. MRI scanning usually discloses multiple white matter lesions that are bright on T2 and FLAIR imaging, and which may show

contrast enhancement. Sometimes gray matter is involved as well as white matter, which may explain the tendency for seizures to occur. However, early in the course of the illness, the MRI scan may be normal. We observed one patient who became comatose during the first few days of a severe attack, but whose MRI scan was normal for another week, at which time it progressed rapidly to diffuse T2 signal throughout the white matter of the brain (Patient 4–4). The diagnosis of acute disseminated encephalomyelitis should be suspected when a patient becomes neurologically ill following a systemic viral infection or vaccination. Evidence of widespread or multifocal nervous system involvement and of mild lymphocytic meningitis supports the diagnosis. An MRI strongly supports the diagnosis when it is consistent with multifocal areas of demyelination.

Acute hemorrhagic leukoencephalopathy is considered a variant of encephalomyelitis.[427] However, a recent report suggests that organisms may be found in the brains of patients who die of the disorder. The organisms, measured by PCR, include herpes simplex virus, herpes zoster virus, and HHV-6. Whether the virus itself or an immune reaction to it was causal was unclear.[428]

This disorder is marked pathologically by inflammation and demyelination similar to disseminated encephalomyelitis, plus widespread hemorrhagic lesions in the cerebral white matter. These latter vary in diameter from microscopic to several centimeters and are accompanied by focal necrosis and edema. The perivascular infiltrations frequently contain many neutrophils, and there is often perivascular fibrinous impregnation. The clinical course is as violent as the pathologic response. The illness may follow a banal viral infection or may complicate septic shock, but often no such history is obtained. The illness begins abruptly with headache, fever, nausea, and vomiting. Affected patients rapidly lapse into coma with high fever but little or no nuchal rigidity. Convulsions and focal neurologic signs, especially hemiparesis, are common. Focal cerebral hemorrhages and edema may produce both the clinical and radiographic signs of a supratentorial mass lesion. The CSF is usually under increased pressure and contains from 10 to 500 mononuclear cells and up to 1,000 red blood cells/mm^3. The CSF protein may be elevated to 100 to 300 mg/dL or more.

As a rule, the problem in the differential diagnosis of coma presented by disseminated and hemorrhagic encephalomyelitis is to distinguish it from viral encephalitis and acute toxic encephalopathy. At times a distinction may be impossible, either clinically or virologically. As a general rule, patients with viral encephalitis tend to be more severely ill and have higher fevers for longer periods of time than patients with disseminated encephalomyelitis, with the exception of the hemorrhagic variety. Acute toxic encephalopathy usually is more acute in onset and is associated with higher ICP and with fewer focal neurologic signs, either clinically or radiographically.

Cerebral Biopsy for Diagnosis of Encephalitis

When faced with a delirious or stuporous patient suspected of suffering acute encephalitis, the physician is often perplexed about how best to proceed. The clinical pictures of the various forms of encephalitis are often so similar that only cerebral biopsy will distinguish them, but the treatment of the various forms differs. Of the acute viral encephalitides, herpes simplex can be effectively treated by antiviral agents, and it is likely that in some immune-suppressed patients other viral infections such as varicella-zoster and cytomegalovirus also respond to antiviral treatment. Acute toxic encephalitis does not respond to antiviral treatment but, at least in Reye's syndrome, meticulous monitoring and control of ICP is effective therapy. Acute parainfectious encephalomyelitis is not reported to respond to either antiviral treatment or control of ICP, but often does respond to steroids or immunosuppressive agents.

Weighing the pros and cons, we tentatively conclude that when noninvasive imaging (MRI, MRS, PET) and other tests (CSF PCR for organisms, cytology, oligoclonal bands, and immune globulins) are unrevealing, the risk of biopsy is often small compared to the risk of missing treatment for a specific diagnosis. If there is a focal lesion, a stereotactic needle biopsy will often suffice.[429,430] If there is no focal lesion, an open biopsy, ensuring that one procures leptomeninges and gray and white matter,[431] is required. The biopsy should be taken either from an involved area, or if the illness is diffuse, from

the right frontal or temporal lobe. Complications of either stereotactic or open biopsy are uncommon. However, nondiagnostic biopsies are common. In one series of 90 brain biopsies for evaluation of dementia, only 57% were diagnostic.[431] However, in this and other studies, the biopsy sometimes identified treatable illnesses such as multiple sclerosis, Whipple's disease, cerebral vasculitis, or paraneoplastic encephalopathy.[431,432]

CEREBRAL VASCULITIS AND OTHER VASCULOPATHIES

Certain inflammatory vascular disorders of the brain are either restricted to CNS vessels (e.g., granulomatous angiitis) or produce such prominent CNS symptoms as to appear to be primarily a brain disorder.[433] Recent reviews classify and detail the clinical and arteriographic findings in a large number of illnesses that produce cerebral or systemic vasculitis (Table 5–21). Only those specific illnesses that may be perplexing causes of stupor or coma are considered here.

Granulomatous Central Nervous System Angiitis

In this acute disorder of the nervous system, the pathologic changes in blood vessels may be limited to the brain or involve other systemic organs. When the disease is limited to the brain, it tends to affect small leptomeningeal and intracerebral blood vessels. When more widespread, it affects larger blood vessels. Even when the disease is extracerebral, it can affect the blood supply of the brain, producing acute neurologic symptomatology including coma.[434] The cause of granulomatous angiitis restricted to the nervous system is unknown and possibly multifactorial. The disorder has been associated with herpes zoster infection, lymphomas, sarcoidosis, amyloid angiopathy, and infections by mycoplasma, rickettsia, viruses, and *Borrelia burgdorferi*.[435] Because the inflammatory lesions can involve blood vessels of any size, the disease can cause large or small infarcts.

Clinically, the onset is usually acute or subacute with headache, mental changes, impair-

Table 5–21 **Classification of Vasculitides That Affect the Nervous System**

Systemic necrotizing arteritis
  Polyarteritis nodosa
  Churg-Strauss syndrome
  Microscopic polyangiitis
Hypersensitivity vasculitis
  Henoch-Schönlein purpura
  Hypocomplementemic vasculitis
  Cryoglobulinemia
Systemic granulomatous vasculitis
  Wegener granulomatosis
  Lymphomatoid granulomatosa
  Lethal midline granuloma
Giant cell arteritis
  Temporal arteritis
  Takayasu arteritis
Granulomatous angiitis of the nervous system
Connective tissue disorders associated with
    vasculitis
  System lupus erythematosus
  Scleroderma
  Rheumatoid arthritis
  Sjögren syndrome
  Mixed connective tissue disease
  Behçet's disease
Inflammatory diabetic vasculopathy
Isolated peripheral nervous system vasculitis
Vasculitis associated with infection
  Varicella zoster virus
  Spirochetes
    Treponema pallidum
    Borrelia burgdorferi
  Fungi
  Rickettsia
  Bacterial meningitis
  Mycobacterium tuberculosis
  HIV-1
Central nervous system vasculitis associated
  with amphetamine abuse
Paraneoplastic vasculitis

From Younger,[433] with permission.

ment of consciousness, focal or generalized seizures, and frequently focal neurologic signs including hemiparesis, visual loss, and extrapyramidal disorders. Patients who are usually alert at onset can rapidly progress to stupor or coma. Untreated, the disease may be fatal. More benign forms of the disorder also exist, including those that are chronic and progressive over months or years, those that recover completely, and those that show a relapsing course.[436,437] In those patients who recover, the original angiographic abnormalities reverse.[437]

The laboratory examination is usually but not always characterized by an elevated blood erythrocyte sedimentation rate (ESR) as opposed to systemic granulomatous angiitis, in which the blood ESR is nearly always elevated. There is mild CSF pleocytosis (20 to 40 lymphocytes/mm^3) with an elevated total protein and an increased gamma-globulin level. MR angiography often fails to identify signs of vascular involvement unless there are irregularities of the larger vessels. Conventional cerebral angiography is more sensitive, but still will only identify irregularity of vessels of 1 mm or larger. In addition, the pattern of irregularity does not verify the underlying pathology, but only indicates areas at which biopsy may be fruitful. The specific diagnosis can only be established by cerebral biopsy, but because the lesions are often multifocal but not diffuse, at times even that fails to demonstrate the pathology. Immunosuppression is sometimes effective, but some patients relapse while on maintenance therapy or when therapy is withdrawn.[436]

Systemic Lupus Erythematosus

Systemic vasculitis occurs in 10% to 15% of patients with systemic lupus erythematosus (SLE) often early in the course of the disease, but there is no evidence of cerebral vasculitis in this condition.[438] Nevertheless, acute neurologic dysfunction, including seizures, delirium, and occasionally cerebral infarcts, stupor or coma, may complicate the course of SLE.[439] The pathophysiology of these disturbances is not well understood, but may reflect the effects of autoantibodies against brain or cerebral blood vessels, or perhaps the effects of cytokines induced by an immune attack on body tissues. For example, antiphospholipid antibodies are common in SLE, and may be a cause of venous thrombi or arterial emboli that produce cerebral infarcts. In addition, the deposition of fibrin-platelet thrombi on heart valves (Libman-Sachs endocarditis) suggests a hypercoagulable state. The CNS disorder may occur early in the course of the systemic disease or even preceding systemic diagnosis.[440]

The clinical onset of CNS lupus is abrupt, often with seizures and/or delirium and sometimes accompanied by focal neurologic signs. Most patients have fever; some have papilledema and elevations of CSF pressure on lumbar puncture. The spinal fluid contents are usually normal, but in about 30% of patients, the CSF is abnormal with a modest pleocytosis and/or an elevated protein concentration (*lupus cerebritis*). The EEG is usually abnormal, with either diffuse or multifocal slow-wave activity. The CT or MRI is usually normal, as is angiography. The diagnosis should be considered in any febrile patient, particularly a young woman with undiagnosed delirium or stupor, especially if complicated by seizures. The diagnosis is supported by systemic findings, particularly a history of arthritis and arthralgia (88%), skin rash (79%), and renal disease (48%), and is established by laboratory evaluation. Ninety percent of patients with nervous system involvement by lupus have antinuclear antibodies in their serum; lupus erythematosus cells are present in 79%, and there is hypocomplementemia in 64%. Anti-DNA antibodies and other autoantibodies are common. However, many of these findings may be absent if the lupus is restricted to the CNS. Even when the diagnosis of systemic lupus erythematosus is established, one must be careful not to attribute all neurologic abnormalities that develop directly to the lupus. In patients with lupus, neurologic disability can be caused by uremia or intercurrent CNS infection.[441] A special concern is that SLE is usually treated with high doses of glucocorticoids, which themselves can produce a delirious state (steroid psychosis). It can be difficult to distinguish this condition from the underlying SLE, but even though the response is more common at doses of prednisone greater than 40 mg/day, there is little if any evidence that decreasing the steroid dose shortens this idiosyncratic response.[442] Hence, the usual recommendation is to treat the SLE as medically necessary, and to give neuroleptic medication to control behavior until the delirium clears. Drugs such as lithium and valproic acid have been used as mood stabilizers, but the underlying illness appears to be self-limited, rarely lasting more than a few weeks even without specific treatment; controlled trials have not been done.

Subacute Diencephalic Angioencephalopathy

DeGirolami and colleagues described a patient with the subacute onset of a confusional state followed by progressive dementia, obtundation, and diffuse myoclonus.[443] The CSF showed a progressive rise in the protein concentration. On postmortem examination, there were extensive destructive lesions of the thalami bilaterally associated with a focal vasculitis of small arteries and veins (20 to 80 microns in diameter). The vascular lesions were characterized by thickening of all layers of the vessel wall, with occasional scattered polymorphonuclear leukocytes in the wall and some collections of mononuclear inflammatory cells in the adventitia. Giant cells were absent. The authors were unable to find similar patients reported in the literature. The disease is so rare, and its clinical signs so nonspecific, as to make it unlikely to be diagnosed in the antemortem state. Since the original report, several other cases have been described.[444] In most instances, imaging revealed patchy contrast enhancement suggesting a brain tumor. In one instance, the diagnosis was made by biopsy prior to the patient's death and then confirmed by autopsy.[445]

Varicella-Zoster Vasculitis

Herpes zoster rarely causes stupor or coma. It usually presents as a cutaneous dermatomal infection, initially with itching and pain, followed by a rash and then vesicular lesions. As many as 40% of patients with uncomplicated herpes zoster have meningitis, usually asymptomatic and characterized only by mild CSF pleocytosis, but sometimes accompanied by fever, headache, and stiff neck.

Less commonly, herpes zoster infection may cause more profound CNS problems by causing a vasculitis.[446] Pathologically, this is a viral infection of the affected cerebral blood vessels, and in immunocompetent patients, this may lead to stroke. This syndrome is especially common with ophthalmic division trigeminal zoster, and typically involves the ipsilateral carotid artery. In an immunocompromised patient, the infectious vasculitis may be more widespread, leading to a diffuse encephalopathy. The diagnosis may be difficult because neurologic features are protean[446] and the disease sometimes occurs months after the cutaneous lesions have cleared. Occasionally there is no history of a zoster rash. The MRI or cerebral angiography suggests a vasculitis. Examination of the spinal fluid looking for a varicella-zoster DNA by PCR or by examination of zoster immunoglobulin establishes the diagnosis. This is important because even months after the rash, antiviral therapy may be effective.[446]

Behçet's Syndrome

Behçet's syndrome is an inflammatory disease of unknown cause, the vasculopathy being largely venous. The patient can present with subacutely developing neurologic symptoms and often on examination has evidence of other systemic disease including recurrent oral ulcerations, recurrent genital ulcerations, anterior or posterior uveitis, and skin lesions including erythema nodosum.[447] The disorder occurs with increased frequency along the "silk road" extending from Japan to the Mediterranean where it is coupled with an HLA-B51 haplotype. It is especially prevalent in Turkey. Neurologic symptoms have been divided into three groups: (1) primary neurologic symptoms include inflammatory disease usually of the brainstem, subacute in onset and tending to remit. Ataxia, diplopia, behavioral changes, and alterations of consciousness are relatively common. The CSF may have a pleocytosis. In fact, meningoencephalitis may be the only finding in the disorder. Characteristic imaging signs include inflammatory lesions of the brainstem sometimes extending into the diencephalon, as well as periventricular subcortical white matter lesions in the hemispheres.[448] Single photon emission computed tomography (SPECT) imaging discloses areas of hypoperfusion localized in the deep basal ganglia or in the frontal temporal cortex.[447] (2) The second neurologic syndrome, characterized by cerebral dural venous sinus thrombosis, may lead to venous infarction. When the dural venous system is involved and there is no venous infarct, headache is the major symptom and there may be no other neurologic signs. (3) Neurologic symptoms may occur as a result of intracranial hypertension from a superior vena cava syndrome or from cerebral emboli resulting from cardiac complications. A combination of parenchymal lesions and dural venous infarction should lead to a careful search for a history of genital or oral ulceration.[449] The long-term outcome is generally fairly good with the disease remitting, and in some cases, burning out.

Corticosteroids often successfully treat acute episodes.[447]

Cerebral Autosomal Dominant Arteriopathy With Subcortical Infarcts and Leukoencephalopathy

Cerebral autosomal dominant arteriopathy with subcortical infarcts and leukoencephalopathy (CADASIL) is an inherited vasculopathy resulting from mutations of the notch-3 gene. It is characterized by recurrent ischemic episodes, cognitive deficits, behavioral disorders, and migraine-type headaches. Encephalopathy and reversible coma have been reported in several patients. Encephalopathy usually begins with a typical migraine headache. The patient may go on to develop focal signs, such as visual field defects or hemiparesis, and then become severely encephalopathic, lapsing into coma.[450–452] In one series, six of 70 patients with the disorder presented with an encephalopathy originally misdiagnosed as acute encephalitis. The patients were febrile and four had convulsions. All had a history of migraine with aura and all the episodes seemed to start with an otherwise typical headache. The patients showed multiple white matter abnormalities on MRI, particularly abnormalities at the anterior temporal pole as well as the external capsule and corpus callosum.[450] A characteristic finding is electron-dense granules in the media of arterioles. Such granules sometimes can be identified on skin biopsy.[453]

MISCELLANEOUS NEURONAL AND GLIAL DISORDERS

This category includes several primary CNS disorders of diverse or unknown cause that usually culminate in stupor or coma. Most primary neuronal and glial disorders cause coma only after a period of profound dementia has led the physician to the appropriate diagnosis. The disorders included below occasionally produce unconsciousness sufficiently early in their course that they may be confused with other conditions described in this book. As a result, a brief discussion of their clinical picture and differential diagnosis seems warranted. Although some of these diseases are caused by transmissible agents (e.g., Creutzfeldt-Jakob disease, progressive multifocal leukoencephalopathy), they are arbitrarily categorized separately from the encephalitides and acute toxic encephalopathies because their onset is less acute and their course not so explosive.

Prion Diseases

Prions are infectious proteinaceous particles (membrane glycoproteins) that, when in certain conformations, can cause infectivity without the presence of nucleic acid.[409] Human prion diseases include the several forms of Creutzfeldt-Jakob disease (CJD) and Gerstmann-Sträussler disease, as well as fatal familial insomnia. The latter group and most cases of Gerstmann-Sträussler disease and some cases of CJD are due to inherited mutations in the prion protein gene. However, most cases of CJD are sporadic. Kuru, one of the first prion disorders to be described, occurred among natives of Papua, New Guinea, who reportedly ate the brains of their relatives as part of a funeral ritual. When this practice was abandoned, the disorder disappeared. The disorder can also be transmitted from infected tissues transplanted to uninfected individuals (iatrogenic CJD) or from the ingestion of meat from cows with bovine spongiform encephalopathy (a variant of CJD that affects primarily young people and causes early psychiatric symptoms). CJD is rare, having an incidence of between 0.5 and 1.5 cases per million people per year. CJD is a subacute disorder producing widespread neuronal degeneration and spongiform pathologic changes in the neocortex and cerebellum.[409]

Clinically, the illness usually affects middle-aged adults. Initial symptoms roughly are divided into thirds. The first third complain of fatigue, anorexia, and insomnia. The second third have behavioral or cognitive changes rapidly progressing to dementia. The final third present with focal signs, particularly visual loss, ataxia, aphasia, and motor defects.

The illness progresses over a period of weeks to months with severe obtundation, stupor, and finally unresponsiveness; 90% of patients die within 1 year and many within a matter of 6 to 8 weeks of diagnosis. The motor system suffers disproportionately with diffuse paratonic rigidity; decorticate posturing and extensor plantar responses develop later. Early in the course, myoclonus appears in response to startle; later the myoclonus occurs spontaneously. Some suffer generalized convulsions. The EEG is characteristic, consisting of a flat, almost isoelectric background with superimposed synchronous periodic sharp waves. The CSF examination is usually normal. A protein called 14-3-3, and particularly its gamma isoform, has been reported to be present in CSF from many patients with CJD,[454] but both false positives and false negatives occur,[455] and a reliable and reproducible version of the test is currently unavailable. The MRI may be characteristic.[456] In some patients there is bilateral symmetric hyperintensity in the caudate nucleus and putamen on FLAIR and diffusion-weighted images. A similar appearance of lesions in the pulvinar is also diagnostic ("pulvinar sign").[457] Additional patients may show cortical hyperintensity on diffusion-weighted imaging, especially in the parietal and occipital regions. Unilateral or asymmetric findings are common early in the course of the disease, but eventually become bilateral and more extensive. The hyperintensity on diffusion-weighted imaging is accompanied by a decrease in the apparent diffusion constant, suggesting restricted water diffusion. The MRI is both more sensitive and specific than EEG. However, when taken together in the appropriate clinical setting, the disorder may be diagnosed without the need for biopsy.[458] In the final stage of the disease, all spontaneous movements cease, and the patients remain in coma until they die of intercurrent infection.

The appearance of subacute dementia with myoclonic twitches in a middle-aged or elderly patient without systemic disease is highly suggestive of the diagnosis. Although there is a tendency to mistake the early symptoms for an involutional depression, the organic nature of the disorder rapidly becomes apparent. A similar picture is produced only by severe metabolic diseases (e.g., hepatic encephalopathy) or CNS syphilis (general paresis).

Fatal insomnia is predominantly familial but can occur in a sporadic form.[410] The onset is disrupted sleep, including loss of sleep spindles and slow-wave sleep. Dementia, myoclonus, ataxia, dysarthria, dysphagia, and pyramidal signs follow. Hypometabolism can be demonstrated by PET in thalamic and limbic areas.

Like the changes in CJD, there is severe neuronal loss and astrogliosis.[410]

Adrenoleukodystrophy (Schilder's Disease)

Adrenoleukodystrophy (ALD; Schilder's disease) is an X-linked disease of white matter inherited as a sex-linked recessive trait that affects male children, adolescents, and rarely adults[459,460]; it occasionally causes coma early in its course.[461] Although Schilder originally described a similar condition in three boys, the exact diagnosis in his cases has been challenged (e.g., one may have been subacute sclerosing panencephalitis) and this eponym is now rarely used. The illness comes in two forms. The first, called pure adrenal myeloneuropathy, affects myelin in the spinal cord and, to a lesser degree, peripheral nerves. It also causes adrenal insufficiency in some patients. There may be abnormalities on MRS in the brain, but cerebral symptoms do not occur. A mild version of this form is also occasionally seen in female carriers (heterozygotes) of the disease. The second form is a rapidly progressive inflammatory myelinopathy beginning in the posterior hemisphere that probably results from an immune response to the very-long-chain fatty acids that accumulate in the disease. MR findings of demyelination in parietal and occipital areas, and the relatively acute onset, may suggest multiple sclerosis, but the presence of very-long-chain fatty acids in the serum establishes the diagnosis.

Many patients have biochemical evidence of adrenocortical failure even in the absence of clinically apparent insufficiency. CSF protein is usually elevated and the gamma globulin is sometimes elevated. The EEG is usually slow, with focal slow and sharp abnormalities.

Marchiafava-Bignami Disease

Marchiafava-Bignami disease is a rare disorder of the white matter that was originally believed to affect predominantly Italian males who were heavy drinkers of red wine. It is now recognized, however, that the disease has no demographic restriction and affects chronic alcoholics no matter what form of alcohol they take;

most of the victims are males.[462] The essential lesion is demyelination of the corpus callosum with extension of the demyelination into the adjacent hemispheres. Axons may either be preserved or destroyed, and there are an abundance of fatty macrophages without evidence of inflammation in the lesion. Presumably, the ultimate cause is a deficiency of some critical nutrient.

About 40% of patients present with the acute onset of stupor or coma, and only half of these have prodromal cognitive or behavioral symptoms.[462] The other 60% present with cognitive and gait dysfunction. Comatose patients may be rigid, with increased reflexes and extensor plantar responses. The diagnosis is established by MRI, with hyperintensity on FLAIR in the corpus callosum, sometimes involving only the splenium. Multiple cortical or subcortical lesions are sometimes present as well.[463,464] About 20% of comatose patients die; the rest recover, often with residual neurologic defects.[462] The disease may be related to central pontine myelinolysis, which is described in Chapter 4 and which may also involve the corpus callosum.

Gliomatosis Cerebri

Gliomatosis cerebri implies diffuse infiltration of the brain by neoplastic glial cells. The term is used if three or more lobes of the brain are involved. Histologically, the tumor can be astrocytic or oligodendroglial and can be low or high grade.[465] Gliomatosis cerebri produces symptoms that begin insidiously and progress slowly with clinical illnesses lasting from less than a month to as long as a decade or more. Mental and personality symptoms predominate with memory loss, lethargy, slowed thinking, and confusion gradually leading into sleepiness, stupor, and often prolonged coma. Hemiparesis is fairly common, but rapidly evolving focal neurologic defects are rare. Less than half the patients have seizures, but focal or generalized seizures may be the presenting complaint. About one-quarter of the patients show signs of direct brainstem involvement. Indirect evidence of increased ICP has marked the course of many cases because continued tumor growth produces simple enlargement of the brain or a narrowing of CSF fluid drainage pathways. The MR scan shows either multiple or diffuse areas of high intensity on FLAIR images involving largely the white matter, but the cortex and often basal ganglia and brainstem as well. Even in the absence of substantial signal abnormality, small ventricles suggest increased brain mass. Abnormalities on the MRI are often much more dramatic than the patient's clinical symptoms. The hyperintense areas may or may not enhance depending on the grade of the lesion. Cerebral biopsy is necessary to make a definitive diagnosis.

The following case description typifies the course and findings.

Patient 5–27

A 61-year-old woman insidiously became disinterested in her surroundings and slow in thought during the early spring of 1978. By June, she was lethargic, forgetful, apathetically incontinent, and could no longer walk unassisted. In another hospital, a ventricular shunt was placed without changing her symptoms. She gradually became mentally unresponsive and was admitted to New York Hospital in September 1978. On examination she was awake but psychologically unresponsive, reacting only to noxious stimuli with an extensor (decerebrate) response. The pupils were 2 mm in diameter, equal, and fixed to light. She had roving eye movements with a gaze preference to the right. Oculocephalic responses were full and conjugate, but caloric irrigation with cold water in the right ear produced irregular upbeat nystagmus, while irrigation in the left ear evoked irregular nystagmus to the right. She had a spastic left hemiparesis and a flaccid right hemiparesis with bilateral extensor plantar responses.

Numerous laboratory tests, including examination of the CSF, CT scan, and arteriogram, were either normal or nonspecifically altered. A brain biopsy taken from the grossly normal-appearing right frontal lobe gave the appearance of a diffuse gemistocytic astrocytoma with considerable variation in the degree of malignant change, as well as areas of normal-looking neurons and astrocytes. The patient died in a nursing home soon afterward.

Comment: The insidious onset of changes in cognition and arousal accompanied by signs of fractional damage to the midbrain (fixed pupils), pontine vestibular complex (abnormal calorics), and corticospinal systems placed the lesion diffusely in the brainstem and perhaps the diencephalon. The CT scan and other tests showed no discrete mass lesions and led to a cerebral biopsy as one of the few possible ways of making a firm diagnosis.

Progressive Multifocal Leukoencephalopathy

Progressive multifocal leukoencephalopathy (PML)[466] (Figure 5–12) is a subacute demyelinating disorder produced when a strain of papovavirus (the JC virus) infects the nervous system. The disorder occurs in patients who are immunosuppressed from AIDS, lymphoma, organ transplants, or various forms of chemotherapy. An outbreak occurred in patients treated with natalizumab, a selective adhesion molecule inhibitor that has been used to treat multiple sclerosis and inflammatory bowel disease.[467] The drug was removed from the market, but has been reintroduced with appropriate safety warnings. PML has rarely been reported in individuals whose immune system appears intact. The neurologic symptoms are implied by the name of the disorder, a progressive asymmetric disorder of white matter with hemiparesis, visual impairment, sensory abnormalities, and ataxia. Headaches and seizures are rare. The course is usually progressive over several months, terminating in coma. Rarely, there may be edema associated with the demyelinating plaques, leading to hemispheral swelling and transtentorial herniation. Patients may have focal cognitive disorders if the areas of leukoencephalopathy affect areas of association cortex, but do not have impairment of consciousness until late in the course. The CSF is usually normal, but PCR for JC virus is positive; the EEG is usually diffusely or multifocally abnormal. The MRI is characterized by multiple discrete areas of white matter with hyperintensity on the FLAIR image, but there is often no enhancement with gadolinium, indicating a minimal inflammatory response; those who do mount an inflammatory response have a better prognosis.[468]

The pathology is one of diffuse multifocal demyelination of white matter, with oligodendroglial nuclei containing eosinophilic inclusions, viral particles, and bizarre giant astrocytes, suggesting neoplastic transformation.

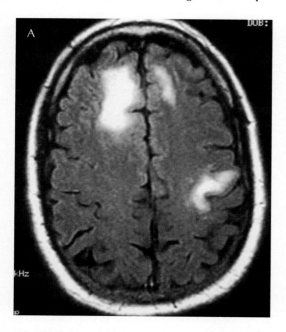

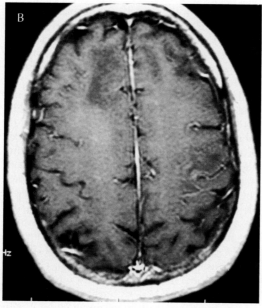

Figure 5–12. Progressive multifocal leukoencephalopathy. This 45-year-old man with AIDS became confused and disoriented. Examination revealed a mild right hemiparesis. Spinal fluid was positive for JC virus. The magnetic resonance image revealed multiple areas hyperintense on the FLAIR image (A) and hypointense on T1 (B). He gradually became more stuporous, went into a coma, and died. Autopsy revealed progressive multifocal leukoencephalopathy.

Epilepsy

Seizures are characterized by intense, repetitive neuronal discharge followed by postictal metabolic cerebral depression of varying degrees and duration. In general, this requires re-entrant neuronal circuits that mainly occur in the forebrain when lesions involve the structures of the cortical mantle. In the experimental animal, one can demonstrate that major seizures produce a 200% to 300% increase in cerebral metabolic demand, a substantial degree of systemic hypertension, and an enormously increased CBF.[469] Repetitive convulsions result in a progressive, abnormal increase in the permeability of the blood-brain barrier.[470] If substrate depletion or a relative decline in blood flow occurs during seizures, the brain maintains its metabolism by the consumption of endogenous substrates. With sustained status epilepticus in such animals, progressive hypoxic-ischemic structural neuronal damage results soon after. Similar but necessarily less comprehensive analyses indicate that seizures cause comparable changes in the human brain.

Postictal coma in humans ranges in intensity from complete unresponsiveness to stupor; protracted deep unresponsiveness lasting more than 15 to 30 minutes suggests continued nonconvulsive seizures or extension of an underlying structural lesion that caused the seizure. Although rare, postictal coma may persist for up to 24 hours without the presence of structural brain injury. In such instances, one should suspect nonconvulsive status epilepticus.[471] Postictal patients in coma usually are hyperpneic until the individual clears the lactic acidemia produced by the repetitive firing of nerves and muscles of the convulsion during a period of impaired breathing; pupillary light reflexes are intact and oculovestibular responses active. The motor system usually is unremarkable except for extensor plantar responses in about half the patients. When a patient is first discovered during the period of postictal unresponsiveness, it is often difficult to determine the cause. However, the diagnosis is clarified quickly because the patient usually rapidly awakens to give his or her history. The problem the physician most frequently faces is retrospective: Was a past, unobserved episode of unconsciousness caused by epilepsy or syncope? In three conditions, coma associated with seizures can be sufficiently prolonged to present diagnostic problems.

The first instance is status epilepticus,[472] a series of generalized convulsions occurring at intervals so closely spaced (i.e., every few minutes) that consciousness is not regained between them. This state strikes about 10% of patients with untreated or inadequately treated epilepsy and often follows the abrupt withdrawal of anticonvulsants. Status epilepticus is a serious medical emergency since the cumulative systemic and cerebral anoxia induced by repeated generalized seizures can produce irreversible brain damage or death; its diagnosis is readily made when repeated convulsions punctuate a state of otherwise nonspecific coma.

A second example of prolonged coma, stupor, or delirium following seizures can occur in elderly patients with an epileptogenic scar or lesion (e.g., from past cerebral infarction) who also suffer from cerebral vascular insufficiency or mild to moderate senile cerebral degeneration with dementia. In these patients, the enormous cerebral metabolic demand imposed by the seizures, plus systemic hypoxemia during the attack, often is sufficient to compromise an already borderline cerebral function and produce several hours of postictal coma followed by several days of delirium. Most such patients ultimately recover their preseizure cerebral function, but each attack risks damaging more and more brain, making effective prevention and prompt treatment important.

A third condition in which sustained coma may be associated with seizures occurs when the loss of consciousness is not simply postictal, but is the result of a cerebral disease that also caused the seizures. Many underlying destructive and metabolic cerebral disorders produce both seizures and coma and must be differentiated by other signs, symptoms, and laboratory studies. If one takes previously healthy patients in our own series, a single or brief series of convulsions was followed by sustained unconsciousness only when caused by acute encephalitis, encephalomyelitis, or acute hyponatremia. However, one may not always have the history available, and many other structural lesions of brain can cause repetitive convulsions followed by a prolonged postictal stupor. It is an axiom of treatment that convulsions should be stopped as promptly as possible, as both the seizures themselves and the accompanying systemic hy-

poxemia are sources of potentially serious brain damage.

Not all patients with epilepsy have convulsions. *Nonconvulsive status epilepticus* is characterized by delirium, stupor, or coma resulting from generalized seizure activity without or with only minor motor activity. In one series of 236 comatose patients with no overt clinical seizure activity, EEG demonstrated that 8% of patients met criteria of nonconvulsive status epilepticus. In this series, the definition included "continuous or nearly continuous electrographic seizure activity lasting at least 30 minutes."[473] The diagnosis can be suspected if the patient has a history of risk factors such as noncompliance with anticonvulsant drugs[474] or a careful neurologic examination reveals particular abnormalities such as subtle motor activity (particularly twitching of the face and distal extremities[474]) or intermittent bouts of nystagmoid eye movements. If the EEG identifies unequivocal continuous epileptic activity,[475] the diagnosis is established. Unfortunately, an electrographic diagnosis is often difficult. Patients may have electrographic activity that suggests seizures but may simply represent diffuse brain damage, or the seizure activity may occur in a part of the brain, such as the medial temporal or orbitofrontal cortex, from which it may be difficult to record electrographic seizure activity. When the diagnosis is strongly suspected, a trial of an intravenous anticonvulsant (usually a benzodiazepine) may be warranted. Improvement in both the EEG and the patient's clinical state confirms the diagnosis. The disorder carries a poor prognosis, probably related more to the underlying cause of the nonconvulsive status rather than the seizure activity itself.[476]

Mixed Metabolic Encephalopathy

All too often, clinical signs and symptoms suggest that a stuporous or comatose patient is suffering from a diffuse metabolic disorder of brain, but laboratory evaluation either reveals a variety of modest abnormalities, none of which appears severe enough to be responsible for the patient's abnormal state of consciousness, or there is no metabolic or toxic abnormality detected. In the first instance, the additive effect of multiple mild metabolic abnormalities may lead to a severe encephalopathy, which can sometimes be remedied by correcting any one of the modest abnormalities.[321]

Patient 5–28

A 74-year-old man with disseminated carcinoma of the prostate was admitted to hospital confused and disoriented. The findings on general physical examination included normal vital signs, cachexia, and an enlarged liver. He was stuporous but arousable by noxious stimuli. When aroused, he was confused and disoriented. His respirations were 16 per minute, his pupils were 2 mm and reactive, and there was a full range of ocular movement to doll's head maneuver. He withdrew all four extremities appropriately, deep tendon reflexes were hyperactive, and plantar responses were flexor. When he was roused to hold his hands outstretched, there was bilateral asterixis. The remainder of the segmental neurologic examination was within normal limits. Laboratory abnormalities included a hemoglobin of 8 g/dL, a calcium of 11.5 mg/dL, a grossly elevated alkaline phosphatase, and modestly elevated liver enzymes. The CT scan showed modest cerebral atrophy. Arterial blood gases revealed an oxygen tension of 55 mm Hg, a pH of 7.49, and a PCO_2 of 30 mm Hg. A small infiltrate was present in the right middle lobe of the lung on chest x-ray. A diagnosis of mixed metabolic encephalopathy was made with anemia, hypoxia, liver metastases, and hypercalcemia all playing a role.

Oxygen given by nasal prongs raised the arterial blood PO_2 but failed to change his clinical state. Two units of blood raised his hemoglobin to 10 g/dL; when this was combined with the oxygen, he awoke and, although disoriented at the time, was otherwise alert and behaved appropriately. At the time he awakened, no change had developed in his serum calcium or abnormal liver function tests.

A more difficult problem arises when no metabolic or toxic abnormalities are detected. In that circumstance, the first step in diagnosis should be to check all medications the patient has received in the past 48 hours. Barring sedative or narcotic drugs, one should check the platelet count and coagulation profile. Some of these patients have subsequently proved to have disseminated intravascular coagulation with neu-

rologic symptoms appearing before coagulation profiles became abnormal. In others, a biochemical defect present prior to the patient's being examined may have left residual brain damage even though the underlying biochemical abnormality has been corrected. Carbon monoxide poisoning and hypoglycemia are examples of this. In still other patients, drug ingestion with chemical substances not detected by usual laboratory tests may be the cause. In some patients, the diagnosis is never established, and one must presume that some unidentified toxin or not understood metabolic abnormality was present. When faced with such a problem, the physician should apply supportive therapy as outlined in Chapter 7 while continuing to search diligently to identify metabolic abnormalities as the illness pursues its course.

ACUTE DELIRIOUS STATES

Delirium and confusional states usually precede metabolic stupor or coma and can be the presenting problem in many of the diseases described in this chapter or listed in Table 5–1. An additional group of disorders cause a severe and acute delirium that is usually self-limited, but may, occasionally, be fatal if not appropriately treated. Because these states usually do not cause stupor or coma, they have not been discussed elsewhere in this text, but they are responsible for acute changes in the state of consciousness that often challenge and perplex the physician. Two such entities, both drug withdrawal syndromes, particularly alcohol, and postoperative delirium, are discussed here.

The clinical picture of these two states can be similar. A patient who was previously alert and oriented (although frequently with some underlying mild dementia) suddenly becomes restless. His or her affect changes such that while previously calm, he or she becomes agitated, fearful, or depressed, and emotionally labile. The patient is less able than previously to give attention to his or her environment; minor defects in cognitive functions can be detected on careful testing if the patient will cooperate. Most of the patients become insomniac, and many are paranoid and misinterpret sensory stimuli, both auditory and visual. They often hallucinate. Autonomic dysfunction including tachycardia, hypertension, diaphoresis, dilated pupils, and at times fever is common. (Fever should never be dismissed simply as a result of delirium until a careful search has ruled out infection, which may contribute to the genesis of the delirium.) In its florid form, the patient is tremulous, extremely restless, and often fearful; asterixis and multifocal myoclonus may be present. Many patients are totally disoriented but may elaborately describe an incorrect environment. When the delirium is severe, such patients are so restless that they cannot lie still, and their thrashing and rolling about in bed may damage a recently operated site and put additional strain on an impaired cardiovascular system. They are so distractible that cognitive testing is impossible. They may engage equally the examiner and imaginary figures in conversation. The speech is so dysarthric that even when the delirious patient does reply correctly to questions, he or she often cannot be understood. If untreated, the agitation of delirium may lead to exhaustion and even death. However, even the most severe of the delirious states, delirium tremens, has only a modest mortality if treated with appropriate sedative therapy. As indicated in Chapter 1, a stroke in the nondominant temporal or parietal lobe can sometimes cause an acute delirious state.

Drug Withdrawal Delirium (Delirium Tremens)

The most common of the acute and florid delirious states is delirium tremens. Although it is caused by withdrawal of alcohol and generally follows complete cessation of drinking, usually by 3 to 4 days, it may occur in a patient still drinking a diminished amount of ethanol. Similar clinical findings may follow benzodiazepine, barbiturate, or other sedative drug withdrawal.[477,478] In each of these withdrawal states generalized convulsions may, independent of the delirium, also occur. Particularly perplexing to the physician are those patients not known to be alcoholics or chronic sedative drug users who enter the hospital for elective surgery and, during the course of workup or shortly following the operation, become acutely delirious. The disease generally runs its course in less than a week. If treated with sedative drugs and good supportive therapy, most patients recover fully, although a mortality ranging from 2% to 15% has been reported from various sources. Much of this mortality is prob-

ably due to other complications of alcoholism, such as liver failure, or to sympathetic activation that commonly accompanies the disorder. The pathogenesis of drug withdrawal syndromes may depend on their effect on receptors, particularly NMDA and GABA$_A$ receptors. NMDA receptors are up-regulated during chronic alcohol exposure and because it is a GABA$_A$ potentiator, GABA$_A$ receptors may be down-regulated. Hence, abrupt cessation increases brain excitability leading to clinically evident anxiety, irritability, agitation, and tremor.[479]

Postoperative Delirium

Postoperative delirium is one of the most florid and frightening postoperative complications to confront the surgeon. Its incidence is unknown, but may affect 20% to 60% of elderly patients after operation for hip fracture or cardiac surgery.[480] The clinical picture may vary from mild cognitive impairment to an acute confusional state resembling delirium tremens (see above). Factors include older age, previous cognitive impairment, anemia, electrolyte abnormalities, a history of alcoholism, narcotic or benzodiazepine use, and a history of cerebral vascular disease.[480] In a group of 818 patients in a surgical intensive care unit, delirium developed in 11%.[481] Cardiac surgery was not a risk factor, but respiratory dysfunction, infections, anemia, hypocalcemia, hyponatremia, azotemia, liver function abnormalities, and metabolic acidosis were.

The pathogenesis is unknown. It is probably multifactorial including cerebral emboli after hip or cardiac surgery,[482] anesthesia, use of opioids or other sedative drugs, sleep deprivation, circadian disorientation in an intensive care unit, and pain. In most instances the outcome is benign, but some patients succumb probably due to their original medical illness while still encephalopathic.

Intensive Care Unit Delirium

Acute delirium frequently occurs in patients hospitalized in intensive care units. Many such patients are postoperative, and all the factors listed under postoperative complications undoubtedly play some causal role. Wilson, however, found that the incidence of postoperative delirium in an intensive care unit without windows was more than double that in patients housed in a unit with windows.[483] He concluded that sensory deprivation, which results in dissociation from normal circadian cues, was a factor in postoperative delirium. The findings stress the importance of environmental stimulation to help potentially confused patients orient themselves.

Drug-Induced Delirium

Myriad drugs, both licit and illicit, can cause acute delirium. Some of these are listed in Tables 5–12 and 5–13, but these are only partial listings. Any patient, particularly an elderly one who develops an unexplained acute delirium, should be considered as having a drug intoxication until proved otherwise. In addition to the supportive care given for delirium, all drugs not essential for maintenance of life should be withdrawn until it can be determined that they are not contributing to the patient's confusion.

REFERENCES

1. Meagher DJ, O'Hanlon D, O'Mahony E, et al. Relationship between symptoms and motoric subtype of delirium. J Neuropsychiatry Clin Neurosci 2000; 12(1), 51–56.
2. Kanard A, Frytak S, Jatoi A. Cognitive dysfunction in patients with small-cell lung cancer: incidence, causes and suggestions on management. J Support Oncol 2004; 2, 127–140.
3. DSM-IV-TR Mental Disorders: Diagnosis, Etiology, and Treatment. Hoboken, NJ: J. Wiley, 2004.
4. Breitbart W, Rosenfeld B, Roth A, et al. The Memorial Delirium Assessment Scale. J Pain Symptom Manage 1997; 13(3), 128–137.
5. Trzepacz PT, Mittal D, Torres R, et al. Validation of the Delirium Rating Scale-revised-98: comparison with the delirium rating scale and the cognitive test for delirium. J Neuropsychiatry Clin Neurosci 2001; 13(2), 229–242.
6. Ely EW, Margolin R, Francis J, et al. Evaluation of delirium in critically ill patients: validation of the Confusion Assessment Method for the Intensive Care Unit (CAM-ICU). Crit Care Med 2001; 29(7), 1370–1379.
7. Ely EW, Inouye SK, Bernard GR, et al. Delirium in mechanically ventilated patients—validity and reliability of the Confusion Assessment Method for the intensive care unit (CAM-ICU). JAMA 2001; 286(21), 2703–2710.
8. Santana SF, Wahlund LO, Varli F, et al. Incidence, clinical features and subtypes of delirium in elderly

9. Camus V, Gonthier R, Dubos G, et al. Etiologic and outcome profiles in hypoactive and hyperactive subtypes of delirium. J Geriatr Psychiatry Neurol 2000; 13(1), 38–42.
10. Caraceni A, Grassi L. Delirium: Acute Confusional States in Palliative Medicine. New York: Oxford University Press, 2003.
11. Norton JW, Corbett JJ. Visual perceptual abnormalities: hallucinations and illusions. Semin Neurol 2000; 20(1), 111–121.
12. Henon H, Lebert F, Durieu I, et al. Confusional state in stroke: relation to preexisting dementia, patient characteristics, and outcome. Stroke 1999; 30(4), 773–779.
13. Behrmann M, Geng JJ, Shomstein S. Parietal cortex and attention. Curr Opin Neurobiol 2004; 14(2), 212–217.
14. Gibb WR, Gorsuch AN, Lees AJ, et al. Reversible coma in Wernicke's encephalopathy. Postgrad Med J 1985; 61(717), 607–610.
15. Hazell AS, Todd KG, Butterworth RF. Mechanisms of neuronal cell death in Wernicke's encephalopathy. Metab Brain Dis 1998; 13(2), 97–122.
16. McEntee WJ. Wernicke's encephalopathy: an excitotoxicity hypothesis. Metab Brain Dis 1997; 12(3), 183–192.
17. Chin K, Ohi M, Fukui M, et al. Inhibitory effect of an intellectual task on breathing after voluntary hyperventilation. J Appl Physiol 1996; 81(3), 1379–1387.
18. Simon RP. Neurogenic pulmonary edema. Neurol Clin 1993; 11(2), 309–323.
19. Fontes RB, Aguiar PH, Zanetti MV, et al. Acute neurogenic pulmonary edema: case reports and literature review. J Neurosurg Anesthesiol 2003; 15(2), 144–150.
20. Swenson ER. Metabolic acidosis. Respir Care 2001; 46(4), 342–353.
21. Zehtabchi S, Sinert R, Baron BJ, et al. Does ethanol explain the acidosis commonly seen in ethanol-intoxicated patients? Clin Toxicol (Phila) 2005; 43(3), 161–166.
22. Depalo VA, Mailer K, Yoburn D, et al. Lactic acidosis: lactic acidosis associated with metformin use in treatment of type 2 diabetes mellitus. Geriatrics 2005; 60(11), 36–41.
23. Purssell RA, Lynd LD, Koga Y. The use of the osmole gap as a screening test for the presence of exogenous substances. Toxicol Rev 2004; 23(3), 189–202.
24. Megarbane B, Borron SW, Baud FJ. Current recommendations for treatment of severe toxic alcohol poisonings. Intensive Care Med 2005; 31(2), 189–195.
25. Alfred S, Coleman P, Harris D, et al. Delayed neurologic sequelae resulting from epidemic diethylene glycol poisoning. Clin Toxicol (Phila) 2005; 43(3), 155–159.
26. Foster GT, Vaziri ND, Sassoon CS. Respiratory alkalosis. Respir Care 2001; 46(4), 384–391.
27. Dale C, Aulaqi AA, Baker J, et al. Assessment of a point-of-care test for paracetamol and salicylate in blood. QJM 2005; 98(2), 113–118.
28. Koulouris Z, Tierney MG, Jones G. Metabolic acidosis and coma following a severe acetaminophen

overdose. Ann Pharmacother 1999; 33(11), 1191–1194.

29. Greene SL, Dargan PI, Jones AL. Acute poisoning: understanding 90% of cases in a nutshell. Postgrad Med J 2005; 81(954), 204–216.

30. Dargan PI, Wallace CI, Jones AL. An evidence based flowchart to guide the management of acute salicylate (aspirin) overdose. Emerg Med J 2002; 19(3), 206–209.

31. Rivers EP, McIntyre L, Morro DC, et al. Early and innovative interventions for severe sepsis and septic shock: taking advantage of a window of opportunity. CMAJ 2005; 173(9), 1054–1065.

32. Khanna A, Kurtzman NA. Metabolic alkalosis. Respir Care 2001; 46(4), 354–365.

33. Bulger RJ, Schrier RW, Arend WP, et al. Spinal-fluid acidosis and the diagnosis of pulmonary encephalopathy. N Engl J Med 1966; 274(8), 433–437.

34. Posner JB, Swanson AG, Plum F. Acid-base balance in cerebrospinal fluid. Arch Neurol 1965; 12, 479–496.

35. Holland AE, Wilson JW, Kotsimbos TC, et al. Metabolic alkalosis contributes to acute hypercapnic respiratory failure in adult cystic fibrosis. Chest 2003; 124(2), 490–493.

36. Epstein SK, Singh N. Respiratory acidosis. Respir Care 2001; 46(4), 366–383.

37. Andrefsky JC, Frank JI, Chyatte D. The ciliospinal reflex in pentobarbital coma. J Neurosurg 1999; 90(4), 644–646.

38. Larson MD, Muhiudeen I. Pupillometric analysis of the 'absent light reflex.' Arch Neurol 1995; 52(4), 369–372.

39. Simon RP. Forced downward ocular deviation. Occurrence during oculovestibular testing in sedative drug-induced coma. Arch Neurol 1978; 35(7), 456–458.

40. Cadranel JF, Lebiez E, Di Martino V, et al. Focal neurological signs in hepatic encephalopathy in cirrhotic patients: an underestimated entity? Am J Gastroenterol 2001; 96(2), 515–518.

41. Huff JS. Stroke mimics and chameleons. Emerg Med Clin North Am 2002; 20(3), 583–595.

42. Adams RD, Foley JM. The neurological disorder associated with liver disease. Res Publ Assoc Res Nerv Ment Dis 1953; 32, 198–237.

43. Rio J, Montalban J, Pujadas F, et al. Asterixis associated with anatomic cerebral lesions: a study of 45 cases. Acta Neurol Scand 1995; 91(5), 377–381.

44. Young RR, Shahani BT. Asterixis: one type of negative myoclonus. Adv Neurol 1986; 43, 137–156.

45. Leavitt S, Tyler HR. Studies in asterixis. I. Arch Neurol 1964; 10, 360–368.

46. Noda S, Ito H, Umezaki H, et al. Hip flexion-abduction to elicit asterixis in unresponsive patients. Ann Neurol 1985; 18(1), 96–97.

47. Shibasaki H. Pathophysiology of negative myoclonus and asterixis. Adv Neurol 1995; 67, 199–209.

48. Shibasaki H, Hallett M. Electrophysiological studies of myoclonus. Muscle Nerve 2005; 31(2), 157–174.

49. Henry JA, Woodruff GH. A diagnostic sign in states of apparent unconsciousness. Lancet 1978; 2(8096), 920–921.

50. Rosenberg ML. The eyes in hysterical states of unconsciousness. J Clin Neuroophthalmol 1982; 2(4), 259–260.

51. Pellerin L, Magistretti PJ. Neuroenergetics: calling upon astrocytes to satisfy hungry neurons. Neuroscientist 2004; 10(1), 53–62.

52. Mulligan SJ, MacVicar BA. Calcium transients in astrocyte endfeet cause cerebrovascular constrictions. Nature 2004; 431(7005), 195–199.

53. Fillenz M. The role of lactate in brain metabolism. Neurochem Int 2005; 47(6), 413–417.

54. Chen Y, Swanson RA. Astrocytes and brain injury. J Cereb Blood Flow Metab 2003; 23(2), 137–149.

55. Ishii K, Sasaki M, Kitagaki H, et al. Regional difference in cerebral blood flow and oxidative metabolism in human cortex. J Nucl Med 1996; 37(7), 1086–1088.

56. Nybo L, Secher NH. Cerebral perturbations provoked by prolonged exercise. Prog Neurobiol 2004; 72(4), 223–261.

57. Nair DG. About being BOLD. Brain Res Brain Res Rev 2005; 50(2), 229–243.

58. Magistretti PJ, Pellerin L. Cellular mechanisms of brain energy metabolism and their relevance to functional brain imaging. Philos Trans R Soc Lond B Biol Sci 1999; 354(1387), 1155–1163.

59. Iadecola C. Neurovascular regulation in the normal brain and in Alzheimer's disease. Nat Rev Neurosci 2004; 5(5), 347–360.

60. Hass WK, Hawkins RA, Ransohoff J. Reduction of cerebral blood flow, glucose utilization, and oxidatvie metabolism after bilateral reticular formation lesions. Trans Am Neurol Assoc 1977; 102, 19–22.

61. Jones TH, Morawetz RB, Crowell RM, et al. Thresholds of focal cerebral ischemia in awake monkeys. J Neurosurg 1981; 54(6), 773–782.

62. Kraig RP, Petito CK, Plum F, et al. Hydrogen ions kill brain at concentrations reached in ischemia. J Cereb Blood Flow Metab 1987; 7(4), 379–386.

63. Clausen T, Khaldi A, Zauner A, et al. Cerebral acid-base homeostasis after severe traumatic brain injury. J Neurosurg 2005; 103(4), 597–607.

64. Zauner A, Daugherty WP, Bullock MR, et al. Brain oxygenation and energy metabolism: part I-biological function and pathophysiology. Neurosurgery 2002; 51(2), 289–301; discussion 302.

65. Banks WA. The source of cerebral insulin. Eur J Pharmacol 2004; 490(1–3), 5–12.

66. Pellerin L. How astrocytes feed hungry neurons. Mol Neurobiol 2005; 32(1), 59–72.

67. Gruetter R. Glycogen: the forgotten cerebral energy store. J Neurosci Res 2003; 74(2), 179–183.

68. Brown AM. Brain glycogen re-awakened. J Neurochem 2004; 89(3), 537–552.

69. Klein JP, Waxman SG. The brain in diabetes: molecular changes in neurons and their implications for end-organ damage. Lancet Neurol 2003; 2(9), 548–554.

70. Payne RS, Tseng MT, Schurr A. The glucose paradox of cerebral ischemia: evidence for corticosterone involvement. Brain Res 2003; 971(1), 9–17.

71. Cox DJ, Kovatchev BP, Gonder-Frederick LA, et al. Relationships between hyperglycemia and cognitive performance among adults with type 1 and type 2 diabetes. Diabetes Care 2005; 28(1), 71–77.

72. Baird TA, Parsons MW, Phanh T, et al. Persistent poststroke hyperglycemia is independently associated with infarct expansion and worse clinical outcome. Stroke 2003; 34(9), 2208–2214.

73. Rady MY, Johnson DJ, Patel BM, et al. Influence of individual characteristics on outcome of glycemic control in intensive care unit patients with or without diabetes mellitus. Mayo Clin Proc 2005; 80(12), 1558–1567.

74. Schurr A, Payne RS, Miller JJ, et al. Preischemic hyperglycemia-aggravated damage: evidence that lactate utilization is beneficial and glucose-induced corticosterone release is detrimental. J Neurosci Res 2001; 66(5), 782–789.

75. Li PA, He QP, Csiszar K, et al. Does long-term glucose infusion reduce brain damage after transient cerebral ischemia? Brain Res 2001; 912(2), 203–205.

76. Jones K. Insulin coma therapy in schizophrenia. J R Soc Med 2000; 93(3), 147–149.

77. Della Porta P, Maiolo AT, Negri VU. Cerebral blood flow and metabolism in therapeutic insulin coma. Metabolism 1964; 13, 131–140.

78. Dieguez G, Fernandez N, Garcia JL, et al. Role of nitric oxide in the effects of hypoglycemia on the cerebral circulation in awake goats. Eur J Pharmacol 1997; 330(2–3), 185–193.

79. Teves D, Videen TO, Cryer PE, et al. Activation of human medial prefrontal cortex during autonomic responses to hypoglycemia. Proc Natl Acad Sci U S A 2004; 101(16), 6217–6221.

80. Choi IY, Lee SP, Kim SG, et al. In vivo measurements of brain glucose transport using the reversible Michaelis-Menten model and simultaneous measurements of cerebral blood flow changes during hypoglycemia. J Cereb Blood Flow Metab 2001; 21(6), 653–663.

81. Blackman JD, Towle VL, Sturis J, et al. Hypoglycemic thresholds for cognitive dysfunction in IDDM. Diabetes 1992; 41(3), 392–399.

82. Choi IY, Seaquist ER, Gruetter R. Effect of hypoglycemia on brain glycogen metabolism in vivo. J Neurosci Res 2003; 72(1), 25–32.

83. Lubow JM, Pinon IG, Avogaro A, et al. Brain oxygen utilization is unchanged by hypoglycemia in normal humans: lactate, alanine, and leucine uptake are not sufficient to offset energy deficit. Am J Physiol Endocrinol Metab 2006; 290, E149–153.

84. Auer RN. Hypoglycemic brain damage. Metab Brain Dis 2004; 19(3–4), 169–175.

85. Ghajar JB, Gibson GE, Duffy TE. Regional acetylcholine metabolism in brain during acute hypoglycemia and recovery. J Neurochem 1985; 44(1), 94–98.

86. Gorell JM, Dolkart PH, Ferrendelli JA. Regional levels of glucose, amino acids, high energy phosphates, and cyclic nucleotides in the central nervous system during hypoglycemic stupor and behavioral recovery. J Neurochem 1976; 27(5), 1043–1049.

87. Ouyang YB, He QP, Li PA, et al. Is neuronal injury caused by hypoglycemic coma of the necrotic or apoptotic type? Neurochem Res 2000; 25(5), 661–667.

88. Mishriki YY. Hypoglycemia-induced neurogenic-type pulmonary edema: an underrecognized association. Endocr Pract 2004; 10(5), 429–431.

89. Berbel-Garcia A, Porta-Etessam J, Martinez-Salio A, et al. [Transient cerebral oedema associated to hypoglycaemia]. Rev Neurol 2004; 39(11), 1030–1033.

90. Jung SL, Kim BS, Lee KS, et al. Magnetic resonance imaging and diffusion-weighted imaging changes after hypoglycemic coma. J Neuroimaging 2005; 15(2), 193–196.

91. Bando N, Watanabe K, Tomotake M, et al. Central pontine myelinolysis associated with a hypoglycemic coma in anorexia nervosa. Gen Hosp Psychiatry 2005; 27(5), 372–374.

92. Clarkson AN, Sutherland BA, Appleton I. The biology and pathology of hypoxia-ischemia: an update. Arch Immunol Ther Exp (Warsz) 2005; 53(3), 213–225.

93. Nelson LE, Guo TZ, Lu J, et al. The sedative component of anesthesia is mediated by GABA(A) receptors in an endogenous sleep pathway. Nat Neurosci 2002; 5(10), 979–984.

94. Mashour GA. Consciousness unbound: toward a paradigm of general anesthesia. Anesthesiology 2004; 100(2), 428–433.

95. Mashour GA, Forman SA, Campagna JA. Mechanisms of general anesthesia: from molecules to mind. Best Pract Res Clin Anaesthesiol 2005; 19(3), 349–364.

96. Campagna JA, Miller KW, Forman SA. Mechanisms of actions of inhaled anesthetics. N Engl J Med 2003; 348(21), 2110–2124.

97. Rudolph U, Mohler H. Analysis of GABAA receptor function and dissection of the pharmacology of benzodiazepines and general anesthetics through mouse genetics. Annu Rev Pharmacol Toxicol 2004; 44, 475–498.

98. Langsjo JW, Maksimow A, Salmi E, et al. S-ketamine anesthesia increases cerebral blood flow in excess of the metabolic needs in humans. Anesthesiology 2005; 103(2), 258–268.

99. Doyle PW, Matta BF. Burst suppression or isoelectric encephalogram for cerebral protection: evidence from metabolic suppression studies. Br J Anaesth 1999; 83(4), 580–584.

100. Nilsson L, Siesjo BK. The effect of anesthetics upon labile phosphates and upon extra- and intracellular lactate, pyruvate and bicarbonate concentrations in the rat brain. Acta Physiol Scand 1970; 80(2), 235–248.

101. Kalviainen R, Eriksson K, Parviainen I. Refractory generalised convulsive status epilepticus: a guide to treatment. CNS Drugs 2005; 19(9), 759–768.

102. Elsersy H, Sheng H, Lynch JR, et al. Effects of isoflurane versus fentanyl-nitrous oxide anesthesia on long-term outcome from severe forebrain ischemia in the rat. Anesthesiology 2004; 100(5), 1160–1166.

103. Bayona NA, Gelb AW, Jiang Z, et al. Propofol neuroprotection in cerebral ischemia and its effects on low-molecular-weight antioxidants and skilled motor tasks. Anesthesiology 2004; 100(5), 1151–1159.

104. Almaas R, Saugstad OD, Pleasure D, et al. Effect of barbiturates on hydroxyl radicals, lipid peroxidation, and hypoxic cell death in human NT2-N neurons. Anesthesiology 2000; 92(3), 764–774.

105. Imaoka S, Osada M, Minamiyama Y, et al. Role of phenobarbital-inducible cytochrome P450s as a source of active oxygen species in DNA-oxidation. Cancer Lett 2004; 203(2), 117–125.

106. Singh D, Kumar P, Majumdar S, et al. Effect of phenobarbital on free radicals in neonates with hypoxic

ischemic encephalopathy—a randomized controlled trial. J Perinat Med 2004; 32(3), 278–281.

107. Vincent JL, Berre J. Primer on medical management of severe brain injury. Crit Care Med 2005; 33(6), 1392–1399.

108. Auer RN, Siesjo BK. Biological differences between ischemia, hypoglycemia, and epilepsy. Ann Neurol 1988; 24(6), 699–707.

109. Maramattom BV, Wijdicks EF. Postresuscitation encephalopathy. Current views, management, and prognostication. Neurologist 2005; 11(4), 234–243.

110. Hossmann KA. Reperfusion of the brain after global ischemia: hemodynamic disturbances. Shock 1997; 8(2), 95–101; discussion 102–103.

111. del Zoppo GJ, Hallenbeck JM. Advances in the vascular pathophysiology of ischemic stroke. Thromb Res 2000; 98(3), 73–81.

112. Hai J, Lin Q, Li ST, et al. Chronic cerebral hypoperfusion and reperfusion injury of restoration of normal perfusion pressure contributes to the neuropathological changes in rat brain. Brain Res Mol Brain Res 2004; 126(2), 137–145.

113. White BC, Sullivan JM, DeGracia DJ, et al. Brain ischemia and reperfusion: molecular mechanisms of neuronal injury. J Neurol Sci 2000; 179(S1–2), 1–33.

114. Miyamoto O, Auer RN. Hypoxia, hyperoxia, ischemia, and brain necrosis. Neurology 2000; 54(2), 362–371.

115. Taraszewska A, Zelman IB, Ogonowska W, et al. The pattern of irreversible brain changes after cardiac arrest in humans. Folia Neuropathol 2002; 40(3), 133–141.

116. Zola-Morgan S, Squire LR. Neuroanatomy of memory. Annu Rev Neurosci 1993; 16, 547–563.

117. Maulaz A, Piechowski-Jozwiak B, Michel P, et al. Selecting patients for early stroke treatment with penumbra images. Cerebrovasc Dis 2005; 20(Suppl 2), 19–24.

118. Schaller B, Graf R. Cerebral ischemia and reperfusion: the pathophysiologic concept as a basis for clinical therapy. J Cereb Blood Flow Metab 2004; 24(4), 351–371.

119. Sharp FR, Ran R, Lu A, et al. Hypoxic preconditioning protects against ischemic brain injury. NeuroRx 2004; 1(1), 26–35.

120. Trzepacz PT. Is there a final common neural pathway in delirium? Focus on acetylcholine and dopamine. Semin Clin Neuropsychiatry 2000; 5(2), 132–148.

121. Perry EK, Perry RH. Neurochemistry of consciousness: cholinergic pathologies in the human brain. Prog Brain Res 2004; 145, 287–299.

122. Tassonyi E, Charpantier E, Muller D, et al. The role of nicotinic acetylcholine receptors in the mechanisms of anesthesia. Brain Res Bull 2002; 57(2), 133–150.

123. Han L, McCusker J, Cole M, et al. Use of medications with anticholinergic effect predicts clinical severity of delirium symptoms in older medical inpatients. Arch Intern Med 2001; 161(8), 1099–1105.

124. Schuck S, tue-Ferrer D, Kleinermans D, et al. Psychomotor and cognitive effects of piribedil, a dopamine agonist, in young healthy volunteers. Fundam Clin Pharmacol 2002; 16(1), 57–65.

125. Tune LE, Bylsma FW. Benzodiazepine-induced and anticholinergic-induced delirium in the elderly. Int Psychogeriatr 1991; 3(2), 397–408.

126. Mouradian MD, Penovich PE. Spindle coma in benzodiazepine toxicity: case report. Clin Electroencephalogr 1985; 16(4), 213–218.

127. Ahboucha S, Pomier-Layrargues G, Butterworth RF. Increased brain concentrations of endogenous (non-benzodiazepine) GABA-A receptor ligands in human hepatic encephalopathy. Metab Brain Dis 2004; 19(3–4), 241–251.

128. Lewis MC, Barnett SR. Postoperative delirium: the tryptophan dysregulation model. Med Hypotheses 2004; 63(3), 402–406.

129. Flacker JM, Lipsitz LA. Neural mechanisms of delirium: current hypotheses and evolving concepts. J Gerontol [A] 1999; 54(6), B239-B246.

130. Van der Mast RC, Fekkes D. Serotonin and amino acids: partners in delirium pathophysiology? Semin Clin Neuropsychiatry 2000; 5(2), 125–131.

131. Markus CR, Jonkman LM, Lammers JH, et al. Evening intake of alpha-lactalbumin increases plasma tryptophan availability and improves morning alertness and brain measures of attention. Am J Clin Nutr 2005; 81(5), 1026–1033.

132. Drugs that may cause psychiatric symptoms. Med Lett Drugs Ther 2002; 44(1134), 59–62.

133. Catalano G, Catalano MC, Alberts VA. Famotidine-associated delirium. A series of six cases. Psychosomatics 1996; 37(4), 349–355.

134. Preuss UW, Koller G, Bahlmann M, et al. No association between metabotropic glutamate receptors 7 and 8 (mGlur7 and mGlur8) gene polymorphisms and withdrawal seizures and delirium tremens in alcohol-dependent individuals. Alcohol Alcohol 2002; 37(2), 174–178.

135. Hawley RJ, Nemeroff CB, Bissette G, et al. Neurochemical correlates of sympathetic activation during severe alcohol withdrawal. Alcohol Clin Exp Res 1994; 18(6), 1312–1316.

136. Koguchi K, Nakatsuji Y, Abe K, et al. Wernicke's encephalopathy after glucose infusion. Neurology 2004; 62(3), 512.

137. Stiefel MF, Heuer GG, Smith MJ, et al. Cerebral oxygenation following decompressive hemicraniectomy for the treatment of refractory intracranial hypertension. J Neurosurg 2004; 101(2), 241–247.

138. Stiefel MF, Spiotta A, Gracias VH, et al. Reduced mortality rate in patients with severe traumatic brain injury treated with brain tissue oxygen monitoring. J Neurosurg 2005; 103(5), 805–811.

139. Smythe PR, Samra SK. Monitors of cerebral oxygenation. Anesthesiol Clin North America 2002; 20(2), 293–313.

140. Siggaard-Andersen O, Ulrich A, Gothgen IH. Classes of tissue hypoxia. Acta Anaesthesiol Scand Suppl 1995; 107, 137–142.

141. Wilson WC, Shapiro B. Perioperative hypoxia. The clinical spectrum and current oxygen monitoring methodology. Anesthesiol Clin North America 2001; 19(4), 769–812.

142. James PB, Calder IM. Anoxic asphyxia—a cause of industrial fatalities: a review. J R Soc Med 1991; 84(8), 493–495.

143. Hossmann KA. The hypoxic brain. Insights from ischemia research. Adv Exp Med Biol 1999; 474, 155–169.

144. Kulik A, Trapp S, Ballanyi K. Ischemia but not anoxia evokes vesicular and Ca(2+)-independent glutamate

release in the dorsal vagal complex in vitro. J Neurophysiol 2000; 83(5), 2905–2915.

145. Fleidervish IA, Gebhardt C, Astman N, et al. Enhanced spontaneous transmitter release is the earliest consequence of neocortical hypoxia that can explain the disruption of normal circuit function. J Neurosci 2001; 21(13), 4600–4608.

146. Kao LW, Nanagas KA. Carbon monoxide poisoning. Med Clin North Am 2005; 89(6), 1161–1194.

147. Ries NL, Dart RC. New developments in antidotes. Med Clin North Am 2005; 89(6), 1379–1397.

148. Miller TH, Kruse JE. Evaluation of syncope. Am Fam Physician 2005; 72(8), 1492–1500.

149. Parry SW, Steen IN, Baptist M, et al. Amnesia for loss of consciousness in carotid sinus syndrome: implications for presentation with falls. J Am Coll Cardiol 2005; 45(11), 1840–1843.

150. Stevens DL, Matthews WB. Cryptogenic drop attacks: an affliction of women. Br Med J 1973; 1(5851), 439–442.

151. Parry SW, Kenny RA. Drop attacks in older adults: systematic assessment has a high diagnostic yield. J Am Geriatr Soc 2005; 53(1), 74–78.

152. Ishiyama G, Ishiyama A, Jacobson K, et al. Drop attacks in older patients secondary to an otologic cause. Neurology 2001; 57(6), 1103–1106.

153. Maurice-Williams RS. Drop attacks from cervical cord compression. Br J Clin Pract 1974; 28(6), 215–216.

154. Ferbert A, Bruckmann H, Drummen R. Clinical features of proven basilar artery occlusion. Stroke 1990; 21(8), 1135–1142.

155. Oguni H, Uehara T, Imai K, et al. Atonic epileptic drop attacks associated with generalized spike-and-slow wave complexes: video-polygraphic study in two patients. Epilepsia 1997; 38(7), 813–818.

156. Fejerman N. Nonepileptic disorders imitating generalized idiopathic epilepsies. Epilepsia 2005; 46(Suppl 9), 80–83.

157. Andermann F, Tenembaum S. Negative motor phenomena in generalized epilepsies. A study of atonic seizures. Adv Neurol 1995; 67, 9–28.

158. Castelli R, Tarsia P, Tantardini C, et al. Syncope in patients with pulmonary embolism: comparison between patients with syncope as the presenting symptom of pulmonary embolism and patients with pulmonary embolism without syncope. Vasc Med 2003; 8(4), 257–261.

159. Marine JE, Goldhaber SZ. Pulmonary embolism presenting as seizures. Chest 1997; 112(3), 840–842.

160. Fred HL, Willerson JT, Alexander JK. Neurological manifestations of pulmonary thromboembolism. Arch Intern Med 1967; 120, 33–37.

161. Cohen-Gadol AA, DiLuna ML, Spencer DD. Partial epilepsy presenting as episodic dyspnea: a specific network involved in limbic seizure propagation. Case report. J Neurosurg 2004; 100(3), 565–567.

162. Munoz X, Marti S, Sumalla J, et al. Acute delirium as a manifestation of obstructive sleep apnea syndrome. Am J Respir Crit Care Med 1998; 158(4), 1306–1307.

163. Basnyat B, Wu T, Gertsch JH. Neurological conditions at altitude that fall outside the usual definition of altitude sickness. High Alt Med Biol 2004; 5(2), 171–179.

164. Basnyat B. Delirium at high altitude. High Alt Med Biol 2002; 3(1), 69–71.

165. Vaughan CJ, Delanty N. Hypertensive emergencies. Lancet 2000; 356(9227), 411–417.

166. Schwartz RB. Hyperperfusion encephalopathies: hypertensive encephalopathy and related conditions. Neurologist 2002; 8(1), 22–34.

167. Hinchey J, Chaves C, Appignani B, et al. A reversible posterior leukoencephalopathy syndrome. N Engl J Med 1996; 334, 494–500.

168. Garg RK. Posterior leukoencephalopathy syndrome. Postgrad Med J 2001; 77(903), 24–28.

169. Stott VL, Hurrell MA, Anderson TJ. Reversible posterior leukoencephalopathy syndrome: a misnomer reviewed. Intern Med J 2005; 35(2), 83–90.

170. Quick AM, Cipolla MJ. Pregnancy-induced upregulation of aquaporin-4 protein in brain and its role in eclampsia. FASEB J 2005; 19(2), 170–175.

171. Schiff D, Lopes MB. Neuropathological correlates of reversible posterior leukoencephalopathy. Neurocrit Care 2005; 2(3), 303–305.

172. Lavigne CM, Shrier DA, Ketkar M, et al. Tacrolimus leukoencephalopathy: a neuropathologic confirmation. Neurology 2004; 63(6), 1132–1133.

173. Mak W, Chan KH, Cheung RT, et al. Hypertensive encephalopathy: BP lowering complicated by posterior circulation ischemic stroke. Neurology 2004; 63(6), 1131–1132.

174. Duley L, Gulmezoglu AM, Henderson-Smart DJ. Magnesium sulphate and other anticonvulsants for women with pre-eclampsia. Cochrane Database Syst Rev 2003; 2, CD000025.

175. Taylor FB Jr, Toh CH, Hoots WK, et al. Towards definition, clinical and laboratory criteria, and a scoring system for disseminated intravascular coagulation. Thromb Haemost 2001; 86(5), 1327–1330.

176. Gogos CA, Lekkou A, Papageorgiou O, et al. Clinical prognostic markers in patients with severe sepsis: a prospective analysis of 139 consecutive cases. J Infect 2003; 47(4), 300–306.

177. Selladurai BM, Vickneswaran M, Duraisamy S, et al. Coagulopathy in acute head injury—a study of its role as a prognostic indicator. Br J Neurosurg 1997; 11(5), 398–404.

178. Morita T, Tei Y, Tsunoda J, et al. Underlying pathologies and their associations with clinical features in terminal delirium of cancer patients. J Pain Symptom Manage 2001; 22(6), 997–1006.

179. Toh CH, Dennis M. Disseminated intravascular coagulation: old disease, new hope. BMJ 2003; 327(7421), 974–977.

180. Levi M. Disseminated intravascular coagulation: what's new? Crit Care Clin 2005; 21(3), 449–467.

181. Idro R, Jenkins NE, Newton CR. Pathogenesis, clinical features, and neurological outcome of cerebral malaria. Lancet Neurol 2005; 4(12), 827–840.

182. Bardana D, Rudan J, Cervenko F, et al. Fat embolism syndrome in a patient demonstrating only neurologic symptoms. Can J Surg 1998; 41(5), 398–402.

183. Guillevin R, Vallee JN, Demeret S, et al. Cerebral fat embolism: usefulness of magnetic resonance spectroscopy. Ann Neurol 2005; 57(3), 434–439.

184. Parizel PM, Demey HE, Veeckmans G, et al. Early diagnosis of cerebral fat embolism syndrome by

diffusion-weighted MRI (starfield pattern). Stroke 2001; 32(12), 2942–2944.

185. Gregorakos L, Sakayianni K, Hroni D, et al. Prolonged coma due to cerebral fat embolism: report of two cases. J Accid Emerg Med 2000; 17(2), 144–146.

186. Schmid A, Tzur A, Leshko L, et al. Silicone embolism syndrome: a case report, review of the literature, and comparison with fat embolism syndrome. Chest 2005; 127(6), 2276–2281.

187. Gao L, Taha R, Gauvin D, et al. Postoperative cognitive dysfunction after cardiac surgery. Chest 2005; 128(5), 3664–3670.

188. McKhann GM, Grega MA, Borowicz LM Jr, et al. Is there cognitive decline 1 year after CABG? Comparison with surgical and nonsurgical controls. Neurology 2005; 65(7), 991–999.

189. Moreillon P, Que YA. Infective endocarditis. Lancet 2004; 363(9403), 139–149.

190. Rogers LR. Cerebrovascular complications in cancer patients. Neurol Clin 2003; 21(1), 167–192.

191. Rivas P, Alonso J, Moya J, et al. The impact of hospital-acquired infections on the microbial etiology and prognosis of late-onset prosthetic valve endocarditis. Chest 2005; 128(2), 764–771.

192. Ekinci EI, Donnan GA. Neurological manifestations of cardiac myxoma: a review of the literature and report of cases. Intern Med J 2004; 34(5), 243–249.

193. Singhal AB, Topcuoglu MA, Buonanno FS. Acute ischemic stroke patterns in infective and nonbacterial thrombotic endocarditis: a diffusion-weighted magnetic resonance imaging study. Stroke 2002; 33(5), 1267–1273.

194. Lee RJ, Bartzokis T, Yeoh T-K, et al. Enhanced detection of intracardiac sources of cerebral emboli by transesophageal echocardiography. Stroke 1991; 22, 734–739.

195. Choi IS. Delayed neurologic sequelae in carbon monoxide intoxication. Arch Neurol 1983; 40(7), 433–435.

196. Kwon OY, Chung SP, Ha YR, et al. Delayed postanoxic encephalopathy after carbon monoxide poisoning. Emerg Med J 2004; 21(2), 250–251.

197. Gilmer B, Kilkenny J, Tomaszewski C, et al. Hyperbaric oxygen does not prevent neurologic sequelae after carbon monoxide poisoning. Acad Emerg Med 2002; 9(1), 1–8.

198. Kim HY, Kim BJ, Moon SY, et al. Serial diffusion-weighted MR imaging in delayed postanoxic encephalopathy. A case study. J Neuroradiol 2002; 29(3), 211–215.

199. Plum F, Posner JB, Hain RF. Delayed neurological deterioration after anoxia. Arch Intern Med 1962; 110, 18–25.

200. Takahashi W, Ohnuki Y, Takizawa S, et al. Neuroimaging on delayed postanoxic encephalopathy with lesions localized in basal ganglia. Clin Imaging 1998; 22(3), 188–191.

201. Weinberger LM, Schmidley JW, Schafer IA, et al. Delayed postanoxic demyelination and arylsulfatase-A pseudodeficiency. Neurology 1994; 44(1), 152–154.

202. Custodio CM, Basford JR. Delayed postanoxic encephalopathy: a case report and literature review. Arch Phys Med Rehabil 2004; 85(3), 502–505.

203. Wijdicks EF, Parisi JE, Sharbrough FW. Prognostic value of myoclonus status in comatose survivors of cardiac arrest. Ann Neurol 1994; 35(2), 239–243.

204. Frucht SJ. The clinical challenge of posthypoxic myoclonus. Adv Neurol 2002; 89, 85–88.

205. Gabriely I, Shamoon H. Hypoglycemia in diabetes: common, often unrecognized. Cleve Clin J Med 2004; 71(4), 335–342.

206. Hart SP, Frier BM. Causes, management and morbidity of acute hypoglycaemia in adults requiring hospital admission. QJM 1998; 91(7), 505–510.

207. Bhasin R, Arce FC, Pasmantier R. Hypoglycemia associated with the use of gatifloxacin. Am J Med Sci 2005; 330(5), 250–253.

208. Park-Wyllie LY, Juurlink DN, Kopp A, et al. Outpatient gatifloxacin therapy and dysglycemia in older adults. N Engl J Med 2006; 354(13), 1352–1361.

209. Pedersen-Bjergaard U, Reubsaet JL, Nielsen SL, et al. Psychoactive drugs, alcohol, and severe hypoglycemia in insulin-treated diabetes: analysis of 141 cases. Am J Med 2005; 118(3), 307–310.

210. Abarbanell NR. Is prehospital blood glucose measurement necessary in suspected cerebrovascular accident patients? Am J Emerg Med 2005; 23(7), 823–827.

211. Izzo JL, Schuster DB, Engel GL. The electroencephalogram of patients with diabetes mellitus. Diabetes 1953; 2(2), 93–99.

212. Kaufman FR, Epport K, Engilman R, et al. Neurocognitive functioning in children diagnosed with diabetes before age 10 years. J Diabetes Complications 1999; 13(1), 31–38.

213. Frier BM. Morbidity of hypoglycemia in type 1 diabetes. Diabetes Res Clin Pract 2004; 65(Suppl 1), S47-S52.

214. Aoki T, Sato T, Hasegawa K, et al. Reversible hyperintensity lesion on diffusion-weighted MRI in hypoglycemic coma. Neurology 2004; 63(2), 392–393.

215. Moore C, Woollard M. Dextrose 10% or 50% in the treatment of hypoglycaemia out of hospital? A randomised controlled trial. Emerg Med J 2005; 22(7), 512–515.

216. Gispen WH, Biessels GJ. Cognition and synaptic plasticity in diabetes mellitus. Trends Neurosci 2000; 23(11), 542–549.

217. Victor M, Adams RD, Collins GH. The Wernicke-Korsakoff syndrome. A clinical and pathological study of 245 patients, 82 with post-mortem examinations. Contemp Neurol Ser 1971; 7, 1–206.

218. Wallis WE, Willoughby E, Baker P. Coma in the Wernicke-Korsakoff syndrome. Lancet 1978; 2(8086), 400–401.

219. Mousseau DD, Rao VL, Butterworth RF. Alterations in serotonin parameters in brain of thiamine-deficient rats are evident prior to the appearance of neurological symptoms. J Neurochem 1996; 67(3), 1113–1123.

220. Waldenlind L. Studies on thiamine and neuromuscular transmission. Acta Physiol Scand Suppl 1978; 459, 1–35.

221. Pepersack T, Garbusinski J, Robberecht J, et al. Clinical relevance of thiamine status amongst hospitalized elderly patients. Gerontology 1999; 45(2), 96–101.

222. Halavaara J, Brander A, Lyytinen J, et al. Wernicke's encephalopathy: is diffusion-weighted MRI useful? Neuroradiology 2003; 45(8), 519–523.

223. Loh Y, Watson WD, Verma A, et al. Restricted diffusion of the splenium in acute Wernicke's encephalopathy. J Neuroimaging 2005; 15(4), 373–375.

224. Lee ST, Jung YM, Na DL, et al. Corpus callosum atrophy in Wernicke's encephalopathy. J Neuroimaging 2005; 15(4), 367–372.

225. Blei AT. The pathophysiology of brain edema in acute liver failure. Neurochem Int 2005; 47(1–2), 71–77.

226. Gerber T, Schomerus H. Hepatic encephalopathy in liver cirrhosis: pathogenesis, diagnosis and management. Drugs 2000; 60(6), 1353–1370.

227. Shawcross D, Jalan R. The pathophysiologic basis of hepatic encephalopathy: central role for ammonia and inflammation. Cell Mol Life Sci 2005; 62(19–20), 2295–2304.

228. Ott P, Larsen FS. Blood-brain barrier permeability to ammonia in liver failure: a critical reappraisal. Neurochem Int 2004; 44(4), 185–198.

229. Caplan LR, Scheiner D. Dysconjugate gaze in hepatic coma. Ann Neurol 1980; 8(3), 328–329.

230. Rai GS, Buxton-Thomas M, Scanlon M. Ocular bobbing in hepatic encephalopathy. Br J Clin Pract 1976; 30(10), 202–205.

231. Weissenborn K, Bokemeyer M, Krause J, et al. Neurological and neuropsychiatric syndromes associated with liver disease. AIDS 2005; 19(Suppl 3), S93-S98.

232. Timmermann L, Gross J, Kircheis G, et al. Cortical origin of mini-asterixis in hepatic encephalopathy. Neurology 2002; 58(2), 295–298.

233. Vergara F, Plum F, Duffy TE. Alpha-ketoglutaramate: increased concentrations in the cerebrospinal fluid of patients in hepatic coma. Science 1974; 183(120), 81–83.

234. Tarasow E, Panasiuk A, Siergiejczyk L, et al. MR and 1H MR spectroscopy of the brain in patients with liver cirrhosis and early stages of hepatic encephalopathy. Hepatogastroenterology 2003; 50(54), 2149–2153.

235. Weissenborn K, Bokemeyer M, Ahl B, et al. Functional imaging of the brain in patients with liver cirrhosis. Metab Brain Dis 2004; 19(3–4), 269–280.

236. Arieff AI, Massry SG. Calcium metabolism of brain in acute renal failure. Effects of uremia, hemodialysis, and parathyroid hormone. J Clin Invest 1974; 53(2), 387–392.

237. Cogan MG, Covey CM, Arieff AI, et al. Central nervous system manifestations of hyperparathyroidism. Am J Med 1978; 65(6), 963–970.

238. Burn DJ, Bates D. Neurology and the kidney. J Neurol Neurosurg Psychiatry 1998; 65(6), 810–821.

239. Topczewska-Bruns J, Pawlak D, Chabielska E, et al. Increased levels of 3-hydroxykynurenine in different brain regions of rats with chronic renal insufficiency. Brain Res Bull 2002; 58(4), 423–428.

240. Vaziri ND. Oxidative stress in uremia: nature, mechanisms, and potential consequences. Semin Nephrol 2004; 24(5), 469–473.

241. Adachi N, Lei B, Deshpande G, et al. Uraemia suppresses central dopaminergic metabolism and impairs motor activity in rats. Intensive Care Med 2001; 27(10), 1655–1660.

242. Chow KM, Wang AY, Hui AC, et al. Nonconvulsive status epilepticus in peritoneal dialysis patients. Am J Kidney Dis 2001; 38(2), 400–405.

243. Abanades S, Nolla J, Rodriguez-Campello A, et al. Reversible coma secondary to cefepime neurotoxicity. Ann Pharmacother 2004; 38(4), 606–608.

244. Lance JW. Action myoclonus, Ramsay Hunt syndrome, and other cerebellar myoclonic syndromes. Adv Neurol 1986; 43, 33–55.

245. Chadwick D, French AT. Uraemic myoclonus: an example of reticular reflex myoclonus? J Neurol Neurosurg Psychiatry 1979; 42(1), 52–55.

246. Palmer CA. Neurologic manifestations of renal disease. Neurol Clin 2002; 20(1), 23–34, v.

247. Oo TN, Smith CL, Swan SK. Does uremia protect against the demyelination associated with correction of hyponatremia during hemodialysis? A case report and literature review. Semin Dial 2003; 16(1), 68–71.

248. Hung SC, Hung SH, Tarng DC, et al. Thiamine deficiency and unexplained encephalopathy in hemodialysis and peritoneal dialysis patients. Am J Kidney Dis 2001; 38(5), 941–947.

249. Bagshaw SM, Peets AD, Hameed M, et al. Dialysis disequilibrium syndrome: brain death following hemodialysis for metabolic acidosis and acute renal failure—a case report. BMC Nephrol 2004; 5, 9.

250. Silver SM, Sterns RH, Halperin ML. Brain swelling after dialysis: old urea or new osmoles? Am J Kidney Dis 1996; 28(1), 1–13.

251. Lien YH, Shapiro JI, Chan L. Study of brain electrolytes and organic osmolytes during correction of chronic hyponatremia. Implications for the pathogenesis of central pontine myelinolysis. J Clin Invest 1991; 88(1), 303–309.

252. Ponticelli C, Campise MR. Neurological complications in kidney transplant recipients. J Nephrol 2005; 18(5), 521–528.

253. Thaisetthawatkul P, Weinstock A, Kerr SL, et al. Muromonab-CD3-induced neurotoxicity: report of two siblings, one of whom had subsequent cyclosporin-induced neurotoxicity. J Child Neurol 2001; 16(11), 825–831.

254. Parizel PM, Snoeck HW, van den HL, et al. Cerebral complications of murine monoclonal CD3 antibody (OKT3): CT and MR findings. AJNR Am J Neuroradiol 1997; 18(10), 1935–1938.

255. Kirsch DB, Jozefowicz RF. Neurologic complications of respiratory disease. Neurol Clin 2002; 20(1), 247–264, viii.

256. Roussos C, Koutsoukou A. Respiratory failure. Eur Respir J Suppl 2003; 47, 3s-14s.

257. Miller A, Bader RA, Bader ME. The neurologic syndrome due to marked hypercapnia, with papilledema. Am J Med 1962; 33, 309–318.

258. Gomersall CD, Joynt GM, Freebairn RC, et al. Oxygen therapy for hypercapnic patients with chronic obstructive pulmonary disease and acute respiratory failure: a randomized, controlled pilot study. Crit Care Med 2002; 30(1), 113–116.

259. Brochard L. Mechanical ventilation: invasive versus noninvasive. Eur Respir J Suppl 2003; 47, 31s–37s.

260. Rotheram EB Jr, Safar P, Robin E. CNS disorder during mechanical ventilation in chronic pulmonary disease. JAMA 1964; 189, 993–996.

261. Faden A. Encephalopathy following treatment of chronic pulmonary failure. Neurology 1976; 26(4), 337–339.

262. Sjaastad O, Gjessing L, Ritland S, et al. Chronic relapsing pancreatitis, encephalopathy with disturbances of consciousness and CSF amino acid aberration. J Neurol 1979; 220(2), 83–94.

263. Estrada RV, Moreno J, Martinez E, et al. Pancreatic encephalopathy. Acta Neurol Scand 1979; 59(2–3), 135–139.

264. Kopieniak M, Wieczorkiewicz-Plaza A, Maciejewski R. Dopamine activity changes in cerebral cortex in the course of experimental acute pancreatitis. Ann Univ Mariae Curie Sklodowska [Med] 2004; 59(1), 382–386.

265. Ohkubo T, Shiojiri T, Matsunaga T. Severe diffuse white matter lesions in a patient with pancreatic encephalopathy. J Neurol 2004; 251(4), 476–478.

266. McMahon MJ, Woodhead JS, Hayward RD. The nature of hypocalcaemia in acute pancreatitis. Br J Surg 1978; 65(3), 216–218.

267. Ruggieri RM, Lupo I, Piccoli F. Pancreatic encephalopathy: a 7-year follow-up case report and review of the literature. Neurol Sci 2002; 23(4), 203–205.

268. Egede LE, Dagogo-Jack S. Epidemiology of type 2 diabetes: focus on ethnic minorities. Med Clin North Am 2005; 89(5), 949–75, viii.

269. Charfen MA, Fernandez-Frackelton M. Diabetic ketoacidosis. Emerg Med Clin North Am 2005; 23(3), 609–628, vii.

270. Nugent BW. Hyperosmolar hyperglycemic state. Emerg Med Clin North Am 2005; 23(3), 629–48, vii.

271. English P, Williams G. Hyperglycaemic crises and lactic acidosis in diabetes mellitus. Postgrad Med J 2004; 80(943), 253–261.

272. Trachtenbarg DE. Diabetic ketoacidosis. Am Fam Physician 2005; 71(9), 1705–1714.

273. Posner JB, Plum F. Spinal fluid pH and neurologic symptoms in systemic acidosis. New Engl J Med 1967; 277, 605–613.

274. Stades AM, Heikens JT, Erkelens DW, et al. Metformin and lactic acidosis: cause or coincidence? A review of case reports. J Intern Med 2004; 255(2), 179–187.

275. Riley LJ Jr, Cooper M, Narins RG. Alkali therapy of diabetic ketoacidosis: biochemical, physiologic, and clinical perspectives. Diabetes Metab Rev 1989; 5(8), 627–636.

276. Troy PJ, Clark RP, Kakarala SG, et al. Cerebral edema during treatment of diabetic ketoacidosis in an adult with new onset diabetes. Neurocrit Care 2005; 2(1), 55–58.

277. Cameron FJ, Kean MJ, Wellard RM, et al. Insights into the acute cerebral metabolic changes associated with childhood diabetes. Diabet Med 2005; 22(5), 648–653.

278. Berner YN, Shike M. Consequences of phosphate imbalance. Annu Rev Nutr 1988; 8, 121–148.

279. Wass CT, Lanier WL. Glucose modulation of ischemic brain injury: review and clinical recommendations. Mayo Clin Proc 1996; 71(8), 801–812.

280. Rovlias A, Kotsou S. The influence of hyperglycemia on neurological outcome in patients with severe head injury. Neurosurgery 2000; 46(2), 335–342; discussion 342–343.

281. Kagansky N, Levy S, Knobler H. The role of hyperglycemia in acute stroke. Arch Neurol 2001; 58(8), 1209–1212.

282. Selvin E, Coresh J, Shahar E, et al. Glycaemia (haemoglobin A(1c)) and incident ischaemic stroke: the Atherosclerosis Risk in Communities (ARIC) Study. Lancet Neurol 2005; 4(12), 821–826.

283. Li PA, Shuaib A, Miyashita H, et al. Hyperglycemia enhances extracellular glutamate accumulation in rats subjected to forebrain ischemia. Stroke 2000; 31(1), 183–192.

284. Kurihara J, Katsura K, Siesjo BK, et al. Hyperglycemia and hypercapnia differently affect post-ischemic changes in protein kinases and protein phosphorylation in the rat cingulate cortex. Brain Res 2004; 995(2), 218–225.

285. Artola A, Kamal A, Ramakers GM, et al. Diabetes mellitus concomitantly facilitates the induction of long-term depression and inhibits that of long-term potentiation in hippocampus. Eur J Neurosci 2005; 22(1), 169–178.

286. Li PA, Rasquinha I, He QP, et al. Hyperglycemia enhances DNA fragmentation after transient cerebral ischemia. J Cereb Blood Flow Metab 2001; 21(5), 568–576.

287. Pramming S, Thorsteinsson B, Bendtson I, et al. Symptomatic hypoglycaemia in 411 type 1 diabetic patients. Diabet Med 1991; 8(3), 217–222.

288. Fanelli CG, Porcellati F, Pampanelli S, et al. Insulin therapy and hypoglycaemia: the size of the problem. Diabetes Metab Res Rev 2004; 20(Suppl 2), S32-S42.

289. Faludi G, Bendersky G, Gerber P. Functional hypoglycemia in early latent diabetes. Ann N Y Acad Sci 1968; 148(3), 868–874.

290. Griffiths MJ, Gama R. Adult spontaneous hypoglycaemia. Hosp Med 2005; 66(5), 277–283.

291. Monami M, Mannucci E, Breschi A, et al. Seizures as the only clinical manifestation of reactive hypoglycemia: a case report. J Endocrinol Invest 2005; 28(10), 940–941.

292. Meijer E, Hoekstra JB, Erkelens DW. Hypoglycaemia unawareness. Presse Med 1994; 23(13), 623–627.

293. Aring AM, Jones DE, Falko JM. Evaluation and prevention of diabetic neuropathy. Am Fam Physician 2005; 71(11), 2123–2128.

294. Torrey SP. Recognition and management of adrenal emergencies. Emerg Med Clin North Am 2005; 23(3), 687–702, viii.

295. Arlt W, Allolio B. Adrenal insufficiency. Lancet 2003; 361(9372), 1881–1893.

296. Ten S, New M, Maclaren N. Clinical review 130: Addison's disease 2001. J Clin Endocrinol Metab 2001; 86(7), 2909–2922.

297. Espinosa G, Santos E, Cervera R, et al. Adrenal involvement in the antiphospholipid syndrome: clinical and immunologic characteristics of 86 patients. Medicine (Baltimore) 2003; 82(2), 106–118.

298. Kaplan PW. The EEG in metabolic encephalopathy and coma. J Clin Neurophysiol 2004; 21(5), 307–318.

299. Patten SB, Neutel CI. Corticosteroid-induced adverse psychiatric effects: incidence, diagnosis and management. Drug Saf 2000; 22(2), 111–122.

300. Beuschlein F, Hammer GD. Ectopic pro-opiomelanocortin syndrome. Endocrinol Metab Clin North Am 2002; 31(1), 191–234.

301. Tews MC, Shah SM, Gossain VV. Hypothyroidism: mimicker of common complaints. Emerg Med Clin North Am 2005; 23(3), 649–67, vii.

302. McKeown NJ, Tews MC, Gossain VV, et al. Hyperthyroidism. Emerg Med Clin North Am 2005; 23(3), 669–685, viii.

303. Konig S, Moura NV. Thyroid hormone actions on neural cells. Cell Mol Neurobiol 2002; 22(5–6), 517–544.

304. Desouza LA, Ladiwala U, Daniel SM, et al. Thyroid hormone regulates hippocampal neurogenesis in the adult rat brain. Mol Cell Neurosci 2005; 29(3), 414–426.

305. Constant EL, de Volder AG, Ivanoiu A, et al. Cerebral blood flow and glucose metabolism in hypothyroidism: a positron emission tomography study. J Clin Endocrinol Metab 2001; 86(8), 3864–3870.

306. Savage MW, Mah PM, Weetman AP, et al. Endocrine emergencies. Postgrad Med J 2004; 80(947), 506–515.

307. Pimentel L, Hansen KN. Thyroid disease in the emergency department: a clinical and laboratory review. J Emerg Med 2005; 28(2), 201–209.

308. Rodriguez I, Fluiters E, Perez-Mendez LF, et al. Factors associated with mortality of patients with myxoedema coma: prospective study in 11 cases treated in a single institution. J Endocrinol 2004; 180(2), 347–350.

309. Pohunkova D, Sulc J, Vana S. Influence of thyroid hormone supply on EEG frequency spectrum. Endocrinol Exp 1989; 23(4), 251–258.

310. River Y, Zelig O. Triphasic waves in myxedema coma. Clin Electroencephalogr 1993; 24(3), 146–150.

311. Chong JY, Rowland LP, Utiger RD. Hashimoto encephalopathy—syndrome or myth? Arch Neurol 2003; 60(2), 164–171.

312. Ferracci F, Bertiato G, Moretto G. Hashimoto's encephalopathy: epidemiologic data and pathogenetic considerations. J Neurol Sci 2004; 217(2), 165–168.

313. Oide T, Tokuda T, Yazaki M, et al. Anti-neuronal autoantibody in Hashimoto's encephalopathy: neuropathological, immunohistochemical, and biochemical analysis of two patients. J Neurol Sci 2004; 217(1), 7–12.

314. Schäuble B, Castillo PR, Boeve BF, et al. EEG findings in steroid-responsive encephalopathy associated with autoimmune thyroiditis. Clin Neurophysiol 2003; 114(1), 32–37.

315. Ghobrial MW, Ruby EB. Coma and thyroid storm in apathetic thyrotoxicosis. South Med J 2002; 95(5), 552–554.

316. Bailes BK. Hyperthyroidism in elderly patients. AORN J 1999; 69(1), 254–258.

317. Randeva HS, Schoebel J, Byrne J, et al. Classical pituitary apoplexy: clinical features, management and outcome. Clin Endocrinol (Oxf) 1999; 51(2), 181–188.

318. Arvanitis ML, Pasquale JL. External causes of metabolic disorders. Emerg Med Clin North Am 2005; 23(3), 827–841, x.

319. Posner JB. Neurologic Complications of Cancer. Philadelphia: F.A. Davis, 1995.

320. Clouston PD, DeAngelis LM, Posner JB. The spectrum of neurologic disease in patients with systemic cancer. Ann Neurol 1992; 31, 268–273.

321. Tuma R, DeAngelis LM. Altered mental status in patients with cancer. Arch Neurol 2000; 57(12), 1727–1731.

322. Maxwell JC. Party drugs: properties, prevalence, patterns, and problems. Subst Use Misuse 2005; 40(9–10), 1203–1240.

323. Fabbri A, Ruggeri S, Marchesini G, et al. A combined HPLC-immunoenzymatic comprehensive screening for suspected drug poisoning in the emergency department. Emerg Med J 2004; 21(3), 317–322.

324. Mokhlesi B, Corbridge T. Toxicology in the critically ill patient. Clin Chest Med 2003; 24(4), 689–711.

325. Judge BS. Metabolic acidosis: differentiating the causes in the poisoned patient. Med Clin North Am 2005; 89(6), 1107–1124.

326. Khom S, Baburin I, Timin EN, et al. Pharmacological properties of GABAA receptors containing gamma1 subunits. Mol Pharmacol 2006; 69, 640–649.

327. Mokhlesi B, Leikin JB, Murray P, et al. Adult toxicology in critical care: part II: specific poisonings. Chest 2003; 123(3), 897–922.

328. Currier GW, Trenton AJ, Walsh PG. Innovations: emergency psychiatry: relative accuracy of breath and serum alcohol readings in the psychiatric emergency service. Psychiatr Serv 2006; 57(1), 34–36.

329. Sterrett C, Brownfield J, Korn CS, et al. Patterns of presentation in heroin overdose resulting in pulmonary edema. Am J Emerg Med 2003; 21(1), 32–34.

330. Reed CE, Driggs MF, Foote CC. Acute barbiturate intoxication: a study of 300 cases based on a physiologic system of classification of the severity of the intoxication. Ann Intern Med 1952; 37(2), 290–303.

331. Young CC, Prielipp RC. Benzodiazepines in the intensive care unit. Crit Care Clin 2001; 17(4), 843–862.

332. Seger DL. Flumazenil—treatment or toxin. J Toxicol Clin Toxicol 2004; 42(2), 209–216.

333. Haimovic IC, Beresford HR. Transient unresponsiveness in the elderly. Report of five cases. Arch Neurol 1992; 49(1), 35–37.

334. Lugaresi E, Montagna P, Tinuper P et al. Endozepine stupor. Recurring stupor linked to endozepine-4 accumulation. Brain 1998; 121(Pt 1), 127–133.

335. Cortelli P, Avallone R, Baraldi M, et al. Endozepines in recurrent stupor. Sleep Med Rev 2005; 9(6), 477–487.

336. Granot R, Berkovic SF, Patterson S, et al. Endozepine stupor: disease or deception? A critical review. Sleep 2004; 27(8), 1597–1599.

337. Lugaresi E, Montagna P, Tinuper P, et al. Suspected covert lorazepam administration misdiagnosed as recurrent endozepine stupor. Brain 1998; 121(Pt 11), 2201.

338. Rowden AK, Norvell J, Eldridge DL, et al. Updates on acetaminophen toxicity. Med Clin North Am 2005; 89(6), 1145–1159.

339. Zimmerman JL. Poisonings and overdoses in the intensive care unit: general and specific management issues. Crit Care Med 2003; 31(12), 2794–2801.

340. Adityanjee, Munshi KR, Thampy A. The syndrome of irreversible lithium-effectuated neurotoxicity. Clin Neuropharmacol 2005; 28(1), 38–49.

341. Rutherford WH. Diagnosis of alcohol ingestion in mild head injuries. Lancet 1977; 1(8020), 1021–1023.
342. McIntosh C, Chick J. Alcohol and the nervous system. J Neurol Neurosurg Psychiatry 2004; 75(Suppl 3), iii16-iii21.
343. Mokhlesi B, Garimella PS, Joffe A, et al. Street drug abuse leading to critical illness. Intensive Care Med 2004; 30(8), 1526–1536.
344. Snead OC III, Gibson KM. Gamma-hydroxybutyric acid. N Engl J Med 2005; 352(26), 2721–2732.
345. Traub SJ, Nelson LS, Hoffman RS. Physostigmine as a treatment for gamma-hydroxybutyrate toxicity: a review. J Toxicol Clin Toxicol 2002; 40(6), 781–787.
346. Bania TC, Chu J. Physostigmine does not effect arousal but produces toxicity in an animal model of severe gamma-hydroxybutyrate intoxication. Acad Emerg Med 2005; 12(3), 185–189.
347. Morris BJ, Cochran SM, Pratt JA. PCP: from pharmacology to modelling schizophrenia. Curr Opin Pharmacol 2005; 5(1), 101–106.
348. Wolff K, Winstock AR. Ketamine: from medicine to misuse. CNS Drugs 2006; 20(3), 199–218.
349. Britt GC, Cance-Katz EF. A brief overview of the clinical pharmacology of "club drugs." Subst Use Misuse 2005; 40(9–10), 1189–1201.
350. Perkin MR, Wey EQ. Emergency drug availability on general paediatric units. Resuscitation 2004; 62(2), 243–247.
351. Christopher MM, Eckfeldt JH, Eaton JW. Propylene glycol ingestion causes D-lactic acidosis. Lab Invest 1990; 62(1), 114–118.
352. Lalive PH, Hadengue A, Mensi N, et al. [Recurrent encephalopathy after small bowel resection. Implication of D-lactate]. Rev Neurol (Paris) 2001; 157(6–7), 679–681.
353. Stacpoole PW, Wright EC, Baumgartner TG, et al. Natural history and course of acquired lactic acidosis in adults. DCA-Lactic Acidosis Study Group. Am J Med 1994; 97(1), 47–54.
354. Xiang Z, Yuan M, Hassen GW, et al. Lactate induced excitotoxicity in hippocampal slice cultures. Exp Neurol 2004; 186(1), 70–77.
355. Lin M, Liu SJ, Lim IT. Disorders of water imbalance. Emerg Med Clin North Am 2005; 23(3), 749–770, ix.
356. Videen JS, Michaelis T, Pinto P, et al. Human cerebral osmolytes during chronic hyponatremia. A proton magnetic resonance spectroscopy study. J Clin Invest 1995; 95(2), 788–793.
357. Fraser CL, Arieff AI. Epidemiology, pathophysiology, and management of hyponatremic encephalopathy. Am J Med 1997; 102(1), 67–77.
358. Moritz ML, Ayus JC. The pathophysiology and treatment of hyponatraemic encephalopathy: an update. Nephrol Dial Transplant 2003; 18(12), 2486–2491.
359. Pasantes-Morales H, Franco R, Ordaz B, et al. Mechanisms counteracting swelling in brain cells during hyponatremia. Arch Med Res 2002; 33(3), 237–244.
360. Massieu L, Montiel T, Robles G, et al. Brain amino acids during hyponatremia in vivo: clinical observations and experimental studies. Neurochem Res 2004; 29(1), 73–81.
361. Hsu YJ, Chiu JS, Lu KC, et al. Biochemical and etiological characteristics of acute hyponatremia in the emergency department. J Emerg Med 2005; 29(4), 369–374.
362. Mooradian AD, Morley GK, McGeachie R, et al. Spontaneous periodic hypothermia. Neurology 1984; 34(1), 79–82.
363. Moon Y, Hong SJ, Shin D, et al. Increased aquaporin-1 expression in choroid plexus epithelium after systemic hyponatremia. Neurosci Lett 2006; 395, 1–6.
364. Vajda Z, Promeneur D, Doczi T, et al. Increased aquaporin-4 immunoreactivity in rat brain in response to systemic hyponatremia. Biochem Biophys Res Commun 2000; 270(2), 495–503.
365. Goh KP. Management of hyponatremia. Am Fam Physician 2004; 69(10), 2387–2394.
366. Torchinsky MY, Deputy S, Rambeau F, et al. Hypokalemia and alkalosis in adipsic hypernatremia are not associated with hyperaldosteronism. Horm Res 2004; 62(4), 187–190.
367. Adrogue HJ, Madias NE. Hypo-Hypernatremia. N Engl J Med 2000; 342, 1493–1499, 1581–1589.
368. Kang SK, Kim W, Oh MS. Pathogenesis and treatment of hypernatremia. Nephron 2002; 92(Suppl 1), 14–17.
369. Gaglia JL, Wyckoff J, Abrahamson MJ. Acute hyperglycemic crisis in the elderly. Med Clin North Am 2004; 88(4), 1063–1084, xii.
370. Ka T, Takahashi S, Tsutsumi Z, et al. Hyperosmolar non-ketotic diabetic syndrome associated with rhabdomyolysis and acute renal failure: a case report and review of literature. Diabetes Nutr Metab 2003; 16(5–6), 317–322.
371. Riggs JE. Neurologic manifestations of electrolyte disturbances. Neurol Clin 2002; 20(1), 227–239, vii.
372. Patten BM, Pages M. Severe neurological disease associated with hyperparathyroidism. Ann Neurol 1984; 15(5), 453–456.
373. Clines GA, Guise TA. Hypercalcaemia of malignancy and basic research on mechanisms responsible for osteolytic and osteoblastic metastasis to bone. Endocr Relat Cancer 2005; 12(3), 549–583.
374. Miller DW, Slovis CM. Hypophosphatemia in the emergency department therapeutics. Am J Emerg Med 2000; 18(4), 457–461.
375. Faden A. Encephalopathy following treatment of chronic pulmonary failure. Neurology 1976; 26(4), 337–339.
376. Kiyatkin EA. Brain hyperthermia as physiological and pathological phenomena. Brain Res Brain Res Rev 2005; 50(1), 27–56.
377. Bazille C, Megarbane B, Bensimhon D, et al. Brain damage after heat stroke. J Neuropathol Exp Neurol 2005; 64(11), 970–975.
378. McCullough L, Arora S. Diagnosis and treatment of hypothermia. Am Fam Physician 2004; 70(12), 2325–2332.
379. Ballester JM, Harchelroad FP. Hypothermia: an easy-to-miss, dangerous disorder in winter weather. Geriatrics 1999; 54(2), 51–57.
380. Foex BA, Butler J. Best evidence topic report. Therapeutic hypothermia after out of hospital cardiac arrest. Emerg Med J 2004; 21(5), 590–591.
381. Shapiro WR, Williams GH, Plum F. Spontaneous recurrent hypothermia accompanying agenesis of the corpus callosum. Brain 1969; 92(2), 423–436.

382. Yeo TP. Heat stroke: a comprehensive review. AACN Clin Issues 2004; 15(2), 280–293.

383. Bouchama A, Knochel JP. Heat stroke 1. N Engl J Med 2002; 346(25), 1978–1988.

384. Thompson HJ, Pinto-Martin J, Bullock MR. Neurogenic fever after traumatic brain injury: an epidemiological study. J Neurol Neurosurg Psychiatry 2003; 74(5), 614–619.

385. Kipps CM, Fung VS, Grattan-Smith P, et al. Movement disorder emergencies. Mov Disord 2005; 20(3), 322–334.

386. Melli G, Chaudhry V, Cornblath DR. Rhabdomyolysis: an evaluation of 475 hospitalized patients. Medicine (Baltimore) 2005; 84(6), 377–385.

387. Rusyniak DE, Sprague JE. Toxin-induced hyperthermic syndromes. Med Clin North Am 2005; 89(6), 1277–1296.

388. Pruitt AA. Nervous system infections in patients with cancer. Neurol Clin 2003; 21(1), 193–219.

389. Cunha BA. Central nervous system infections in the compromised host: a diagnostic approach. Infect Dis Clin North Am 2001; 15(2), 567–590.

390. van de BD, De Gans J, Spanjaard L, et al. Clinical features and prognostic factors in adults with bacterial meningitis. N Engl J Med 2004; 351(18), 1849–1859.

391. Mylonakis E, Hohmann EL, Caderwood SB. Central nervous system infection with *Listeria monocytogenes*—33 years' experience at a general hospital and review of 776 episodes from the literature. Medicine 1998; 77(5), 313–336.

392. Nau R, Brück W. Neuronal injury in bacterial meningitis: mechanisms and implications for therapy. Trends Neurosci 2002; 25(1), 38–45.

393. Kastenbauer S, Pfister HW. Pneumococcal meningitis in adults: spectrum of complications and prognostic factors in a series of 87 cases. Brain 2003; 126(Pt 5), 1015–1025.

394. Gerner-Smidt P, Ethelberg S, Schiellerup P, et al. Invasive listeriosis in Denmark 1994–2003: a review of 299 cases with special emphasis on risk factors for mortality. Clin Microbiol Infect 2005; 11(8), 618–624.

395. Drevets DA, Leenen PJ, Greenfield RA. Invasion of the central nervous system by intracellular bacteria. Clin Microbiol Rev 2004; 17(2), 323–347.

396. Van Crevel H, Hijdra A, De Gans J. Lumbar puncture and the risk of herniation: when should we first perform CT? J Neurol 2002; 249(2), 129–137.

397. Romer FK. Difficulties in the diagnosis of bacterial meningitis. Evaluation of antibiotic pretreatment and causes of admission to hospital. Lancet 1977; 2(8033), 345–347.

398. Romer FK. Bacterial meningitis: a 15-year review of bacterial meningitis from departments of internal medicine. Dan Med Bull 1977; 24(1), 35–40.

399. Rennick G, Shann F, de Campo J. Cerebral herniation during bacterial meningitis in children. BMJ 1993; 306, 953–955.

400. Carpenter RR, Petersdorf RG. The clinical spectrum of bacterial meningitis. Am J Med 1962; 33, 262–275.

401. Roos KL. Mycobacterium tuberculosis meningitis and other etiologies of the aseptic meningitis syndrome. Semin Neurol 2000; 20(3), 329–335.

402. Ratnaike RN. Whipple's disease. Postgrad Med J 2000; 76(902), 760–766.

403. Mohm J, Naumann R, Schuler U, et al. Abdominal lymphomas, convulsive seizure and coma: a case of successfully treated, advanced Whipple's disease with cerebral involvement. Eur J Gastroenterol Hepatol 1998; 10(10), 893–895.

404. Mendel E, Khoo LT, Go JL, et al. Intracerebral Whipple's disease diagnosed by stereotactic biopsy: a case report and review of the literature. Neurosurgery 1999; 44(1), 203–209.

405. Bratton RL, Corey R. Tick-borne disease. Am Fam Physician 2005; 71(12), 2323–2330.

406. Davies NWS, Brown LJ, Gonde J, et al. Factors influencing PCR detection of viruses in cerebrospinal fluid of patients with suspected CNS infections. J Neurol Neurosurg Psychiatry 2005; 76(1), 82–87.

407. Johnson RT. The pathogenesis of acute viral encephalitis and postinfectious encephalomyelitis. J Infect Dis 1987; 155(3), 359–364.

408. Collinge J. Molecular neurology of prion disease. J Neurol Neurosurg Psychiatry 2005; 76(7), 906–919.

409. Johnson RT. Prion diseases. Lancet Neurol 2005; 4(10), 635–642.

410. Montagna P, Gambetti P, Cortelli P, et al. Familial and sporadic fatal insomnia. Lancet Neurol 2003; 2(3), 167–176.

411. Omalu BI, Shakir AA, Wang G, et al. Fatal fulminant pan-meningo-polioencephalitis due to West Nile virus. Brain Pathol 2003; 13(4), 465–472.

412. Sejvar JJ, Haddad MB, Tierney BC, et al. Neurologic manifestations and outcome of West Nile virus infection. JAMA 2003; 290(4), 511–515.

413. Olival KJ, Daszak P. The ecology of emerging neurotropic viruses. J Neurovirol 2005; 11(5), 441–446.

414. Kamei S, Sekizawa T, Shiota H, et al. Evaluation of combination therapy using aciclovir and corticosteroid in adult patients with herpes simplex virus encephalitis. J Neurol Neurosurg Psychiatry 2005; 76(11), 1544–1549.

415. Jereb M, Lainscak M, Marin J, et al. Herpes simplex virus infection limited to the brainstem. Wien Klin Wochenschr 2005; 117(13–14), 495–499.

416. Chu K, Kang DW, Lee JJ, et al. Atypical brainstem encephalitis caused by herpes simplex virus 2. Arch Neurol 2002; 59(3), 460–463.

417. Chaudhuri A, Kennedy PG. Diagnosis and treatment of viral encephalitis. Postgrad Med J 2002; 78(924), 575–583.

418. Kennedy PGE. Viral encephalitis: causes, differential diagnosis, and management. J Neurol Neurosurg Psychiatry 2004; 75(Supp 1), 10–15.

419. Wasay M, Mekan SF, Khelaeni B, et al. Extra temporal involvement in herpes simplex encephalitis. Eur J Neurol 2005; 12(6), 475–479.

420. De Marcaida JA, Reik L Jr. Disorders that mimic central nervous system infections. Neurol Clin 1999; 17(4), 901–941.

421. Yao D, Kuwajima M, Kido H. Pathologic mechanisms of influenza encephalitis with an abnormal expression of inflammatory cytokines and accumulation of miniplasmin. J Med Invest 2003; 50(1–2), 1–8.

422. Togashi T, Matsuzono Y, Narita M, et al. Influenza-associated acute encephalopathy in Japanese children in 1994–2002. Virus Res 2004; 103(1–2), 75–78.
423. Orlowski JP, Hanhan UA, Fiallos MR. Is aspirin a cause of Reye's syndrome? A case against. Drug Saf 2002; 25(4), 225–231.
424. Menge T, Hemmer B, Nessler S, et al. Acute disseminated encephalomyelitis: an update. Arch Neurol 2005; 62(11), 1673–1680.
425. Garg RK. Acute disseminated encephalomyelitis. Postgrad Med J 2003; 79(927), 11–17.
426. Schwarz S, Mohr A, Knauth M, et al. Acute disseminated encephalomyelitis: a follow-up study of 40 adult patients. Neurology 2001; 56(10), 1313–1318.
427. Gibbs WN, Kreidie MA, Kim RC, et al. Acute hemorrhagic leukoencephalitis: neuroimaging features and neuropathologic diagnosis. J Comput Assist Tomogr 2005; 29(5), 689–693.
428. An SF, Groves M, Martinian L, et al. Detection of infectious agents in brain of patients with acute hemorrhagic leukoencephalitis. J Neurovirol 2002; 8(5), 439–446.
429. Whiting DM, Barnett GH, Estes ML, et al. Stereotactic biopsy of non-neoplastic lesions in adults. Cleve Clin J Med 1992; 59(1), 48–55.
430. Hornef MW, Iten A, Maeder P, et al. Brain biopsy in patients with acquired immunodeficiency syndrome: diagnostic value, clinical performance, and survival time. Arch Intern Med 1999; 159(21), 2590–2596.
431. Warren JD, Schott JM, Fox NC, et al. Brain biopsy in dementia. Brain 2005; 128(Pt 9), 2016–2025.
432. Gray F, N'guyen JP. [Brain biopsy in systemic diseases]. Ann Pathol 2002; 22(3), 194–205.
433. Younger DS. Vasculitis of the nervous system. Curr Opin Neurol 2004; 17(3), 317–336.
434. Ruegg S, Engelter S, Jeanneret C, et al. Bilateral vertebral artery occlusion resulting from giant cell arteritis: report of 3 cases and review of the literature. Medicine (Baltimore) 2003; 82(1), 1–12.
435. Heinrich A, Khaw AV, Ahrens N, et al. Cerebral vasculitis as the only manifestation of Borrelia burgdorferi infection in a 17-year-old patient with basal ganglia infarction. Eur Neurol 2003; 50(2), 109–112.
436. MacLaren K, Gillespie J, Shrestha S, et al. Primary angiitis of the central nervous system: emerging variants. QJM 2005; 98(9), 643–654.
437. Hajj-Ali RA, Furlan A, Abou-Chebel A, et al. Benign angiopathy of the central nervous system: cohort of 16 patients with clinical course and long-term followup. Arthritis Rheum 2002; 47(6), 662–669.
438. Devinsky O, Petito CK, Alonso DR. Clinical and neuropathological findings in systemic lupus erythematosus: the role of vasculitis, heart emboli, and thrombotic thrombocytopenic purpura. Ann Neurol 1988; 23(4), 380–384.
439. Nived O, Sturfelt G, Liang MH, et al. The ACR nomenclature for CNS lupus revisited. Lupus 2003; 12(12), 872–876.
440. Meroni PL, Tincani A, Sepp N, et al. Endothelium and the brain in CNS lupus. Lupus 2003; 12(12), 919–928.
441. Hung JJ, Ou LS, Lee WI, et al. Central nervous system infections in patients with systemic lupus erythematosus. J Rheumatol 2005; 32(1), 40–43.
442. Sirois F. Steroid psychosis: a review. Gen Hosp Psychiatry 2003; 25(1), 27–33.
443. DeGirolami U, Haas ML, Richardson EP Jr. Subacute diencephalic angioencephalopathy. A clinicopathological case study. J Neurol Sci 1974; 22(2), 197–210.
444. Rauschka H, Retzl J, Baumhackl U, et al. Subacute brainstem angioencephalopathy: a case report and review of the literature. J Neurol Sci 2003; 208(1–2), 101–104.
445. Tihan T, Burger PC, Pomper M, et al. Subacute diencephalic angioencephalopathy: biopsy diagnosis and radiological features of a rare entity. Clin Neurol Neurosurg 2001; 103(3), 160–167.
446. Gilden DH, Mahalingam R, Cohrs RJ, et al. The protean manifestations of varicella-zoster virus vasculopathy. J Neurovirol 2002; 8(Suppl 2), 75–79.
447. Siva A, Altintas A, Saip S. Behcet's syndrome and the nervous system. Curr Opin Neurol 2004; 17(3), 347–357.
448. Kidd D, Steuer A, Denman AM, et al. Neurological complications in Behcet's syndrome. Brain 1999; 122(Pt 11), 2183–2194.
449. Siva A, Kantarci OH, Saip S, et al. Behcet's disease: diagnostic and prognostic aspects of neurological involvement. J Neurol 2001; 248(2), 95–103.
450. Schon F, Martin RJ, Prevett M, et al. "CADASIL coma": an underdiagnosed acute encephalopathy. J Neurol Neurosurg Psychiatry 2003; 74(2), 249–252.
451. Feuerhake F, Volk B, Ostertag CB, et al. Reversible coma with raised intracranial pressure: an unusual clinical manifestation of CADASIL. Acta Neuropathol (Berl) 2002; 103(2), 188–192.
452. Le BI, Carluer L, Derache N, et al. Unusual presentation of CADASIL with reversible coma and confusion. Neurology 2002; 59(7), 1115–1116.
453. Federico A, Bianchi S, Dotti MT. The spectrum of mutations for CADASIL diagnosis. Neurol Sci 2005; 26(2), 117–124.
454. Van Everbroeck BRJ, Boons J, Cras P. 14–3–3 gamma-isoform detection distinguishes sporadic Creutzfeldt-Jakob disease from other dementias. J Neurol Neurosurg Psychiatry 2005; 76(1), 100–102.
455. Geschwind MD, Martindale J, Miller D, et al. Challenging the clinical utility of the 14-3-3 protein for the diagnosis of sporadic Creutzfeldt-Jakob disease. Arch Neurol 2003; 60(6), 813–816.
456. Tschampa HJ, Murtz P, Flacke S, et al. Thalamic involvement in sporadic Creutzfeldt-Jakob disease: a diffusion-weighted MR imaging study. AJNR Am J Neuroradiol 2003; 24(5), 908–915.
457. Summers DM, Collie DA, Zeidler M, et al. The pulvinar sign in variant Creutzfeldt-Jakob disease. Arch Neurol 2004; 61(3), 446–447.
458. Mendonca RA, Martins G, Lugokenski R, et al. Subacute spongiform encephalopathies. Top Magn Reson Imaging 2005; 16(2), 213–219.
459. Moser HW, Loes DJ, Melhem ER, et al. X-Linked adrenoleukodystrophy: overview and prognosis as a function of age and brain magnetic resonance imaging abnormality. A study involving 372 patients. Neuropediatrics 2000; 31(5), 227–239.

460. Moser H, Dubey P, Fatemi A. Progress in X-linked adrenoleukodystrophy. Curr Opin Neurol 2004; 17(3), 263–269.

461. Ravid S, Diamond AS, Eviatar L. Coma as an acute presentation of adrenoleukodystrophy. Pediatr Neurol 2000; 22(3), 237–239.

462. Heinrich A, Runge U, Khaw AV. Clinicoradiologic subtypes of Marchiafava-Bignami disease. J Neurol 2004; 251(9), 1050–1059.

463. Kawarabuki K, Sakakibara T, Hirai M, et al. Marchiafava-Bignami disease: magnetic resonance imaging findings in corpus callosum and subcortical white matter. Eur J Radiol 2003; 48(2), 175–177.

464. Johkura K, Naito M, Naka T. Cortical involvement in Marchiafava-Bignami disease. AJNR Am J Neuroradiol 2005; 26(3), 670–673.

465. Taillibert S, Chodkiewicz C, Laigle-Donadey F, et al. Gliomatosis cerebri: a review of 296 cases from the ANOCEF database and the literature. J Neurooncol 2006; 76(2), 201–205.

466. Koralnik IJ. New insights into progressive multifocal leukoencephalopathy. Curr Opin Neurol 2004; 17(3), 365–370.

467. Keeley KA, Rivey MP, Allington DR. Natalizumab for the treatment of multiple sclerosis and Crohn's disease. Ann Pharmacother 2005; 39 (11), 1833–1843.

468. Du Pasquier RA, Koralnik IJ. Inflammatory reaction in progressive multifocal leukoencephalopathy: harmful or beneficial? J Neurovirol 2003; 9(Suppl 1):25–31.

469. Ingvar M. Cerebral blood flow and metabolic rate during seizures. Relationship to epileptic brain damage. Ann N Y Acad Sci 1986; 462, 194–206.

470. Uzum G, Sarper DA, Bahcekapili N, et al. Erythropoietin prevents the increase in blood-brain barrier permeability during pentylentetrazol induced seizures. Life Sci 2006; 78(22), 2571–2576.

471. Langheinrich TC, Chattopadhyay A, Kuc S, et al. Prolonged postictal stupor: nonconvulsive status epilepticus, medication effect, or postictal state? Epilepsy Behav 2005; 7(3), 548–551.

472. Shorvon S, Walker M. Status epilepticus in idiopathic generalized epilepsy. Epilepsia 2005; 46(Suppl 9): 73–79.

473. Towne AR, Waterhouse EJ, Boggs JG, et al. Prevalence of nonconvulsive status epilepticus in comatose patients. Neurology 2000; 54(2), 340–345.

474. Husain AM, Horn GJ, Jacobson MP. Non-convulsive status epilepticus: usefulness of clinical features in selecting patients for urgent EEG. J Neurol Neurosurg Psychiatry 2003; 74(2), 189–191.

475. Brenner RP. EEG in convulsive and nonconvulsive status epilepticus. J Clin Neurophysiol 2004; 21(5), 319–331.

476. Kaplan PW. Assessing the outcomes in patients with nonconvulsive status epilepticus: nonconvulsive status epilepticus is underdiagnosed, potentially overtreated, and confounded by comorbidity. J Clin Neurophysiol 1999; 16(4), 341–352; discussion 353.

477. Griffiths RR, Johnson MW. Relative abuse liability of hypnotic drugs: a conceptual framework and algorithm for differentiating among compounds. J Clin Psychiatry 2005; 66(Suppl 9):31–41.

478. Sellers EM. Alcohol, barbiturate and benzodiazepine withdrawal syndromes: clinical management. CMAJ 1988; 139(2), 113–120.

479. Bayard M, McIntyre J, Hill KR, et al. Alcohol withdrawal syndrome. Am Fam Physician 2004; 69(6), 1443–1450.

480. Amador LF, Goodwin JS. Postoperative delirium in the older patient. J Am Coll Surg 2005; 200(5), 767–773.

481. Aldemir M, Ozen S, Kara IH, et al. Predisposing factors for delirium in the surgical intensive care unit. Crit Care 2001; 5(5), 265–270.

482. Bitsch M, Foss N, Kristensen B, et al. Pathogenesis of and management strategies for postoperative delirium after hip fracture: a review. Acta Orthop Scand 2004; 75(4), 378–389.

483. Wilson LM. Intensive care delirium. The effect of outside deprivation in a windowless unit. Arch Intern Med 1972; 130, 225–226.

Chapter 6

Psychogenic Unresponsiveness

CONVERSION REACTIONS

CATATONIA

PSYCHOGENIC SEIZURES

CEREBELLAR COGNITIVE AFFECTIVE SYNDROME

"AMYTAL INTERVIEW"

Differentiating psychogenic neurologic symptoms from those caused by structural disease is often very difficult. The difficulty arises in part because many patients are very accurate in mimicking neurologic signs (actors are often used to train medical students in the diagnosis of neurologic illnesses) and, in part, because many patients with psychogenic neurologic disorders (conversion reactions) also have somatic disease, the somatic illness representing a stressor that causes psychologic problems. Examples abound: approximately one-half of patients with psychogenic seizures also have epilepsy.[1] Of those who do not have epilepsy, over 20% show evidence of a brain disorder characterized either by epileptiform activity on electroencephalogram (EEG), magnetic resonance imaging (MRI) abnormalities, or neuropsychologic deficits.[2] Psychogenic neurologic symptoms sometimes complicate the course of multiple sclerosis.[3] Merskey and Buhrich studied 89 patients with classic motor conversion symptoms and found that 48% had a cerebral disorder.[4] Of all the psychogenic illnesses that mimic structural disease, psychogenic unresponsiveness is among the most difficult to diagnose. With most psychogenic illnesses that mimic structural neurologic disease, the physician pursues a two-pronged diagnostic attack. He must first determine by the neurologic examination that the patient's neurologic signs and symptoms are not in keeping with the anatomy and physiology of the nervous system (i.e., they are anatomically or physiologically impossible). Secondly, he must discern from the history and mental status examination that the patient's emotional make-up and current psychologic problems are sufficient to explain the abnormal findings on a psychologic basis. Because in psychogenic unresponsiveness no history or mental status examination from the patient is possible (a history should be obtained from relatives or friends), the physician is left with only the first portion of his diagnostic armamentarium (i.e., the demonstration that despite apparent unconsciousness, the patient is in fact physiologically awake). Thus, the diagnosis of psychogenic unresponsiveness must be approached with the greatest care. A careful neurologic examination, sometimes supplemented by caloric tests, EEG, and an "Amytal interview," as described below, will usually establish the diagnosis and obviate the need for extensive, potentially harmful laboratory investigations. However, if after such a meticulous examination of a patient with suspected psychogenic unresponsiveness any question remains about the diagnosis, a careful search for other causes of coma is obligatory.

Psychogenic unresponsiveness is uncommon; it was the final diagnosis in only eight of our original 500 patients (Table 1–1). We have, however, encountered the condition as a challenging diagnostic problem in several further patients at

a rate of about one every other year since that time. In one study of conversion symptoms in 500 psychiatric outpatients, "unconsciousness" occurred in 17.[5] Two older series from London each report six patients with psychogenic unresponsiveness who were initially puzzling diagnostically.[6,7] Over how long a period of time these cases were collected, or from how wide a patient population, is not stated. More recently, Lempert and colleagues found that 405 (9%) of 4,470 consecutive neurologic inpatients were found to have psychogenic rather than neurologic disorders[8] (Table 6–1). Among these only

Table 6–1 Signs and Symptoms (*N* = 717) of 405 Patients With Psychogenic Dysfunction of the Nervous System*

Pain			*Ocular Symptoms*	
Trunk and extremities	89		Amblyopia	10
Headache	61		Amaurosis	6
Atypical facial pain	13		Visual field defects	6
			Color blindness	2
Motor Symptoms			Double vision	2
Astasia/abasia	52		Other visual phenomena	6
Monoparesis	31		Ptosis	1
Hemiparesis	20		Convergence spasm	1
Tetraparesis	18		Unilateral gaze paresis	1
Paraparesis	10			
Paresis of both arms	2		*Alimentary Symptoms*	
Recurrent head drop	1		Dysphagia	4
Tremor	11		Vomiting	4
Localized jerking	1			
Stereotyped motor behavior	1		*Speech Disturbances*	
Hypokinesia	1		Dysarthria	9
Akinesia	1		Slow speech	1
Foot contracture	1		Aphonia	2
Isolated ataxia of the upper extremities			Mutism	1
Sensory Symptoms			*Neuropsychologic Symptoms*	
Hypesthesia/anesthesia	81		Cognitive impairment	2
Paresthesia/dysesthesia	63		Amnestic aphasia	1
Sensation of generalized vibration	1		Apathy	2
Sensation of fever	1		Coma	1
Pressure in the ears	1			
			Other Symptoms	
Seizures			Bladder dysfunction	11
With motor phenomena	47		Stool incontinence	1
Other (amnestic episodes, mental and emotional alterations)	34		Cough	1
Vertigo/Sizziness				
Attacks of phobic postural vertigo	47			
Continuous dizziness	38			

From Lempert et al.,[8] with permission.

one was comatose, although 34 had seizures described as consisting of "amnestic episodes, mental and emotional alterations." How many of these had disorders of consciousness is unclear. Another study conducted in the 566-bed tertiary care hospital identified a conversion disorder in 42 patients over 10 years.[9] In 17 patients, the presenting complaints were "seizure activity, syncope, or loss of consciousness." Patients admitted directly to the hospital without a definitive diagnosis were not included among the 42; how many there were was not stated.

Because the diagnosis of psychogenic neurologic symptoms is often difficult, mistakes are sometimes made. Sometimes a structural disorder is initially diagnosed as psychogenic,[10,11] but sometimes the opposite occurs. The latter is typically true when psychogenic coma complicates a physical illness.[12,13] Although errors were common in the past, a recent systematic review of misdiagnosis of conversion symptoms suggests an error rate of only 4% since 1970.[14] Among the 390 patients with a diagnosis of nonepileptic seizures and/or loss of consciousness, only nine were misdiagnosed.

Several psychiatric disorders can result in psychogenic unresponsiveness. These include (1) conversion reaction, which may in turn be secondary to a personality disorder, severe depression, anxiety, or an acute situational reaction[15]; (2) catatonic stupor, often a manifestation of schizophrenia; (3) a dissociative or "fugue" state; and (4) factitious disorder or malingering.

The two major categories of psychogenic unresponsiveness are those that result from a conversion disorder (often called conversion hysteria) and those that are part of the syndrome of catatonia (often thought to be a manifestation of schizophrenia). The two clinical pictures differ somewhat, but both may closely simulate delirium, stupor, or coma caused by structural or metabolic brain disease. The diagnosis of psychogenic unresponsiveness of either variety is made by demonstrating that both the cerebral hemispheres and the brainstem-activating pathways can be made to function in a physiologically normal way, even though the patient will seemingly not respond to his or her environment.

The physician must recognize that with the exception of factitious disorders and malingering, psychologically produced neurologic symptoms are not "imaginary." The disorders are associated with measurable changes in brain function. Although routine tests including MRI, evoked potentials, and EEG are usually normal, measurement of cerebral metabolism is regionally abnormal.[16] Using single photon emission computed tomography (SPECT), Vuilleumier and colleagues conducted a study in which seven patients with conversion symptoms mimicking motor or sensory dysfunction revealed a consistent decrease of blood flow in the thalamus and basal ganglia contralateral to the deficit. These abnormalities resolved in those patients who recovered.[17] Spence and colleagues studied two patients with psychogenic weakness affecting their left arms. They compared positron emission tomography (PET) scans of these patients with normal individuals, and also with normal individuals who feigned paralysis of the left arm. The left dorsolateral prefrontal cortex was activated in the normal individuals and those feigning paralysis, but was hypofunctional in the patient's with the conversion reaction. Interestingly, those feigning paralysis exhibited hypofunction of the right anterior prefrontal cortex when compared with controls.[18] A study of four patients with "hysterical anesthesia" using functional MRI revealed that stimuli to the anesthetic parts of the body did not activate areas in the thalamus, posterior region of the anterior cingulate cortex, or Brodmann's areas 44 and 45. These are the areas activated by individuals who perceived the stimuli. A patient studied during catatonic stupor showed hypometabolism in a large area of the prefrontal cortex including anterior cingulate, medial prefrontal, and dorsolateral cortices when compared with controls.[16] The few other studies of functional imaging in patients with catatonia also showed hypometabolism in the frontal lobes.[19–21] Although no patients with psychogenic coma have been studied by these techniques (the catatonic patient was stuporous), the data from patients with other conversion reactions suggests that one would find abnormalities of brain metabolism in these patients as well.

CONVERSION REACTIONS

A conversion reaction is the cause of most psychogenic comas. As used here, the term conversion reaction describes a psychogenic or nonphysiologic loss or disorder of neurologic function involving the special senses or the voluntary nervous system. Many physicians associate conversion reactions with a hysterical personality (conversion hysteria) but, in fact, conversion reactions may occur as a psychologic defense against a wide range of psychiatric syndromes, including depressive states and neuroses.[22] Furthermore, as indicated on page 297, conversion symptoms, including psychogenic unresponsiveness, may be a reaction to organic disease, and thus occur in a patient already seriously ill. We find it impossible to differentiate conversion reactions, presumably representing involuntary responses by patients to stress, from voluntary malingering except by the direct statement of the subject involved and perhaps by PET.[18]

Patients suffering from psychogenic unresponsiveness, owing to either a conversion reaction or to malingering, usually lie with their eyes closed and do not attend to their surroundings. The respiratory rate and depth are usually normal, but in some instances the patient may be overbreathing as another manifestation of the psychologic dysfunction (hyperventilation syndrome). The pupils may be slightly widened, but are equal and reactive except in the instance of the individual who self-instills mydriatic agents. Oculocephalic responses may or may not be present, but caloric testing invariably produces quick-phase nystagmus away from the ice water irrigation rather than either tonic deviation of the eyes toward the irrigated ear or no response at all. *It is the presence of normal nystagmus in response to caloric testing that firmly indicates that the patient is physiologically awake and that the unresponsive state cannot be caused by structural or metabolic disease of the nervous system.* (A rare patient with pre-existing vestibular dysfunction may be awake, but not have caloric responses.) Henry and Woodruff described six patients with psychogenic unresponsiveness in whom the eyes deviated tonically toward the floor when the patient lay on his side.[6] The authors postulate that the deviation of the eyes was psychologically mediated as a way of avoiding eye contact with the examiner. In some patients, the eyes deviate upward (or sometimes downward) when the eyelids are passively opened. Upward eye deviation also occurs during syncopal attacks.[23] When one attempts to open the closed lids of a patient suffering from psychogenic unresponsiveness, the lids often resist actively and usually close rap-

idly when they are released. The slow, steady closure of passively opened eyelids that occurs in many comatose patients cannot be mimicked voluntarily. Similarly, slow roving eye movements cannot be mimicked voluntarily. Patients suffering from psychogenic unresponsiveness as a conversion symptom usually offer no resistance to passive movements of the extremities although normal tone is present; if an extremity is moved suddenly, momentary resistance may be felt. The patient usually does not withdraw from noxious stimuli. Dropping the passively raised arm toward the face is a maneuver said to be positive when the patient's hand avoids hitting the face. However, the weight of the upper arm sometimes pulls the hand away from the face, giving the appearance of voluntary avoidance.[24] The deep tendon reflexes are usually normal, but they can be voluntarily suppressed in some subjects and thus may be absent or, rarely, asymmetric. The abdominal reflexes are usually present and plantar responses are invariably absent or flexor. The EEG is that of an awake patient, rather than one in coma.

Patient 6–1

A 26-year-old nurse with a history of generalized convulsions was admitted to the hospital after a night of alcoholic drinking ostensibly followed by generalized convulsions. She had been given 50% glucose and 500 mg sodium amobarbital intravenously. Upon admission she was reportedly unresponsive to verbal command, but when noxious stimuli were administered she withdrew, repetitively thrust her extremities in both flexion and extension, and on one occasion spat at the examiner. Her respirations were normal. The remainder of the general physical and neurologic examination was normal. She was given 10 mg of diazepam intravenously and 500 mg of phenytoin intravenously in two doses 3 hours apart. Eight hours later, because she was still unresponsive, a neurologic consultation was requested. She lay quietly in bed, unresponsive to verbal commands and not withdrawing from noxious stimuli. Her respirations were normal; her eyelids resisted opening actively and, when they were opened, closed rapidly. The eyes did not move spontaneously, the doll's eye responses were absent, and the pupils were 3 mm and reactive. Her extremities were flaccid with normal deep tendon reflexes, normal superficial abdominal reflexes, and flexor plantar responses. When 20 mL of ice water was irrigated against the left tympanum, nystagmus with a quick component to the right was produced. The examiner indicated to a colleague that the production of nystagmus indicated that she was conscious and an EEG would establish that fact. She immediately "awoke." Her speech was dysarthric and she was unsteady on her feet when she arose from bed. An EEG was marked by low- and medium-voltage fast activity in all leads with some 8-Hz alpha activity and intermittent 6- to 7-Hz activity, a recording suggesting sedation owing to drugs. She recovered full alertness later in the day and was discharged a day later with her neurologic examination having been entirely normal. An EEG done at a subsequent time showed background alpha activity of 8 to 10 Hz with a moderate amount of fast activity and little or no 5- to 7-Hz slow activity.

Comment: This patient illustrates a common problem in differentiating "organic" from psychogenic unresponsiveness. She had been sedated and had a mild metabolic encephalopathy, but the preponderance of her signs was a result of psychogenic unresponsiveness. The presence of nystagmus on oculovestibular stimulation, and an EEG that was only mildly slowed without other signs of neurologic abnormality, effectively ruled out organic coma.

The converse of Patient 6–1 is illustrated by Patient 5–3 (see page 194). In the latter, the initial examination suggested psychogenic unresponsiveness, but vestibular testing elicited tonic deviation of the eyes without nystagmus. The tonic eye deviation clearly indicated physiologic rather than psychologic unresponsiveness. A rare patient with psychogenic unresponsiveness is able to inhibit nystagmus induced by caloric testing (probably by intense visual fixation), but in that instance there is no tonic deviation of the eyes and the combination of other signs can establish the diagnosis.

When a patient with severe organic illness, whether systemic or neurologic, becomes unresponsive, the physician sometimes fails to entertain the possibility that the unresponsiveness is psychogenic and represents a conversion reaction to a difficult psychologic situation. Patient 6–2 illustrates this.

Patient 6–2

A 69-year-old woman was admitted to the coronary care unit complaining of chest pain. On examination she was diaphoretic and the electrocardiogram (ECG) showed changes suggestive of an acute anterior wall myocardial infarction. She was awake and alert at the time of admission and had a normal neurologic examination. The following morning she was found to be unresponsive. On examination her respiratory rate was 16 and regular, pulse 92, temperature 37.5, and blood pressure 120/80. The general physical examination was unremarkable, revealing no changes from the day before. On neurologic examination she failed to respond to either verbal or noxious stimuli. She held her eyes in a tightly closed position and actively resisted passive eye opening, and the lids, after being passively opened, sprung closed when released. Oculocephalic responses were absent. Cold caloric responses yielded normal, brisk nystagmus. Pupils were 4 mm and reactive. Tone in the extremities was normal. The deep tendon reflexes were equal throughout and plantar responses were flexor. The neurologist who examined the patient suggested to the cardiologist that the unresponsiveness was psychogenic and that psychiatric consultation be secured. At the patient's bedside the incredulous cardiologist began to discuss how the diagnosis of psychogenic unresponsiveness was made. When the decision was finally made to consult a psychiatrist, the patient, without opening her eyes, responded with the words, "No psychiatrist."

In this instance, the presence of severe heart disease led the patient's physicians to refuse initially to entertain a diagnosis of psychogenic unresponsiveness. In Patient 6–3, the presence of severe organic neurologic disease masked the diagnosis for a considerable period.

Patient 6–3

A 28-year-old man with hepatic carcinoma metastatic to the lungs was admitted to the hospital complaining of abdominal pain. His behavior was noted to be inappropriate a few days after admission, but this was believed secondary to the opioids given for pain. The inappropriate behavior progressed to lethargy and then stupor. When first examined by a neurologist, he was unresponsive to verbal stimuli but grimaced when stimulated noxiously. He held his eyes open and blinked in response to a bright light. Nuchal rigidity and bilateral extensor plantar responses were present, but there were no other positive neurologic signs. A lumbar puncture revealed bloody cerebrospinal fluid (CSF) with xanthochromic supernatant fluid and a CSF glucose concentration of 15 mg/dL. The EEG consisted of a mixture of theta and delta activity, which was bilaterally symmetric. Carotid arteriography failed to reveal the cause of his symptoms, which were believed to be caused by leptomeningeal metastases. For the next 2 weeks his state of consciousness waxed and waned. When awake he continued to act oddly. Two weeks after the initial neurologic examination, he was noted to be lying in bed staring at the ceiling with no responses to verbal stimuli and with 6-mm pupils, which responded actively to light. Bilateral extensor plantar responses persisted. The EEG now was within normal limits, showing good alpha activity, which blocked with eye opening. Because of the confusion about the exact cause of his diminished state of consciousness, an "Amytal interview" was carried out (see page 307). After 300 mg of intravenous Amytal was given slowly over several minutes, the patient awoke, was fully oriented, and was able to perform the serial sevens test without error. During the course of the discussion, when the problems of his cancer were broached, he broke into tears. Further history indicated that the patient's brother had a history of hospitalizations for both mania and depression. A diagnosis of psychogenic unresponsiveness superimposed on metastatic disease of the nervous system was made. The patient was started on psychotropic drugs and he remained alert and responsive throughout the remainder of his hospital stay.

The two patients above illustrate the difficulties in making a diagnosis of psychogenic unresponsiveness in patients with organic disease. Merskey and Buhrich have stressed the frequency of conversion hysteria in patients suffering from structural disease.[4] Of 89 patients with hysterical conversion symptoms, 67% had some organic diagnosis; 48% of the group with organic diagnoses had either an organic cerebral disorder or a systemic illness affecting the brain. The authors believe that organic cere-

bral disease predisposes patients to the development of conversion reactions.

CATATONIA

The second major category of psychogenic unresponsiveness is catatonia. Catatonia is a symptom complex characterized by either stupor or excitement accompanied by behavioral disturbances that include, among others, mutism, posturing, rigidity, grimacing, waxy flexibility (a mild but steady resistance to passive motion, which gives the examiner the sensation that he is bending a wax rod), and catalepsy (the tonic maintenance for a long period of time of a limb in a potentially uncomfortable posture where it has been placed by an examiner). Tables 6–2 and 6–3 list the signs of catatonia and some of its causes.

In a retroprospective clinical study of patients admitted to a psychiatric unit with catatonic symptoms, only four of 55 were schizophrenic; 39 had affective disorders, three had reactive psychoses, and nine suffered from organic brain diseases, which included toxic psychosis, encephalitis, alcoholic degeneration, and drug-induced psychosis.[27] Patients with catatonic stupor usually give the appearance of being obtunded or semi-stuporous rather than comatose. This state is compatible with normal pupillary and oculovestibular function even when the obtundation has a structural origin. In addition, catatonic stupor is accompanied by a variety of autonomic and endocrine abnormalities that give the patient a particularly strong appearance of organic neurologic disease.

Catatonia occurs in two forms: retarded and excited. The patient in a catatonic stupor who presents a problem in the differential diagnosis of stupor or coma usually appears unresponsive to his or her environment. Severe and prolonged catatonic stupor, as described below, is uncommon, since such patients are usually treated early with psychotropic medications before the full picture develops. The patient in catatonic stupor usually lies with the eyes open, apparently unseeing. The skin is pale and frequently marred by acne and has an oily or greasy appearance. The patient's pulse is rapid, usually between 90 and 120, and may be hypertensive. Respirations are normal or rapid. The body temperature is often elevated 1.0°C to 1.5°C above normal. Such patients usually do not

Table 6–2 **Signs of Catatonia**

Excitement	Nonpurposeful hyperactivity or motor unrest
Immobility	Extreme hypoactivity, reduced response to stimuli
Mutism	Reduced or absent speech
Stupor/coma	Unresponsive to all stimuli; eyes closed, flaccid, or rigid
Staring	Fixed, nonreactive gaze, reduced blinking
Posturing	Spontaneous maintenance of posture (the posture itself may or may not be abnormal) for longer than is usual
Grimacing	Maintenance of odd facial expressions
Echolalia	Mimicking of examiner's speech (may be delayed)
Echopraxia	Mimicking of examiner's movements (may be delayed)
Stereotypy	Repetitive, non-goal-directed movements
Mannerisms	Odd, purposeful voluntary movements
Verbigeration	Repetition of meaningless phrases or sentences
Rigidity	Maintenance of position despite efforts to be moved
Negativism	Apparently motiveless resistance to instructions or attempts to make contact
Waxy flexibility	During reposturing there is initial resistance, then the new posture is maintained
Withdrawal	Refusal to eat, drink, or make eye contact
Impulsivity	Sudden inappropriate behaviors with no explanation
Automatic	Exaggerated cooperation with request or continuation of obedience movement requested
Mitgehen	Raising of arm in response to light finger pressure (like an angle-poise lamp) despite instructions to the contrary
Gegenhalten	Resistance to passive movement in proportion to strength of stimulus
Ambitendency	Indecisive, hesitant movement
Grasp reflex	Reflex grasping movement of hand in response to stroking palm
Perseveration	Repeatedly returns to same topic or persists with movement
Combativeness	Usually undirected aggression or violent behavior

Modified from Bush et al.[25]

Table 6–3 **Some Reported Causes of Catatonia**

Category	Association
Idiopathic	Perhaps nearly 50% of patients
Psychiatric	Affective disorders, dissociative disorders, schizophrenia, drug-induced and other psychoses, obsessive compulsive disorder, personality disorder
Neurologic	Cerebral tumors, subarachnoid hemorrhage, subdural hemorrhage, hemorrhagic infarcts, closed head injury, multiple sclerosis, narcolepsy, tuberous sclerosis, epilepsy, Wernicke's encephalopathy, Parkinsonism, systemic lupus erythematosus
Metabolic	Addison's disease, Cushing's disease, diabetic ketoacidosis, hypercalcemia, acute intermittent porphyria, Wilson's disease
Drugs and toxins	Alcohol, anticonvulsants, disulfiram, neuroleptics, amphetamines, mescaline, phencyclidine, aspirin, L-dopa, steroids
Infections	Encephalitis (especially herpes), malaria, syphilis, tuberculosis, typhoid, acquired immuno-deficiency mononucleosis, viral hepatitis

Modified from Philbrick and Rummans.[26]

move spontaneously and appear to be unaware of their surroundings. They may not blink to visual threat, although optokinetic responses are usually present. The pupils are dilated and there is frequently alternating anisocoria; they are, however, reactive to light. Some patients hold their eyes tightly closed and will not permit passive eye opening. Doll's eye movements are absent and caloric testing produces normal ocular nystagmus rather than tonic deviation. At times there is increased salivation, the patient allowing the saliva either to drool from the mouth or to accumulate in the back of the pharynx without being swallowed. Such subjects may be incontinent of urine or feces or, on the contrary, may retain urine requiring catheterization. Their extremities may be relaxed, but more commonly are held in rigid positions and are resistant to passive motion. Many patients demonstrate waxy flexibility. Catalepsy is present in about 30% of retarded catatonics. Choreiform jerks of the extremities and grimaces are common. The deep tendon reflexes are usually present and there are no pathologic reflexes.

Although appearing comatose, the patient is fully conscious. This normal level of consciousness is attested to both by a normal neurologic examination at the time the patient appears stuporous and by the fact that when he or she recovers, the patient is often (but not always) able to recall all the events that took place during the "stuporous" state (Patient 6–4).

Patient 6–4

A 74-year-old woman with a history of hypertension and hypothyroidism, but otherwise in good health, was admitted to the hospital for replacement of her left hip. She had a previous replacement of the right hip several years before. She recovered well from the surgery, but 3 days later at 4:30 a.m., she was found unresponsive in bed. She lay quietly with eyes closed but did not respond to voice or noxious stimuli. She was seen by a neurologist at 7:30 a.m. She was unresponsive to voice, her eyes were open, and she would direct her eyes to sound and would blink to threat, but would not follow commands and did not respond to noxious stimuli. Tone was normal, as was the remainder of the neurologic exam. Ninety minutes later she "awoke" and responded entirely appropriately. She reported that at 4:30 a.m., unable to sleep, she had the sudden feeling that she had died. Physicians whom she recognized entered the room, but she was unable to respond to them. She reported that the noxious stimuli were very painful, but she could not move, nor could she respond to questions. She continued to think that she was dead until somewhat later in the morning, when a nurse whom she knew well sat by the bedside and talked to her gently. Because the nurse was being so nice she thought she had to respond and she began to talk. There had been no history of previous psychologic disorder nor was there any hint during the rest of her hospitalization of a psychologic abnormality.

Comment: It is hard to classify this patient with psychogenic coma, but the patient's mutism and inability or unwillingness to move suggest a *form fruste* of catatonia. That this disorder can be transient and occur in people without other underlying psychologic difficulty is well known and is perhaps illustrated by this patient.

While the patient with the retarded form of catatonia may be difficult to distinguish from a patient with stupor caused by structural disease, the patient with the excited type of catatonia may be difficult to distinguish from a patient with an acute delirium. Both may be wildly agitated and combative, and such behavior may make it impossible to test for orientation and alertness. Hallucinatory activity can be caused by either organic or psychologic disease, although pure visual hallucinations are usually due to structural or metabolic disease, and pure auditory hallucinations to psychologic disease. The segmental neurologic examination, insofar as it can be tested in a delirious or excited patient, may be normal with either structural or organic disease. Grimacing, stereotypic motor behavior, and posturing suggest catatonia rather than metabolic delirium.

Although the passage of time usually resolves the diagnostic problem, the only immediately distinguishing feature between psychogenic and organic delirious reactions is seen on the EEG. In patients with an acute toxic delirium caused by hepatic encephalopathy, encephalitis, alcohol, or other sedative drugs, slow EEG activity predominates. The EEG of the patient with the delirium of withdrawal from alcohol or barbiturates is dominated by low-voltage fast activity. The EEG is usually normal in patients with catatonia unless there is an underlying medical illness.[28,29] Thus, an entirely normal EEG with good background alpha activity that responds to eye opening and noise suggests that an either unresponsive or excessively excited patient is suffering from catatonia rather than structural or metabolic disease of the nervous system. If the EEG is dominated by high-voltage slow activity in the case of a stuporous patient, or low-voltage fast activity in the case of an excited patient, the likelihood is that the disorder is metabolic or structural rather than psychogenic.

PSYCHOGENIC SEIZURES

More difficult than identifying psychogenic coma is differentiating a psychogenic seizure from an epileptic seizure.[30] Psychogenic seizures are common; in one population study, psychogenic seizures affected 4% of the population.[1] The patient often presents in the emergency room having symptoms that may mimic a generalized tonic-clonic seizure or a complex partial seizure.[31] There is often no history available and the patient may be unresponsive, or appear to be stuporous or comatose. Because 50% of such patients also have epilepsy, differentiating a psychogenic from an epileptic seizure in a particular episode may be very difficult. Some clues both from the history and examination are given in Table 6–4. As indicated in the table, the physician should suspect a psychogenic seizure when the patient's

motor movements are unusual, particularly when the seizure lasts a long time. An EEG is usually unavailable and even if available, is often so marred by movement artifact as to not be interpretable. Furthermore, some EEGs in patients with complex partial seizures are normal. The physician should draw a prolactin level. An elevated prolactin level strongly suggests that a generalized tonic-clonic or complex partial seizure is epileptic.[32] A normal prolactin level does not rule out a nongeneralized seizure. Because the diagnosis is often uncertain and because, as indicated below, intravenous benzodiazepines treat psychogenic alterations of consciousness as well as epilepsy,

Table 6–4 **Findings That Can Help Distinguish Psychogenic From Epileptic Seizures**

	Psychogenic Seizures	Epileptic Seizures
History		
Started <10 years of life	Unusual	Common
Seizures in presence of doctors	Common	Unusual
Recurrent "status"	Common	Rare
Multiple unexplained physical symptoms	Common	Rare
Multiple operations/invasive tests	Common	Rare
Psychiatric treatment	Common	Rare
Sexual and physical abuse	Common	Rare
Observation		
Situational onset	Occasional	Rare
Gradual onset	Common	Rare
Precipitated by stimuli (noise, light)	Occasional	Rare
Purposeful movements	Occasional	Very rare
Opisthotonus, "arc de cercle"	Occasional	Very rare
Tongue biting (tip)	Occasional	Rare
Tongue biting (side)	Rare	Common
Prolonged ictal atonia	Occasional	Very rare
Vocalization during "tonic-clonic" phase	Occasional	Very rare
Reactivity during "unconsciousness"	Occasional	Very rare
Rapid postictal reorientation	Common	Unusual
Undulating motor activity	Common	Very rare
Asynchronous limb movements	Common	Rare
Rhythmic pelvic movements	Occasional	Rare
Side-to-side head shaking	Common	Rare
Ictal crying	Occasional	Very rare
Closed mouth in "tonic phase"	Occasional	Very rare
Closed eyelids	Very common	Rare
Convulsion >2 minutes	Common	Very rare
Resisted lid opening	Common	Very rare
Pupillary light reflex	Usually retained	Commonly absent
Lack of cyanosis	Common	Rare

Modified from Reuber and Elger.[31]

one can often stop the episode with intravenous benzodiazepines. However, if there is a strong suspicion that the seizures are psychogenic, anticonvulsants should not be given. In most instances, a definitive diagnosis will require evaluation in an epilepsy unit, often with a video-EEG.

CEREBELLAR COGNITIVE AFFECTIVE SYNDROME

At times mistaken for catatonia, the cerebellar cognitive affective syndrome[33] was originally described in children following surgery to the vermis of the cerebellum. Because the children were awake but mute, the disorder was called the cerebellar mutism syndrome.[34] Cerebellar mutism also occurs in adults either after surgery involving the posterior fossa or as a result of lesions affecting the vermis and posterior lobes of the cerebellum. Such patients are awake, but may be somnolent. Whatever their level of alertness, they do not speak and often behave abnormally, either by not responding to the examiner or by behaving inappropriately. Patients may refuse to swallow food although they are not dysphagic. In children the syndrome characteristically occurs after a period of normality in the postoperative period. The mutism begins hours to days after awakening from anesthesia. The syndrome is largely reversible, but neuropsychologic tests given long after apparent recovery demonstrate defects in executive function, affect, and language.[34]

Patient 6–5

A 32-year-old man with a cerebellar ependymoma complained of headache and mild imbalance. He had been operated on twice 2 years before with a vermis splitting operation that removed most of the lesion, but left residual tumor in the lateral wall of the fourth ventricle. An operation was undertaken to remove the residual tumor. The surgeon did not invade the vermis but lifted the cerebellar tonsil to successfully resect the residual tumor. Neurologic consultation was sought in the immediate postoperative period when the patient appeared to be "unresponsive." He was lying in bed with his eyes open. He was still intubated, so that he could not speak, but he did not appear to re-

spond to any verbal commands. He moved spontaneously and sometimes appeared to withdraw from noxious stimuli but never would look at the examiner or regard the examiner in any way. When the patient was extubated he did not speak. Gradually over the next 24 to 36 hours, the patient began to respond by closing his eyes to command, but rarely looking at the examiner. He would carry out some commands, particularly grasping the examiner's hand. However, he had difficulty with commands involving the lips or tongue (oral buccal apraxia). Transiently, he demonstrated catalepsy. He would say his name, but to other questions he would only repeat his name. Later, when one of us asked him his name he responded "George Bush." It turned out that the nurse had asked him who the president was about 10 minutes before and he had responded appropriately.

Over time he made a good recovery and was discharged from the hospital. However, even at discharge his affect seemed flat and he himself reported that he was not the same as prior to surgery,

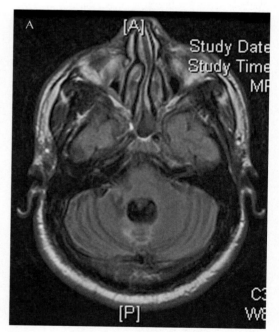

Figure 6–1. (A) A fluid-attenuated inversion recovery sequence demonstrating hyperintensity in the vermis, a result of the first two operations, with residual tumor. (B) A 24-hour postoperative film done during the time when the patient was responding poorly. The hyperintensity in the vermis is more marked and there is new hyperintensity in the right posterior lobe of the cerebellum.

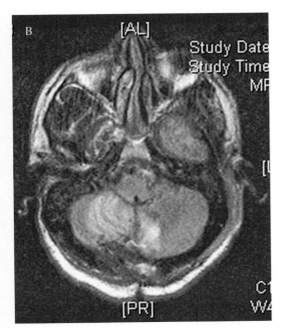

Figure 6–1. (B) (*continued*).

although he could not describe what the changes were.

Comment: The cerebellar cognitive affective syndrome is rare in adults and can easily be mistaken for catatonia or psychogenic unresponsiveness. This patient had suffered modest damage to the vermis of the cerebellum from the first two operations (Figure 6–1A), and suffered further transient damage to both a vermis and the right posterior lobe of the cerebellum as a result of the trauma of the third operation (Figure 6–1B). Interestingly, the surgeon noted that when she first interviewed him his affect seemed "flat." She referred him to a psychiatrist, who noted that his behavior had changed after the first operation in that he found himself "apathetic" and "not happy with the way I am." She found impaired memory, and language "adequate, but not descriptive of his feelings and emotions." These changes were probably a result of the vermis damage from the first two operations.

"AMYTAL INTERVIEW"

In many instances, an immediate distinction between organic and psychologic delirium or stupor cannot be made on the basis of the neu-rologic examination or the EEG, and in these instances an Amytal interview is often helpful. Although historically we have used Amytal, clinical evidence suggests that a benzodiazepine such as lorazepam works just as well and is more available.[35] We use the term *Amytal interview* loosely to describe the slow intravenous injection of an anxiolytic agent. The Amytal interview is conducted by injecting the drug intravenously at a slow rate while talking to the patient and doing repeated neurologic examinations. It is important that the discussion remain fairly neutral and not represent a direct challenge of the patient's veracity. Patients with structural or metabolic disease of the nervous system usually show immediately increasing neurologic dysfunction as the drug is injected. Neurologic signs not present prior to the injection of amobarbital (such as extensor plantar responses or hemiparesis) may appear after only a small dose has been introduced, and behavioral abnormalities, especially confusion and disorientation, grow worse. On the other hand, patients with psychogenic unresponsiveness or psychogenic excitement frequently require large doses of amobarbital before developing any change in their behavior, and the initial change is toward improvement in behavioral function rather than worsening of abnormal findings. Thus, a patient apparently stuporous may fully awaken after several hundred milligrams of Amytal and carry out a rational conversation (see Patient 6–3). A stuporous and withdrawn patient who is catatonic may become fully rational. An excited patient may calm down and demonstrate that he or she is alert, is oriented, and has normal cognitive functions. Patients in nonconvulsive status epilepticus may also awaken (see page 281).

In a few instances, even the Amytal interview does not make a distinction between organic and psychologic delirium. In such instances, the patient must be hospitalized for observation while a meticulous search for a metabolic cause of the delirium is made. In one of our patients, a diagnosis of catatonic stupor, although strongly suspected, did not make itself certain until the patient fully awoke after a thorough diagnostic evaluation had proved uninformative and electroshock therapy was initiated.[35] Once a psychogenic basis for unresponsiveness is established, a more extensive developmental and psychiatric history must be obtained to determine the type of psychiatric disturbance. The exact psychiatric diagnosis will determine the treatment. While the Amytal interview is a relatively safe procedure for diagnostic purposes, and is the first line treatment for catatonia,[35] most psychiatrists do not recommend it for treatment if the patient relapses into psychogenic unresponsiveness after the diagnosis has been made. Intravenous barbiturates given with the assumption that they will remove a symptom can be hazardous, because the patient who has resolved his or her conflict by developing the conversion symptom may develop more serious psychologic disturbances should the symptom abruptly be removed.[36]

REFERENCES

1. Sigurdardottir KR, Olafsson E. Incidence of psychogenic seizures in adults: a population-based study in Iceland. Epilepsia 1998; 39, 749–752.
2. Reuber M, Fernandez G, Helmstaedter C, et al. Evidence of brain abnormality in patients with psychogenic nonepileptic seizures. Epilepsy Behav 2002; 3, 249–254.
3. Caplan LR, Nadelson T. Multiple sclerosis and hysteria. Lessons learned from their association. JAMA 1980; 243, 2418–2421.
4. Merskey H, Buhrich NA. Hysteria and organic brain disease. Br J Med Psychol 1975; 48, 359–366.
5. Guze SB, Woodrugg RA, Clayton PJ. A study of conversion symptoms in psychiatric outpatients. Am J Psychiatry 1971; 128, 643–646.
6. Henry JA, Woodruff GH. A diagnostic sign in states of apparent unconsciousness. Lancet 1978; 2, 920–921.
7. Hopkins A. Pretending to be unconscious. Lancet 1973; 2, 312–314.
8. Lempert T, Dieterich M, Huppert D, et al. Psychogenic disorders in neurology: frequency and clinical spectrum. Acta Neurol Scand 1990; 82, 335–340.
9. Dula DJ, DeNaples L. Emergency department presentation of patients with conversion disorder. Acad Emerg Med 1995; 2, 120–123.
10. Slater E. Diagnosis of "hysteria." Br Med J 1965; 5447, 1395–1399.
11. Shraberg D, D'Souza T. Coma vigil masquerading as psychiatric illness. J Clin Psychiatry 1982; 43, 375–376.
12. Meyers TJ, Jafek BW, Meyers AD. Recurrent psychogenic coma following tracheal stenosis repair. Arch Otolaryngol Head Neck Surg 1999; 125, 1267–1269.
13. Reuber M, Kral T, Kurthen M, et al. New-onset psychogenic seizures after intracranial neurosurgery. Acta Neurochir (Wien) 2002; 144, 901–907.
14. Stone J, Smyth R, Carson A, et al. Systematic review of misdiagnosis of conversion symptoms and "hysteria." BMJ 2005; 331, 989.
15. Binzer M, Andersen PM, Kullgren G. Clinical characteristics of patients with motor disability due to conversion disorder: a prospective control group study. J Neurol Neurosurg Psychiatry 1997; 63, 83–88.
16. De T, X, Bier JC, Massat I, et al. Regional cerebral glucose metabolism in akinetic catatonia and after remission. J Neurol Neurosurg Psychiatry 2003; 74, 1003–1004.
17. Vuilleumier P, Chicherio C, Assal F, et al. Functional neuroanatomical correlates of hysterical sensorimotor loss. Brain 2001; 124, 1077–1090.
18. Spence SA, Crimlisk HL, Cope H, et al. Discrete neurophysiological correlates in prefrontal cortex during hysterical and feigned disorder of movement. Lancet 2000; 355, 1243–1244.
19. Atre-Vaidya N. Significance of abnormal brain perfusion in catatonia: a case report. Neuropsychiatry Neuropsychol Behav Neurol 2000; 13, 136–139.
20. Lauer M, Schirrmeister H, Gerhard A, et al. Disturbed neural circuits in a subtype of chronic catatonic schizophrenia demonstrated by F-18-FDG-PET and F-18-DOPA-PET. J Neural Transm 2001; 108, 661–670.
21. Northoff G, Kotter R, Baumgart F, et al. Orbitofrontal cortical dysfunction in akinetic catatonia: a functional magnetic resonance imaging study during negative emotional stimulation. Schizophr Bull 2004; 30, 405–427.
22. Hurwitz TA. Somatization and conversion disorder. Can J Psychiatry 2004; 49, 172–178.
23. Lempert T, von BM. The eye movements of syncope. Neurology 1996; 46, 1086–1088.
24. Jackson AO. Faking unconsciousness. Anaesthesia 2000; 55, 409.
25. Bush G, Fink M, Petrides G, et al. Catatonia. I. Rating scale and standardized examination. Acta Psychiatr Scand 1996; 93, 129–136.
26. Philbrick KL, Rummans TA. Malignant catatonia. J Neuropsychiatry Clin Neurosci 1994; 6, 1–13.
27. Gelenberg AJ. The catatonic syndrome. Lancet 1976; 1, 1339–1341.
28. Louis ED, Pflaster NL. Catatonia mimicking nonconvulsive status epilepticus. Epilepsia 1995; 36, 943–945.
29. Carroll BT, Boutros NN. Clinical electroencephalograms in patients with catatonic disorders. Clin Electroencephalogr 1995; 26, 60–64.
30. Devinsky O, Thacker K. Nonepileptic seizures. Neurol Clin 1995; 13, 299–319.
31. Reuber M, Elger CE. Psychogenic nonepileptic seizures: review and update. Epilepsy Behav 2003; 4, 205–216.
32. Chen DK, So YT, Fisher RS. Use of serum prolactin in diagnosing epileptic seizures: report of the Therapeutics and Technology Assessment Subcommittee of the American Academy of Neurology. Neurology 2005; 65, 668–675.
33. Schmahmann JD, Sherman JC. The cerebellar cognitive affective syndrome. Brain 1998; 121, 561–579.
34. Robertson PL, Muraszko KM, Holmes EJ, et al. Incidence and severity of postoperative cerebellar mutism syndrome in children with medulloblastoma: a prospective study by the Children's Oncology Group. J Neurosurg 2006; 105, 444–451.
35. Bush G, Fink M, Petrides G, et al. Catatonia. II. Treatment with lorazepam and electroconvulsive therapy. Acta Psychiatr Scand 1996; 93, 137–143.
36. Menza MA. A suicide attempt following removal of conversion paralysis with amobarbital. Gen Hosp Psychiatry 1989; 11, 137–138.

Chapter 7

Approach to Management of the Unconscious Patient

A CLINICAL REGIMEN FOR DIAGNOSIS AND MANAGEMENT

Of the acute problems in clinical medicine, none is more challenging than the prompt diagnosis and effective management of the patient in coma. The challenge exists in part because the causes of coma are so many and the physician possesses only a limited time in which to make the appropriate diagnostic and therapeutic judgments. Coma caused by a subdural or epidural hematoma may be fully reversible when the patient is first seen, but if treatment is not promptly undertaken, the brain injury may become either irreparable or fatal within a very short period of time. A comatose patient suffering from diabetic ketoacidosis or hypoglycemia may rapidly return to normal if appropriate treatment is begun immediately, but may die or be rendered permanently brain damaged if treatment is delayed. In extradural hematoma, meticulous evaluation of acid-base balance and substrate availability is not only useless, but it is also dangerous, because precious time may be lost. In untreated diabetic coma, time spent performing imaging is meddlesome, fruitless, and potentially dangerous.

The physician evaluating a comatose patient requires a systematic approach that will allow directing the diagnostic and therapeutic endeavors along appropriate pathways. The preceding chapters of this text presented what may appear to be a bewildering variety of disease states that cause stupor or coma. However, these chapters have also indicated that for any disease or functional abnormality of the brain to cause unconsciousness, it must either (1) produce bilateral dysfunction of the cerebral hemispheres, (2) damage or depress the physiologic activating mechanisms that lie along the central core of the upper brainstem and diencephalon, or (3) metabolically or physiologically damage or depress the brain globally. Conditions that can produce these effects can be divided into (1) supratentorial mass lesions that compress or displace the diencephalon and brainstem, (2) infratentorial destructive or expanding lesions that damage or compress the reticular formation, or (3) metabolic, diffuse, or multifocal encephalopathies that affect the brain in a widespread or diffuse fashion. In addition, the clinician must be alert to unresponsiveness of psychiatric causes. Conditions associated with loss of motor response but intact cognition must be excluded as etiologies (e.g., brainstem infarction, degenerative loss of motor nerves, or acute peripheral neuropathy [Guillain-Barré syndrome] producing a locked-in state[1]). Using these physiologic principles, one may considerably narrow the diagnostic possibilities and start specific treatment rapidly enough to make a difference in outcome. This chapter outlines a clinical approach that in most instances allows the physician to assign the cause of unresponsiveness promptly into one of the above four main categories while preventing irreversible damage to the patient's brain.

The key to making a categorical clinical diagnosis in coma consists of two steps: first, the accurate interpretation of a limited number of physical signs that reflect the integrity or impairment of various levels of the brain, and second, the determination of whether structural or metabolic dysfunction best explains the pattern and evolution of these signs. As Table 7–1

Table 7–1 Differential Characteristics of States Causing Sustained Unresponsiveness

I. *Supratentorial mass lesions compressing or displacing the diencephalon or brainstem*
   Signs of focal cerebral dysfunction present at onset
   Signs of dysfunction progress rostral to caudal
   Neurologic signs at any given time point to one anatomic area (e.g., diencephalon, midbrain-pons, medulla)
   Motor signs often asymmetric

II. *Subtentorial masses or destruction causing coma*
   History of preceding brainstem dysfunction or sudden onset of coma
   Localizing brainstem signs precede or accompany onset of coma
   Pupillary and oculomotor abnormal findings usually present
   Abnormal respiratory patterns common and usually appear at onset

III. *Metabolic, diffuse, or multifocal coma*
   Confusion and stupor commonly precede motor signs
   Motor signs are usually symmetric
   Pupillary reactions are usually preserved
   Asterixis, myoclonus, tremor, and seizures are common
   Acid-base imbalance with hyper- or hypoventilation is frequent

IV. *Psychiatric unresponsiveness*
   Lids close actively
   Pupils reactive or dilated (cycloplegics)
   Oculocephalic responses are unpredictable; oculovestibular responses physiologic for wakefulness (i.e., nystagmus is present)
   Motor tone is inconsistent or normal
   Eupnea or hyperventilation is usual
   No pathologic reflexes are present
   Electroencephalogram is normal

indicates, each of these pathophysiologic categories causes a characteristic group of symptoms and signs that usually evolve in a predictable manner. Once the patient's disease can be assigned to one of the three main categories, specific radiographic, electrophysiologic, or chemical laboratory studies can be employed to make disease-specific diagnoses or detect conditions that potentially complicate the patient's management. Once diagnosis is made and treatment started, changes in these same clinical signs and laboratory tests can be used serially to extend or supplement treatment (medical or surgical), to judge its effect, and, as indicated in Chapter 9, to estimate recovery and prognosis.

Many efforts have been made to find an ideal clinical approach to the unconscious patient. Most such approaches repeat or even enlarge upon the complete neurologic examination, which makes them too time consuming for practical daily use. A few are admirably brief and to the point (Chapter 2) (e.g., Glasgow Coma Scale), but have been designed for limited purposes, such as following patients with head injury; generally they provide too little information to allow diagnosis or the monitoring of metabolic problems. The recently described FOUR score scale (Chapter 2) gives more information, but is still limited.[2] The clinical profile described in Chapter 2, which has been employed extensively by ourselves and others, has advantages. The examination judges the normal and abnormal physiology of functions described earlier in Chapter 2: arousal, pupillary responses, eye movements, corneal responses, the breathing pattern, skeletal muscle motor function, and deep tendon reflexes. Most of these functions undergo predictable changes in association with localizable brain abnormalities that can locate the lesion or lesions. The constellation and evolution of these abnormal functions in a given patient can determine the cause of altered consciousness, whether supratentorial (focal findings start rostrally and evolve caudally), infratentorial (focal findings start in the brainstem), metabolic (lacks focal findings, but evidence of diffuse forebrain dysfunction), or psychiatric (lacks focal or diffuse signs of brain dysfunction).

PRINCIPLES OF EMERGENCY MANAGEMENT

No matter what the diagnosis or the cause of coma, certain general principles of management apply to all patients and should be addressed as one pursues the examination and undertakes definitive therapy (Table 7–2). Algorithms describing the initial management of the comatose patient have also been published (Figure 7–1).

Table 7–2 **Principles of Management of Comatose Patients**

1. Ensure oxygenation
2. Maintain circulation
3. Control glucose
4. Lower intracranial pressure
5. Stop seizures
6. Treat infection
7. Restore acid-base balance and electrolyte balance
8. Adjust body temperature
9. Administer thiamine
10. Consider specific antidotes (e.g., naloxone, flumazenil, etc.)
11. Control agitation

Ensure Oxygenation, Airway, and Ventilation

The brain must have a continuous supply of oxygen, and adequate blood oxygenation depends on sufficient respiration. Scrupulous attention must be given to the airway and the lungs themselves. *Check the airway.* If the airway is obstructed, attempt to clear it by suctioning and then arrange for a cuffed endotracheal tube to be placed by a skilled practitioner. Prior to placing the tube, extend the head gently, elevate the jaw, and ventilate the patient with 100% oxygen using a mask and bag to ensure maximal possible blood oxygenation during the procedure. Tracheal irritation usually produces a sympathetic discharge with hypertension, tachycardia, and occasional premature ventricular contractions. The increase in heart rate and mean arterial pressure transiently raises intracranial pressure, possibly worsening outcome,[4] an effect that can be mitigated by lidocaine administration (either topically or IV), IV thiopental, or propofol. Detailed reviews of rapid sequence intubation address these and several other pharmacologic agents used to ease intubation and prevent complications.[5–7] The choice depends on the specific clinical situation.[8,9] Rarely, particularly in hypoxemic patients, a vagal discharge leading to bradycardia or cardiac arrest occurs. Maximal oxygenation helps prevent cardiac arrhythmias that otherwise may result from the vagal stimulation. To place an endotracheal tube usually requires the physician to extend the neck, raising concern that the procedure may

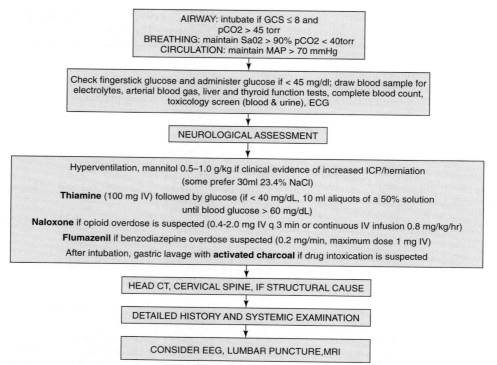

Figure 7–1. Algorithm for initial emergent management of the comatose patient. CT, computed tomography; ECG, electrocardiograph; EEG, electroencephalograph; GCS, Glasgow Coma Scale; ICP, intracranial pressure; MAP, mean

further damage an already injured cervical spine. In any patient who may have suffered a traumatic injury (obvious or suspected) requiring intubation, the neck should be manipulated as little as possible and fixed in a cervical collar. (The same principle applies to testing oculocephalic reflexes.) Several techniques exist for intubating patients with suspected cervical cord injuries. These include nasotracheal intubation, the use of a laryngeal mask,[10] and fiberoptic endoscopic intubation.[11] However, in one series, as many as 12% (37 of 308) of patients intubated by physicians in one emergency department were subsequently shown to have cervical spine injuries,[12] but none suffered worsening neurologic injury.[13] Whatever technique is used, the most important point is that a skilled physician should perform the procedure.

EVALUATE RESPIRATORY EXCURSIONS

Arterial blood gas measurement is the most reliable method of determining adequate ventilation but, as a rule of thumb, if breath sounds can be heard at both lung bases, and if the respiratory rate is greater than 8 per minute, ventilation is probably adequate. A pulse oximeter placed on the finger allows continuous recording of blood oxygenation and pulse rate, but may slightly overestimate oxygen saturation in dark-skinned individuals and is falsely elevated with carbon monoxide intoxication. Noninvasive CO_2 monitoring, if available, is also useful. Patients comatose from drug overdose or who are hypothermic have depressed metabolism and require less ventilation than awake individuals. The comatose patient ideally should maintain a PaO_2 greater than 100 mm Hg and a $PaCO_2$ between 35 and 40 mm Hg.

After initial management, patients with metabolic coma who are not intubated should be kept in a semiprone Trendelenburg position and turned from side to side each hour. Others, particularly those with increased intracranial pressure (ICP), are kept supine with the head of the bed elevated 15 to 30 degrees. It is necessary to perform chest physical therapy frequently and to suction the airway using a sterile technique. The inspissation of dried mucus in the tube can be minimized by attaching a freely vented hose to the endotracheal tube and delivering humidified air (or oxygen, if necessary). Because prolonged intubation can cause laryngeal[14] or middle ear damage[15] or sinusitis, some have suggested early tracheostomy in critically ill trauma patients.[16] However, most patients can be safely maintained for approximately 2 weeks. If prolonged coma seems likely, a tracheostomy should be performed after several days.

Maintain the Circulation

The circulation must be maintained if the brain is to receive adequate oxygen. *Check the blood pressure and pulse.* Insert an intravenous and an intra-arterial line (a radial artery line is as accurate as a central arterial line[17]), replace blood volume loss, and infuse vasoactive agents as needed. Dopamine, dobutamine, adrenaline, norepinephrine, and vasopressin are the most commonly used drugs. Current evidence does not indicate which vasopressor is superior[18]; however, vasopressin is becoming increasingly popular.[19] *Monitor the cardiac rate and rhythm and treat unstable vital signs and cardiac arrhythmias.* If the patient is in shock, seek an extracerebral source. Damage to the brain above the level of the medulla does not cause systemic hypotension (see Chapter 2).

Maintain the mean arterial pressure (MAP) between 70 and 80 mm Hg[20] using hypertensive and/or hypotensive agents as necessary (MAP = 1/3 systolic + 2/3 diastolic). In general, hypertension should not be immediately treated unless diastolic pressure exceeds 120 mm Hg. A number of intravenous agents are available to treat hypertensive emergencies.[21] These include sodium nitroprusside (0.25 to 10 µg/kg/minute), labetalol (20 to 80 mg bolus over 10 minutes), nicardipine (2 to 10 mg/hour), and others.[21] In an older patient with known chronic hypertension, do not allow the blood pressure to fall below previously accustomed levels, because the relative hypotension may cause cerebral hypoxia. In young, previously healthy patients, particularly those with depressant drug poisoning, a systolic blood pressure of 70 to 80 mm Hg is usually adequate. However, if ICP is elevated, a higher MAP may be necessary to maintain cerebral perfusion pressure (e.g., MAP 65 mm Hg > ICP).

Measure the Glucose

The brain depends not only on oxygen and blood flow, but also on an obligate use of glucose for its homeostasis (see Chapter 5). Both hypoglycemia and hyperglycemia have deleterious effects on the brain (see Chapter 5). If the bedside blood glucose test reveals hypoglycemia, glucose should be given. (Glucose is often given empirically along with thiamine and naloxone [see below] by paramedics, before the patient arrives at the hospital.) Some investigators give 25 g of glucose as a 50% solution; others give glucose in 5 g increments as a 10% solution (50 mL). The latter technique results in lower posttreatment blood glucose levels preventing the development of hyperglycemia.[22] Increasing evidence suggests that tight control of hyperglycemia using insulin decreases morbidity in severely ill hyperglycemic patients. Glucose should be maintained between 80 and 110 mg/dL.[23] Even after a hypoglycemic patient has been treated with glucose, care must be taken to prevent recurrent hypoglycemia. Therefore, infuse glucose and water intravenously until the situation has stabilized.

ADMINISTER THIAMINE

Wernicke's encephalopathy is a rare cause of coma.[33] However, many patients admitted as emergencies in stupor or coma are chronic alcoholics or otherwise malnourished.[34,35] In such a patient, a glucose load may precipitate acute Wernicke's encephalopathy.[36] Therefore, it is important to administer 50 to 100 mg thiamine at the time glucose is given or shortly thereafter.

Lower the Intracranial Pressure

The methods are described under *supratentorial mass lesions*, page 320.

Stop Seizures

Repeated seizures of whatever etiology cause brain damage and must be stopped.[24] Treat generalized convulsions with intravenous

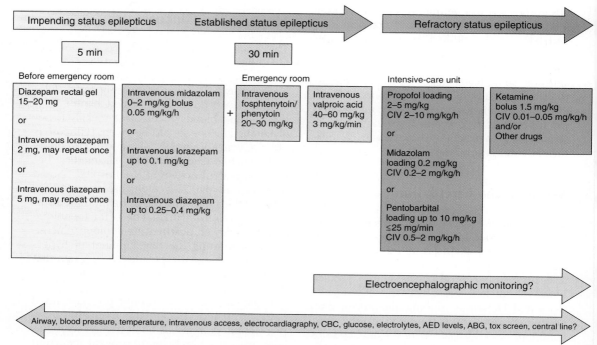

Figure 7–2. Management of status epilepticus. Impending or established status epilepticus: start with 20 mg/kg of fos-phenytoin or phenytoin, and if status epilepticus persists, give an additional 10 mg/kg. Follow the flow chart UNLESS there is a history of drug intolerance (e.g., allergy to phenytoin or benzodiazepine)—then replace by IV valproic acid 40 to 60 mg/kg or IV phenobarbital 20 mg/kg; UNLESS treatment-induced hypotension slows rate of delivery, or UNLESS history of progressive (PME) or juvenile (JME) myoclonus epilepsy (phenytoin/fosphenytoin harmful in PME, ineffective in JME)—replace with IV valproic or IV phenobarbital; UNLESS tonic status epilepticus with Lennox-Gastaut syndrome (might be worsened by benzodiazepines)—replace with IV valproic acid or IV phenobarbital; UNLESS acute intermit-tent porphyria—avoid P450 inducers, replace by nasogastric (NG) gabapentin (is possible) or by IV valproic acid; UNLESS, focal status epilepticus without impairment of consciousness—IV treatment not indicated, load anticonvulsants orally or rectally. Refractory status epilepticus: IV valproic acid: start with 40 mg/kg and, if status epilepticus persists, give an additional 20 mg/kg. Continuous intravenous infusion (CIV) usually starts with the lower dose, which is titrated to achieve seizure suppression and is increased as tolerated if tachyphylaxis develops. Ketamine: rule out increased intracranial pressure before administration. Other drugs: felbamate, topiramate, levetiracetam, lidocaine, inhalation an-esthetics, etc.: dosage and pharmacokinetics of most anticonvulsants must be adjusted appropriately in patients with hepatic or renal failure, or with drug interactions. Some patients in refractory status epilepticus will need systemic and pulmonary artery catheterization, with fluid and vasopressors as indicated to maintain blood pressure. ABG, arterial blood gas; AED, antiepileptic drug; CBC, complete blood count. (From Chen and Wasterlain,[24] with permission.)

lorazepam (up to 0.1 mg/kg). Figure 7–2 is a recently published algorithm for the treatment of status epilepticus. A ventilator must be avail-able, since large doses of the drug may depress breathing. Once the seizures have stopped, give intravenous phenytoin 15 mg/kg at 50 mg/minute or fosphenytoin at the same dosage of phenytoin equivalents, but at 100 to 150 mg/minute. Intravenous valproic acid may also be used at 40 to 60 mg/kg at a rate of 20 mg/minute to maintain seizure control. However, at these rates, it takes at least 20 minutes to administer 1,000 mg of phenytoin and more than an hour

to give doses of valproate above 1,200 mg. Hence, it is not unusual for seizures to recur during the administration of the antiepileptic drug, and this may require additional loraze-pam. At times, generalized seizures cannot be stopped with the above agents and anesthesia with propofol, midazolam, or pentobarbital is necessary. Because these drugs further suppress respiration, the patient should be intubated at this point as well if this has not been done al-ready. All of these drugs have short half-lives, and are given at dosages that produce elec-troencephalographic (EEG) burst suppression.

Alternatively, some physicians prefer intravenous boluses of phenobarbital 65 mg every 3 to 5 minutes (which has a longer half-life) until seizures cease. Typically, the patient must remain in a deeply drug-induced coma for at least 24 hours, followed by attempts to wean the patient off the anesthetic doses of medication. Importantly, approximately 10% to 20% of patients presenting with impaired consciousness show nonconvulsive status epilepticus on EEG examination (Chapter 5).[25,26] Nonconvulsive status epilepticus also causes brain injury and requires the same treatment as generalized motor seizures. Focal continuous epilepsy, by contrast, frequently occurs with metabolic brain disease, but is less threatening to the brain, and does not require the use of anesthetic doses of anticonvulsant drugs.

Treat Infection

Many different infections cause delirium or coma, and infection may exacerbate coma from other causes. Draw blood cultures on all febrile patients and those who are hypothermic without obvious cause. As indicated in Chapter 3, if there is a strong suspicion of bacterial meningitis, empiric antibiotic therapy should begin immediately after blood cultures are drawn. In one large series of patients with sepsis treated in intensive care units, cultures were positive in only 60% of patients.[27] *Staphylococcus aureus*, *Pseudomonas* species, and *Escherichia coli* were the most common organisms. A third-generation cephalosporin (cefotaxime, 2 g every 6 hours or ceftriaxone 2 g every 12 hours) should be started.[28,29] Some physicians add vancomycin 2 g every 12 hours to cover cephalosporin-resistant *S. pneumoniae*. In elderly or obviously immunosuppressed patients, ampicillin should be added to cover *Listeria monocytogenes*. Current evidence suggests that dexamethasone added to the regimen decreases long-term complications of the infection.[30] Because herpes simplex encephalitis is a relatively common infectious cause of coma (page 156), an antiviral agent (e.g., acyclovir 10 mg/kg every 8 hours) should be started if clinically indicated. In immunosuppressed patients, fungal and parasitic infections must also be considered, but because they tend to be less acute, they can await evaluation by imaging and spinal fluid examination. Other infections causing coma (Chapter 5) must

be considered and, in appropriate circumstances, treated.

As discussed in Chapter 3, it is generally necessary in a comatose patient to obtain a computed tomography (CT) scan prior to attempting lumbar puncture (Figure 7–3). If there is no evidence of a mass lesion, or if cerebrospinal fluid (CSF) cultures can be obtained within the first hour or two after antibiotics are administered, it may still be possible to identify the organism and its antibiotic sensitivities.

Restore Acid-Base Balance

With severe metabolic acidosis or alkalosis, the pH should be returned to a normal level by treating the cause, as metabolic acidosis can lead to cardiovascular abnormalities and metabolic alkalosis can depress respiration. Respiratory acidosis presages respiratory failure and warns the physician that ventilatory assistance may soon be needed. The elevated CO_2 also raises ICP. Respiratory alkalosis can cause cardiac arrhythmias and hinders weaning from ventilatory support.

Adjust Body Temperature

Several metabolic and structural abnormalities lead to either hyperthermia or hypothermia, and these states may exacerbate abnormalities of cerebral metabolism.[31] Hyperthermia is dangerous because it increases cerebral metabolic demands and, at extreme levels, can denature brain cellular proteins.[32] The body temperature above 38.5°C of hyperthermic patients should be reduced using antipyretics and, if necessary, physical cooling (e.g., cooling blanket). Significant hypothermia (below 34°C) can lead to pneumonia, cardiac arrhythmias, electrolyte disorders, hypovolemia, metabolic acidosis, impaired coagulation, and thrombocytopenia and leukopenia.[31] Patients should be gradually warmed to maintain a body temperature above 35°C.

Administer Specific Antidotes

Many patients entering an emergency room in coma are suffering from drug overdose. Any of the gamut of sedative drugs, alcohol, opioids,

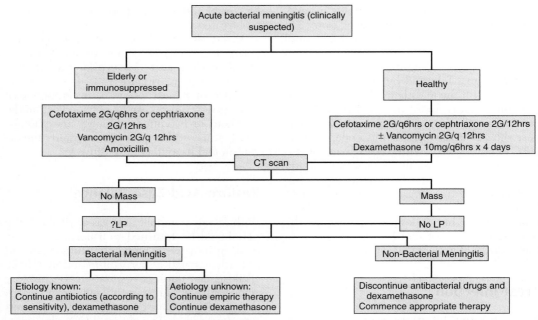

Figure 7–3. Therapeutic approach to a patient with acute bacterial meningitis. Empiric addition of amoxicillin is indicated for meningitis caused by *Listeria monocytogenes*. Continuation or change of antibiotics is guided by the results of cerebrospinal fluid analysis, blood culture, bacterial sensitivity to antibiotics, and clinical status of the patient. Steroid treatment in meningitis is unlikely to be of benefit if the diagnosis is delayed, if antibiotics have not been given, or if meningitis is Gram-negative bacillar or requires aminoglycoside antibiotics. Unless pneumococcal meningitis is proven or strongly suspected, dexamethasone use is not recommended in immunosuppressed or malnourished patients and in patients with other system infections. HSE, herpes simplex encephalitis; LP, lumbar puncture. (Modified from Chaudhuri.[102])

tranquilizers, and hallucinogens may have been ingested singly or in combination. Most drug overdoses are best treated by the supportive measures considered in a subsequent section. Because these patients have ingested multiple agents, specific antagonists are often not useful.[38] Even the so-called coma cocktail[3] (dextrose, thiamine, naloxone, and flumazenil) is rarely helpful and may be harmful.[39] However, when there is a strong suspicion that a specific agent has been ingested, certain antagonists specifically reverse the effects of several coma-producing drugs.

For opioid overdose, naloxone may be given at 0.4 to 2.0 mg IV every 3 minutes or by continuous IV infusion at 0.8 mg/kg/hour until consciousness is restored. This drug must be used with great care, because in a patient physically dependent on opioids, the drug may cause acute withdrawal symptoms requiring opioid therapy.[40] (If the patient is a known or suspected opioid addict, 0.4 mg naloxone should be diluted in 10 mL of saline and given slowly.

One should use the minimum amount necessary to establish the diagnosis by pupillary dilation and reverse the comatose state.) Naloxone has a duration of action from 2 to 3 hours, much shorter than the action of several opioid drugs, especially methadone. Thus, patients who have taken an overdose of opioids, and whose toxic reactions are reversed by naloxone, may lapse back into coma after a few hours and require further treatment.

Benzodiazepine overdose can be treated with flumazenil, a specific competitive benzodiazepine receptor antagonist[41] (0.2 mg/minute to a maximum dose of 1 mg IV). Flumazenil acts within minutes and has a half-life of about 40 to 75 minutes. However, the drug is not often used because it can precipitate acute withdrawal in chronic users and blockade of the benzodiazepine receptor may unmask epileptogenic features of common medications such as tricyclic antidepressants or theophylline.[41] Specific clinical features of benzodiazepine intoxication should be present (see Chapter 5).

Table 7–3 **Specific Antidotes for Agents Causing Delirium and Coma**

Antidote	Indication
Naloxone	Opioid overdose
Flumazenil	Benzodiazepine overdose
Physostigmine	Anticholinergic overdose (? gamma-hydroxybutyrate toxicity)
Fomepizole	Methanol, ethylene glycol toxicity
Glucagon	? Tricyclic overdose
Hydroxocobalamin	Cyanide overdose
Octreotide	Sulfonylurea hypoglycemia

Data from Ries and Dart.[37]

Certain effects of sedative drugs that have anticholinergic properties, particularly the tricyclic antidepressants and possibly gamma-hydroxybutyrate, can be reversed by the intravenous injection of 1 mg physostigmine. However, its use is controversial as it may cause seizures and cardiac arrhythmias; because of its potential side effects and short duration of action, it is rarely used.[37] Specific antidotes for several other agents are discussed in Chapter 5 and indicated in Table 7–3.

Control Agitation

Many patients who are delirious or stuporous are grossly agitated. The hyperactivity is distressing to patients and family and may lead to self-injury. Sedative dosages of drugs should be avoided until the diagnosis is clear and one is certain that the problem is metabolic rather than structural. Agitation can be controlled by keeping the patient in a lighted room and asking a relative or staff member to sit at the bedside and talk reassuringly to the patient. Small doses of lorazepam 0.5 to 1.0 mg orally with additional doses every 4 hours as needed may control agitation. If this proves insufficient,[42] haloperidol 0.5 to 1.0 mg twice daily orally or intramuscularly may be used; additional doses can be given every 4 hours as needed. In patients who have habitually ingested alcohol or sedative drugs, larger doses may be necessary because of cross-tolerance. A recent report suggests that valproate, benzodiazepine, and/or antipsychotics may relieve agitation when the primary drugs have failed.[43] For very short-term sedation, as might be necessary to perform a CT scan, intravenous sedation with propofol or midazolam may be used,[44] as these are short acting and midazolam can be reversed at the end of the procedure.

Physical restraints should be avoided whenever possible, but sometimes they are necessary for severely agitated patients. Take care to ensure that body restraints do not interfere with breathing and that limb restraints do not occlude blood flow or damage peripheral nerves. The restraints should be removed as soon as the agitation is controlled.

Protect the Eyes

Corneal erosions can occur within 4 to 6 hours if the eyes of comatose patients remain partially or fully opened. Exposure keratitis may lead to secondary bacterial corneal ulcerations. To prevent such changes, lubricate the eyes with a lubricating artificial tears ointment every 4 hours[45] or apply a polyethylene corneal bandage.[46] Repeated testing of the corneal reflex with cotton can also damage the cornea. A safer technique is to drip sterile saline onto the cornea from a distance of 4 to 6 inches.[2]

EXAMINATION OF THE PATIENT

Once the vital functions have been protected, proceed with the history and examination. The examination of the unconscious patient is covered in detail in Chapter 2, but a brief reprise is included here with emphasis on the elements that need to be covered quickly while initiating therapy in a clinical setting.

The history should, to whatever extent possible, be obtained from relatives, friends, paramedics, or sometimes even the police. If it has not already been done, search the patient's belongings and check for a medical alert bracelet. Implanted computer chips that give full medical information are currently available, but are not yet in common use.

The history of onset is important. Coma of sudden onset in a previously healthy patient usually turns out to be self-induced drug poisoning, subarachnoid hemorrhage, head trauma, or, in older persons, brainstem hemorrhage or infarction. Most examples of supratentorial mass lesions produce a more gradual impairment of consciousness, as do the metabolic encephalopathies.

In the general physical examination, after assessing and dealing with abnormalities of vital signs, look for evidence of trauma or signs that might suggest an acute or chronic systemic medical illness or the ingestion of self-administered drugs. Evaluate nuchal rigidity, but take care

first to ensure that the cervical spine has not been injured.[47]

It is the neurologic examination that is most helpful in assessing the nature of the patient's unconsciousness. Table 7–4 outlines the clinical neurologic functions that provide the most useful information in making a categoric diagnosis. These clinical indices have been extensively tested and applied to patients. They have

Table 7–4 **A Score Sheet for Examination of the Comatose Patient**

HISTORY (from Relatives or Friends)
Onset of coma (abrupt, gradual)
Recent complaints (headache, depression, focal weakness, vertigo)
Recent injury
Previous medical illnesses (diabetes, uremia, heart disease)
Previous psychiatric history
Access to drugs (sedatives, psychotropic drugs)
Occupation (pesticides, CO exposure)
Exposure to pathogens (ticks, mosquitoes)

General Physical Examination
Vital signs
Evidence of trauma
Evidence of acute or chronic systemic illness
Evidence of drug ingestion (needle marks, alcohol on breath)
Nuchal rigidity (examine with care)

NEUROLOGIC PROFILE
Verbal responses
 Oriented speech
 Confused conversation
 Inappropriate speech
 Incomprehensible speech
 No speech
Respiratory pattern
 Regular
 Periodic
 Ataxic
Eye opening
 Spontaneous
 Response to verbal stimuli
 Response to noxious stimuli
 None
Pupillary reactions
 Present
 Asymmetric (describe)
 Absent

Spontaneous eye movements
 Orienting
 Roving conjugate
 Roving dysconjugate
 Abnormal movements (describe)
 None
Oculocephalic responses
 Normal awake
 Full comatose
 Abnormal (describe)
 Minimal
 None
Oculovestibular responses
 Normal awake (nystagmus)
 Tonic conjugate
 Abnormal (describe)
 Minimal
 None
Corneal responses
 Present
 Absent
Motor responses
 Obeying commands
 Localizing
 Withdrawal
 Abnormal flexion posturing
 Abnormal extension posturing
 None
Deep tendon reflexes
 Normal
 Increased
 Absent
Skeletal muscle tone
 Normal
 Paratonic
 Flexor
 Extensor
 Flaccid

proved themselves to be easily and quickly obtained and to have a high degree of consistency from examiner to examiner.[2,48–50] Furthermore, they give valuable information upon which to base both diagnosis and prognosis. When serially recorded on a vital signs sheet as best-worst changes during each 24 hours, the result reflects accurately the patient's clinical course. The following paragraphs give the detailed description of each clinical sign.

Verbal Responses

The best response, oriented speech, implies awareness of self and the environment. The patient knows who he or she is, where he or she is, why he or she is there, and the year, season, and month. Confused conversation describes conversational speech with syntactically correct phrases but with disorientation and confusion in the content. Inappropriate speech means intelligible but with isolated words. The content can include profanity but no sustained conversation. Incomprehensible speech refers to the production of word-like mutterings or groans. The worst verbal response, no speech, applies to total mutism.

Respiratory Pattern

The pattern is recorded as regular, periodic, ataxic, or a combination of these. Respiratory rate should be determined in patients not being mechanically ventilated.

Eye Opening

Patients with spontaneous eye opening have some tone in the eyelids and generally demonstrate spontaneous blinking, which differentiates them from completely unresponsive patients whose eyes sometimes remain passively open. Though spontaneous eye opening rules out coma by our definition, it does not guarantee awareness. Some vegetative patients with eye opening have been shown postmortem to have total loss of the cerebral cortex (see Chapter 9). Eye opening in response to verbal stimuli means that any verbal stimulus, whether an appropriate command or not, produces eye opening. More severely damaged patients demonstrate eye opening only in response to a noxious stimulus applied to the trunk or an extremity. (A noxious stimulus to the head commonly evokes eye closing.) The worst response, no eye opening, applies to all remaining patients except when local changes such as periorbital edema preclude examination.

Pupillary Reactions

Pupillary reactions to an intense flashlight beam are evaluated for both eyes, and the better response is recorded; use a hand lens or the plus 20 lens on the ophthalmoscope to evaluate questionable responses. Record pupillary diameters and note the presence of any somatic third nerve paresis.

Spontaneous Eye Movement

The best response is spontaneous orienting eye movements in which the patient looks toward environmental stimuli. Record roving conjugate and roving dysconjugate eye movements when present, and reserve a miscellaneous movement category for patients without orienting eye movements who have spontaneous nystagmus, opsoclonus, ocular bobbing, or other abnormal eye movement. Absent spontaneous eye movements should be noted, as should the presence of lateral deviation to either side or dysconjugate gaze at rest (e.g., skew).

Oculocephalic Responses

These are evaluated in conjunction with passive, brisk, horizontal head turning. When appropriate, the response to vertical head movement should also be recorded. Patients with normal waking responses retain orienting eye movements and do not have consistent oculocephalic responses. Full oculocephalic responses are brisk and tonic and generally include conjugate eye movements opposite to the direction of turning. Minimal responses are defined as conjugate movements of less than 30 degrees or bilateral inability to adduct the eyes. Absence of response is the poorest level of function. *Remember, do not test oculocephalic reflexes in patients suspected of having sustained a neck injury.*

Caloric Vestibulo-Ocular Responses

These are tested by irrigating each external auditory canal with up to 50 mL ice water with the head 30 degrees above the horizontal plane (Chapter 2). A normal (awake) response includes rapid nystagmus toward the nonirrigated ear and minimal, if any, tonic deviation. Do not use ice water (use tap water) in an awake patient. An intact response in an unconscious patient consists of tonic responses with conjugate deviation toward the irrigated ear.

Corneal Responses

Responses to a cotton wisp drawn fully across the cornea or, safer, sterile saline dripped onto the cornea are recorded as present or absent for the eye with the better response.

Motor Responses

These should be tested and recorded in all extremities and strength noted as normal or weak. The best score is given to patients who obey commands; care should be taken to avoid interpreting reflex grasping as obedience. If a command evokes no responses, apply a noxious stimulus gently but firmly to each extremity (compression of finger or toenail beds, or of Achilles tendon) and to the supraorbital notches or temporomandibular joints. Localizing responses designate the use of an extremity to locate or resist a remote noxious stimulus (e.g., the arm crossing the midline toward a cranial stimulus or reaching above shoulder level toward a cranial stimulus). A more primitive response consists of a nonstereotyped, rapid withdrawal from a noxious stimulus; this response often incorporates hip or shoulder adduction. An abnormal flexion response in the upper extremities is stereotyped, slow, and dystonic, and the thumb is often held between the second and third fingers. Abnormal flexion in the lower extremities (the reflex triple flexion response) sometimes can be difficult to distinguish from withdrawal. An abnormal extension response in the upper extremity consists of adduction and internal rotation of the shoulder and pronation of the forearm. No response is recorded only when strong stimuli are applied to more than

one site and when muscle relaxants have not recently been administered.

Tendon Reflexes

These reflexes are recorded for the best limb as normal, increased, or absent; minimal responses are best regarded as normal.

Skeletal Muscle Tone

This should be recorded as normal, paratonic (diffuse resistance throughout the range of passive motion), flexor (spasticity), extensor (rigidity), or flaccid.

GUIDES TO SPECIFIC MANAGEMENT

Supratentorial Mass Lesions

The differential characteristics that suggest a supratentorial mass lesion producing stupor or coma are outlined in Table 7–1. The laboratory tests useful for the differential diagnosis of stupor and coma are listed in Table 7–5.

If the physician elicits a history of headache or prior head trauma, no matter how trivial, he or she should consider a supratentorial mass lesion. At times, the historian will be able to describe symptoms or signs (facial asymmetry, weakness of one arm, dragging of the leg, or complaints of unilateral sensory loss) that existed prior to coma and suggest the presence of a supratentorial lesion. The presence at the initial examination of strikingly asymmetric motor signs, or of dysfunction progressing in a rostral-caudal fashion, provides strong presumptive evidence of a supratentorial mass. The combination of neurologic signs should point to a single plane of diencephalic or brainstem dysfunction as illustrated in Chapter 3. The combination of third nerve motor dysfunction and impaired pupillary responses evolving as coma deepens suggest a supratentorial mass. The major problem in differential diagnosis arises when supratentorial mass lesions, either extracerebral or in "silent" areas of the forebrain that do not produce obvious focal signs, cause stupor or coma at the diencephalic stage

Table 7–5 **Emergency Laboratory Evaluation of Metabolic Coma**

1. Stat tests
   A. Venous blood
      1. Glucose
      2. Electrolytes
      3. Urea or creatinine
      4. Osmolality
      5. Complete blood count
      6. Coagulation studies
   B. Arterial blood
      1. Check color
      2. pH
      3. PO_2
      4. PCO_2
      5. Carboxyhemoglobin (if available, especially if blood is bright red)
   C. Cerebrospinal fluid
      1. Cells
      2. Gram stain
      3. Glucose
   D. Electrocardiogram
2. Additional tests°
   A. Venous blood
      1. Liver function tests
      2. Thyroid and adrenal function
      3. Blood cultures
      4. Viral titers
   B. Urine
      1. Culture
   C. Cerebrospinal fluid
      1. Protein
      2. Culture
      3. Viral and fungal antibodies, polymerase chain reaction

°These tests are "additional," because in most hospitals it will take hours to days to get the results. The blood and cerebrospinal fluid for these tests, however, is drawn at the same time as the stat tests.

without producing preceding or accompanying focal motor signs. Because such patients often have reactive pupils, intact oculocephalic and oculovestibular responses, and abnormal motor signs that are symmetric or only mildly asymmetric, the physician may suspect metabolic encephalopathy rather than a supratentorial mass. Unless there is a clear history to help one differentiate, the physician should consider both diagnostic categories and obtain an immediate brain CT or magnetic resonance imaging (MRI) scan.

If the patient is suspected to be suffering from a supratentorial mass, determine how se-

vere the symptoms are and estimate how rapidly they are worsening. If the patient is stuporous or comatose but relatively stable, procure an emergency CT scan. A CT will rule out all significant mass lesions and usually identify subarachnoid hemorrhages. However, MRI, when available, is more sensitive and may be required to identify recent cerebral infarcts, particularly in the brainstem, and focal inflammatory lesions.

If the patient is deeply comatose, or if transtentorial herniation is evolving rapidly in a stuporous patient, it is necessary to *treat intracranial hypertension first*. The patient may initially be hyperventilated by a mask and Ambu bag while waiting for appropriate personnel and equipment to intubate the patient. An arterial sample for blood gas analysis should also be taken after hyperventilation is begun. Hyperventilation is the most rapid technique for lowering ICP,[51] and may effectively withdraw a patient from the edge of herniation within a minute or two. The resulting decrease in $PaCO_2$ causes cerebral vasoconstriction, thus decreasing cerebral blood flow (CBF). Although this may also decrease CBF,[52] risking further brain ischemia, lowering ICP is mandatory in patients who are herniating and hyperventilation is the fastest way to do it. In the absence of direct measurement of ICP, one cannot be certain of the best $PaCO_2$ level. We suggest the airway be secured and the patient hyperventilated to a $PaCO_2$ between 25 and 30 mm Hg. The higher the ICP, and the lower the intracranial CSF compensatory reserve, the more a given decrease in $PaCO_2$ will lower the ICP.[53] After other treatment is under way, the $PaCO_2$ can be increased to approximately 35 mm Hg. This technique lowers ICP rapidly, but its effect is transient. Hence, it is necessary to use the time that is bought by hyperventilation to begin more long-lasting efforts to reduce ICP.

Some evidence suggests that raising the head of the bed to 30 degrees reduces ICP without affecting mean arterial blood pressure (but see page 43). On the other hand, this method raises the differential between mean arterial pressure and cerebral perfusion pressure,[54] and the net effect on brain perfusion is difficult to measure and may vary among patients.[55,56] Thus, eventually the position must be chosen based on measurements of ICP.

Hyperosmolar agents should be administered at the same time; they decrease the water content of the brain by creating an osmolar gradient between the blood and that portion of the brain with an intact blood-brain barrier. Because most brain lesions cause local breakdown of the blood-brain barrier, hyperosmolar agents pull water from normal brain, which may lower ICP,[57] but do not reduce the size of such lesions. Fortunately, this does not appear to deleteriously affect brain shifts.[57] Mannitol is the agent most used; it is given in a 20% solution at a dose of 1.5 to 2 g/kg by bolus injection. Its effects are rapid and last several hours. Mannitol also lowers blood viscosity, increasing cerebral perfusion, and may also act as a free radical scavenger. However, repeated doses of mannitol increase the risk of renal failure. Recently, hypertonic saline has gained favor as an alternative to mannitol. Doses in the range of 7 to 10 g of NaCl, in concentrations from 3% to 23.4%, have been administered by rapid injection, or in some cases by continuous intravenous infusion titrated to ICP.[58,59] The results in general were comparable to mannitol; the brain dehydration could be maintained for several days and there have been few complications.

In patients with brain tumors, whether primary or metastatic, subdural or epidural hematomas and empyemas, or other mass lesions that incite neovascularization with blood vessels that lack a blood-brain barrier, adrenal corticosteroids dramatically reverse signs and symptoms of herniation. Substantial clinical improvement is seen within 6 to 12 hours even though changes in water content of the brain may not be seen for days.[60,61] The dose required to reverse herniation in patients with brain tumors is unknown, but given the seriousness of the situation, high doses are desirable. The typical initial dose is 10 mg of dexamethasone, although as much as 100 mg of dexamethasone can be given safely as an intravenous bolus. (In awake patients, the bolus may cause severe genital paresthesias[62]; the agent can be dripped in over 10 to 15 minutes.)

The exact mechanism of the salutary response is unknown. Steroids decrease the transfer constant of substances across a disrupted blood-brain barrier within an hour, and they may increase clearance of edema fluid in the extracellular space, but substantial changes in brain water are not seen for many hours or days.[60,61] They also improve compliance of brain tissue and diminish the plateau waves (sudden transient increase in ICP that may increase transtentorial herniation).[63]

Corticosteroids are also indicated in patients with suspected bacterial meningitis.[64] The drug should be started prior to or at the time antibiotics are given. A dose of 10 mg every 6 hours is standard.[64] The role of corticosteroids in cerebral vascular disease is controversial.[65,66] Most current evidence suggests that steroids do not improve the course of patients with cerebral infarction or cerebral hemorrhage. The brain edema in stroke is largely cytotoxic, rather than vasogenic, and steroids do not produce the dramatic amelioration of the symptoms of brain edema seen in patients with tumors. Furthermore, the hyperglycemic effects of steroids may actually deleteriously affect the outcome. Corticosteroids are contraindicated in patients with head injury.[67]

The above steps should require no more than a few minutes to bring the ICP under control. Once it is controlled, procure a CT or, if available, an MRI. The scan will demonstrate the nature of the supratentorial mass lesion and often determines the degree of transtentorial herniation as well. If a subdural or epidural hematoma is identified, it should be evacuated immediately.[68,69] Similarly, a brain abscess requires urgent surgery to decompress the lesion and establish cultures. If one of these lesions is suspected clinically and the patient is deteriorating rapidly, a neurosurgeon should be contacted at the time of imaging. For brain tumors, it is sometimes best to allow the steroids to reduce the level of edema for several days prior to surgery. Intraparenchymal hemorrhages, traumatic brain injury, or infarctions are best treated by careful supportive care if the ICP can be controlled and the patient is not in danger of herniation.[70,71]

Monitor the patient's vital signs and the neurologic examination constantly during therapy. An endotracheal tube should be in place, and the patient ventilated to PaO_2 at greater than 100 mm Hg. After initial hyperventilation, adjust the $PaCO_2$ between 35 and 40 mm Hg. Mannitol may be repeated as often as every 4 to 6 hours, depending on the patient's clinical state, but it is important to maintain intravascular volume by monitoring the inputs and outputs, and to watch for rebound increased ICP. In patients suffering from cerebral tumors or abscess, continue dexamethasone (typically 4 mg every 6 hours, although doses up to 24 mg every 6 hours may be used if clinically necessary) or an equivalent steroid. The head of the bed should probably be slightly elevated. Insert a Foley catheter and record urine output each hour. Measure electrolytes frequently if mannitol or saline is being given, because the use of these drugs can result in severe electrolyte imbalance. Once in the intensive care unit, ICP should be monitored.

Some investigators have advocated barbiturate anesthesia to treat severe intracranial hypertension from head injury.[72] The drug usually employed is pentobarbital (although thiopental works faster) given intravenously. In one protocol, a loading dose of 10 mg/kg is given over 30 minutes followed by 5 mg/kg over 60 minutes for three doses. The patient is then maintained at 1 to 3 mg/kg/hour to maintain the pentobarbital level at 3 to 4 mg/dL.[73] The level of coma is also monitored by EEG, to produce a burst suppression pattern at about three to five bursts per minute.[74] The effect of this treatment on long-term outcome is not dramatic and the frequent monitoring of EEG, drug levels, and potential cardiopulmonary complications make it extremely labor intensive. With such therapy, the ICP decreases rapidly and usually remains low as long as the patient is anesthetized. This technique requires extremely careful monitoring of vital signs and should be carried out only in an intensive care unit. There are reports of decreases in mortality with the use of barbiturate anesthesia in head injuries, drownings, cerebral infarction, and other supratentorial mass lesions.[75] How barbiturates act to reduce the ICP is unknown. It is not simply through anesthesia, since in experimental animals gas anesthesia appears to have no such salutary effect. The clinical usefulness of barbiturate therapy for coma must be regarded as still in the stage of experimental evaluation.

Midazolam and propofol are also used to lower ICP, but like barbiturate coma, it is unclear if they result in an improved outcome.[76] Another second-tier therapy to control intractable intracranial hypertension is decompressive craniectomy.[77] The procedure is being used in patients with severe traumatic brain injury and also those with massive cerebral infarction. It may improve outcome in the former,[77] but while it may be lifesaving in the latter, functional outcome is often poor especially in the elderly.[78]

Infratentorial Mass Lesions

Infratentorial lesions fall into two groups: those that are intrinsic to the brainstem and those that compress it. In patients with infratentorial mass or destructive lesions causing coma, one may elicit a history of occipital headache or complaints of vertigo, diplopia, or other symptoms and signs suggesting brainstem dysfunction. Frequently, however, the onset of the coma is sudden and headache occurs only moments before the patient loses consciousness. If the onset of the headache is accompanied by vomiting, one should suspect an infratentorial lesion, as acute vomiting is less common with supratentorial masses in adults. Characteristic oculovestibular abnormalities including skew deviation, dysconjugate gaze, fixed gaze palsies, or dysconjugate responses to oculocephalic and oculovestibular testing are strong presumptive evidence of an infratentorial lesion. Cranial nerve palsies are often present and abnormal respiratory patterns usually are present from onset. The major problem in differential diagnosis arises when a patient with a supratentorial mass lesion has progressed far enough to arrive at the pontine or medullary level of coma. In this instance, it is virtually impossible to distinguish by physical examination between the effects of supratentorial and infratentorial masses. Metabolic coma can usually be distinguished from destructive or compressive lesions because the pupils remain reactive. A CT scan distinguishes between supra- and infratentorial masses and often establishes the diagnosis definitively. A hyperdense basilar artery strongly suggests brainstem infarction even when the infarct cannot be seen on CT. MRI, particularly with diffusion-weighted imaging, is much better at identifying brainstem infarcts.

At times it is impossible to distinguish on clinical grounds an intrinsic brainstem lesion (such as infarction from basilar artery occlusion) from an extrinsic compressive lesion (such as cerebellar hematoma), but the treatment is different: surgery for compressive lesions[73] and thrombolysis for acute vascular occlusions.[79] Hematomas of the cerebellum or the subdural space should be evacuated if the patient is stuporous or comatose, if the state of consciousness is progressively becoming impaired, or if other signs indicate progressive brainstem compression (see Chapter 4).[80] A cerebellar infarct causing stupor or coma from brainstem compression appears on CT scan as a hypodense area and likewise may require surgical decompression by removal of infarcted tissue. Some reports describe successful surgical evacuation of brainstem hematomas,[81] particularly when the hemorrhage is due to a cavernous angioma. Primary pontine hemorrhages (those due to hypertension) usually are not treated surgically, particularly when the patient is comatose.[82]

The principles of treatment of infratentorial masses are similar to those for supratentorial masses, discussed above.

Metabolic Encephalopathy

Metabolic coma (Table 7–1) is usually characterized by a history of confusion and disorientation having preceded the onset of stupor or coma, usually in the absence of any motor signs. When motor signs (decorticate or decerebrate rigidity) appear, they are usually symmetric. If the patient is stuporous rather than comatose, asterixis, myoclonus, and tremor are common, and in comatose patients the presence of repetitive seizures, either focal or generalized, provide presumptive evidence of metabolic dysfunction. Many patients with metabolic coma either hyper- or hypoventilate, but it is rare to see the abnormal respiratory patterns that characterize infratentorial mass or destructive lesions (see page 50). There are two major errors in the diagnosis of metabolic coma. The first is in differentiating patients with the diencephalic stage of supratentorial masses from those with metabolic coma. In the absence of focal motor signs, one may initially suspect metabolic coma even in patients who have a supratentorial mass lesion with early central herniation. The second error occurs in those occasional patients with metabolic coma (e.g., hepatic coma or hypoglycemia) who have strikingly asymmetric motor signs with hyperventilation and deep coma. In this instance, the preservation of intact and symmetric pupillary and oculovestibular responses provides strong presumptive evidence for metabolic rather than structural disease.

It is stupor and coma caused by metabolic brain disease that most challenges the internist, neurologist, or general physician likely to be reading this monograph. If patients suffer from major damage caused by supra- or infratentorial mass lesions or destructive lesions, specific treatment often involves a surgical or intravascular procedure. If psychogenic unresponsiveness is the problem, the ultimate management of the patient rests with a psychiatrist. In metabolic brain disease, however, the task of preserving the brain from permanent damage rests with the physician of first contact. The physician should first evaluate the vital signs, provide adequate ventilation and arterial pressure, and then draw blood for metabolic studies. Metabolic studies that should be secured from the first blood drawing are indicated in Table 7–5. Because drug ingestion is a common cause of coma, procure blood and urine for toxicologic study on all patients (see Table 7–6). Those metabolic encephalopathies that are most likely to produce either irreversible brain damage or a quick demise but are potentially treatable include drug overdose, hypoglycemia, metabolic or respiratory acidosis (from several causes), hyperosmolar states, hypoxia, bacterial meningitis or sepsis, and severe electrolyte imbalance.

It is important to secure an arterial sample for blood gas analysis, although emergency management may have to begin even before laboratory results are returned. Both acidosis and alkalosis can cause cardiac arrhythmias, but acute metabolic acidosis is more likely to be lethal; however, pH is not an independent predictor of mortality in critically ill patients with metabolic acidosis.[83] Whether sodium bicarbonate should be given to treat severe acidosis is controversial.[84–86] The agent is not indicated in the treatment of diabetic acidosis and may not be helpful in treating acidosis from other causes. Instead, urgent treatment of the underlying cause of the acidosis is probably the best approach. Relieve hypoxia immediately by ensuring an adequate airway and delivering sufficient oxygen to keep the blood fully oxygenated. Even in the presence of a normal PaO_2, blood oxygen content may be insufficient to supply the brain's needs for several reasons: (1) the hemoglobin may be abnormal (carboxyhemoglobinemia, methemoglobinemia, or sulfhemoglobinemia). Methemoglobin or sulfhemoglobin are diagnosed by the typical chocolate appearance of oxygenated blood, and patients are treated with methylene blue (1 to 2 mg/kg IV over 5 minutes).[87,88] Topical anesthetic agents such as benzocaine used in endoscopy can cause acute methemoglobi-

Table 7–6 **Stat Toxicology Assays Required to Support an Emergency Department**

Quantitative Serum Toxicology Assays	Qualitative Urine Toxicology Assays
Acetaminophen (paracetamol)	Cocaine
Lithium	Opiates
Salicylate	Barbiturates
Co-oximetry for oxygen saturation, carboxyhemoglobin, and methemoglobin	Amphetamines
	Propoxyphene
Theophylline	Phencyclidine (PCP)
Valproic acid	Tricyclic antidepressants (TCAs)
Carbamazepine	
Digoxin	
Phenobarbital (if urine barbiturates are positive)	
Iron	
Transferrin (or unsaturated iron-binding capacity [UIBC] assay if transferrin is not available)	
Ethyl alcohol	
Methyl alcohol	
Ethylene glycol	

From Wu et al.,[93] with permission.

nemia.[89] (2) Carbon monoxide binds hemoglobin with 200 times the affinity of oxygen and thus displaces oxygen and yields carboxyhemoglobin. The PaO_2 is normal and the patient's color is pink or "cherry red," but he or she is hypoxic because insufficient hemoglobin is available to deliver oxygen to the tissue. Such patients should be given 100% oxygen and hyperventilated to increase blood oxygenation. Hyperbaric oxygenation may improve the situation, and if a hyperbaric chamber is available, it should probably be utilized for patients with life-threatening exposure.[90] (3) Severe anemia itself will not cause coma, but lowers the oxygen-carrying capacity of the blood even when the PaO_2 is normal, and thus decreases the oxygen supply to the brain. In patients with other forms of hypoxia, anemia may exacerbate the symptoms. Severe anemia (hematocrit less than 25) in a comatose patient should be treated with transfusion of whole blood or packed red cells. (4) Tissues can be hypoxic even when the PaO_2 and O_2 content is normal if they cannot metabolize the oxygen (e.g., cyanide poisoning). Hydroxocobalamin administered as a one-time dose of 4 to 5 g IV is a safe and effective method of treating poisoning.[91]

In any comatose or stuporous patient who is febrile, whether or not nuchal rigidity and/or other signs of meningeal irritation (e.g., positive Kernig or Brudzinski signs or jolt accentuation; see page 133) are present, consider *acute bacterial meningitis*. As described above, initial treatment includes antibiotic and steroid administration, followed as soon as possible by CT scan and lumbar puncture if no mass is seen that would threaten herniation. It is often useful to do a Gram stain of the centrifuged sediment, as this may yield an organism that can guide therapy; additional CSF should be sent for culture; polymerase chain reaction (PCR) analysis for bacteria and viruses, especially herpes viruses; and additional tests as may be dictated by the clinical situation. The absence of cells in the spinal fluid does not rule out acute bacterial meningitis; if there is a high index of suspicion, the lumbar puncture can be repeated in 6 to 12 hours. The centrifuged sediment should also be examined by Gram stain, as occasionally organisms may be seen even before there is pleocytosis.

Severe *potassium imbalance* usually affects the heart more than the brain. Accordingly, an electrocardiogram often suggests the diagnosis before serum electrolytes are returned from the laboratory. It usually is advisable to adjust both electrolyte and acid-base imbalances slowly, since too rapid correction often leads to overshoot or intracellular-extracellular imbalances and worsens the clinical situation.[92]

Drug overdose is a common cause of coma in patients brought to an emergency room. Many emergency departments can provide a rapid assessment of toxic drugs (Table 7–6).[93] Most of these drugs are not rapidly lethal but, because they are respiratory depressants, they risk producing respiratory arrest or circulatory depression at any time. Therefore, no stuporous or comatose patient suspected of having ingested sedative drugs should ever be left alone. This is particularly true in the minutes immediately following the initial examination; the stimulation delivered by the examining physician may arouse the patient to a state in which he or she appears relatively alert or his or her respiratory function appears normal, only to lapse into coma with depressed breathing when external stimulation ceases. The management of specific drug poisonings is beyond the scope of this chapter,[88,94] but certain general principles apply to all patients suspected of having ingested sedative drugs. The type of medication influences the treatment and its duration. Accordingly, search the patient and ask relatives or the police to search the patient's living quarters for potentially toxic agents, or empty medication vials that might have contained sedative drugs. Both respiratory and cardiovascular failure may occur with massive sedative drug overdose. Anticipation and early treatment of these complications often smooth the clinical course. Insert an endotracheal tube in any stuporous or comatose patient suspected of drug overdose and be certain that an apparatus for respiratory support is available in case of acute respiratory failure. The placement of a central venous line allows one to maintain an adequate blood volume without overloading the patient. Give generous amounts of fluid to maintain blood volume and blood pressure, but avoid overhydrating oliguric patients. Place a pulse oximeter on the finger, but also measure arterial blood gases; a difference between the two (oxygen saturation gap) may indicate poisoning. Carbon monoxide, methemoglobin, cyanide, and hydrogen sulfide cause an increased oxygen saturation gap.

Once the vital signs have been stabilized, one should attempt to remove, neutralize, or reverse the effects of the drug. Attempts to remove poison from the gastrointestinal tract and thus prevent absorption have included inducing vomiting with syrup of ipecac,[95] gastric lavage,[96] cathartics,[97] activated charcoal ingestion,[98] and whole bowel irrigation.[99] Position papers from the American Academy of Clinical Toxicology and the European Association of Poison Centers and Clinical Toxicologists indicate a lack of evidence that inducing vomiting is helpful; it is contraindicated in patients with a decreased level or impending loss of consciousness.[95] They concluded that gastric lavage should not be employed routinely, but could be considered in patients who have ingested a potentially life-threatening amount of a poison within an hour of the time they are to be treated.[96] However, aspiration is a common complication, and so patients with impaired consciousness should be intubated first. Cathartics have no role in the management of the poisoned patient.[97] A single dose of activated charcoal (50 g) can be administered to a patient with an intact or protected airway but it will not efficiently adsorb acid, alkali, ethanol, ethylene glycol, iron, lithium, or methanol. Multiple doses of charcoal administered at an initial dose of 50 to 100 g, and then at a rate of not less than 12.5 g/hour via nasogastric tube, may be indicated when patients have ingested a life-threatening amount of carbamazepine, dapsone, phenobarbital, quinine, or theophylline. In addition to eliminating drugs from the small bowel, the agents may interrupt the enteroenteric and, in some cases, the enterohepatic circulation of drugs.[100] Whole bowel irrigation using polyethylene glycol electrolyte solutions may decrease the bioavailability of ingested drugs, particularly enteric-coated or sustained-release drugs.[99]

Intravenous sodium bicarbonate in amounts sufficient to produce a urine pH of 7.5 promotes the elimination of salicylate, phenobarbital, and chlorpropamide.[101] For very severe poisoning with barbiturates, glutethimide, salicylates, or alcohol, hemodialysis or hemoperfusion may be necessary.[100,101] Although acetaminophen does not by itself cause impaired consciousness, it may be included in opioid combinations (e.g., acetaminophen with codeine or oxycodone), and is often included in polydrug overdoses. Doses above 5 g in adults may cause acute hepatic injury, especially if combined with other hepatotoxins such as ethanol, and when acetaminophen overdose is suspected, the patient should be treated with N-acetylcysteine as well.[103]

Psychogenic Unresponsiveness

Psychogenic unresponsiveness is characterized by a normal neurologic examination, including normal waking oculocephalic and oculovestibular responses. Once one has considered the possibility of psychogenic unresponsiveness and performed the appropriate neurologic examination, little difficulty arises in making the definitive diagnosis. If the patient meets the clinical criteria for psychogenic unresponsiveness, no further laboratory tests are required. If, however, there is still some question after the examination, an EEG is the most helpful diagnostic test. An EEG that shows normal alpha activity inhibited by eye opening and other stimuli strongly supports the diagnosis of psychogenic unresponsiveness. The Amytal interview (see Chapter 6) may be both diagnostic and therapeutic. In emergency evaluation of the unresponsive patient, the Amytal interview may establish the diagnosis and "wake the patient up," so that one may begin more definitive treatment. However, it also breaks down a major psychologic defense, and should only be done in conjunction with definitive psychiatric treatment. Hence, it is necessary to secure emergency psychiatric consultation, and often the patient must be admitted to the psychiatric service. The physician must evaluate thoroughly the patient's physical state to rule out coexisting organic disease; psychogenic unresponsiveness often occurs in a setting of serious medical illness.

A FINAL WORD

This chapter has presented a physiologic approach to the differential diagnosis and the emergency management of the stuporous and comatose patient. The approach is based on the belief that after a history and a general physical and neurologic examination, the informed physician can, with reasonable confidence, place the patient into one of four major groups of illnesses that cause coma. The specific group into which the patient is placed directs the rest of the diagnostic evaluation and treatment. At times, however, the diagnosis is uncertain even after the examination is completed, and it is necessary to defer even the preliminary categorization of patients until the imaging or metabolic tests are carried out and the most serious infections or metabolic abnormalities have been considered. If there is any suspicion of a mass lesion, immediate imaging is mandatory despite the absence of focal signs. Conversely, the presence of hemiplegia or other focal signs does not rule out metabolic disease, especially hypoglycemia. At all times during the diagnostic evaluation and treatment of a patient who is stuporous or comatose, the physician must ask him- or herself whether the diagnosis could possibly be wrong and whether he or she needs to seek consultation or undertake other diagnostic or therapeutic measures. Fortunately, with constant attention to the changing state of consciousness and a willingness to reconsider the situation minute by minute, few mistakes should be made.

REFERENCES

1. Laureys S, Pellas F, Van Eeckhout P, et al. The locked-in syndrome: what is it like to be conscious but paralyzed and voiceless? Prog Brain Res 2005; 150, 495–511.
2. Wijdicks EF, Bamlet WR, Maramattom BV, et al. Validation of a new coma scale: the FOUR score. Ann Neurol 2005; 58, 585–593.
3. Stevens RD, Bhardwaj A. Approach to the comatose patient. Crit Care Med 2006; 34, 31–41.
4. Yanagawa Y, Sakamoto T, Okada Y, et al. Intubation without premedication may worsen outcome for unconsciousness patients with intracranial hemorrhage. Am J Emerg Med 2005; 23, 182–185.
5. Wadbrook PS. Advances in airway pharmacology. Emerging trends and evolving controversy. Emerg Med Clin North Am 2000; 18, 767–788.
6. Reynolds SF, Heffner J. Airway management of the critically ill patient: rapid-sequence intubation. Chest 2005; 127, 1397–1412.
7. Marik PE, Varon J, Trask T. Management of head trauma. Chest 2002; 122, 699–711.
8. Roppolo LP, Walters K. Airway management in neurological emergencies. Neurocrit Care 2004; 1(4), 405–141.
9. Hamill JF, Bedford RF, Weaver DC, et al. Lidocaine before endotracheal intubation: intravenous or laryngotracheal? Anesthesiology 1981; 55, 578–581.
10. Komatsu R, Nagata O, Kamata K, et al. Intubating laryngeal mask airway allows tracheal intubation when the cervical spine is immobilized by a rigid collar. Br J Anaesth 2004; 3, 655–659.
11. Koerner IP, Brambrink AM. Fiberoptic techniques. Best Pract Res Clin Anaesthesiol 2005; 19, 611–621.
12. Patterson, H. Emergency department intubation of trauma patients with undiagnosed cervical spine injury. Emerg Med J 2004; 21, 302–305.
13. Muckart DJ, Bhagwanjee S, van der Merwe R. Spinal cord injury as a result of endotracheal intubation in patients with undiagnosed cervical spine fractures. Anesthesiology 1997; 87, 418–420.

14. Chung YH, Chao TY, Chiu CT, et al. The cuff-leak test is a simple tool to verify severe laryngeal edema in patients undergoing long-term mechanical ventilation. Crit Care Med 2006; 34, 409–414.

15. Lin CC, Lin CD, Cheng YK, et al. Middle ear effusion in intensive care unit patients with prolonged endotracheal intubation. Am J Otolaryngol 2006; 27, 109–111.

16. Shirawi N, Arabi Y. Bench-to-bedside review: early tracheostomy in critically ill trauma patients. Crit Care 2005; 10, 201–205.

17. Mignini MA, Piacentini E, Dubin A. Peripheral arterial blood pressure monitoring adequately tracks central arterial blood pressure in critically ill patients: an observational study. Crit Care 2006; 10, R43.

18. Mullner M, Urbanek B, Havel C, et al. Vasopressors for shock. Cochrane Database Syst Rev 2004; 3, CD003709.

19. Asfar P, Hauser B, Radermacher P, et al. Catecholamines and vasopressin during critical illness. Crit Care Clin 2006; 22, 131–149.

20. Seguin P, Laviolle B, Guinet P, et al. Dopexamine and norepinephrine versus epinephrine on gastric perfusion in patients with septic shock: a randomized study [NCT00134212]. Crit Care 2006; 10, R32.

21. Aggarwal M, Khan IA. Hypertensive crisis: hypertensive emergencies and urgencies. Cardiol Clin 2006; 24, 135–146.

22. Moore C, Woollard M. Dextrose 10% or 50% in the treatment of hypoglycaemia out of hospital? A randomised controlled trial. Emerg Med J 2005; 22, 512–515.

23. Van den BG, Wilmer A, Hermans G, et al. Intensive insulin therapy in the medical ICU. N Engl J Med 2006; 354, 449–461.

24. Chen JW, Wasterlain CG. Status epilepticus: pathophysiology and management in adults. Lancet Neurol 2006; 5, 246–256.

25. Towne AR, Waterhouse EJ, Boggs JG, et al. Prevalence of nonconvulsive status epilepticus in comatose patients. Neurology 2000; 54, 340–345.

26. Claassen J, Mayer SA, Kowalski RG, et al. Detection of electrographic seizures with continuous EEG monitoring in critically ill patients. Neurology 2004; 62, 1743–1748.

27. Vincent JL, Sakr Y, Sprung CL, et al. Sepsis in European intensive care units: results of the SOAP study. Crit Care Med 2006; 34, 344–353.

28. Paul M, Silbiger I, Grozinsky S, et al. Beta lactam antibiotic monotherapy versus beta lactam-aminoglycoside antibiotic combination therapy for sepsis. Cochrane Database Syst Rev 2006; CD003344.

29. Begg N, Cartwright KA, Cohen J, et al. Consensus statement on diagnosis, investigation, treatment and prevention of acute bacterial meningitis in immunocompetent adults. British Infection Society Working Party. J Infect 1999; 39, 1–15.

30. van de Beek D, De Gans J, McIntyre P, et al. Steroids in adults with acute bacterial meningitis: a systematic review. Lancet Infect Dis 2004; 4, 139–143.

31. Mcilvoy LH. The effect of hypothermia and hyperthermia on acute brain injury. AACN Clin Issues 2005; 16, 488–500.

32. Minamisawa H, Smith ML, Siesjo BK. The effect of mild hyperthermia and hypothermia on brain damage following 5, 10, and 15 minutes of forebrain ischemia. Ann Neurol 1990; 28, 26–33.

33. De KJ, Deleu D, Solheid C, et al. Coma as presenting manifestation of Wernicke's encephalopathy. J Emerg Med 1985; 3, 361–363.

34. Bleggi-Torres LF, De Medeiros BC, Ogasawara VSA, et al. Iatrogenic Wernicke's encephalopathy in allogeneic bone marrow transplantation: a study of eight cases. Bone Marrow Transplant 1997; 20, 391–395.

35. Omer SM, al Kawi MZ, al Watban J, et al. Acute Wernicke's encephalopathy associated with hyperemesis gravidarum: magnetic resonance imaging findings. J Neuroimaging 1995; 5, 251–253.

36. Koguchi K, Nakatsuji Y, Abe K, et al. Wernicke's encephalopathy after glucose infusion. Neurology 2004; 62, 512.

37. Ries NL, Dart RC. New developments in antidotes. Med Clin North Am 2005; 89, 1379–1397.

38. Barnett R, Grace M, Boothe P, et al. Flumazenil in drug overdose: randomized, placebo-controlled study to assess cost effectiveness. Crit Care Med 1999; 27, 78–81.

39. Bledsoe BE. No more coma cocktails. Using science to dispel myths & improve patient care. JEMS 2002; 27, 54–60.

40. Clarke SF, Dargan PI, Jones AL. Naloxone in opioid poisoning: walking the tightrope. Emerg Med J 2005; 22, 612–616.

41. Weinbroum AA, Flaishon R, Sorkine P, et al. A risk-benefit assessment of flumazenil in the management of benzodiazepine overdose. Drug Saf 1997; 17, 181–196.

42. Inouye SK. Delirium in older persons. N Engl J Med 2006; 354, 1157–1165.

43. Bourgeois JA, Koike AK, Simmons JE, et al. Adjunctive valproic acid for delirium and/or agitation on a consultation-liaison service: a report of six cases. J Neuropsychiatry Clin Neurosci 2005; 17, 232–238.

44. Krauss B, Zurakowski D. Sedation patterns in pediatric and general community hospital emergency departments. Pediatr Emerg Care 1998; 14, 99–103.

45. Lenart SB, Garrity JA. Eye care for patients receiving neuromuscular blocking agents or propofol during mechanical ventilation. Am J Crit Care 2000; 9, 188–191.

46. Koroloff N, Boots R, Lipman J, et al. A randomised controlled study of the efficacy of hypromellose and Lacri-Lube combination versus polyethylene/Cling wrap to prevent corneal epithelial breakdown in the semiconscious intensive care patient. Intensive Care Med 2004; 30, 1122–1126.

47. Piatt Jr JH. Detected and overlooked cervical spine injury in comatose victims of trauma: report from the Pennsylvania Trauma Outcomes Study. J Neurosurg Spine 2006; 5, 210–216.

48. Teasdale G, Knill-Jones R, van der Sande J. Observer variability in assessing impaired consciousness and coma. J Neurol Neurosurg Psychiatry 1978; 41, 603–610.

49. Lagares A, Gomez PA, Alen JF, et al. A comparison of different grading scales for predicting outcome after subarachnoid haemorrhage. Acta Neurochir (Wien) 2005; 147, 5–16.

50. Diringer MN, Edwards DF. Does modification of the Innsbruck and the Glasgow coma scales improve their ability to predict functional outcome? Arch Neurol 1997; 54, 606–611.

51. Stocchetti N, Maas AI, Chieregato A, et al. Hyperventilation in head injury: a review. Chest 2005; 127, 1812–1827.
52. Diringer MN, Yundt K, Videen TO, et al. No reduction in cerebral metabolism as a result of early moderate hyperventilation following severe traumatic brain injury. J Neurosurg 2000; 92, 7–13.
53. Steiner LA, Balestreri M, Johnston AJ, et al. Predicting the response of intracranial pressure to moderate hyperventilation. Acta Neurochir (Wien) 2005; 147, 477–483.
54. Ng I, Lim J, Wong HB. Effects of head posture on cerebral hemodynamics: its influences on intracranial pressure, cerebral perfusion pressure, and cerebral oxygenation. Neurosurgery 2005; 54, 593–598.
55. Schneider GH, von Helden GH, Franke R, et al. Influence of body position on jugular venous oxygen saturation, intracranial pressure and cerebral perfusion pressure. Acta Neurochir Suppl (Wien) 1993; 59, 107–112.
56. Ropper AH, O'Rourke D, Kennedy SK. Head position, intracranial pressure, and compliance. Neurology 1982; 32, 1288–1291.
57. Videen TO, Zazulia AR, Manno EM, et al. Mannitol bolus preferentially shrinks non-infarcted brain in patients with ischemic stroke. Neurology 2001; 57, 2120–2122.
58. Huang SJ, Chang L, Han YY, et al. Efficacy and safety of hypertonic saline solutions in the treatment of severe head injury. Surg Neurol 2006; 65, 539–546.
59. Vialet R, Albanese J, Thomachot L, et al. Isovolume hypertonic solutes (sodium chloride or mannitol) in the treatment of refractory posttraumatic intracranial hypertension: 2 mL/kg 7.5% saline is more effective than 2 mL/kg 20% mannitol. Crit Care Med 2003; 31, 1683–1687.
60. Sinha S, Bastin ME, Wardlaw JM, et al. Effects of dexamethasone on peritumoural oedematous brain: a DT-MRI study. J Neurol Neurosurg Psychiatry 2004; 75, 1632–1635.
61. Rabinstein AA. Treatment of cerebral edema. Neurologist 2006; 12, 59–73.
62. Czerwinski AW, Czerwinski AB, Whitsett TL, et al. Effects of a single, large intravenous injection of dexamethasone. Clin Pharmacol Ther 1972; 13, 638–642.
63. Alberti E, Hartmann A, Schutz HJ, et al. The effect of large doses of dexamethasone on the cerebrospinal fluid pressure in patients with supratentorial tumors. J Neurol 1978; 217, 173–181.
64. De Gans J, van de Beek D. European dexamethasone AB dexamethasone in adults with bacterial meningitis. N Engl J Med 2002; 347, 1549–1556.
65. Norris JW. Steroids may have a role in stroke therapy. Stroke 2004; 35, 228–229.
66. Poungvarin N. Steroids have no role in stroke therapy. Stroke 2004; 35, 229–230.
67. Roberts I, Yates D, Sandercock P, et al. Effect of intravenous corticosteroids on death within 14 days in 10008 adults with clinically significant head injury (MRC CRASH trial): randomised placebo-controlled trial. Lancet 2004; 364, 1321–1328.
68. Bullock MR, Chesnut R, Ghajar J, et al. Surgical management of acute subdural hematomas. Neurosurgery 2006; 58, 16–24.
69. Bullock MR, Chesnut R, Ghajar J, et al. Surgical management of acute epidural hematomas. Neurosurgery 2006; 58, 7–15.
70. Bullock MR, Chesnut R, Ghajar J, et al. Surgical management of traumatic parenchymal lesions. Neurosurgery 2006; 58, S25-S46.
71. Subramaniam S, Hill MD. Controversies in medical management of intracerebral hemorrhage. Can J Neurol Sci 2005; 32(Suppl 2), S13–S21.
72. The Brain Trauma Foundation. The American Association of Neurological Surgeons. The Joint Section on Neurotrauma and Critical Care. Use of barbiturates in the control of intracranial hypertension. J Neurotrauma 2000; 17, 527–530.
73. Chesnut RM. Management of brain and spine injuries. Crit Care Clin 2004; 20, 25–55.
74. Bader MK, Arbour R, Palmer S. Refractory increased intracranial pressure in severe traumatic brain injury: barbiturate coma and bispectral index monitoring. AACN Clin Issues 2005; 16, 526–541.
75. Schalen W, Sonesson B, Messeter K, et al. Clinical outcome and cognitive impairment in patients with severe head injuries treated with barbiturate coma. Acta Neurochir (Wien) 1992; 117, 153–159.
76. Cremer OL, Van Dijk GW, van WE, et al. Effect of intracranial pressure monitoring and targeted intensive care on functional outcome after severe head injury. Crit Care Med 2005; 33, 2207–2213.
77. Albanese J, Leone M, Alliez JR, et al. Decompressive craniectomy for severe traumatic brain injury: evaluation of the effects at one year. Crit Care Med 2003; 31, 2535–2538.
78. Subramaniam S, Hill MD. Massive cerebral infarction. Neurologist 2005; 11, 150–160.
79. Arnold M, Nedeltchev K, Schroth G, et al. Clinical and radiological predictors of recanalisation and outcome of 40 patients with acute basilar artery occlusion treated with intra-arterial thrombolysis. J Neurol Neurosurg Psychiatry 2004; 75, 857–862.
80. Bullock MR, Chesnut R, Ghajar J, et al. Surgical management of posterior fossa mass lesions. Neurosurgery 2006; 58, S47–S55.
81. Wang CC, Liu A, Zhang JT, et al. Surgical management of brain-stem cavernous malformations: report of 137 cases. Surg Neurol 2003; 59, 444–454.
82. Rabinstein AA, Tisch SH, McClelland RL, et al. Cause is the main predictor of outcome in patients with pontine hemorrhage. Cerebrovasc Dis 2004; 17, 66–71.
83. Gunnerson KJ, Saul M, He S, et al. Lactate versus non-lactate metabolic acidosis: a retrospective outcome evaluation of critically ill patients. Crit Care 2006; 10, R22.
84. Forsythe SM, Schmidt GA. Sodium bicarbonate for the treatment of lactic acidosis. Chest 2000; 117, 260–267.
85. Gunnerson KJ, Kellum JA. Acid-base and electrolyte analysis in critically ill patients: are we ready for the new millennium? Curr Opin Crit Care 2003; 9, 468–473.
86. Swenson ER. Metabolic acidosis. Respir Care 2001; 46, 342–353.
87. Clifton J, Leikin JB. Methylene blue. Am J Ther 2003; 10, 289–291.
88. Mokhlesi B, Corbridge T. Toxicology in the critically ill patient. Clin Chest Med 2003; 24, 689–711.

89. Bayard M, Farrow J, Tudiver F. Acute methemoglobinemia after endoscopy. J Am Board Fam Pract 2004; 17, 227–229.

90. Weaver LK, Hopkins RO, Chan KJ, et al. Hyperbaric oxygen for acute carbon monoxide poisoning. N Engl J Med 2002; 347, 1057–1067.

91. Sauer SW, Keim ME. Hydroxocobalamin: improved public health readiness for cyanide disasters. Ann Emerg Med 2001; 37, 635–641.

92. Weiss-Guillet EM, Takala J, Jakob SM. Diagnosis and management of electrolyte emergencies. Best Pract Res Clin Endocrinol Metab 2003; 17, 623–651.

93. Wu AH, McKay C, Broussard LA, et al. National academy of clinical biochemistry laboratory medicine practice guidelines: recommendations for the use of laboratory tests to support poisoned patients who present to the emergency department. Clin Chem 2003; 49, 357–379.

94. Critical Care Toxicology: Diagnosis and Management of the Critically Poisoned Patient, 2005, 1–1690.

95. Position paper: ipecac syrup. J Toxicol Clin Toxicol 2004; 42, 133–143.

96. Vale JA, Kulig K. Position paper: gastric lavage. J Toxicol Clin Toxicol 2004; 42, 933–943.

97. Barceloux D, McGuigan M, Hartigan-Go K. Position statement: cathartics. American Academy of Clinical Toxicology; European Association of Poisons Centres and Clinical Toxicologists. J Toxicol Clin Toxicol 1997; 35, 743–752.

98. Chyka PA, Seger D, Krenzelok EP, et al. Position paper: single-dose activated charcoal. Clin Toxicol (Phila) 2005; 43, 61–87.

99. Tenenbein M. Position statement: whole bowel irrigation. American Academy of Clinical Toxicology; European Association of Poisons Centres and Clinical Toxicologists. J Toxicol Clin Toxicol 1997; 35, 753–762.

100. Bradberry SM, Vale JA. Poisons. Initial assessment and management. Clin Med 2003; 107–110.

101. Proudfoot AT, Krenzelok EP, Vale JA. Position paper on urine alkalinization. J Toxicol Clin Toxicol 2004; 42, 1–26.

102. Megarbane B, Borron SW, Baud FJ. Current recommendations for treatment of severe toxic alcohol poisonings. Intensive Care Med 2005; 31, 189–195.

103. Rowden AK, Norvell J, Eldridge DL, Kirk MA. Updates on acetaminophen toxicity. Med Clin North Am 2005; 89, 1145–1159.

Chapter 8

Brain Death

DETERMINATION OF BRAIN DEATH

Since Mollaret and Goulon[1] first examined the question in 1959, investigators have tried to establish criteria that would accurately and unequivocally determine that the brain is dead or about to die no matter what therapeutic measures one might undertake. Since that time, several committees and reviewers have sought to establish appropriate clinical and laboratory criteria for brain death based on retrospective analyses. The earliest widely known definition is that of the 1968 Ad Hoc Committee of the Harvard Medical School to examine the criteria of brain death (called, at the time, "irreversible coma"[2]) (Table 8–1). At present, in the United States the principle that brain death is equivalent to the death of the person is established under the Uniform Determination of Death Act.[3] (In fact, all death is brain death. An artificial heart can keep a patient alive. If all the organs, save the brain, were artificial, that individual would still be alive. Conversely, when the brain is dead, sustaining the other organs by artificial means is simply preserving a dead body and not keeping the individual alive. Thus, although this chapter uses the term brain death, the term as we use it carries the same import as death.) Detailed evidence-based guidelines and practice parameters for the clinical diagnosis of brain death are available from the American Academy of Neurology online (http://www.aan.com).

Three medical considerations emphasize the importance of the concept of brain death: (1) transplant programs require the donation of healthy peripheral organs for success. The early diagnosis of brain death before the systemic circulation fails allows the salvage of such organs. However, ethical and legal considerations demand that if one is to declare the brain dead, the criteria must be clear and unassailable. (2) Even if there were no transplant programs, the ability of modern medicine to keep a body functioning for extended periods often leads to prolonged, expensive, and futile procedures accompanied by great emotional strain on family and medical staff. Conversely, the recuperative powers of the brain sometimes can seem

331

Table 8–1 **Harvard Criteria for Brain Death (1968)**

1. Unresponsive coma
2. Apnea
3. Absence of cephalic reflexes
4. Absence of spinal reflexes
5. Isoelectric electroencephalogram
6. Persistence of conditions for at least 24 hours
7. Absence of drug intoxication or hypothermia

From Ad Hoc Committee of the Harvard Medical School.[2]

Table 8–2 **Clinical Criteria for Brain Death in Adults and Children in the United States**

A. Coma of established cause
  1. No potentially anesthetizing amounts of either toxins or therapeutic drugs can be present; hypothermia below 30°C or other physiologic abnormalities must be corrected to the extent medically possible.
  2. Irreversible structural disease or a known and irreversible endogenous metabolic cause due to organ failure must be present.

B. Absence of motor responses
  1. Absence of pupillary responses to light and pupils at midposition with respect to dilation (4–6 mm)
  2. Absence of corneal reflexes
  3. Absence of caloric vestibulo-ocular responses
  4. Absence of gag reflex
  5. Absence of coughing in response to tracheal suctioning
  6. Absence of sucking and rooting reflexes
  7. Absence of respiratory drive at a $PaCO_2$ that is 60 mm Hg or 20 mm Hg above normal baseline values (apnea testing)

C. Interval between two evaluations, by patient's age
  1. Term to 2 months old, 48 hours
  2. >2 months to 1 year old, 24 hours
  3. >1 year to <18 years old, 12 hour
  4. ≥18 years old, optional

D. Confirmatory tests
  1. Term to 2 months old, two confirmatory tests
  2. >2 months to 1 year old, one confirmatory test
  3. >1 year to <18 years old, optional
  4. ≥18 years old, optional

astounding to the uninitiated, and individual patients whom uninformed physicians might give up for hopelessly brain damaged or dead sometimes make unexpectedly good recoveries (see *pitfalls*, page 338). It is even more important to know when to fight for life than to be willing to diagnose death. (3) Critical care facilities are limited and expensive and inevitably place a drain on other medical resources. Their best use demands that one identify and select patients who are most likely to benefit from intensive techniques, so that these units are not overloaded with individuals who can never recover cerebral function.

The cornerstone of the diagnosis of brain death remains a careful and sure clinical neurologic examination (Table 8–2). In addition, a thorough evaluation of clinical history, neuroradiologic studies, and laboratory tests must be done to rule out potential confounding variables. The diagnosis of brain death rests on two major and indispensable tenets. The first is that the cause of brain nonfunction must be inherently irreversible. This means that damage must be due to either known structural injury (e.g., cerebral hemorrhage or infarction, brain trauma, abscess) or known irreversible metabolic injury such as prolonged asphyxia. The second indispensable tenet is that the vital structures of the brain necessary to maintain consciousness and independent vegetative survival are damaged beyond all possible recovery.

The cause of brain damage must be known irreversible structural or metabolic disease. This first criterion is crucial, and the diagnosis of brain death cannot be considered until it is fulfilled. The reason for stressing this point is that both in the United States and abroad often "coma of unknown origin" arising outside of a hospital is due to depressant drug poisoning. Witnesses cannot be relied upon for accurate

histories under such circumstances because efforts at suicide or homicide can readily induce false testimony by companions or family. Even in patients already in the hospital for the treatment of other illnesses, drug poisoning administered by self or others sometimes occurs and at least temporarily can deceive the medical staff. Accordingly, the diagnosis of an irreversible lesion by clinical and laboratory means must be fully documented and unequivocally accurate before considering a diagnosis of brain death. The ease of being mistaken in such a diagnosis is illustrated by some of the results of a collaborative study sponsored several years ago by the National Institutes of

Table 8–3 **Most Common Etiologies of Brain Death**

1. Traumatic brain injury
2. Aneurysmal subarachnoid hemorrhage
3. Intracerebral hemorrhage
4. Ischemic stroke with cerebral edema and herniation
5. Hypoxic-ischemic encephalopathy
6. Fulminant hepatic necrosis with cerebral edema and increased intracranial pressure

From Wijdicks,[6] with permission.

Health.[5] The findings of toxicologic analyses revealed many more cases in which drug poisoning caused deep coma than had been suspected clinically by physicians, not all of whom had previous experiences with the ubiquity and subtlety of sedative-induced coma. The most common underlying causes of brain death are listed in Table 8–3. Documentation of structural injury explaining loss of brainstem function by computed tomography (CT) or magnetic resonance imaging (MRI) is possible in almost all patients. If scans are normal and clinical history is equivocal for the origin of cerebral demise, an examination of the cerebral spinal fluid is indicated.

A prospective study[7] evaluated 310 patients with cardiac arrest or other forms of acute medical coma who met the clinical criteria of brain death for 6 hours; none improved despite maximal treatment. Asystole occurred in all within a matter of hours or days. Jorgenson and Malchow-Moller[8] systematically examined the time required for recovery of neurologic functions in 54 patients following cardiopulmonary arrest, and plotted these times against eventual outcomes. For respiratory movements, pupillary light reflexes, coughing, swallowing, and ciliospinal reflexes, the longest respective times of reappearance compatible with any cerebral recovery were 15, 28, 58, and 52 minutes. In other words, if no recognizable brain function returned within an hour, the brain never recovered.

Time periods for repeated evaluations of brain death criteria may vary and are influenced by the etiology of injury. Several guidelines suggest a minimum time period of 24 hours over which human subjects must show signs of brain death following anoxic injury (or other diffuse toxic-metabolic insult, e.g. air, fat

embolism, endocrine derangement) before the final diagnosis can be reached.[9] Evaluation times for identified structural injuries of the brainstem are typically shorter. Since time is so strong a safeguard, and few brain-damaged patients escape receiving at least an initial dose of a drug (alcohol or sedative outside of hospital, sedatives or anticonvulsants inside), guidelines suggest a 6-hour period of observation before making a clinical diagnosis of brain death (https://www.aan.com/professionals/practice/guidelines/pda/Brain_death_adults.pdf). This seems a reasonable time interval for cases where all circumstances of onset, diagnosis, and treatment can be fully identified.

CLINICAL SIGNS OF BRAIN DEATH

All observers agree that in order to conclude that the vital functions of the brain have ceased, no behavioral or clinical reflex responses that depend on structures innervated from the supraspinal nervous system can exist. In a practical sense, because forebrain function depends on the integrity of the brainstem, the brain death examination primarily focuses on functional brainstem activity (Table 8–2). These observations may be accompanied by confirmatory tests providing evidence of absence of cerebral hemispheric and upper brainstem function, discussed below.

Brainstem Function

PUPILS

The pupils must be nonreactive to light. In the period immediately following brain death, the agonal release of adrenal catecholamines into the bloodstream may cause the pupils to become dilated. However, as the catecholamines are metabolized, the pupils return to a midposition. Hence, although the Harvard criteria required that the pupils be dilated as well as fixed, midposition fixed pupils are a more reliable sign of brain death, and failure of the pupils to return to midposition within several hours after brain death suggests residual sympathetic activation arising from the medulla. The pupils should be tested with a bright light and the physician should be certain that mydriatic agents, including intravenous atropine, have not been used (although conventional doses of atropine used in treating patients with cardiac arrest will not block the direct light response). Neuromuscular blocking agents, however, should not affect pupillary size as nicotinic receptors are not present in the iris. One recent report has described an unusual observation of persistent asynchronous light-independent pupillary activity (2.5 seconds constriction/10 seconds dilation) in an otherwise "brain-dead" patient.[10]

OCULAR MOVEMENTS

Failure of brainstem function should be determined by the inability to find either oculocephalic or caloric vestibulo-ocular responses (see Chapter 2). In patients in whom a history of possible trauma has not been eliminated, cervical spine injury must be excluded before testing oculocephalic responses. Care should be taken when performing cold water caloric testing to ensure that the stimulus reaches the tympanic membrane. Up to 1 minute of observation for eye movement should follow irrigation of each side with a 5-minute interval between each examination.

MOTOR, SENSORY, AND REFLEX ACTIVITY

The initial Harvard criteria demanded that there be an absence of all voluntary and reflex movements, including absence of corneal responses and other brainstem reflexes; no postural activity, including decerebrate rigidity; and no stretch reflexes in the extremities. Reflex responses mediated by the brainstem (e.g., corneal and jaw jerk reflexes as well as cutaneous reflexes such as snout and rooting reflexes) must be absent before making the diagnosis of brain death. The absence of a gag reflex should be tested by stimulation of the posterior pharynx, but may be difficult to elicit or observe in intubated patients. Additionally, response to noxious stimulation of the supraorbital nerve or temporomandibular joints[11] should be tested during the examination. However, spinal reflex activity, in response to both noxious stimuli and tendon stretch, often can be shown to persist in experimental animals whose brains have been destroyed above the spinal level. The same reflexes can be found in the isolated spinal cord of humans following high spinal cord transection.

A variety of unusual, spinally mediated movements can appear and persist for prolonged periods during artificial life support.[12–18] Such phenomena include spontaneous movements in synchrony with the mechanical ventilator; slow body movements producing flexion at the waist, causing the body to rise to a sitting position ("Lazarus sign"); "stepping movements"; and preservation of lower body reflexes.[4] The consensus view is that in a patient in whom apneic oxygenation shows no return of breathing, such movements are generated by the spinal cord and the vital functions of the brainstem have no chance of recovery, making the diagnosis of brain death appropriate. It is important to note that spontaneous hypoxic or hypotensive events and apnea testing may precipitate these movements. Surprisingly, extensor plantar responses are not found in brain-dead patients.[14] Instead, plantar responses are either flexor, absent, or consistent with undulations of toe flexion.[19]

APNEA

Spontaneous respiration must be absent. Most patients on a mechanical ventilator will have a PaO_2 above and a $PaCO_2$ below normal levels. However, the threshold for stimulation of respiratory movements by the blood gases usually is elevated in patients in deep coma, sometimes to $PaCO_2$ values as high as 50 to 55 mm Hg. As a result, such patients may be apneic for several minutes when removed from the ventilator, even if they have a structurally normal brainstem. To test brainstem function without concurrently inducing severe hypoxemia under such circumstances, respiratory activity should be tested by the technique of apneic oxygenation. With this technique, the patient is ventilated with 100% oxygen for a period of 10 to 20 minutes. The respirator is then disconnected to avoid false readings and oxygen is delivered through a catheter to the trachea at a rate of about 6 L/minute. The resulting tension of oxygen in the alveoli will remain high enough to maintain the arterial blood at adequate oxygen tensions for as long as an hour or more. The $PaCO_2$ rises by about 3 mm Hg/minute during apneic oxygenation in a deeply comatose or clinically brain-dead patient.[20] Apneic oxygenation of 8 to 10 minutes thus allows the $PaCO_2$ to rise without danger of further hypoxia and ensures that one exceeds the respiratory threshold. A $PaCO_2$ that rises above 60 mm Hg without concomitant breathing efforts provides unequivocal evidence of nonfunctioning respiratory centers. The American Academy of Neurology guidelines for brain death (https://www.aan.com/professionals/practice/guidelines/pda/Brain_death_adults.pdf) accept either a $PaCO_2$ of 60 mm Hg or a value 20 mm Hg higher than baseline as the threshold for maximum stimulation of the respiratory centers of the medulla oblongata. Chronic pulmonary disease producing baseline hypercapnia may complicate the apnea testing and can be identified in initial blood gas examination by elevated serum bicarbonate concentration. In such cases, ancillary testing is recommended by current guidelines. Alternatively, hypocapnia often arises in the setting of hyperventilation to manage increased intracranial pressure (ICP). Since it is important to start the examination near a target PCO_2 of 40 mm Hg, hypocapnia should be corrected by adjusting the minute volume of ventilation through either a reduction of the tidal volume or a resetting of the respiratory rate.

During testing the patient should be observed for respiration defined as abdominal or chest excursions.[6] If respiration occurs during apnea testing, it is usually early into the testing. After 8 minutes have elapsed, arterial blood gases should be sampled and the ventilator reconnected. The absence of respiratory movements and rise of PCO_2 past 60 mm Hg indicates a positive apnea test. Alternatively, if respiratory movements are seen, the test is negative and retesting at a later time is indicated. Prior to initiating apnea testing the absence of brainstem reflexes should have already been established. Additionally, several other prerequisites must be established, as indicated in Table 8–4. Hypothermia must be excluded; if core temperatures obtained by rectal measurement are below 36.5°C, the patient should be warmed with a blanket. A systolic blood pressure of greater than 90 mm Hg should be maintained using dopamine infusion if required. If hypotension (systolic blood pressure less than 90 mm Hg) arises during the examination, blood samples should be promptly drawn and the ventilator immediately reconnected. Conversely, any elevation

Table 8–4 **Prerequisites for Apnea Testing**

1. Core temperature >36.5°C or 97°F
2. Systolic blood pressure >90 mm Hg
3. Euvolemia. *Option*: positive fluid balance in the previous 6 hours
4. Normal PCO_2. *Option*: arterial PCO_2 >40 mm Hg
5. Normal PO_2. *Option*: preoxygenation to obtain arterial PO_2 >200 mm Hg

Adapted from Wijdicks.[6]

of blood pressure during testing is evidence of lower brainstem function. As diabetes insipidus is a common complication of severe brain injuries, this should be recognized if present and managed. Accordingly, efforts should ensure euvolemia or positive fluid balance for at least 6 hours prior to testing. Finally, arterial gas pressures should reflect PO_2 greater than 200 mm Hg and PCO_2 greater than or equal to 40 mm Hg prior to testing as discussed above.

Confirmatory Laboratory Tests and Diagnosis

When the clinical examination is unequivocal, no additional tests are required. However, if there is any question, clinical practice guidelines suggest the potential use of four modalities of confirmatory testing in the determination of brain death[4,6]: conventional angiography, electroencephalography (EEG)/evoked potential (EP) studies, transcranial Doppler sonography (TCD), and cerebral scintigraphy. Consensus criteria for brain death determination are only available for EEG/EP studies.

STUDIES TO ESTABLISH CESSATION OF CEREBRAL BLOOD FLOW: CEREBRAL ANGIOGRAPHY, TRANSCRANIAL DOPPLER SONOGRAPHY, AND CEREBRAL SCINTIGRAPHY

Cerebral angiography is a widely accepted procedure for determination of brain death and can be used to overcome the limitation of the clinical neurologic examination due to facial trauma, baseline pulmonary disease, and other confounding factors. This procedure also has the advantage, when positive, of establishing a structural cause of brain death (i.e., absence of blood flow to the brain). In cases where the original cause of cerebral injury is not known, the absence of blood flow provides the crucial information necessary to declare brain death with certainty.

Physiologically, two events may produce failure of the cerebral circulation. First, a sudden and massive increase in ICP (e.g., during subarachnoid hemorrhage) may cause it to rise to the level of arterial perfusion pressure at which point cerebral circulation ceases. The second, and probably more common, occurrence is a progressive loss of blood flow that accompanies death of the brain. As the dead tissue becomes edematous, the local tissue pressure exceeds capillary perfusion pressure, resulting in stasis of blood flow, further edema, and further vascular stasis. If the respiratory and cardiovascular systems are kept functioning for many hours or days after brain circulation has ceased, the brain undergoes autolysis at body temperature, resulting in a soft and necrotic organ at autopsy referred to by pathologists as a "respirator brain."[21]

Demonstration of the failure of intracerebral filling at the level of entry of the carotid and vertebral arteries indicates brain death. Recently, magnetic resonance angiography (MRA) has been reported for diagnosis of brain death, but this technique is less reliable, as MRA often fails to demonstrate slow flow. Additional MRI criteria for brain death include loss of the subarachnoid spaces, slow flow in the intracavernous and cervical internal carotid arteries, loss of flow void in both small and large intracranial arteries and venous sinuses, and loss of gray-white matter distinction on T1-weighted images, but "supranormal" distinction on T2-weighted images.[22] However, until additional data are available on the reliability of these indicators for determining brain death, the presence of complete cessation of brain function on examination, or complete loss of blood flow, must remain the gold standards for diagnosis. In addition, the rarity of ventilators that are compatible with MR scanners continues to limit the availability of this mode of diagnosis.

Bilateral insonation of the intracranial arteries using a portable 2-MHz pulsed Doppler device (*transcranial Doppler ultrasonograph*

[*TCD*]) is now a widely used confirmatory test for brain death.[23] The middle cerebral arteries are insonated on both sides through the temporal bone above the zygomatic arch (of note, up to 10% of patients may not have temporal insonation windows, limiting use of this method) and the vertebral arteries or basilar artery through a suboccipital transcranial window. Two types of abnormalities have been correlated with brain death: (1) an absence of diastolic or reverberating flow, indicating the loss of arterial contractive force, and (2) the appearance of small systolic peaks early in systole, indicative of high vascular resistance. Both abnormalities are associated with significant elevations of ICP. The technique is limited by the requirement of skill in the operation of the equipment and has a potentially high error rate for missing blood flow because of incorrect placement of the transducer. Recent studies report a sensitivity of 77% and a specificity of 100% of diagnosing brain death if both the middle cerebral arteries and the basilar artery were insonated; sensitivity improved with increasing time of evaluation following initial clinical diagnosis.[24]

Cerebral scintigraphy measures the failure of uptake of the radioisotope nuclide technetium (Tc) 99m hexametazime in brain parenchyma. This technique has shown good correlation with cerebral angiography. The test can be done at the bedside using a portable gamma camera after injection of isotope, which should be used within 30 minutes after its reconstitution. A static image of 500,000 counts obtained at several time points is recommended (taken immediately, 30 to 60 minutes after injection, and at 2 hours past injection time[25]). A recent prospective study using 99m Tc-hexamethyl-propylamineoxime (HMPAO) single photon emission tomography (SPECT) in 50 comatose and brain-dead patients to examine cerebral perfusion found the characteristic "empty skull" image indicating arrest of cerebral perfusion in 45 of 47 brain-dead patients.[26] The bedside nuclide brain scan test is probably the best adjunct test to confirm the diagnosis in unclear cases. It is inexpensive, can be done without moving a patient on a ventilator, and is extremely reliable when it shows an empty skull (see Figure 8–1). This test can be considered a gold standard for use in difficult cases.

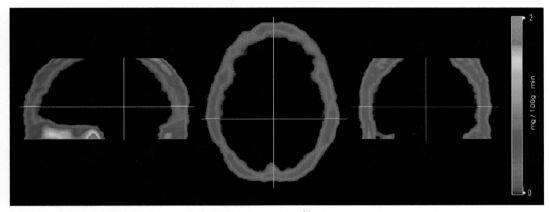

Figure 8–1. Cerebral metabolism in brain death measured by ^{18}F-fluorodeoxyglucose-positron emission tomography demonstrating the unequivocal finding of an "empty skull." (Sequence of images: sagittal [left]; transverse [middle]; and coronal [right]). (From Laureys et al.,[42] with permission.)

ELECTROENCEPHALOGRAPHY/ EVOKED POTENTIAL MEASUREMENTS

The EEG has little place in the determination of brain death, except perhaps in those rare cases where other clinical evidence is equivocal. An isoelectric EEG, often termed *electrocerebral inactivity* by electroencephalographers that lasts for a period of 6 to 12 hours in a patient who is not hypothermic and has not ingested or been given depressant drugs, identifies forebrain death (because the EEG does not demonstrate brainstem activity, it can be isoelectric in patients with brainstem reflexes who are clearly not brain dead). Silverman and associates reported on a survey of 2,650 isoelectric EEGs that lasted up to 24 hours.[27] Only three patients in this group, each in coma caused by overdose of central nervous system depressant drugs, recovered cerebral function. However, Heckmann and colleagues[28] have reported a patient with an isoelectric EEG following cardiac arrest who showed residual brainstem function, including spontaneous breathing and SPECT evidence of cerebral blood flow, for 7 weeks prior to death.

Electrical interference makes artifact-free EEG or evoked potential records exceedingly difficult to obtain in the intensive care setting. Moreover, technical recording errors can simulate electrocerebral activity as well as electrocerebral inactivity and several ostensibly isoelectric tracings must be discarded because of faulty technique. A national cooperative group has published technical requirements necessary to establish electrocerebral silence (Table 8–5), and has produced an atlas illustrating potential problems of interpretation of the EEG in coma.[29] It should be noted that the EEG is not infallible, even with anoxic-ischemic injury. Cerebral activity may be absent on the EEG for up to several hours following cardiac arrest, only to return later.[30] A prolonged vegetative existence is occasionally possible in such cases despite the presence of an initially silent EEG. After depressive drug poisoning, total loss of cerebral hemispheric function and electrocerebral silence have been observed for as long as 50 hours with full clinical recovery.

Physicians have appropriately raised questions as to whether a few fragments of cerebral electrical activity mean anything when they arise from a body that has totally lost all capacity for the brain to regulate internal and external homeostasis. Death is a process in which different organs and parts of organs lose their living properties at widely varying rates. Death of the brain occurs when the organ irreversibly loses its capacity to maintain the vital integrative functions regulated by the vegetative and consciousness-mediating centers of the brainstem. Not surprisingly, the time when the state of brain death is reached often precedes the final demise of small collections of electrically generating cells in the cerebral hemispheres,

Table 8–5 **Electroencephalographic Recording for Diagnosing Cerebral Death**

1. A minimum of eight scalp electrodes and ear reference electrodes
2. Interelectrode impedances under 10,000 ohms, but over 100 ohms
3. Test of integrity of recording system by deliberate creation of electrode artifact by manipulation
4. Interelectrode distances of at least 10 cm
5. No activity with a sensitivity increased to at least 2 μV/mm for 30 minutes with inclusion of appropriate calibrations
6. The use of 0.3- or 0.4-second time constants during part of the recording
7. Recording with an electrocardiogram and other monitoring devices, such as a pair of electrodes on the dorsum of the right hand, to detect extracerebral responses
8. Tests for reactivity to pain, loud noises, or light
9. Recording by a qualified technician
10. Repeat record if doubt about electrocerebral silence (ECS)
11. Telephonic transmitted electroencephalograms are not appropriate for determination of ECS

From Bennett et al.[29]

as evidenced by the observation that 20% of 56 patients meeting other clinical criteria for brain death had residual EEG activity lasting up to 168 hours.[31] Thus, EEG examinations may pick up a few patients with brainstem death who have not yet progressed to full brain death. Given the extremely poor prognosis of such individuals, using EEG as a criterion for prolonging the period of futile life support is not a service to them.

Diagnosis of Brain Death in Profound Anesthesia or Coma of Undetermined Etiology

It must be repeatedly emphasized that patients with very deep but reversible anesthesia due to sedative drug ingestion can give the clinical appearance of brain death, and even can have an electrically silent EEG. Furthermore, recovery in such instances has been observed even when the EEG showed no physiologic activity for as

long as 50 hours. Given such evidence, when and how is one to decide in such cases that anesthesia has slipped into death and further cardiopulmonary support is futile? Unfortunately, few empirical data provide an answer to the question, particularly if faced with the complex problem of a patient with a coma of undetermined origin. In such cases, the combination of a prolonged period of observation (more than 24 hours), loss of cerebral perfusion, and exclusion of other potential confounds is required.[32] It is important to test drug levels and follow the patient until the drug is eliminated. A general guideline proposed for known intoxications is the following: an observation period greater than four times the half-life of the pharmacologic agent should be used.[4] Of course, the presence of unmeasured metabolites, potentiation by additional medications, and impaired renal or hepatic clearance are likely to complicate individual evaluations.

Pitfalls in the Diagnosis of Brain Death

Potential pitfalls accompany the diagnosis of brain death, particularly when coma occurs in hospitalized patients or those who have been chronically ill. Almost none of these will lead to serious error in diagnosis if the examining physician is aware of them and attends to them when examining individual patients who are considered brain dead. In fact, there are no reported cases of "recovery" from correctly diagnosed brain death.

With meticulous efforts, other organs (e.g. heart, kidney, etc.) can be sustained, but usually only for hours or days.[33,34] Prolonged survival of peripheral organs is quite rare,[35,36] so much so that in the few reported cases, one must question whether the clinical criteria were correctly met. Conversely, there are several reported cases of recovery from "cardiac" death,[37] the Lazarus phenomenon (not to be confused with Lazarus sign, a spinal reflex [see page 334]). A number of case reports describe patients with clinical and electrocardiographic cardiac arrest who, after failed attempts at resuscitation, are pronounced dead, only to be discovered to be alive later, sometimes in the mortuary.[38] Some of these pitfalls are outlined in Table 8–6.

Table 8–6 **Some Pitfalls in the Diagnosis of Brain Death**

Findings	Possible Causes
1. Pupils fixed	Anticholinergic drugs, tricyclic antidepressants Neuromuscular blockers Pre-existing disease
2. No oculovestibular reflexes	Ototoxic agents Vestibular suppression Pre-existing disease Basal skull fracture
3. No respiration	Posthyperventilation apnea Neuromuscular blockers
4. No motor activity	Neuromuscular blockers "Locked-in" state Sedative drugs
5. Isoelectric electroencephalogram	Sedative drugs Anoxia Hypothermia Encephalitis Trauma

Adapted from Wijdicks.[4]

In comatose patients, pupillary fixation does not always mean absence of brainstem function. In rare instances, the pupils may have been fixed by pre-existing ocular or neurologic disease. More commonly, particularly in a patient who has suffered cardiac arrest, atropine has been injected during the resuscitation process and pupils are widely dilated; fixed pupils may result without indicating the absence of brainstem function. Neuromuscular blocking agents also can produce pupillary fixation, although in these instances the pupils are usually midposition or small rather than widely dilated.

Similarly, the absence of vestibulo-ocular responses does not necessarily indicate absence of brainstem vestibular function. Like pupillary responses, vestibulo-ocular reflexes may be absent if the end organ is either poisoned or damaged. For example, traumatic injury producing basal fractures of the petrous bone may cause unilateral loss of caloric response. Some otherwise neurologically normal patients suffer labyrinthine dysfunction from peripheral disease that predates the onset of coma. Other patients with chronic illnesses have suffered ototoxicity from a variety of drugs, including antibiotics such as gentamicin. In these patients, vestibulo-ocular responses may be absent even

though other brainstem processes are still functioning. Finally, a variety of drugs, including sedatives, anticholinergics, anticonvulsants, chemotherapeutic agents, and tricyclic antidepressants, may suppress vestibular and/or oculomotor function to the point where oculovestibular reflexes disappear.

Pitfalls in the diagnosis of apnea in comatose patients maintained on respirators have been discussed above.

The absence of motor activity also does not guarantee loss of brainstem function. Neuromuscular blockers are often used early in the course of artificial respiration when the patient is resisting the respirator; if suspected brain death subsequently occurs, there may still be enough circulating neuromuscular blocking agent to produce absence of motor function when the examination is carried out. One report has described the simulation of brain death by excessive sensitivity to succinylcholine[39]; in this case the presence of activity in the EEG established cerebral viability. If neuromuscular blockade has been recently withdrawn, guidelines require that a peripheral nerve stimulator be used to demonstrate transmission (e.g., a train of four stimulation pulses produces four thumb twitches).

Therapeutic overdoses of sedative drugs to treat anoxia or seizures likewise may abolish reflexes and motor responses to noxious stimuli. At least two reports document formal brain death examinations in reversible intoxications with tricyclic antidepressant and barbiturate agents.[40,41]

There are pitfalls in using the EEG as an ancillary technique in the diagnosis of cerebral death. Isoelectric EEGs with subsequent recovery have been reported with sedative drug overdoses, after anoxia, during hypothermia, following cerebral trauma, and after encephalitis, especially cases of diffuse acute disseminated encephalomyelitis.[5]

REFERENCES

1. Mollaret P, Goulon M. [The depassed coma (preliminary memoir).]. Rev Neurol (Paris) 1959; 101, 3–15.
2. A definition of irreversible coma. Report of the Ad Hoc Committee of the Harvard Medical School to Examine the Definition of Brain Death. JAMA 1968; 205, 337–340.
3. Uniform Laws Annotated 320 Uniform Determination of Death Act. 1990.

4. Wijdicks EF. The diagnosis of brain death. N Engl J Med 2001; 344, 1215–1221.

5. An appraisal of the criteria of cerebral death. A summary statement. A collaborative study. JAMA 1977; 237, 982–986.

6. Wijdicks EF. Determining brain death in adults. Neurology 1995; 45, 1003–1011.

7. Bates D, Caronna JJ, Cartlidge NE, et al. A prospective study of nontraumatic coma: methods and results in 310 patients. Ann Neurol 1977; 2, 211–220.

8. Jorgensen EO. Spinal man after brain death. The unilateral extension-pronation reflex of the upper limb as an indication of brain death. Acta Neurochir (Wien) 1973; 28, 259–273.

9. President's Commission for the Study of Ethical Problems in Medicine and Biomedical Behavioral Research Defining Death: Medical, Legal and Ethical Issues in the Determination of Death. 1981.

10. Shlugman D, Parulekar M, Elston JS, et al. Abnormal pupillary activity in a brainstem-dead patient. Br J Anaesth 2001; 86, 717–720.

11. Wijdicks EFM. Temporomandibular joint compression in coma. Neurology 1996; 46, 1774–1774.

12. Christie JM, O'Lenic TD, Cane RD. Head turning in brain death. J Clin Anesth 1996; 8, 141–143.

13. Hanna JP, Frank JI. Automatic stepping in the pontomedullary stage of central herniation. Neurology 1995; 45, 985–986.

14. de Freitas GR, Andre C. Absence of the Babinski sign in brain death: a prospective study of 144 cases. J Neurol 2005; 252, 106–107.

15. Martí-Fàbregas J, López-Navidad A, Caballero F, et al. Decerebrate-like posturing with mechanical ventilation in brain death. Neurology 2000; 54, 224–227.

16. Ropper AH. Unusual spontaneous movements in brain-dead patients. Neurology 1984; 34, 1089–1092.

17. Saposnik G, Bueri JA, Mauriño J, et al. Spontaneous and reflex movements in brain death. Neurology 2000; 54, 221–223.

18. Saposnik G, Maurino J, Saizar R, et al. Spontaneous and reflex movements in 107 patients with brain death. Am J Med 2005; 118(3), 311–314.

19. McNair NL, Meador KJ. The undulating toe flexion sign in brain death. Mov Disord 1992; 7, 345–347.

20. Schafer JA, Caronna JJ. Duration of apnea needed to confirm brain death. Neurology 1978; 28, 661–666.

21. Walker AE, Diamond EL, Moseley J. The neuropathological findings in irreversible coma. A critique of the "respirator." J Neuropathol Exp Neurol 1975; 34, 295–323.

22. Lee DH, Nathanson JA, Fox AJ, et al. Magnetic resonance imaging of brain death. Can Assoc Radiol J 1995; 46, 174–178.

23. Sloan MA, Alexandrov AV, Tegeler CH, et al. Assessment: transcranial Doppler ultrasonography: report of the Therapeutics and Technology Assessment Subcommittee of the American Academy of Neurology. Neurology 2004; 62, 1468–1481.

24. Kuo JR, Chen CF, Chio CC, et al. Time dependent validity in the diagnosis of brain death using transcra-

nial Doppler sonography. J Neurol Neurosurg Psychiatry 2006; 77, 646–649.

25. Bonetti MG, Ciritella P, Valle G, et al. 99mTc HM-PAO brain perfusion SPECT in brain death. Neuroradiology 1995; 37, 365–369.

26. Facco E, Zucchetta P, Munari M, et al. 99mTc-HMPAO SPECT in the diagnosis of brain death. Intensive Care Med 1998; 24, 911–917.

27. Silverman D, Masland RL, Saunders MG, et al. Irreversible coma associated with electrocerebral silence. Neurology 1970; 20, 525–533.

28. Heckmann JG, Lang CJ, Pfau M, et al. Electrocerebral silence with preserved but reduced cortical brain perfusion. Eur J Emerg Med 2003; 10, 241–243.

29. Bennett DR, Hughes JR, Korein J. Atlas of Electroencephalography in Coma and Cerebral Death. EEG at the Bedside or in the Intensive Care Unit. San Diego: Raven Press, 1976.

30. Jorgensen EO. Clinical note. EEG without detectable cortical activity and cranial nerve areflexia as parameters of brain death. Electroencephalogr Clin Neurophysiol 1974; 36, 70–75.

31. Grigg MM, Kelly MA, Celesia GG, et al. Electroencephalographic activity after brain death. Arch Neurol 1987; 44, 948–954.

32. Practice parameters for determining brain death in adults (summary statement). The Quality Standards Subcommittee of the American Academy of Neurology. Neurology 1995; 45, 1012–1014.

33. Yoshioka T, Sugimoto H, Uenishi M, et al. Prolonged hemodynamic maintenance by the combined administration of vasopressin and epinephrine in brain death: a clinical study. Neurosurgery 1986; 18, 565–567.

34. Hung TP, Chen ST. Prognosis of deeply comatose patients on ventilators. J Neurol Neurosurg Psychiatry 1995; 58, 75–80.

35. Shewmon DA. Chronic "brain death": meta-analysis and conceptual consequences. Neurology 1998; 51, 1538–1545.

36. Repertinger S, Fitzgibbons WP, Omojola MF, et al. Long survival following bacterial meningitis-associated brain destruction. J Child Neurol 2006; 21, 591–595.

37. Maleck WH, Piper SN, Triem J, et al. Unexpected return of spontaneous circulation after cessation of resuscitation (Lazarus phenomenon). Resuscitation 1998; 39, 125–128.

38. Mullie A, Miranda D. A premature referral to the mortuary. Cerebral recovery with barbiturate therapy. Acta Anaesthesiol Belg 1979; 30, 145–148.

39. Tyson RN. Simulation of cerebral death by succinylcholine sensitivity. Arch Neurol 1974; 30, 409–411.

40. Grattan-Smith PJ, Butt W. Suppression of brainstem reflexes in barbiturate coma. Arch Dis Child 1993; 69, 151–152.

41. Yang KL, Dantzker DR. Reversible brain death. A manifestation of amitriptyline overdose. Chest 1991; 99, 1037–1038.

42. Laureys S, Owen AM, Schiff ND. Brain function in coma, vegetative state, and related disorders. Lancet Neurol 2004; 3, 537–546.

Chapter 9

Prognosis in Coma and Related Disorders of Consciousness, Mechanisms Underlying Outcomes, and Ethical Considerations

341

INTRODUCTION

It is much more difficult to predict the outcome for patients with severe brain damage than to make the usually straightforward diagnosis of brain death. Brain death is a single biologic state with an unequivocal future, while severe brain injuries span a wide range of outcomes (Figure 9–1) depending on a number of variables that include not only the degree of neurologic injury, but also the presence and severity of medical complications. Scientific, philosophic, and emotional uncertainties that attend predictions of outcome from brain damage can intimidate even the most experienced physicians. Nevertheless, the problem must be faced; physicians are frequently called upon to treat patients with severe degrees of neurologic dysfunction. To do the job responsibly, the physician must organize available information to anticipate as accurately as possible the likelihood that the patient will either recover or remain permanently disabled. The physician's role as a translator of

medical knowledge is essential in counseling families who must make the ultimate decisions concerning the care of an unconscious patient. The financial and emotional costs of caring for those left hopelessly damaged can exhaust both family and medical staff. Physicians must attempt to reduce those burdens, while at the same time retaining an unwavering commitment to do everything possible to treat those who can benefit.

In the 26 years since the publication of the third edition of *Stupor and Coma*, several groups of neurologists and neurosurgeons have initiated studies to identify and quantify early clinical, neurophysiologic, radiologic, and biochemical indicants that might predict outcome in comatose patients. These studies have identified the etiology of injury, the clinical depth of coma, and the length of time that a patient remains comatose as the most critical factors. Additional important factors include the age of the patient, the neurologic findings, and concurrent medical complications (particularly the complications of increased intracranial pressure [ICP] and hypoxia in the setting of traumatic in-

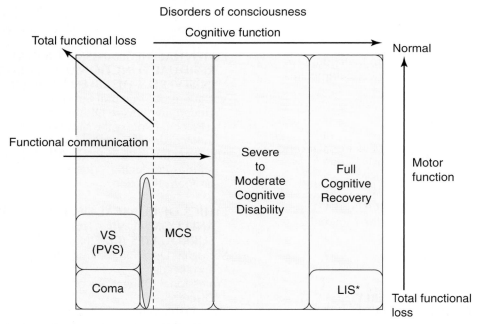

Figure 9–1. Conceptual overview of functional outcomes following severe brain injuries. Gray zone between vegetative state (VS) and minimally conscious state (MCS) reflects rare patients with fragments of behavior that arise spontaneously and not in response to stimulation. By nosologic criteria, these patients remain in VS (see page 365). The bold black line indicates emergence from the minimally conscious state, defined by reliable functional communication. LIS, locked-in state; PVS, persistent vegetative state. °LIS is not a disorder of consciousness. (Adapted from Schiff.[193])

juries). Several limitations, as discussed below, place stringent demands on physicians to carefully consider all available historical details and the reliability of clinical and laboratory evaluations in their consideration of prognosis for an individual patient.

Prospective studies of prognosis in adults and children indicate that within a few hours or days after the onset of coma, neurologic signs and electrophysiologic markers in many patients differentiate, with a high degree of probability, the extremes of no improvement or good recovery. Unfortunately, radiologic and biochemical indicators have generally provided less accurate predictions of outcome, with some exceptions discussed below. Accurate prognostication improves over time, but it is still unclear how early one can make accurate predictions within different diagnostic categories (e.g., vegetative state [VS] vs. minimally conscious state [MCS]). The first section of this chapter details what we now know about prognosis, emphasizing broad outcome categories and short-term outcomes rather than outcomes beyond a year or longer, although we recognize that rarely, even severely brain-injured patients may improve after many years (see page 371). We use the scheme in Table 9–1 to assess the reliability of the data presented in this section.

The second section addresses mechanisms that may underlie recovery, or lack thereof, from coma. Severe cognitive disabilities can arise from at least two fairly different anatomic injuries: (1) extensive, relatively uniform diffuse axonal injury or hypoxic-ischemic damage causing widespread neuronal death and (2) focal cerebral injuries causing functional alteration of integrative systems in the upper brainstem and thalamus. New studies suggest that physiologic correlates of brain function in some severely disabled patients with relatively intact cerebral structures may ultimately lead to identification of residual cerebral capacities.

Figure 9–1 shows a conceptual organization of functional outcomes following severe brain injuries and indicates that a very wide range of cognitive capacities may be present in the setting of impaired motor function, including normal cognition in the locked-in state (LIS). In this section we discuss advances in neuroimaging aimed at uncovering the biologic distinctions that underlie VS, persistent vegetative state (PVS), MCS, and related enduring disorders of consciousness following coma. Despite the relatively small number of studies in this area to date, functional imaging has added to our general understanding of pathophysiologic mechanisms in VS. Ongoing work in MCS patients suggests that significant physiologic differences in brain function will generally separate these categories.

The third section addresses important ethical considerations in dealing with comatose patients and their families and caregivers.

PROGNOSIS IN COMA

Coma has a grave prognosis. For the two most carefully studied etiologies of coma, traumatic brain injury and cardiopulmonary arrest, mortality ranges from 40% to 50% and 54% to 88%,[2] respectively. These statistics have actually improved since the last edition of *Stupor and Coma*, because of better acute management both in the field and in intensive care. Beyond mortality statistics, very few studies of prognosis in coma have looked at large numbers of patients for careful evaluation of outcomes other than survival or death. These indicate that patients comatose from traumatic brain injury have a significantly better prognosis than patients with anoxic injuries. For example, of 1,000 trauma patients in coma for at least 6 hours, 39% recovered independent function at 6 months,[3] whereas only 16% of 500 patients suffering nontraumatic coma made similar recoveries at 1 year.[4]

Statistics such as the above, however, are too coarse to guide individual patient management.

Table 9–1 **Levels of Evidence**

Level I	Data from randomized trials with low false-positive (alpha) and low false-negative (beta) errors
Level II	Data from randomized trials with high false-positive (alpha) or high false-negative (beta) errors
Level III	Data from nonrandomized concurrent cohort studies
Level IV	Data from nonrandomized cohort studies using historical controls
Level V	Data from anecdotal case series

Modified from Broderick et al.[1]

That step requires clinical judgment combined with accurate knowledge of the medical literature, as applied specifically to the patient's history and awareness of common diagnostic pitfalls. This section reviews efforts to predict outcome from coma for different etiologies. The reader will find that the literature continues to provide little specific information about the kind of outcome enjoyed or suffered by patients.[5] As a result, except where specified, descriptions of recovery from coma often connote little more than survival and fail to tell one about the social, vocational, or emotional outcome (i.e., the human qualities) of the life that followed.

The Glasgow Outcome Scale (GOS; Table 9–2) originates from a study of outcome following nontraumatic coma in 500 patients. The definitions attempted to identify fairly precisely what was meant by each grade of outcome. Only a small number of outcomes were chosen in the hope that sufficient numbers of patients would fall into each class to allow statistical analysis, but that important differences in medical and social recovery would not be excessively blurred. A shortcoming of this classification is that the category of severe disability (3) is too broad in that it includes all patients who cannot

Table 9–2 Glasgow Outcome Scale (GOS)

Good recovery (5)	Patients who regain the ability to conduct a normal life or, if a pre-existing disability exists, to resume the previous level of activity
Moderate disability (4)	Patients who achieve independence in daily living but retain either physical or mental limitations that preclude resuming their previous level of function
Severe disability (3)	Patients who regain at least some cognitive function but depend on others for daily support
Vegetative state (2)	Patients who awaken but give no sign of cognitive awareness
No recovery (1)	Patients who remain in coma until death

From Jennett and Bond,[5] with permission.

function independently, from those minimally conscious to those almost independent. There still exists a need for further subdivision and consideration of outcomes in the severely disabled group, as discussed below. An important limitation in evaluating the prognostic data in the literature is that some studies conflate death, VS, and severely disabled but conscious outcomes of coma survivors. For example, when using the prognostic data provided below, care should be taken to distinguish indicators of death from those indicating outcomes including severe disability, which remains a very broad category. Moreover, many outcome studies do not provide sufficient follow-up of subjects to assess outcomes of permanent VS. To allow comparisons across studies, this chapter indicates the GOS cutoff score used in each report below and does not categorize outcomes as "good," "bad," "favorable," or "unfavorable."

Another fundamental issue in determining a prognosis for any individual patient is the etiology of injury. It must be recognized that the overwhelming weight of medical knowledge for prognosis in coma falls into two large categories: traumatic brain injury (TBI) and anoxic-ischemic encephalopathy (AIE). Unfortunately, there are many additional etiologies that can produce coma and related disorders of consciousness, and it is often not possible simply to place an individual patient with another etiology into the context of TBI or AIE. Where possible, information specific to other etiologies is provided below, but the physician should recognize this general limitation when formulating a prognosis for a comatose patient who has not suffered a traumatic brain injury or cardiac arrest.

PROGNOSIS BY DISEASE STATE

Traumatic Brain Injury

More effort has been directed at trying to predict outcome from TBI than from any other cause of coma. This emphasis reflects the high prevalence of TBI (estimated at 1.5 to 2.0 million persons per year in the United States[6]), the young age of most patients (peak 15 to 24 years old), and the enormous financial, social, and emotional impact of the illness that may persist for decades. Coma arising from TBI has a better prognosis than nontraumatic coma, possibly because patients are usually younger and the pathophysiology differs from other types of coma. Recovery after prolonged traumatic coma is well described and, unlike nontraumatic causes, unconsciousness for 1 month does not necessarily preclude significant recovery. Severe head injury causing 6 hours or more of coma still carries a 40% probability of recovering to a level of moderate disability or better.[7] A comprehensive literature review by the Brain Trauma Foundation in 2000[8] organizes evidence-based data for early prognostic signs in TBI; class I prognostic evidence is listed in Table 9–3.

The Glasgow Coma Scale (GCS) score has at least a 70% positive predictive value (PPV) for an outcome less than 4 on the GOS, if evaluations done after cardiopulmonary resuscitation were performed after sedative and paralytic agents had been metabolized. Gennarelli and colleagues[9] found a progressive increase in mortality for patients with descending GCS scores in the 3 to 8 range in 46,977 head-injured patients. Two studies provide class I evidence for the predictive value of the GCS. Narayan and associates[10] prospectively studied

Table 9–3 Class I Evidence for Early Prognosis in Coma Due to Traumatic Brain Injury

I. Glasgow Coma Scale (see Chapter 1): worsening outcome grades in continuous stepwise manner with lower GCS score

II. Age: 70% positive predictive value (PPV) with increasingly worse outcome in continuous and stepwise manner associated with increasing age

III. Absent pupillary responses: 70% PPV of an outcome <4 on the GOS

IV. Hypotension/hypoxia: systolic blood pressure <90 mm Hg has a 67% PPV for an outcome <4 on the GOS outcome, and 79% PPV when combined with evidence of hypoxia

V. Computed tomography imaging abnormalities: 70% PPV of an outcome <4 on the GOS with initial abnormalities including compression, effacement, or blood within the basal cisterns, or extensive traumatic subarachnoid hemorrhage

Developed from the Brain Trauma Foundation Management and Prognosis of Severe Traumatic Brain Injury.[8]

133 patients of all age ranges and found that 62% of patients with a GCS of 3 to 5, when examined either in the emergency room or on admission to an intensive care unit, at later evaluation had a GOS of 1 (Table 9–1). Braakman and colleagues[11] prospectively studied 305 patients and correlated GOS level 1 outcomes in 100% of patients with a GCS of 3, 80% with a GCS of 4, and 68% with a GCS of 5. The several studies examined in the Brain Trauma Foundation review support a survival rate of 20% for patients with the lowest GCS scores and an outcome above the level of severe disability (GOS 4 or 5) in 8% to 10% of the patients, limiting the use of the GCS alone for prognosis.

MOTOR FINDINGS

A reasonably good indication of outcome can be obtained by testing motor responses to noxious stimulation.[12,13] Abnormal flexor (decorticate), abnormal extensor (decerebrate), or predominantly flaccid responses in patients with severe head injury denote an outcome of less than 4 on the GOS in every reported series. By 6 hours, motor responses no better than abnormal flexor were associated with a mortality of 63%, while abnormal extensor or flaccid responses predicted an 83% mortality.[7] Unfortunately, the European Brain Injury Consortium found that the motor score of the GCS was untestable in 28% of 1,005 patients at the time of admission to a neurosurgery service, and that the full GCS score could not be assessed in 44% patients due to prehospital medications and management with intubation.[12] Testing of the motor response by application of nail-bed or supraorbital pressure is considered most reliable but may be complicated by tissue injury (e.g., periorbital swelling or quadriplegia).[14,15]

AGE

Advanced age unfavorably influences outcome in traumatic coma. Paradoxically, elderly patients may require a much longer recovery time, so it is risky to predict ultimate recovery early in the course. Of 600 patients with severe head injury causing coma, 56% of those younger than age 20 recovered to a GOS of 4 or 5. This number fell to 39% between age 20 and 59 years and to only 5% among those older than

60 years.[16] In a prospective study of 372 patients with a GCS score of less than 13, age older than 50 years and lower GCS scores correlated with higher mortality.[16] A prospective series with 2,664 patients found an essentially linear correlation of age and outcome following severe brain injury.[17] The odds of an outcome less than 4 on the GOS increased 40% to 50% for every 10 years of age as a continuous variable. A meta-analysis of 5,600 patients identified a continuously worsening prognosis with increasing age without a sharp stepwise drop at any point.[17] Several factors, other than age alone, may play a role in the association of age with outcome in TBI. Data from the Traumatic Coma Data Bank[8] reveal an increased incidence of intracranial hemorrhage with age and premorbid medical illnesses, but did not demonstrate a significant statistical association.

NEURO-OPHTHALMOLOGIC SIGNS

The Brain Trauma Foundation review identified class I evidence that loss of pupillary light reflexes has at least a 70% PPV for a poor prognosis following TBI. Bilateral absence of pupillary or oculocephalic responses or both at any point in the illness predicts an outcome less than 4 on the GOS. In one series, 95% of patients who had either bilaterally nonreactive pupils or absent oculocephalic responses at 6 hours after injury died.[18]

SECONDARY INJURIES

Hypotension, hypoxia, and uncontrolled intracranial hypertension are independent predictors of poor outcome. Class I evidence supports a high likelihood of an outcome less than 4 on the GOS in comatose TBI patients who suffer either hypoxia or hypotension (defined as a systolic blood pressure of less than 90 mm Hg) early in the course. A single episode of hypotension (arterial line reading) is associated with a doubling of mortality and a significant increase in morbidity.[8]

NEUROIMAGING

Several neuroimaging findings correlate with outcome following TBI. Class I and strong class II evidence identifies several computed tomography (CT) findings that predict outcome[8]; accurate interpretation requires consideration of

the type of brain injury (e.g., focal brain injuries vs. diffuse axonal injury). The majority of patients with TBI have an abnormal CT scan, but certain findings carry a stronger predictive value for an outcome less than 4 on the GOS. Compression of the basal cisterns, a reliable indicator of increased ICP, is a strong negative predictor in several studies[19] (see [8] for review). Midline shift of brain structures, another indicator of increased ICP, is also a predictor of an outcome less than 4 on the GOS.[20] A midline shift of greater than 1.5 cm has a 70% PPV of death.[8] Other CT findings that predict an outcome less than 4 on the GOS include traumatic subarachnoid hemorrhage in the suprasellar or ambient cisterns, and mass lesions (intracerebral hematoma, variable density CT abnormalities, epidural and subdural hematomas).

DURATION OF COMA

Figure 9–2 reproduces Carlsson and colleagues'[21] classic diagram (1968) of the effect of duration of TBI-induced coma on outcomes at different ages. Not surprisingly, the longer the coma lasts, the worse the outcome is. Although length of coma provides a good indication of severity of brain damage, it can be determined only retrospectively when the patient awakens and thus cannot be used for early prognosis of outcome. On the other hand, it can be predicted with some confidence that a patient in prolonged coma is unlikely to recover. The same limitation applies to efforts to correlate outcomes of recovery of cognitive functions with the duration of posttraumatic amnesia.

ELECTROPHYSIOLOGIC MARKERS

Electrophysiologic measures have limited effectiveness in assessing TBI outcome. Several electroencephalographic (EEG) abnormalities are seen following TBI,[22] and although EEG is useful for the identification of treatable complications of head trauma such as seizures, it does not predict outcome. Somatosensory-evoked potentials (SSEPs) are a better indicator.[23] Bilateral absence of cortical components of SSEPs strongly correlates with a GOS below 4[24]; in one small study, bilateral loss of SSEPs predicted outcomes of death or VS in all patients,[25] but other reports indicate that bilateral loss of cortical response in posttraumatic coma may, on rare occasions, be associated with

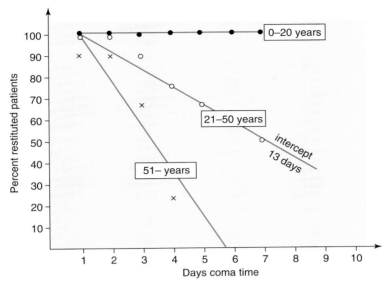

Figure 9–2. Percentage of patients who recovered full consciousness as a function of duration of coma for several age groups. (From Carlsson et al.,[21] with permission.)

favorable outcome.[26,27] In these published reports, the measurements may have been confounded by sedating medications or the very early testing of the evoked potentials. Logi and associates[24] prospectively studied 131 comatose patients of varying etiologies, including head trauma patients ($N = 22$), and found 100% specificity for bilateral absence of cortical responses predicting nonawakening when sedating medications had been withdrawn and there were no other metabolic disturbances. Other electrophysiologic markers, including cognitive event-related potentials,[28] might provide better prognostic value in future studies. Lew and colleagues[25] suggested that the P300 response elicited by spoken words such as "mommy" may find use as an early predictor of outcomes greater than 3 on the GOS for comatose TBI patients. However, Perrin and associates[29] found that similar P300 paradigms could not differentiate patients remaining in VS studied months after injury from other patients recovering to higher functional levels.

BIOCHEMICAL MARKERS

Elevated serum levels of glial fibrillary acidic protein (GFAP), part of the astroglial skeleton, and S100B, an astroglial protein, have been reported to predict mortality.[30] In 42 severely injured adults studied within 7 days of injury, the ratio of glutamate/glutamine (Glx) and choline (Cho) was significantly elevated in occipital gray and parietal white matter in patients who showed long-term (6- to 12-month) outcomes of less than 4 on the GOS.[31]

Nontraumatic Coma

PROSPECTIVE ANALYSES OF OUTCOME FROM NONTRAUMATIC COMA

In the late 1960s, a team of investigators at The New York Hospital, led by Dr. Plum and coworkers, in close association with Dr. Jennett and colleagues in Glasgow, undertook prospective studies of the outcome from coma as caused by medical disorders.[4] Collaborating with the Royal Victoria Hospital, Newcastle-upon-Tyne, United Kingdom, and the San Francisco General Hospital, the investigators ultimately evaluated 500 patients in acute nontraumatic coma. All patients over 12 years old, save those with head trauma or exogenous intoxication in acute coma, were identified and repeatedly examined. Meticulous efforts were made to examine every patient in coma using examining techniques that guaranteed consistency of observation. To avoid bias, the

examiners refrained from either making recommendations for therapy or disclosing preliminary results to the treating staffs. The patients were followed for a minimum of 12
months (unless death occurred first) and many
for much longer (only two of the 500 patients
were lost to follow-up). This large population
provided landmark data on substantial numbers of individuals in each of the major disease
categories, permitting correlations between
outcome and both the severity of early signs of
neurologic dysfunction and the specific etiology of coma. Subsequent studies have largely
confirmed the conclusions drawn from this
patient population, including larger prospective studies of coma following cardiac arrest.[2]

The results of the medical coma study indicate that loss of consciousness lasting 6 hours
or more bestows a poor prognosis. Of the 500
patients, 379 (76%) died within the first month
and 88% had died by the end of a year. Three-
quarters of those dying by 1 month never regained consciousness, and within that month,
only 15% of the entire 500 recovered to a GOS
of 4 or 5.

Table 9–4 charts the *best* 1-month recovery
by disease state. Some of the patients died during that first month of nonneurologic causes,
but the table is constructed so as to indicate the
highest possible chance of recovery by the brain.
(*Actual outcome* from the illness in many instances was worse than this best neurologic
state, because some patients who temporarily
recovered neurologically died from complications, such as recurrent cardiac arrhythmias,
infections, and pulmonary embolism.)

Nontraumatic coma, while always serious,
has a better outcome in some diseases than in
others. About 30% of patients with hepatic and
miscellaneous causes of coma recovered to a
GOS of 4 or 5, three times the recovery rate
of patients with vascular-ischemic neurologic
injuries (subarachnoid hemorrhage, cerebral
vascular diseases, and hypoxia-ischemia). The
difference is explained by most of the hepatic and miscellaneous patients having reversible biochemical, infectious, or extracerebral intracranial (e.g., subdural hematoma)
lesions that may have transiently depressed
brain function, but nevertheless left the structure of the brain intact. By contrast, many patients with stroke or global cerebral ischemia
suffered destruction of brain structures crucial
for consciousness. Reflecting this difference,
the metabolic-miscellaneous group of patients
showed significantly fewer signs of severe
brainstem dysfunction than did those with
vascular-ischemic disorders. For example, corneal responses were absent in fewer than 20%
of the metabolic group, but in more than 30%
of the remaining patients. Furthermore, when
patients with hepatic-miscellaneous causes of
coma did show abnormal neuro-ophthalmologic signs (see below), their prognosis was as
poor as that of patients in the other disease
groups with similar signs.

Patients who survived medical coma had
achieved most of their improvement by the end
of the first month. Among the 121 patients still
living at 1 month, 61 died within the next year,
usually from progression or complication of
the illness that caused coma in the first place.

Table 9–4 Best One-Month Outcome Related to Cause of Coma

Cause of Coma	Best One-Month Outcome (%)				
	No Recovery	Vegetative State	Severe Disability	Moderate Disability	Good Recovery
All patients (500)	61	12	12	5	10
Subarachnoid hemorrhage (38)	74	5	13	5	3
Other cerebrovascular disease (143)°	74	7	11	4	4
Hypoxia-ischemia (210)°	58	20	11	3	8
Hepatic encephalopathy (51)	49	2	16	10	23
Miscellaneous (58)°	45	10	14	5	6

°Hypoxia-ischemia includes 150 patients with cardiac arrest, 38 with profound hypotension, and 22 with respiratory arrest.
Other cerebrovascular diseases include 76 with brain infarcts and 67 with brain hemorrhage. Miscellaneous includes 19
patients with mixed metabolic disturbances and 16 with infection.

There were seven moderately disabled patients who improved to a good recovery. Of 39 patients severely disabled at 1 month, nine later improved to a good recovery or moderate disability rating. At the end of the year, three patients remained vegetative and four severely disabled. While current patients may have a greater chance of survival with modern therapies, it is unfortunately not likely that they would have a significantly different natural history after 1 month, suggesting that the data from this series remain relevant.

The outcome was influenced by three major clinical factors: the duration of coma, neuro-ophthalmologic signs, and motor function. Of somewhat lesser importance was the course of recovery; a history of steady improvement was generally more favorable than was initially better function that remained unchanged for the next several days. Only one patient who remained in coma for a week recovered to a GOS of 5 at 1 month. Conversely, the earlier consciousness returned, the better was the outcome. Among patients who awakened and regained their mental faculties within 1 day, nearly one-half achieved a GOS of 4 or 5, compared with only 14% among those who at 1 day remained vegetative or in coma. Among patients who survived three days, 60% who were awake and talked made a satisfactory recovery within the first month, compared with only 5% of those still vegetative or in a coma. Contrary to initial expectations, no consistent relationship emerged between age and prognosis either for the study as a whole or for individual illnesses. The sex of the patient had no apparent influence on outcome. Coma of 6 hours or more turned out to be such an innately serious state that in most cases it became difficult to predict accurately who would do well (i.e., make a moderate or good recovery) much before the third day of illness. By contrast, about one-third of patients destined to achieve a GOS of 1 or 2 showed overwhelmingly strong indications of that outcome on admission.

As Table 9–5 immediately discloses, a potentially bewildering amount of early clinical information showed an association with outcomes in patients with medical coma. To reduce this mass of data to manageable proportions and thereby sharpen the accuracy of prognosis for physicians working at the bedside, Levy and associates[32] constructed logic diagrams based on the actual outcomes of patients showing

certain signs at various time intervals (Figure 9–3). In constructing these decision trees, which give an estimate of prognosis based on actual experience, the most important concern was to be sure that signs denoted as implying a GOS prognosis of 1 or 2 described virtually no one (less than 3%) who achieved an ultimate GOS of 4 or 5. One can immediately recognize that an inaccurate estimate of prognosis could result in the curtailing of potentially useful treatment, a step to be avoided at almost all costs. Chi-square testing of the decision criteria given in Figure 9–3 against the actual findings and outcomes of the 500 patients indicates that all the discriminations have an accuracy of association with $p < 0.001$.

Even as early as 6 hours after the onset of coma, clinical signs identified 120 patients as having virtually no chance of regaining independent function (Figure 9–3A). Only one of 120 patients achieved even a brief functional return equivalent to a moderate level of disability, a 19-year-old woman with cardiac arrest associated with uremia who briefly improved before dying the following week. The remaining 380 patients could be divided on the basis of their clinical findings into groups with relatively better prognoses, the best having a 41% chance of attaining independent function. Similar discrimination was possible at 1 day (Figure 9–3B). At this time, 29 of the 87 patients with the poorest prognosis survived 2 more days and 10 survived at least a week; on the other hand, 24 patients could be predicted as recovering to an outcome of GOS 4 or 5, and two-thirds of these actually regained independent function. With the further passage of time (Figure 9–3C, D), success at identifying patients with a prognosis of GOS 4 or 5 improved even further.

Subsequent prospective evaluations of outcome in medical coma have generally confirmed the accuracy of these original studies. A prospective cohort study of 596 patients with nontraumatic coma identified five clinical variables that predicted 2-month mortality (Table 9–6).[33] This population reflected mostly patients in coma following cardiac arrest (31%), cerebral infarction, or intracerebral hemorrhage (36%) (other etiologies included subarachnoid hemorrhage, sepsis, neoplasm, and infections). Patients with four of five clinical findings of abnormal brainstem responses (absent pupillary responses, absent corneal

Table 9–5 **Best One-Month Outcome in 500 Patients in Medical Coma Versus Early Neurologic Signs—Original**

Time (and Number) of Subjects in Categories	Number (and Percentage) of Patients Having Poor Outcome (i.e., No Recovery or Vegetative State)	Number (and Percentage) of Patients Having Good Outcome (i.e., Moderate Disability or Good Recovery)
Admission		
a. All patients (500)	365 (73)	75 (15)
b. Any two absent: corneals, pupils, OC-OV (119)	117 (98)	1 (0.8)°
c. Remaining patients (381)	250 (66)	71 (19)
One day		
a. Surviving patients (387)	256 (66)	74 (19)
b. Any two absent: corneals, pupils, OV-OC, motor (86)	85 (99)	1 (1)°
c. OC or OV normal, or roving eye movements, or orienting eye movements (159)	64 (40)	58 (36)
d. Comprehensible words (25)		15 (60)
e. Voluntary motor responses (40)		20 (50)
Three Days		
a. Surviving patients (261)	135 (52)	71 (27)
b. Absence of any: corneals, pupils, OV-OC, spontaneous eye movements (63)	61 (97)	0
c. Presence of any of the following: (106)		
Comprehensive words (68)	1 (2)	47 (69)
Obeys commands (55)	0	36 (65)
Orienting eye movements (69)	3 (4)	48 (70)
Normal OC or OV (64)	5 (8)	43 (67)
Localizing motor response (93)	3 (3)	56 (60)
Seven Days		
a. Surviving patients (179)	63 (35)	63 (35)
b. Absence of any: corneals, pupils, OC-OV, spontaneous eye movements, motor response (24)	20 (83)	0
c. Presence of any of the following: (111)		
Comprehensive words (86)	0	62 (72)
Obeys commands (74)	0	49 (66)
Orienting eye movements (84)	3 (4)	59 (70)
Normal OC or OV (70)	4 (5.7)	60 (86)
Localizing motor response (100)	3 (3)	66 (66)

°This patient died within a month.

reflexes, and absent or dysconjugate roving eye movements), absent verbal response, absent withdrawal to pain, age older than 70 years, or a creatinine of greater than or equal to 1.5 mg/dL (132 μmol/L) had a 97% mortality at 2 months. An age-related worsening of prognosis was identified in distinction from the Plum and Levy study,[4] but may be partly confounded by comorbid systemic conditions. A prospective study of 169 patients older than 10 years with nontraumatic coma admitted to an intensive care unit found that 75% of those with hypoxic or ischemic injuries had died or remained comatose at 2 weeks[34] (Table 9–7).

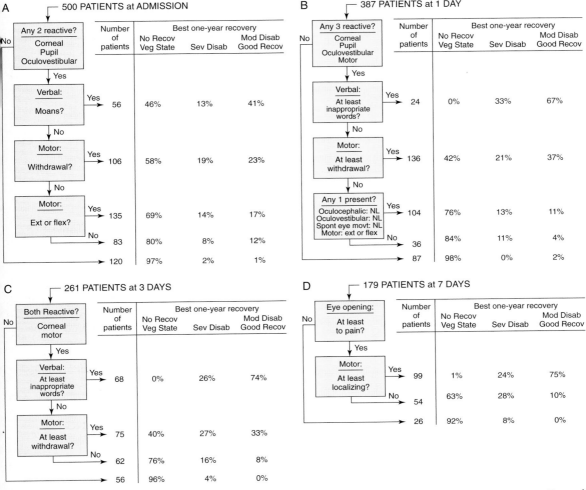

Figure 9–3. (A-D) The best 1-year outcome for 500 conventionally treated patients in coma from nontraumatic causes. For each time period following onset, the diagram correlates the degree of recovery with clinical signs. The numbers are, in most instances, sufficiently large to provide a basis for estimating prognosis among similarly affected patients in the future. (From Levy et al.,[4] with permission.)

How is one to act on these predictions? The physician, together with the patient's health care proxy and family, must decide. A patient who has been in coma for 6 hours from a known nonpharmacologic cause, without pupillary responses or eye movements, has essentially no chance of making a satisfactory recovery. Knowledge of this prognosis will deter many physicians from applying heroic and extraordinary measures of care. (Nevertheless, such patients may be candidates for well-controlled new or unconventional treatments, as conventional therapy offers such a dismal outcome.) Conversely, a seriously ill and still unresponsive patient who shows normal eye or motor signs at 1 to 3 days following cardiac arrest has about a 30% chance of recovering to a GOS of 4 or 5. This information should provide strong encouragement to intensive care staff members. The latter individuals often feel they are working blindly and with little chance of success when caring for patients who have suffered brain injury. Knowledge of a potentially favorable outcome greatly improves morale and the associated level of care.

Table 9–6 **Variables Correlated With Two-Month Mortality**

Risk Factor Present on Day Three	Two-Month Mortality, Number (%)	
	If Factor Present	If Factor Not Present
Abnormal brainstem function	88/99 (89)	83/136 (61)
Absent verbal response	151/175 (86)	23/57 (40)
Absent withdrawal to pain	122/136 (90)	52/96 (54)
Creatinine ≥132.6 μmol/L (1.5 mg/dL)	82/94 (87)	99/153 (65)
Age ≥70	93/111 (84)	88/136 (65)

From Hamel et al.,[33] with permission.

CARDIOPULMONARY ARREST/ HYPOXIC-ISCHEMIC ENCEPHALOPATHY

Several large studies have examined outcome in coma specifically following cardiac arrest. Data from 942 patients prospectively enrolled in the Brain Resuscitation Clinical Trials[35] (circa 1979 to 1994) demonstrated that loss of any of the cranial nerve reflexes following cardiac arrest significantly predicted poor outcome. Booth and associates[2] reviewed all available large studies of coma following cardiac arrest from 1966 to 2003 to assess the precision and accuracy of the physical examination in prognosis. They found that five clinical signs were strongly predictive of death, VS, or severe disability (GOS 1, 2, or 3): absent corneal reflexes, absent pupillary reflexes, absent withdrawal to painful stimuli, absent motor response at 24 hours, and absent motor response at 72 hours. Notably, no clinical examination finding strongly predicted a GOS of 4 or 5. In

the aggregate, the data shown in Table 9–8 support the algorithms shown in Figure 9–3 and add further details as well as time points. It should be recognized that the Booth et al. predictors aggregate severely disabled outcomes (GOS 3) with outcomes of death or permanent VS (GOS 1 and 2). Thus, careful explanation of the predicted outcomes is required if the physician uses these data to counsel families, as choices concerning severe disability may differ widely (see *family dynamics and philosophic considerations*, page 379).

ELECTROPHYSIOLOGIC TESTING IN HYPOXIC-ISCHEMIC ENCEPHALOPATHY

Although the physical examination gives a strong prediction of poor outcome, it does not accurately assess the extent of cortical injury. Electrophysiologic testing adds valuable data. SSEPs provide the best predictors of poor

Table 9–7 **Two-Week Outcome of Nontraumatic Coma and Coma Etiology**

Coma Etiology	Two-Week Outcome			
	No. (%)	% Awake	% Dead	% Coma
Hypoxic/ischemic	61 (36.1)	21.3	54.1	24.6
Metabolic or septic	37 (21.8)	32.4	48.7	18.9
Focal cerebral injury	38 (22.5)	34.2	47.4	18.4
Generalized cerebral injury	22 (13.0)	45.4	36.4	18.2
Drug induced	11 (6.5)	72.7	0	27.3
All	169 (100)	33.1	44.4	21.5

Modified from Sacco et al.,[34] with permission.

Table 9–8 Useful Clinical Findings in the Prognosis of Postcardiac Arrest Coma Organized by Time After Onset of Coma

Clinical Finding	LR* of Poor Neurologic Outcome (95% Confidence Interval)	
	Positive	Negative
Absent pupillary reflex	7.2 (1.9–28.0)	0.5 (0.4–0.6)
Absent motor response	3.5 (1.4–8.6)	0.6 (0.4–0.7)
Absent corneal reflex	3.2 (1.1–9.5)	0.7 (0.6–0.8)
Absent oculocephalic reflex	2.5 (1.3–4.8)	0.4 (0.3–0.6)
Absent spontaneous eye movement	2.2 (1.3–4.0)	0.4 (0.3–0.6)
ICS <4	2.2 (1.1–4.5)	0.2 (0.1–0.6)
GCS <5	1.4 (1.1–1.6)	0.3 (0.2–0.5)
Absent verbal effort	1.2 (0.9–1.6)	0.1 (0.0–0.7)
At 12 Hours		
Absent cough reflex	13.4 (4.4–40.3)	0.3 (0.2.-0.4)
Absent corneal reflex	9.1 (3.9–21.1)	0.3 (0.2–0.4)
Absent gag reflex	8.7 (4.0–18.9)	0.4 (0.4–0.5)
Absent pupillary reflex	4.0 (2.5–6.6)	0.5 (0.5–0.6)
GCS <5	3.5 (2.4–5.2)	0.4 (0.3–0.4)
Absent motor response	3.2 (2.2–4.6)	0.4 (0.3–0.5)
Absent withdrawal to pain	2.3 (1.9–3.1)	0.2 (0.1–0.2)
Absent verbal effort	1.6 (1.4–1.9)	0.1 (0.0–0.1)
At 24 Hours		
Absent cough reflex	84.6 (5.3–1342.0)	0.4 (0.3–0.5)
Absent gag reflex	24.9 (6.3–98.3)	0.5 (0.4–0.5)
GCS <5	8.8 (5.1–15.1)	0.4 (0.3–0.4)
Absent eye opening to pain	5.9 (3.9–9.0)	0.3 (0.3–0.4)
Absent spontaneous eye movement	3.5 (1.4–8.8)	0.5 (0.4–0.7)
Absent eye opening to pain	3.0 (1.5–6.2)	0.4 (0.3–0.5)
Absent oculocephalic reflex	2.9 (1.8–4.6)	0.5 (0.5–0.6)
Absent spontaneous eye movement	2.7 (2.1–3.4)	0.3 (0.2–0.3)
Absent verbal effort	2.4 (2.0–2.9)	0.1 (0.0–0.1)
At 48 Hours		
GCS <6	2.8 (1.3–5.9)	0.3 (0.1–0.5)
GCS <10	1.3 (1.0–1.7)	0.0 (0.0–0.7)
At 72 Hours		
Absent withdrawal to pain	36.5 (2.3–569.9)	0.3 (0.2–0.4)
Absent spontaneous eye movement	11.5 (1.7–79.0)	0.6 (0.5–0.7)
Absent verbal effort	7.4 (2.0–28.0)	0.3 (0.2–0.5)
Absent eye opening to pain	6.9 (1.8–27.0)	0.5 (0.4–0.6)
At 7 Days		
Absent withdrawal to pain	29.7 (1.9–466.0)	0.4 (0.3–0.6)
Absent verbal effort	14.1 (2.0–97.7)	0.4 (0.2–0.6)

GCS, Glasgow Coma Scale; ICS, Innsbruck Coma Scale; LR, likelihood ratio.
*Clinical findings that have a positive LR >2 and a lower confidence interval boundary >1 are presented with the corresponding negative LR.

Modified from Booth et al.,[2] with permission.

Table 9–9 **Somatosensory-Evoked Potentials in Anoxic-Ischemic Encephalopathy: Absent N20 Response**

Series	Day	Proportion With Sign	Proportion Recovering
Brunko and Zegers De Byl, 1987	<8 hours	30/50	0/30
Rothstein, 2000	<2 hours	19/40	0/19
Madl et al., 2000	<2 hours	22/66	0/22
Chen et al., 2000	1–3	12/34	0/12
Total	<3	83/190	0/83

From Young et al.,[23] with permission.

outcomes and are relatively insensitive to metabolic derangements and drug effects.[36] Bilateral loss of primary cortical somatosensory responses has been repeatedly confirmed to have a 100% specificity for outcomes no better than a permanent VS following anoxic injuries.[37,38] A recent review[23] found that of 176 patients with absent bilateral primary somatosensory responses (N20), none recovered past a permanent VS (Table 9–9). The robust correlation of bilateral loss of SSEPs and poor outcome reflects a close connection with the underlying degree of anoxic injury as indicated by autopsy studies.[39] Of 10 patients examined at autopsy who had SSEP measurements obtained within 48 hours of cardiac arrest, all seven with bilateral absence of the SSEPs had extensive anoxic-ischemic destruction of the cerebral cortex (with acute ischemic changes in patients with short survival, and frank necrosis of the pseudolaminar type in those patients with longer survival times). Two additional patients (one with delayed SSEPs and one with normal-latency SSEPs) showed patchy neuronal loss in the cerebral cortex. Importantly, although an index of better outcomes, preservation of normal-latency SSEPs following cardiac arrest is not a definite predictor of positive outcomes. Death or vegetative outcomes may occur in as many as 40% of cases where a normal N20 response is measured.[38]

Other electrophysiologic techniques, including EEG, brainstem auditory-evoked responses (BAERs), and transcranial motor-evoked responses, also have predictive value (see [23] for detailed review). EEG patterns are often suppressed early following anoxic injuries and a variety of signal abnormalities[22] correlate with poor outcomes; these include burst suppression, alpha-theta patterns, and generalized suppression or periodic patterns. The BAER test can identify severe brainstem injury, but does not address the outcome of cerebral cortical injury. Preservation of longer latency auditory-evoked responses that involve contributions from larger cerebral cortical networks may predict recovery of cerebral function with greater specificity. Both a late auditory response (N100) and the mismatch negativity (MMN) response have value in predicting outcome from coma following anoxic injury.[40] Other longer latency evoked responses such as the P300 and N400 have also been studied (see [22] for review).

PITFALLS IN THE EVALUATION OF COMA FOLLOWING CARDIOPULMONARY ARREST

Although prognosis in coma following cardiopulmonary arrest is generally accurate, pitfalls do exist. The following case illustrates an extreme, although not isolated, example from the literature.[41]

Patient 9–1

A 25-year-old asthmatic man collapsed at home and stopped breathing. The patient received cardiopulmonary resuscitation (CPR) from a family member for 6 minutes until emergency medical personnel arrived to find the patient without respiratory effort or palpable pulse. Electrocardiogram (ECG) showed a rate of 24 bpm; CPR and tracheal intubation were performed. Three minutes later the pulse was 107 bpm and spontaneous respirations were noted. Initial GCS was 3. In the emergency room the patient was unresponsive with dilated pupils that were responsive to light; spontaneous decorticate posturing was noted. The patient was sedated with propofol, given atracurium, and transferred to the intensive care unit (ICU). In the ICU the patient required mild pressor support and was noted to exhibit frequent myoclonic jerks of the head and all four limbs. EEG recordings revealed generalized status epilepticus. Theophylline levels were within the normal therapeutic range. Seizures were uncontrolled with phenytoin, midazolam, clonazepam, valproate, and $MgSO_4$, so that thiopental infusion producing burst suppression was required. After cessation of the thiopental drip, generalized alpha frequency activity was noted. On the sixth day the patient was extubated, given a Do Not Resuscitate (DNR) status, and transferred to the general neurology floor still with a GCS of 3. He subsequently gradually improved and had a GCS of 10 by day 16 with the recovery of head nodding and verbalization. His GCS reached 15 by the 19th week following the respiratory arrest. While EEG examinations showed progressive improvements, the patient continued to exhibit frequent myoclonic jerks and epileptiform activity despite multiple antiepileptic medication trials. Ultimately, this patient regained independent function.

This patient's case highlights the potential complexity of prognosis in coma even in circumstances that appear to predict poor outcome following cardiac arrest and severe hypoxic injury. A retrospective review of the history suggests several points for consideration. While the patient's young age, initial presence of pupillary light responses, and early return of spontaneous respiration were positive predictors, the presence of myoclonus and seizures with no history of epilepsy suggested severe hypoxic injury. As reviewed above, postanoxic myoclonus usually predicts a dismal prognosis,[42] but this is not invariably the case.[43] The early sedation and paralysis of the patient due to the seizure activity may have masked improvement in level of consciousness within the first 6 hours, and the extensive use of different antiepileptic medications may have mimicked the pattern of alpha coma, a finding that otherwise carries a greater than 90% mortality in the setting of anoxic injury.[44]

This patient demonstrates the limitations of obtaining complete information from events in the field and unequivocal separation of the effects of primary injury versus potential confounds introduced by methods of treatment. A pulseless patient may still have some undetected circulatory activity, or have lost perfusion just prior to evaluation, making accurate estimate of duration of hypoxia problematic. A similar case involving seizures and myoclonus following a cardiac arrest has been reported, with late improvement on day 16 after remaining at a GCS of 5 until that point.[45]

Finally, a postictal state can severely depress brainstem function, and tonic seizures can simulate flexion or extension posturing, whereas single epileptic jerks can be difficult to distinguish from myoclonus. Cardiac arrest from a seizure-induced cardiac arrhythmia[46] can further complicate the picture.

Vascular Disease

STROKE

Prognosis in coma following stroke depends on the arterial territory affected by the stroke that produces bilateral hemispheric dysfunction as detailed in Chapter 4. Wijdicks and Rabinstein[47] surveyed the literature of prognostic factors for severe stroke from 1966 to 2003. They found no evidence-based studies better than class III to indicate prognosis, although several suggestive clinical and radiologic features were identified. Large proximal vessel occlusions causing diffuse hemispheric edema and midline shift carry a grave prognosis with a nearly 90% mortality when the shift of the septum pellucidum was greater than 12 mm.[48] Patients with coma caused by acute basilar occlusions may recover[49] (see Chapter 2), whereas those with coma due to hypertensive pontine hemorrhages usually do not.[50]

SUBARACHNOID HEMORRHAGE

Coma resulting from spontaneous subarachnoid hemorrhage (SAH) has a grave prognosis. The World Federation of Neurological Surgeons (WFNS) grades SAH using the GCS[51] (see also [52]) (Table 9–10). Although brief loss of consciousness is common, coma is a relatively uncommon sign in patients who reach the hospital with SAH; two-thirds present with WFNS grade III examinations or better.

Table 9–10 **Grading System for Subarachnoid Hemorrhage**

Grade	GCS Score	Presence of any Motor Deficit
I	15	None
II	14–15	None
III	14–13	Present
IV	12–7	Present or absent
V	6–3	Present or absent

World Federation of Neurological Surgeons score is indexed by Glasgow Coma Scale (GCS) and evidence of identifiable motor deficits.

From the World Federation of Neurological Surgeons,[51] with permission

However, as many as one-half of the patients presenting with grades I or II deteriorate from vasospasm, rebleeding, hydrocephalus, or brain edema. About 10% (range 3% to 17%) of patients die before reaching medical attention and another 10% prior to hospital evaluation. The overall mortality is 40% to 50%.[53]

GCS is a good predictor of outcome from SAH if the patient's age, the amount of blood on CT scan, the location of the aneurysm (worse for posterior circulation sites compared with anterior circulation),[53] and secondary complications following the initial rupture are also factored in. A high percentage of patients with grades IV and V die from secondary complications if they remain in coma for 2 weeks or more.

Rebleeding of an aneurysm causing coma and depression or loss of brainstem reflexes carries a mortality rate of 50%. In one study, bilateral loss of pupillary responses carried a 95% mortality rate. Electrophysiologic measurements have also shown some utility in the prognosis of SAH; loss of BAERs and SSEPs correlate with poor grades on examination.[54,55]

Central Nervous System Infection

Coma was present on admission in 14% of 696 patients with bacterial meningitis[56] (see also page 262). Obtundation on admission was a significant risk factor for death or a GOS less than 4, as were age older than 60 years, hypotension, seizures within 24 hours (often associated with a low serum sodium), and cere-brospinal fluid (CSF) abnormalities including decreased glucose concentration or elevation of the CSF protein (greater than or equal to 250 mg/dL). In most cases, death was a result of herniation, occasionally following an ill-advised lumbar puncture. Some investigators have suggested that the presence of coma is the best predictor of morbidity from acute meningitis.[57] Coma is often the result of increased ICP resulting from alteration of the blood-barrier by toxins (vasogenic edema), impaired resorption of CSF (interstitial edema), or venous or arterial occlusions (infarction with cytotoxic edema).[58] A brain abscess causing coma also has a poor prognosis (GOS less than 4)[59]; herniation is the principal cause of coma with a 60% mortality rate.[60]

Acute Disseminated Encephalomyelitis

Acute disseminated encephalomyelitis (ADEM) (see also page 366) is a monophasic autoimmune demyelinating disease most commonly affecting children and young adults that follows viral or bacterial illnesses or may arise postvaccination.[61] Although prognosis for ADEM has historically been considered poor, current experience reflects that most patients (range 55% to 90% across studies) will recover fully or with minor neurologic disabilities. The improved prognosis may reflect either the increased frequency of diagnosis of relatively mild cases, which often can be demonstrated on magnetic resonance imaging (MRI), or perhaps the tendency to treat patients with corticosteroids. Most patients with ADEM improve within 6 months, although many documented cases showed longer recovery times.

Hepatic Coma

Hepatic coma develops either as an inexorable stage in progressive hepatic failure or as a more reversible process in patients with portal systemic shunts when increased loads of nitrogenous substances are suddenly presented into the circulation (see Chapter 5). Prognosis in hepatic coma depends on the cause, the acuteness and severity of the liver failure, and the presence or absence of dysfunction of other organs. The prognosis is far worse in fulminant hepatic failure than in coma associated with chronic cirrhosis or portacaval shunting. Among patients with nontraumatic coma, those with hepatic encephalopathy demonstrated the best chance for recovery (33%).[4]

Survival also correlates with age in patients with infectious and serum hepatitis. Patients with chronic hepatocellular disease often drift in and out of encephalopathy, a situation that can be managed by correction of intercurrent processes such as infection or reduction of circulating nitrogenous load. If no exogenous factor can be identified, the presence of encephalopathy is far more ominous and correlates with high mortality; approximately 50% of patients with cirrhosis die within 1 year of demonstrating encephalopathy.[62]

Depressant Drug Poisoning

Most fatal intentional depressant drug poisonings occur outside the hospital. Once such patients reach treatment, experienced centers worldwide generally report an overall mortality among patients with altered consciousness of less than 1% (Table 9–7). The death rate climbs to approximately 5% in those with grade 3 to 4 coma. The mortality can be substantially higher when institutions treat only small numbers of patients or lack experience or proper facilities. Adverse prognostic factors in depressant drug coma include an advanced age, the presence of complicating medical illnesses (especially systemic infections, hepatic insufficiency, and heart failure), and lengthy coma. Alkaline diuresis (for phenobarbital), hemodialysis, and charcoal hemoperfusion all have been reported to shorten coma and improve prognosis for patients with severe poisoning, especially from phenobarbital. Barring unexpected complications, patients recovering from depressant drug poisoning suffer no residual brain damage even after prolonged coma lasting 5 days or more. Rare exceptions to this rule occur in overdose patients who suffer aspiration pneumonia or cardiac arrest (e.g., during tracheal or gastric intubation). A small number of patients develop cutaneous pressure sores or pressure neuropathies from prolonged periods of immobility during the period of immobile coma before the victim is found and brought to hospital; this may be particularly common with barbiturate overdoses.

VEGETATIVE STATE

The *vegetative state* (also called *coma vigil* or *apallic state*) denotes the recovery of a crude cycling of arousal states heralded by the appearance of "eyes-open" periods in an unresponsive patient.[63] Very few patients remain in eyes-closed coma for more than 10 to 14 days; vegetative behavior usually replaces coma by that time. Patients in VS, like comatose patients, show no evidence of awareness of self or their environment, but do retain brainstem regulation of cardiopulmonary function and visceral autonomic regulation. The term *persistent vegetative state* is now commonly reserved for patients remaining in that state for at least 30 days (see ANA Committee on Ethical Affairs 1993). As indicated in the paragraphs below, there are no clear criteria for determining when PVS becomes permanent.

One reason for the inability to predict permanence early in the course of PVS is that patients usually have badly damaged cerebral hemispheres combined with a relatively intact brainstem. Such a combination during the early days of illness causes coma with relatively good brainstem function, a picture similar to patients with reversible cerebral injury.

Since the publication of the third edition of *Stupor and Coma*, guidelines to aid construction of prognosis in VS have advanced greatly.[64–66] The Multisociety Task Force on PVS,[64,65] a joint commission composed of neurologists, neurosurgeons, and other specialists, organized a comprehensive review of outcomes of patients with prolonged VS using GOS criteria. Outcomes of 434 adult and 106 pediatric patients with TBI and 169 adult and 45 pediatric patients with nontraumatic etiologies were assessed. Figure 9–4 displays data from the TBI group for adults. For patients in VS for at least 1 month, 52% had recovered consciousness at 1 year postinjury (some 33% of the patients had recovered earlier than 3 months from the time of injury). If adult TBI patients remained in VS at 3 months, the percentage recovering consciousness at 1 year dropped to 35%, and to 16% for VS lasting at least 6 months. For pediatric patients with a TBI-induced VS for 1 month, 62% recovered consciousness at 1 year; if VS persisted for 3 months, this percentage dropped only to 56%, and to 32% for patients in VS for at least 6

Table 9–11. **Prognosis of Vegetative State (VS) in Traumatic and Anoxic Brain Injury**

Age	N TBI*	N ABI*	Dead (%) CI (99%) TBI	ABI	VS (%) CI (99%) TBI	ABI	Conscious (%) CI (99%) TBI	ABI	Independent (%) CI (99%) TBI	ABI
VS at 1 Month										
Adults	434	169	33	53	15	32	52	15	24	4
Children	106	45	9	22	29	65	62	13	27	6
VS at 3 Months										
Adults	218	77	35 (27–43)	46 (31–61)	30 (22–38)	47 (32–62)	35 (27–44)	8 (2–19)	16 (10–22)	1 (0–4)
Children	50	31	14 (1–27)	3 (0–11)	30 (13–47)	94 (82–100)	56 (37–74)	3 (0–11)	32 (15–49)	0
VS at 6 Months										
Adults	123	50	32 (40–64)	28 (12–44)	52 (40–64)	72 (56–88)	16 (9–27)	0	4 (0–9)	0
Children	28	30	14 (30–78)	0	54 (30–78)	97 (89–100)	32 (12–58)	3 (0–11)	11 (0–26)	0

°TBI, traumatic brain injury; ABI, anoxic brain injury.
Adapted from Jennet[66] and the Multisociety Task Force.[65]

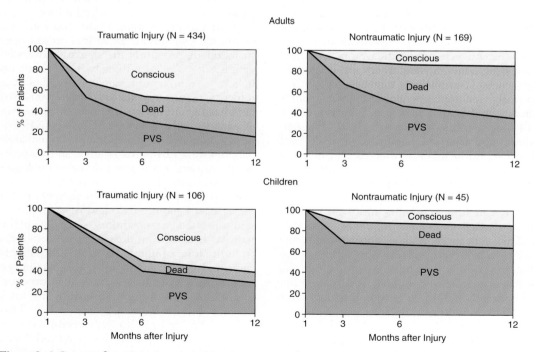

Figure 9–4. Outcome for patients in a persistent vegetative state after a traumatic or nontraumatic injury. See also Table 9–11. (From the Multisociety Task Force,[64] with permission.)

months. The outcome of "conscious" per se does not reflect level of disability. However, the Task Force review indicated that for adults, within the 52% of patients recovering consciousness after 1 month in VS, only 24% became independent by GOS criteria. This figure dropped to 16% for VS lasting 3 months and to only 4% if taken out to at least 6 months.

Not surprisingly, nontraumatic VS carries a far less optimistic prognosis. Figure 9–4 shows comparison percentages for adult and pediatric patients with nontraumatic VS. For adult VS patients remaining in VS at 1 month, only 15% regained consciousness (with only 4% independent by GOS). These percentages worsened to 8% and 0% for patients remaining in a nontraumatic VS for 3 and 6 months, respectively.

Based on these data, the Task Force paper suggested that VS after 12 months following TBI, or 3 months following an anoxic injury, should be considered essentially permanent. However, it is important to recognize that a small number of patients may recover from VS beyond these time points.[67–69] Such late recovery past the cutoffs for permanent VS from both anoxic and traumatic etiologies has generally been to levels of severe disability, including the minimally conscious state.[66] Nevertheless, application of these statistics to individual cases can be risky, unless independent evidence of the mechanism of brain injury is available, as rare cases of late recovery continue to be reported. The uncertainty in prognosis in such cases highlights the need for better methods, such as direct measurements of cerebral function, to help identify cases where recovery is likely.

Mortality is very high within the first year; approximately one-third of patients die.[64,65] If patients remain alive after a year, mortality per year is low and some patients may continue to live for many years.[66] Plum and Schiff studied one patient who had remained in PVS for 25 years (see Figure 9–8). Most patients in VS die from infection of the pulmonary system or urinary tract.

Clinical, Imaging, and Electrodiagnostic Correlates of Prognosis in the Vegetative State

A few clinical signs or confirmatory tests, including those negative predictors for coma in general (as reviewed previously), help predict the prognosis of VS. As noted, abnormal SSEPs reliably indicate cortical damage and a high probability of remaining in VS following anoxic and traumatic brain injuries. However, normal evoked responses do not predict recovery. In a study of 124 patients in VS or MCS following TBI, three variables predicted recovery of ability to follow commands: (1) initial score on the Disability Rating Scale (DRS), (2) rate of change on the DRS measure in the first 2 weeks of observation, and (3) the time of admission to a rehabilitation program following injury.[70]

Several structural and functional correlates of VS have been examined. A prospective study of MRI imaging correlates of 80 patients remaining in VS following TBI at 6 to 8 weeks (with MRI and clinical follow-up at 2, 3, 6, 9, and 12 months) found that 42 patients who remained in VS at 1 year showed that structural injuries within the corpus callosum and dorsolateral brainstem significantly predicted nonrecovery (214-fold and sevenfold higher probability of nonrecovery from VS, respectively, based on adjusted odds ratios accounting for age, GCS, pupillary dysfunction, and number of brain lesions).[71] Overall, this model achieved a classification rate of 87.5% for identifying patients who would not recover past VS.

Quantitative fluorodeoxyglucose-positron emission tomography (FDG-PET) studies measuring resting cerebral metabolism have consistently demonstrated that global cerebral metabolism is markedly reduced to 40% to 50% of normal metabolic rates in most VS patients (see page 365). Unfortunately, early identification of low metabolic activity is not a clear predictor of outcome and some patients have recovered consciousness despite significant remaining abnormalities in resting metabolic level.[72] The N-acetylaspartate (NAA)-to-creatine (Cr) ratio on magnetic resonance spectroscopy (MRS) of the thalamus is low in all patients in VS, but lower in those who do not recover[73]; however, only a few patients have been studied.

Efforts to predict outcome or characterize VS using EEG have been disappointing. EEG studies may remain abnormal as patients improve or, conversely, improve when patients do not.[74] Event-related potentials (ERPs) may hold more promise. These potentials require cortical processing of stimuli that can be passively presented to subjects in VS. The responses are long latency with peak activation usually several hundred milliseconds after stimulation and are not strictly time locked to the stimulus onset. Long-latency auditory cortical potentials (N100, P150), the P300 response, and the mismatch negativity (MMN) ERPs have each shown some potential for providing evidence of recovery. The P300 response can be elicited by inclusion of an "oddball" tone in an otherwise monotonous presentation of repeated identical tones. The MMN is an early component of the auditory response to the oddball stimulus that is attention independent and reliably induced following the N100 auditory cortex potential, an early primary auditory evoked response. In a study of 346 patients in coma for 12 months with outcomes divided into VS versus all categories better than VS (including MCS), N100 and MMN were strong predictors of recovery past VS; no patient with MMN in this cohort remained in VS. If the electrophysiologic variables were combined with information about the pupillary light reflex, the probability of recovery past VS reached 89.9%.[40] However, other studies have raised questions about the specificity of preserved ERP responses[75] in VS.

MINIMALLY CONSCIOUS STATE

The minimally conscious state[76] identifies a condition of severely impaired consciousness with minimal but definite behavioral evidence of self or environmental awareness. Table 9–12 provides the criteria for the diagnosis of MCS. Like VS, MCS often exists as a transitional state arising during recovery from coma or during the worsening of progressive neurologic disease. In some patients, however, it may be a permanent condition. A few studies have examined differences in outcome between VS and MCS. Giacino and Kalmar reported retrospective findings in 55 VS patients and 49 MCS patients evaluated at 1, 3, 6, and 12 months following either traumatic or nontraumatic injuries.[77] Both presented with similar levels of disability at 1 month postinjury. The MCS patients, however, had significantly better outcomes as measured by the Disability Rating Scale compared with outcomes for VS patients at 1 year, particularly in the TBI patients. Strauss and colleagues[78] retrospectively studied life expectancy of a large number of children (ages 3 to 15) in VS ($N = 564$) and

Table 9–12 Aspen Working Group Criteria for the Clinical Diagnosis of the Minimally Conscious State

Evidence of limited but clearly discernible self or environmental awareness on a reproducible or sustained basis, as demonstrated by one or more of the following behaviors:

1. Simple command following
2. Gestural or verbal "yes/no" responses (independent of accuracy)
3. Intelligible verbalization
4. Purposeful behavior including movements or affective behaviors in contingent relation to relevant stimuli. Examples include:
   a. Appropriate smiling or crying to relevant visual or linguistic stimuli
   b. Response to linguistic content of questions by vocalization or gesture
   c. Reaching for objects in appropriate direction and location
   d. Touching or holding objects by accommodating to size and shape
   e. Sustained visual fixation or tracking as response to moving stimuli

From Giacino et al.,[76] with permission.

MCS, dividing the latter into two groups: immobile MCS ($N = 705$) and mobile MCS (3,806). A significant increase in the percentage of patients still alive at 8 years was noted for the mobile MCS group (81%) compared to the immobile MCS (65%) or the VS (63%) group; the latter two were statistically indistinguishable. Lammi and associates[79] examined 18 MCS patients 2 to 5 years after injury and found a marked heterogeneity of outcome despite prolonged duration of MCS after TBI. Most of their patients regained functional independence, but there was a poor correlation between duration of MCS and outcome. In general, clinical and electrodiagnostic tests have not yet been developed for use in the diagnosis and prognosis of MCS outside of a research context (see below for discussion).

MCS also includes some forms of the clinical syndrome of *akinetic mutism* (Box 9–1) and other less well-characterized disorders of consciousness. At least two different identifiable groups of patients are considered exemplars of akinetic mutism. Although occasionally confused with VS, classical akinetic mutism resembles a state of constant hypervigilance. The patients appear attentive and vigilant but

Box 9–1 Akinetic Mutism Versus "Slow Syndrome"

The term *akinetic mutism* originated with Cairns and colleagues.[80] They described a young woman who, although appearing wakeful, became mute and rigidly motionless when a craniopharyngiomatous cyst expanded to compress the walls of her third ventricle and the posterior medial-ventral surface of the frontal lobe. The patient appeared to be unconscious; there was no spasticity. After the cyst was drained, she recovered full awareness but possessed no memory of the "unconscious" period. Eye movements were not described in this woman but most documented cases of this type reveal seemingly attentive, conjugate eye movements. Oculocephalic stimulation may elicit some lateral gaze.

Subsequent observations have shown that similar findings can be produced by lesions of the medial-basal prefrontal area, the anterior cingulate cortex, the medial prefrontal regions supplied by the anterior cerebral arteries, and the rostral basal ganglia. A similar syndrome can rarely be a feature of untreated, rigid Parkinson's disease or prion disease.[81]

The hyperattentive form of akinetic mutism is typically seen in patients with bilateral lesions of the anterior cingulate and medial prefrontal cortices, as occurs after rupture of an anterior communicating artery aneurysm.[82] The associated injury may sometimes be accompanied by injury to the hypothalamus and anterior pallidum. Castaigne and associates[83] and Segarra[84] introduced "akinetic mutism" to describe the behavior of patients suffering structural injuries affecting the medial-dorsal thalamus extending into the mesencephalic tegmentum. The patients suffered severe memory loss and demonstrated apathetic behavior. Although such patients exhibit severe global disturbances of consciousness, they are not categorized as minimally conscious because they are capable of communication. To mitigate confusion, we use the term *slow syndrome*[85] to describe patients who appear apathetic and hypersomnolent but are able to move and may speak with understandable words.[86] Unlike akinetic mute patients, they are not semi-rigid and lack the appearance of vigilance. Subcortical lesions that may produce the slow syndrome include bilateral lesions of the paramedian anterior or posterior thalamus and basal forebrain; the mesencephalic reticular formation including periaqueductal gray matter, caudate nuclei (or either caudate in isolation), and globus pallidus interna; or selective interruption of the medial forebrain bundle.

A common denominator of akinetic mute states may be damage to the cortico-striato-pallidal-thalamocortical loops that are critical for the function of the frontal lobes.[87] The prefrontal cortex is served by a loop including the ventral striatum, ventral pallidum, and mediodorsal nucleus of the thalamus; akinetic mutism can result from bilateral damage at any level of this system.[87] Similarly, bilateral injury to the nigrostriatal bundle in the lateral hypothalamus may produce a state of akinetic mutism that is reversible with dopaminergic agonists.[88] At least partial cognitive function can be recovered following restricted bilateral injuries to the paramedian thalamus and mesencephalon.[83,84,89,90] remain motionless with robust preservation of visual tracking in the form of smooth pursuit movements (or optokinetic responses). Limited preservation of brief visual fixation can be accepted in VS, but robust and consistent visual tracking as seen in *akinetic mutism* is absent in VS.[66]

Patient 9–2

A 47-year-old right-handed man was brought to the ICU with progressive somnolence and unresponsiveness. Neurologic examination revealed bilateral third nerve palsy, fluctuating bradycardia with hypertension, and extensor posturing to pain. The initial CT scan (Figure 9–5A) revealed a large mass lesion centered on the mesencephalon with surrounding edema. Intracranial lymphoma was suspected and confirmed by biopsy. The patient received cranial irradiation, IV steroids, and chemotherapy. A posttreatment MRI (Figure 9–5B) demonstrated resolution of mass effect with high signal abnormalities within the upper mesencephalon and hypothalamus. The patient appeared alert but did not initiate communication. He occasionally displayed sudden periods of agitated behavior. Responses to simple questions were markedly delayed, but correct using yes and no answers. Physical examination was notable for waxy flexibility as well as rigidity, and spontaneous movements were minimal and limited to the left upper extremity.

EEG showed periods of frontal intermittent rhythmic delta activity and mild generalized slowing. An HmPAO single photon emission computed tomography (SPECT) scan revealed diffuse profound frontal bihemispheric hypoperfusion (left greater than right, see Figure 9–5C). The patient's clinical state did not improve prior to death from a systemic infection.

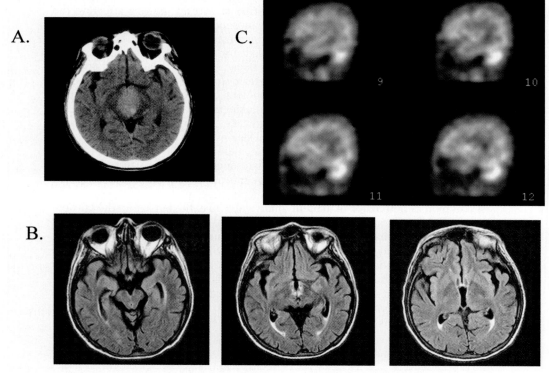

Figure 9–5. Akinetic mutism seen in Patient 9–2. (A) Computed tomography scan demonstrating large mesencephalic mass with surrounding edema. (B) Series of magnetic resonance axial images following treatment with steroids and reduction of mesencephalic lesion. Middle image shows high-signal abnormalities in the ventral midbrain. (C) Single photon emission tomography imaging demonstrates diffuse cerebral hypoperfusion with relative sparing of cerebellar blood flow. (Images courtesy of Drs. Ayeesha Kamal and N. Schiff.)

Autopsy of brain was normal except for the midbrain, hypothalamus, and left paramedian thalamus, which showed infiltration of lymphoma cells and necrosis in the midline of the midbrain extending rostrally into the left thalamus to involve the intralaminar nuclei and surrounding tissue.

Late Recoveries From the Minimally Conscious State

Word-of-mouth stories and news reports sometimes claim dramatic recovery from prolonged coma or VS. Invariably, these reports generate wide public interest and much confusion concerning the difference between coma and VS, as well as between diagnosis and prognosis. The Multisociety Task Force[64,65] examined 14 cases from the media and found that the majority of these "late" recoveries from VS fell within their guidelines (i.e., less than 3 months following an anoxic injury or 12 months following a traumatic brain injury in an adult). Nonetheless, as noted above, a few rare, well-documented late recoveries underscore the statistical nature of the guidelines for prognosis of permanent VS. However, most reports of late recovery from "coma" involve very late transition of MCS patients to emergence (see page 373). There are no data to allow guidelines for the expected duration of MCS. Some MCS patients harbor significant residual capacities as demonstrated by wide fluctuation of cognitive function.[91] The term *minimally conscious state* seems most appropriate; alternatives include *minimal, responsive state* and *minimal awareness state*.[92] Minimal responsiveness as assessed at the bedside may belie considerable cognitive capacities without further evaluation of etiologic mechanisms, including normal cognitive function as present in the locked-in state, discussed below.

LOCKED-IN STATE

A related and important issue is late recovery of consciousness in patients with severe motor and sensory impairment leading to the locked-in or partial locked-in state (condition with severe motor disability approximating the traditional definition). The locked-in state is not

a disorder of consciousness, as reviewed in Chapter 1. Nonetheless, because most cases of the locked-in state are due to a pontine injury, it is common for patients to experience an initial coma (see [93] for an example) or to respond inconsistently during the initial period of the injury similar to MCS. In a survey of 44 locked-in patients, the mean time of diagnosis was 2.5 months after onset; in more than one-half of these cases, a family member and not a physician first recognized the condition.[94] Furthermore, investigators working with locked-in patients often report early counseling of withdrawal of care either because of an incorrect diagnosis or based on physician attitudes without a careful and vetted informed consent process that includes a review of the available information on quality of life obtained from surveys of patients in this condition.[94,95] While it is quite reasonable to doubt that most people would want to trade a normal existence for that of a locked-in patient, the important question is whether a locked-in patient would rather live or die. Quality-of-life assessments administered to locked-in patients provide a source of information for patients and families as do written first-person accounts, several of which have become well known.[96] Doble and colleagues[95] reported on 5-, 10-, and 20-year survival (83%, 83%, and 40%, respectively) and quality of life in 29 patients. Among several notable findings, these investigators found that 12 patients remained living 11 years after the study onset; seven of these patients described "satisfaction with life," five were noted to exhibit occasional depressive symptoms, but none held a DNR order. Leon-Carrion and associates[94] described quality-of-life measures in more detail in their survey of 44 locked-in patients (Table 9–13). The majority of these patients (86%) described a good capacity to maintain attention, nearly half (47%) described their mood as "good," most (81%) met with friends at least twice a month, and 30% could maintain sexual relations (Table 9–13).

Quality of life was also assessed in 17 chronic (i.e., more than 1 year) locked-in patients who used eye movements or blinking as a principal mode of communication, lived at home, and had a mean duration of locked-in state of 6 years (range 2 to 16 years).[97,98] Self-scored perception of mental health (evaluating mental well-being and psychologic distress) and personal general health were not significantly

Table 9–13 **Functional Measurements in a Cohort of Locked-in Patients (N = 44)**

Variable	%
Cognitive Functioning	
Level of attention	
• Good	86.0
• Tends to sleep	9.0
• Normally awake	2.3
• Sleeps most of the time	2.3
Can pay attention >15 minutes	95.3
Can watch and follow a film on TV	95.3
Can say what day it is	97.6
Can read	76.7
Has a visual deficit	14.0
Has memory problems	18.6
Emotions and Feelings	
Mood state	
• Good	47.5
• Bad	5.0
• Depressed	12.5
• Other	35.0
Is more sensitive since onset	85.0
Laughs or cries more easily	87.8
Sexuality	
Has sexual desire	61.1
Can maintain sexual relations	30.0
Communication	
Can emit sounds	78.0
Can communicate with or without technical aid	65.8
Social Activities	
Enjoys going out	73.2
Participates in social activities	14.3
Watches television normally	23.8
Participates in other family activities	61.9
Is accompanied out once or twice a week	61.9
Meets with friends at least twice a month	81.0

lower than values from age-matched French control subjects. Importantly, perception of mental health and the presence of physical pain correlated with the frequency of suicidal thoughts (r = −0.67 and 0.56, respectively, $p < 0.05$), indicating the importance of proper pain management in chronic locked-in patients who are frequently undertreated. At present,

there are three European societies for locked-in-patients with a membership exceeding 300 persons (http://alis-asso.fr/).

MECHANISMS UNDERLYING OUTCOMES OF SEVERE BRAIN INJURY: NEUROIMAGING STUDIES AND CONCEPTUAL FRAMEWORKS

The above discussion details the problems of diagnostic accuracy and prognosis for disorders of consciousness. At present, careful clinical evaluations combined in some instances with structural imaging criteria, or measurements of early cortical sensory responses, remain the foundation for decision making. Available guidelines invariably indicate likelihoods of death or VS as outcomes rather than providing reliable indices of potential for functional recoveries with or without persistent disabilities. In large part this is a consequence of the fact that preserved brainstem function may only herald PVS. Moreover, it is clear that in the aggregate, the clinical neurologic examination and assessments of structural brain integrity provide only limited insight into the neurophysiologic mechanisms of coma, VS, or MCS. This is because the functional impairment of distributed neuronal populations of the cerebral cortex, basal ganglia, and thalamus underlying the conditions often cannot be adequately assessed by these methods. Neuroimaging techniques that can directly assess functional changes within these cerebral networks hold significant promise to ultimately improve diagnostic accuracy and understanding of the pathophysiology of the severely injured brain (see [99] for review).

Expanded use of neuroimaging techniques for evaluating functional outcomes of patients recovering from coma will likely have the greatest impact on the category of severe disability. This broad category includes within its limits patients who, while not permanently unconscious, as in the chronic VS, may nonetheless never regain a capacity to communicate, as well as other patients near the functional borderline of independence in activities of daily living. More than 20 years ago, the third edition of *Stupor and Coma* commented that the overly broad definition of severe disability needed significant refinement. As discussed above, recent efforts to define MCS are a step in this direction. The significance of identifying the physiologic mechanisms underlying different functional outcomes within the category of severe disability is that this knowledge will lead to a better understanding of the necessary and sufficient neurologic substrates to recover consciousness and varying levels of cognitive capacity. Just as the concept of brain death clarified the concept of death, MCS and other future subdivisions of the category of severe disability will force us to consider the concept of consciousness more precisely.

FUNCTIONAL IMAGING OF THE PERSISTENT VEGETATIVE STATE

Levy and associates[100] provided the first experimental evidence supporting the clinical hypothesis that patients in VS were unconscious. Using FDG-PET, seven patients in PVS were compared to three patients in the locked-in state and 18 normal subjects. In PVS patients, cerebral metabolic rates were globally reduced by 50% or more. Regional cerebral blood flow measurements showed a similar but more variable pattern of global reduction. Subsequent studies have confirmed these findings, with an average of less than 50% of normal metabolic rates in most VS patients studied (reduced further to 30% to 40% in cases of hypoxic-ischemic etiology).[101–105] Comparable reductions are identified during generalized anesthesia[106,107] and in stage IV sleep in normal individuals.[108] The small number of patients in the locked-in state (three) in the Levy study had a low average metabolic rate, but recent quantitative FDG-PET studies have demonstrated essentially normal resting metabolic rates in the cerebrum, even acutely.[99] Cerebellar metabolic rates were low, consistent with the lack of motor outflow in the locked-in state.[98]

More sensitive imaging techniques have recently been applied to the evaluation of PVS patients. They reveal a marked loss of distributed network processing in VS.[99,104,109] Elementary auditory and somatosensory stimuli fail to produce brain activation outside of primary sensory cortices (Figure 9–6). The data suggest multiple functional disconnections along the auditory or somatosensory cortical pathways and support the inference that the residual cortical activity seen in PVS patients does not reflect awareness. The findings are consistent with evidence of early sensory processing in PVS patients as measured by evoked potential studies, but loss of later components[39]; they suggest that VS/PVS correlates with failure of sensory information to propagate beyond the earliest stages of cortical processing. Preliminary studies discussed below indicate that MCS patients show wider activation of cortical networks, findings that may help ultimately distinguish the conditions among patients with severe sensory and motor impairments limiting behavioral assessments (e.g., spastic contractions and blindness).

Atypical Behavioral Features in the Persistent Vegetative State

Stereotyped behavior, typically limbic displays of crying, smiling, or other emotional patterns that are not related to environmental stimuli, occur in some VS patients. Occasionally, other fragments of behavior that may appear semi-purposeful, or inconsistently related to environmental stimuli, arise in VS/PVS patients. Neuroimaging studies, including FDG-PET, magnetoencephalography (MEG), and functional MRI (fMRI), have identified residual cerebral circuits underlying such isolated behavioral fragments.[105,110,117] One remarkable patient studied had remained in the PVS for 20 years but infrequently expressed single words (typically epithets) not related to environmental stimulation (Figure 9–7C). Two other patients in this group revealed similar isolated metabolic activity that could be correlated with unusual behavioral patterns.[105] These data provide novel evidence for the modular organization of the brain and suggest that preservation of residual cerebral activity following severe brain injuries is not random. Regional preservation of cerebral metabolic activity likely reflects both preservation of anatomic connectivity and endogenous neuronal firing patterns of remnant but incomplete networks.

Further study of this patient showed that islands of higher resting brain metabolism included Heschl's gyrus (Figure 9–8), Broca's area, Wernicke's area, and the left anterior basal ganglia (caudate nucleus, possibly putamen). Despite limited amounts of remaining left thalamus identified by MRI that expressed

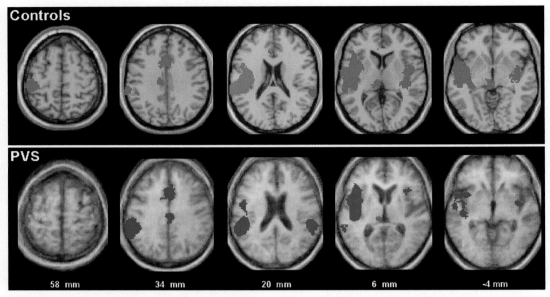

Figure 9–6. Somatosensory stimulation in the vegetative state. Top row: Brain activation patterns from normal subjects, shown in red, that were elicited by noxious stimulation (super-threshold electrical stimulation experienced as "painful"; subtraction stimulation-rest). Bottom row: Brain activation patterns from the persistent vegetative state (PVS), again shown in red, that were elicited by same noxious stimulation method (subtraction stimulation-rest). Blue regions indicate areal differences in network activation showing region less active in patients than in controls (interaction [stimulation vs. rest] × [patient vs. control]). All regions of activation are projected onto transverse sections of a normalized brain magnetic resonance imaging (MRI) template in controls and on the mean MRI of the patients (distances are relative to the bicommissural plane). (From Laureys et al.,[109] with permission.)

a very low metabolic rate, incompletely preserved MEG patterns of spontaneous and evoked gamma-band responses were seen. Taken together, these imaging data suggest the modular sparing of cortical networks associated with language functions.[117] Nevertheless, despite this patient, any verbal output suggests function better than vegetative until proved otherwise.

Another patient, a 26-year-old man, remained in a behaviorally unremarkable VS for 6 years following a motor vehicle accident (Figure 9–8A). MRI T1 images revealed bilateral paramedian thalamic injury, severe bilateral infarction of the tegmental mesencephalon, and diffuse white matter injury. However, nearly normal cerebral cortical metabolism was measured by quantitative FDG-PET in the brain. EEG showed diffuse low-voltage, low-frequency activity that did not change with arousal patterns correlating with the marked loss of metabolic signal in the paramedian mesencephalon and thalami. Isolated damage to the paramedian thalamus and mesencephalon alone

may cause PVS,[112,113] so that in this patient, the preserved cortical metabolism may reflect multiple preserved but isolated networks that fail to integrate because of the overwhelming injury to the paramedian mesencephalon and thalamus.[105]

Neuroimaging of Isolated Cortical Responses in Persistent Vegetative State Patients

In a widely discussed *Lancet* paper, Menon and colleagues[114] described selective cortical activation patterns using a ^{15}O-PET subtraction paradigm in a 26-year-old woman described as being in PVS 4 months following an attack of ADEM. MRI studies of the patient's brain showed evidence of both diffuse cortical and subcortical (brainstem and thalamic) lesions. Although the patient inconsistently demonstrated visual tracking (leading to some debate as to whether her condition at the

Multi-focal brain injury

Anoxia

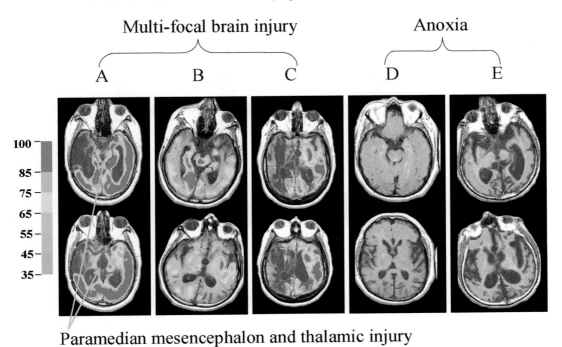

Paramedian mesencephalon and thalamic injury

Figure 9–7. An overview of coregistered magnetic resonance imaging and fluorodeoxyglucose-positron emission tomography (FDG-PET) images in five chronic persistent vegetative state (PVS) patients.[105] The PET data are normalized by region and expressed on a color scale ranging from 35% to 100% of normal. The brackets segregate three patients who suffered focal brain injuries due to trauma (A, B) or deep brain hemorrhage (C), and two patients in PVS due to anoxic injuries (D, E). As seen in the marked difference in overall brain metabolism, patients in PVS following anoxic injuries demonstrate global reductions of cerebral metabolism in all brain regions. Patient C is a 49-year-old woman who suffered successive hemorrhages from a deep, central arteriovenous malformation of her brain. Despite a 20-year period of PVS, this patient infrequently expressed isolated words (typically epithets) not related to environmental stimulation. (From Schiff, et al.,[105] with permission.)

time of study reflected PVS or MCS), no other features of her examination were inconsistent with the diagnosis of VS. Improvements in responsiveness unequivocally consistent with the MCS level were noted by 6 months, with emergence from MCS occurring some time after 8 months. As noted above, it is now generally recognized that prognosis in ADEM includes later recoveries at time periods 6 months or longer after the injury. Thus, patients with ADEM may harbor residual integrative capacities despite a long convalescence. By contrast, similar clinical examination findings in a patient 6 months following cardiac arrest would not portend such a cerebral reserve. The patient eventually made a full cognitive recovery.[115] Imaging studies in this patient at 4 months, when described as being in PVS, demonstrated selective activations of right occipital-temporal regions (in a subtraction paradigm

comparing familiar faces and scrambled images). The investigators interpreted activation of the right fusiform gyrus and extrastriate visual association areas as indicating a recovery of minimal awareness without behavioral manifestation. The findings in this patient, however, point out a significant limitation of brain imaging techniques in this clinical context and have been extensively debated.[111,116]

The selective identification of relatively complex information processing associated with visual processing of faces as shown here may not alone provide an index of recovery of cognitive function or even potential for recovery. Specific cortical responses to faces are obtainable in anesthetized animals[118] and, if found in isolation of any other imaging evidence or bedside demonstration of awareness, do not guarantee that these patterns of activation represent cognitive function per se. Without

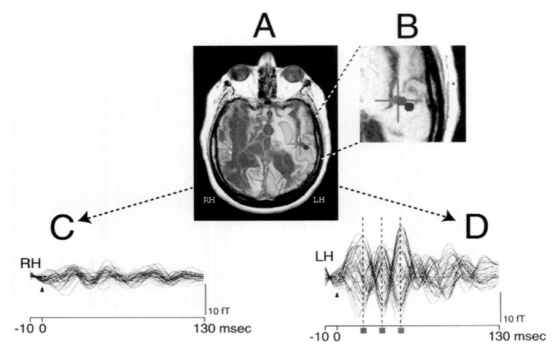

Figure 9–8. (A) A magnetic resonance image (1.5T) from the same patient illustrated in Figure 9–7C reveals destruction of the right basal ganglia and thalamus as well as severe damage to most of the cerebral cortex of the right hemisphere. Additional areas of damage include the left posterior thalamus and posterior parietal cortex with moderately severe atrophy of the rest of the left hemisphere. Resting fluorodeoxyglucose-positron emission tomography measurements of the patient's brain demonstrated a widespread and marked reduction in cerebral metabolism to less than 50% of normal across most brain regions. Several isolated and relatively small regions in the left hemisphere, however, expressed higher levels of metabolism (yellow color indicates values greater than 55% of normal). Magnetoencephalographic analysis of responses to bilateral auditory stimulation (C, D) demonstrated a time-locked response in the high-frequency (20 to 50 Hz) range restricted to the left hemisphere reduced in amplitude, coherence, and duration compared with normal controls.[194] Source localization of the time-varying magnetic field obtained from the averaged response identified sources in the left (D) but not right (C) temporal lobe, consistent with preservation of a response from Heschl's gyrus. (From Schiff et al.,[117] with permission.)

further clinical evidence, the present state of imaging technologies cannot provide alternative markers of awareness. While neuroimaging studies hold the promise of elucidating underlying differences between VS/PVS and MCS patients, at present no techniques are able to identify awareness in such patients unambiguously.

Owen and colleagues[119] have subsequently developed a new imaging framework to evaluate volitional responses in VS and MCS patients that address the ambiguities of the methods used in the Menon study.[114] Applying these new methods,[120] they identified unequivocal neuroimaging evidence of a patient remaining in VS at 5 months following a severe traumatic brain injury being able to follow commands to imagine various visual scenes. The

commands were associated with activation of appropriate areas of the cerebral cortex, despite lack of an external motor response. At the time of examination the patient showed evidence of brief visual fixation, a possible transitional sign for evolution into MCS.[76] Another examination 11 months later revealed visual tracking to a mirror, another transitional sign, but no evidence of object manipulation or behavioral manifestations of command following. Figure 9–9 shows the main result of the study. The imaging findings demonstrated preservation of cognitive function for this particular patient that the clinical bedside examination failed to reveal, and indicated a cognitive level at least consistent with MCS. It is important to recognize that command following is a cardinal feature of MCS that does imply

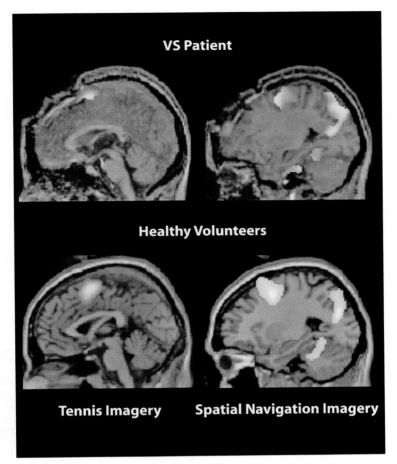

Figure 9–9. Command following in posttraumatic brain injury vegetative state (VS) at 5 months. A 23-year-old woman with clinical examination consistent with VS, with the exception of brief periods of visual fixation, following severe traumatic brain injury was asked to imagine playing tennis or walking throughout her own house. The regionally selective brain activation patterns obtained from functional magnetic resonance imaging measurements for each condition were identical to those of normal controls. (From Owen et al.,[120] with permission.)

communication. MCS patients may show consistent evidence of command following with visible motor responses that cannot be used to establish communication. Neuroimaging studies in such MCS patients also show preservation of large-scale cerebral networks (see below). As a result, it is unclear from the methods used in the Owen study whether or not the patient's level of consciousness was consistent with MCS or a higher level of recovery.

FUNCTIONAL IMAGING OF MINIMALLY CONSCIOUS STATES

Only a few studies have examined brain activity in MCS.[121] In five MCS patients,[15] O-PET identified activation of auditory association regions in the superior temporal gyrus not seen in PVS patients.[122] In addition, stronger correlation of the auditory cortical responses with frontal cortical regions was observed in both MCS patients and control subjects than in PVS patients. Median nerve electrical stimulation activated the entire pain network, similar to the response in normal subjects[123] (see Figure 9–6). These findings stress the need for analgesic medications when MCS patients undergo painful procedures.

Multimodal imaging studies using functional MRI activation paradigms and FDG-PET in two MCS patients near emergence from MCS uncovered unexpected evidence of widely

Minimally Conscious State Patient   Normal Subject

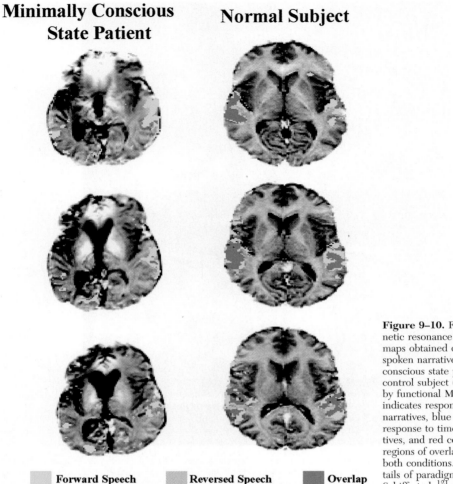

Forward Speech   **Reversed Speech**   **Overlap**

Figure 9–10. Functional magnetic resonance imaging (MRI) maps obtained during listening to spoken narratives, in a minimally conscious state patient (left) and control subject (right) measured by functional MRI. Yellow color indicates response to spoken narratives, blue color indicates response to time-reversed narratives, and red color indicates regions of overlapping response to both conditions. See text for details of paradigm. (Adapted from Schiff et al.,[121] with permission.)

preserved large-scale cerebral network responses[121] (Figure 9–10). Both patients suffered sudden brain injuries (blunt trauma, spontaneous intracerebral hemorrhage) leaving them in MCS for longer than 18 months. The acute phase of injury of each patient included herniation to a midbrain level. This historical feature is commonly associated with MCS and other poor outcomes following traumatic brain injuries as a result of focal infarction or indirect (axonal shearing, ischemic) damage.[124] Neither patient demonstrated consistent command following or functional communication (either gestural or verbal) on repeated examinations. Both patients, however, did demonstrate best responses that included command following or occasional verbal output (single words).

Significant fluctuations in their responsiveness occurred across examinations. Figure 9–10 shows cortical activity for one patient and one normal control associated with receptive language comprehension during presentation of 40-second narratives prerecorded by a familiar relative, presented as normal speech, and also played as time reversed (backward). Brain activations in response to normal speech are shown in yellow. Selective responses to backward presentations are shown in blue. Normal speech generated robust activity in language-related areas of the superior and middle temporal gyri for both the control subject and the MCS patient. In addition, the normal speech stimuli produced brain activations in the MCS patient's brain in the inferior and middle frontal

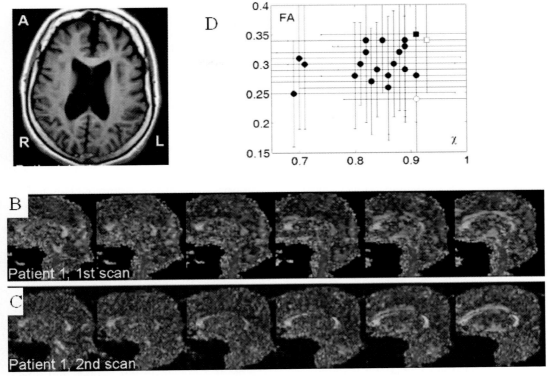

Figure 9–11. Diffusion tensor imaging studies of a patient with late recovery (19 years) from the minimally conscious state. (A) Magnetic resonance imaging demonstrating diffuse atrophy. (B) Fractional anisotropy maps showing fiber tracks: red, fibers with left-right directionality; blue, fibers with up-down directionality; green, fibers with anterior-posterior directionality. Images show volume loss of the corpus callosum throughout the medial component and regions in parieto-occipital white matter with prominent left-right directionality. (C) Fractional anisotropy maps obtained 18 months after studies shown in (B) demonstrate reduction of left-right direction in parieto-occipital regions with increased anisotropy noted in the midline cerebellum (see text). (D) Quantitative comparison of midline cerebellum fractional anisotropy versus left-right directionality. Open circle, values obtained from patient's first scan; open square, values obtained from second scan; filled circles, values from 20 normal subjects. (From Voss et al.,[132] with permission.)

gyri, primary and secondary visual areas including the calcarine sulcus, and precuneus. The pattern of brain activations for normal speech in this patient overlapped with that in the normal controls. However, different from the normals, neither patient activated in response to reversed speech. The findings also indicate that the functional MRI technique alone is insufficient to characterize the presumably wide differences in brain function that separate the patients and the control subjects. In addition, unlike PVS patients who fail to produce activation of polymodal association cortices in response to natural stimuli, the two MCS patients retain potentially recruitable cerebral networks that underlie language comprehension and expression despite their inability to

execute motor commands or communicate reliably. The preservation of large-scale forebrain networks associated with higher cognitive functions such as language provides a clinical foundation for wide fluctuations sometimes observed in MCS patients. Other investigators have obtained similar neuroimaging findings from single MCS patients.[99,125]

The same limitations of imaging techniques for determining awareness in VS/PVS patients also limit assessment in MCS patients. One cannot determine whether or not the functional MRI activations indicate awareness without communication, and by definition these patients cannot communicate. In addition, when they do awaken, they typically are amnestic for this period of time. Neuroimaging studies of visual awareness in patients and normal subjects implicate certain patterns of coactivation across cortical networks as the principal correlates of awareness, including coactivation of prefrontal and parietal cortices along with the occipital-temporal cortex.[126] Although the activation patterns identified in the MCS patient shown in Figure 9–10 include several of these specific regions, the patient is unable to communicate reliably to indicate whether visual or self-reflective awareness is present. The coactivation of prefrontal, parietal, and occipital regions suggests awareness but is potentially consistent with other interpretations. Similar concerns arise in the interpretation of the Owen[120] findings shown in Figure 9–9.

In the future, functional brain imaging techniques in combination with electrodiagnostics may identify patients with rehabilitative potential, and conversely, those in whom further recovery is not expected. The introduction of the MCS nosologic category is aimed at directing efforts to identify patients who may have some substrate for further recovery despite very limited behavioral evidence of awareness. On the other hand, fragmentary cortical networks may remain in VS patients without heralding further recovery or signifying awareness. The "gray zone" between VS and the lower functional boundary of MCS in Figure 9–1 reflects a probable overlap region where patients may acquire a reliable sensory-motor loop response of very limited cerebral systems that, despite contingency with environmental stimuli, may not reflect awareness or potential for further recovery. It is critical, then, to identify residual capacity as opposed to isolated functional activity in the cortex. This will require prospective studies of large numbers of patients with early VS, to determine if there are indices on functional imaging that can predict eventual improvement.

POTENTIAL MECHANISMS UNDERLYING RESIDUAL FUNCTIONAL CAPACITY IN SEVERELY DISABLED PATIENTS

The neuroimaging studies reviewed above raise the question of what mechanisms might limit further recovery in MCS patients who harbor widely connected and responsive cerebral networks. Fluctuations of cognitive function in MCS patients[91,127] (and occasional late spontaneous emergence from MCS [see below]) demonstrate an underlying residual cognitive capacity in some severely injured brains. At present, no studies have addressed this question by systematically correlating brain structural integrity, cerebral metabolism, and electrophysiology across a large sample of patients with severe disability. Nonetheless, several careful observations of variations in structural injury patterns, patterns of normal resting metabolic activity, and abnormal brain dynamics provide potentially important clues and directions for future research.

Variations of Structural Substrates Underlying Severe Disability

Clinical observations and quantitative measurements of neuronal loss following complex brain injuries do not support an invariably straightforward relationship of recovery of cognitive function that is simply graded by the degree of vascular, diffuse axonal, and direct ischemic brain damage. Although indirectly measured volumetric indices do offer some prediction of long-term outcome in PVS following overwhelming traumatic[71] or anoxic brain injury,[38] pathologic studies comparing patients remaining severely disabled following brain injuries to those remaining in VS demonstrate that severely disabled and some MCS patients may have only focal brain damage, whereas PVS patients suffer diffuse axonal injury.[128] Severely disabled patients with diffuse axonal injury appeared to have lesser quantitative damage than PVS patients. These findings suggest that significant variations in underlying mechanisms of cognitive disabilities and residual brain function accompany MCS and other severe but less disabling brain injuries.

It is also well known that enduring global disorders of consciousness can arise in the setting of only focal injuries.[129] These injuries are typically concentrated in the rostral tegmental mesencephalon and paramedian thalamus.[112,130] Patients with moderate, diffuse axonal injury combined with limited focal damage to these paramedian structures have not been systematically studied, but this pathology probably plays an important role in causing severe disability.[128,131] The paramedian thalamic and upper brainstem structures are specifically vulnerable to injury during periods of acute cerebral edema produced by traumatic brain injuries, infarctions, hemorrhages, infections, and brain tumors, as reviewed in Chapters 3 and 4.

Recent studies suggest that slowly developing structural remodeling may be a potential source of late recovery following severe brain injury. Voss and associates[132] longitudinally characterized brain structural connectivity and resting metabolism in a 40-year-old man who recovered expressive and receptive language after remaining in MCS for 19 years after a traumatic brain injury. The patient continued to improve over the next 2 years. MRI revealed extensive cerebral and subcortical atrophy particularly affecting the brainstem and frontal lobes; there was marked volume loss throughout the brain with ventricular dilation (Figure 9–11A). Diffusion tensor imaging (DTI) data revealed severe diffuse axonal injury, as indicated by volume loss in the medial corpus callosum (Figure 9–11B, C). In contrast to the overall severe reduction of brain connectivity demonstrated by DTI fractional anisotropy maps, measurements also revealed large regions of increased connectivity in posterior brain white matter not seen in 20 normal subjects (Figure 9–11B). These large, bilateral regions of posterior white matter anisotropy were reduced in directionality when measured in a second DTI study 18 months later (Figure 9–11C). At this time, repeat imaging identified significant increases in anisotropy within the midline cerebellar white matter that correlated with significant clinical improvements in motor control over the intervening time period.[132] Figure 9–11D shows the quantitative changes in an index of fractional anisotropy and left-right fiber directions; the open circle shows measurements at the time of the first scan (Figure 9–11B), and the open square shows the marked increase in fractional anisotropy corresponding to the increased intensity of the red region within the midline cerebellum (Figure 9–11C). These findings suggest the possibility of structural changes within the patients' white matter playing a role in their functional recovery. Recent experimental studies provide some support for such a mechanism of late remodeling of white matter connections after structural injuries[133,134] and in normal human adults.[135]

Although suggestive and fascinating, individual case studies of this sort must be interpreted cautiously. Nevertheless, such findings indicate the need for larger prospective studies examining whether slow structural changes do arise in the setting of severe traumatic brain injuries and, if present, whether they influence functional outcomes.

The Potential Role of the Metabolic "Baseline" in Recovery of Cognitive Function

As discussed on page 370 and illustrated in the example shown in Figure 9–10, the abnormal response to speech reversal in some MCS patients provides a potentially important clue to the mechanisms underlying their profound cognitive impairment. Control subjects were instructed to listen passively to the sounds; however, the time-reversed narratives elicited an involuntary attempt to decode the speech. The failure of the time-reversed narratives to activate the large-scale language-responsive networks identified by the forward presentations in MCS patients suggests a significant difference in the resting state of the brain in MCS patients and control subjects. The recruitment of a normal network activation pattern suggests that MCS patients may require very salient stimuli to activate these language systems (e.g., clear human speech, familiar voice, emotional content, etc.).

Raichle and colleagues have proposed that the normal human brain has a "baseline" state of metabolic activation (as reflected by oxygen uptake) reflecting "default self-monitoring."[136–138] Specific areas of brain that are active at rest (e.g., posterior cingulate cortex and ventral anterior cingulate cortex[139]) form a network that deactivates during tasks that activate other areas of the brain. Data obtained from these investigators provide some evidence supporting a functional role of a resting state of monitoring environmental factors and an internal state that might be sensitive to salient events such as emotionally meaningful human speech.[138–141] Loss of signal in these regions is a common finding in VS and partial recovery of this metabolic signal is seen in MCS.[141,99]

The very low overall resting cerebral metabolic rates in MCS patients generally include the posterior and ventroanterior cingulate regions associated by Raichle with self-awareness. This may account for the failure to engage functional network activation with presentation of time-reversed narratives (Figure 9–10). Specifically, a lack of a metabolically expensive ongoing self and environmental monitoring process may leave the MCS brain stimulus bound and limited to activations provoked by extremely salient events. This interpretation is supported by direct comparisons of changes in cerebral metabolism, functional MRI signal activation, and neuronal activity that indicate a linear correlation of these measures.[142,143] The dissociation of low resting cerebral metabolism and recruitable cerebral networks in MCS invites speculation that patients who remain near the border of emergence from MCS (see red line in Figure 9–1) may show fluctuation of recruitment of these large-scale networks under varying internal conditions of arousal and appearance of environmentally salient stimuli, leading to the occasional surprisingly high level of response.

A further consideration is whether injuries incurred by compression of the thalamus and brainstem during acute herniation may underlie the chronically low metabolic rates in patients remaining in MCS despite connected and recruitable cerebral networks (both MCS patients studied[121] had herniated with midbrain signs of third nerve palsies during the acute phase of their injuries). As discussed in Chapter 1, the paramedian mesencephalon and thalamus contain several interconnected brain systems that interact closely with the brainstem arousal systems. Although these structures were originally identified as the primary arousal systems, the thalamic intralaminar nuclei (ILN) (and paralaminar regions of the thalamus rich in neurons that preferentially project to layer I of the cerebral cortex), the mesencephalic reticular formation (MRF), and their connections with the thalamic reticular nucleus appear to play a key role linking arousal states to the control of moment-to-moment intention or attentional gating (reviewed in [144]). These structures are well positioned to control interactions of the cerebral cortex, basal ganglia, and thalamus through their patterns of innervation within the cortex as well as rich innervation from the brainstem arousal systems.[145,146] Even incomplete injuries to these networks may produce unique deficits in maintaining adequate cerebral activation and patterns of brain dynamics necessary to establish, maintain, and complete complex behaviors.

The Potential Role of Regionally Selective Injuries Producing Widespread Effects on Brain Function

At least three different mechanisms may lead to marked alteration of integrative brain activity following relatively focal or regionally restricted brain lesions: (1) a form of passive inhibition of a brain area following deafferentation of remote but strongly connected areas, (2) active inhibitory phenomena resulting from altered connectivity and neuronal function following injury, and (3) persistent or paroxysmal functional activity producing excess excitation of distributed neuronal networks.[121] Whether such processes underlie partially reversible impairment of cognitive function in severely disabled patients is unknown. It is likely, however, that transient changes in distributed network function underlie the wide fluctuations in cognitive performance in some MCS patients and patients who emerge from MCS. These phenomena are well known but not frequently described in the medical literature.[91,127] We briefly discuss potentially relevant sources of variations of brain dynamics within the wakeful state of the injured brain.

A relatively common finding following focal ischemia or traumatic brain injury is a reduction in cerebral metabolism in brain regions remote from the site of injury. This transsynaptic (or "crossed") down-regulation of distant neuronal populations results from the loss of excitatory inputs from the damaged regions.[147] The clinical significance of these changes is unclear, although electrophysiologic correlates have been identified. A recent study by Gold and Lauritzen[148] showed that although changes in blood flow may be modest in remote cortical regions, the transsynaptic down-regulation produces dramatic decreases in neuronal firing rates (e.g., a neuronal firing rate decreased by 80% with only a 20% reduction in regional blood flow). Thus, stable down-regulation of cortical, thalamic, or basal ganglia neuronal populations through passive inhibition secondary to deafferentation is a possible source of functionally reversible alteration of cerebral network function. Intrinsic neuronal membrane properties allow nonlinear state changes on the basis of small deviations in excitation. In vivo experimental studies demonstrate that the loss of excitatory drive to neuronal populations as a result of transsynaptic down-regulation produces a powerful form of inhibition that hyperpolarizes the neuronal membrane potential.[149] In cerebral cortex[150] and basal ganglia,[151] up and down states have been identified in in vitro studies comparable to burst and tonic mode firing in the thalamus (Chapter 1). The potential interplay of these mechanisms in the setting of brain injury remains to be unraveled, but the observations suggest mechanisms by which large connected networks of potentially functional systems might remain dormant despite a balance of neuromodulators producing a wakeful EEG and arousal pattern.[152]

Other types of alteration of the balance of excitation and inhibition, particularly hypersynchronous discharges, may play a key role. Experimental studies have shown increased excitability following even modest brain trauma that may promote epileptiform activity in both cortical and subcortical regions.[153,154] Hypersynchronous activity within relatively restricted networks may underlie several different clinical phenomena following structural brain injuries. For example, a patient fluctuating from classic akinetic mutism to interactive awareness following an encephalitic injury[155] had epileptiform activity in the thalamus that appeared only as surface slow waves in the EEG. Such a mechanism might also explain a reported case of episodic remission of akinetic mutism.[91] A 52-year-old man remained in an akinetic mute state following the rupture of a basilar artery aneurysm with infarcts in the thalamus and basal ganglia. This behavioral state persisted without change for 17 months, at which time a spontaneous fluctuation in behavioral state occurred, described as a return to his "premorbid state, with full return of his demeanor and affect." The patient's functional recovery lasted 1 day and then he relapsed. One year after this event, the patient had a second "awakening" following a grand mal seizure. Electroconvulsive therapy, tried empirically, also reproduced the change.

A related mechanism may explain the late emergence from MCS reported by Clauss and colleagues.[127] A 28-year-old man suffered a diffuse axonal injury (presumably grade III with subcortical hemorrhages in the basal ganglia, thalamus, and brainstem). Spontaneous eye opening with a GCS of 9 persisted for 3 years following injury until 10 mg of zolpidem (a $GABA_A$ potentiator that binds to many of the same sites as benzodiazepines) was administered. Within 15 minutes of administration, the patient began to speak and was able to respond to questions with "yes or no" answers and ultimately demonstrated intact remote and immediate memory. Temporary remission of chronic aphasia in a 52-year-old woman 3 years following administration of zolpidem has also been reported.[156] In this patient, regional cerebral blood flow (CBF) measurements using SPECT demonstrated a 35% to 40% increase in the medial frontal cortex bilaterally, and left middle frontal and supramarginal gyri (Broca's area) 30 minutes after zolpidem ingestion. Similar mechanisms most likely underlie the well-publicized cases of Gary Dockery ("The Coma Cop") and Donald Herbert, a fireman who made international headlines in 2005 with a marked recovery of speech and cognitive function after 9 years of remaining in MCS following traumatic brain injury.

Injury to the paramedian thalamus (intralaminar and related thalamic nuclei) and upper brainstem alone can produce widespread hemispheric transsynaptic down-regulation,[157,158] as well as a variety of paroxysmal disturbances. Most common among the types of paroxysmal alterations in brain dynamics following injury to the paramedian thalamus are generalized epileptic seizures, typically variations of the 3/s spike-and-wave form.[90,159] Other less well-known phenomena, such as oculogyric crises, are also associated with injuries to this region.[160] Hypersynchronous discharges restricted to the thalamostriatal system might also account for forms of catatonia[161,162] and the obsessive-compulsive disorder infrequently observed after brain injuries.[163] Thus, damage to the upper brainstem and medial thalamus, in combination with other cerebral injuries, may lead to a variety of partially reversible mechanisms of dysfunction that could contribute to a reduced baseline activity in severely disabled patients and provide a structural basis for wide variation in functional performance. Overreliance on clinical examination features and structural imaging may fail to identify such changes in brain dynamics arising in the setting of abnormal connective topologies induced by severe injuries.

ETHICS OF CLINICAL DECISION MAKING AND COMMUNICATION WITH SURROGATES (J.J. FINS)

Decisions concerning care for patients with severe disorders of consciousness necessarily involve surrogates. Family members, friends, or other intimates must make decisions about care or its withdrawal. In this section, we consider the special challenges faced by those decision makers entrusted with the care of a patient with a disorder of consciousness and describe what practitioners might do to ease their burden by improving communication.

Surrogate Decision Making, Perceptions, and Needs

A surrogate decision maker is a person, other than the patient, who directs care when the patient is unable to provide consent. Under prevailing legal and ethical norms, surrogate decisions should be based on what is known about the patient's expressed choices when he or she was able to give informed consent.[164] Thus, surrogates should follow *expressed wishes* of the patient when they are known and invoke *substituted judgment*, what is believed or inferred about patient choices, when actual preferences are unknown. In the absence of evidence of prior wishes or known patient values, surrogates should invoke a *best interests standard*, intended to represent what an average person would do when confronted by prevailing circumstances.

When working with surrogates, the physician must determine who among many has standing and priority.[165] A surrogate designated by the patient through an advance directive has precedence over other potential decision makers because he or she was expressly chosen by the patient. This exercise of patient self-determination can take place through an advance directive, variably called a durable power

attorney for health care, health care agent, or health care proxy.[166] Alternately, a patient without a designated surrogate can express preferences in a living will. A living will details patient wishes, but does not authorize a designated spokesperson. If there is no designated surrogate, family members and close friends are selected in order of their relationship to the patient (spouse > parents > children > siblings > other relatives > friends).

The importance of advance care planning, or the use of living wills or health care proxies, has been inextricably linked to prominent legal cases involving patients in a VS. In the Cruzan case, which considered the withdrawal of artificial nutrition and hydration in a young woman in a persistent VS, Justice Sandra Day O'Connor first suggested a greater role for advance care planning, a mechanism for patients to express their wishes before decisional incapacity. The lack of such an advance directive became part of the conflict in the now well-known case of Terri Schiavo, who remained in a permanent VS following a cardiac arrest and anoxic brain injury in 1990.[167] Her case gained national prominence in 2003 and again in 2005 when family members disputed the propriety of removing her feeding tube. Multiple courts ruled that her prior wishes were known and that her husband, who advocated the removal of her percutaneous gastrostomy, was the appropriate surrogate decision maker under state law. Nonetheless, the tragedy of that family dispute illustrated the utility of talking about preferences in advance and sharing wishes with one's family and friends. Prompting discussions ahead of incapacity is a lesson for the general medical and neurology outpatient clinics as much as it is for the neurology ICU.[168,169]

Even without an advance directive surrogate designate, the ethical challenge of determining the best course of action remains. Surrogates balance their knowledge of the patient's preferences with their own sense of prognosis and likely outcome,[170] as it is unusual for the patient to have anticipated the precise set of circumstances in advance. When the patient is comatose, surrogates may step forward and authorize a DNR order and pursue a less aggressive course of care than in an awake patient. However, in one study, only 32% of patients had consented to their own DNR orders; in the remaining cases, 64% had been put in place by a surrogate, and 5% by physicians alone.[171] This figure is comparable to a study a decade earlier in which only 30% of patients discussed resuscitation with a physician prior to a cardiac arrest.[172] Thus, the decision on DNR orders frequently rests on the shoulders of the surrogate.

Because perception of outcome hinges so strongly on the question of recovery of consciousness, the physician must communicate to surrogates the best estimate of the likelihood and degree of recovery, or conversely the inevitability of death or permanent VS. This is easier said than done as indicated in previous sections of this chapter. Moreover, it is important to recognize that the right to die (i.e., the negative right to be left alone) was established through cases involving patients in the VS.[173] In addressing the case of Karen Anne Quinlan in 1976, the New Jersey Supreme Court asserted that the justification of the removal of her ventilator was predicated upon her irreversible loss of a "cognitive sapient state."[174,175] The identification of VS with medical futility allowed surrogates to be granted the discretion to withdraw life-sustaining therapy.[176]

This historical legacy may lead in some cases to a diagnostic and therapeutic nihilism, in which diagnostic categories that are relevant are conflated and confused. VS is but one of many disorders of consciousness; patients who are vegetative may progress to permanence or move on to the minimally conscious state or another level of brain function. Because of the importance of consciousness to surrogate decision makers and the value placed on the "cognitive sapient state," it is important to strive toward diagnostic accuracy and precision. This is particularly important as evolving knowledge indicates that obtaining an accurate diagnosis of MCS may strongly alter prognosis for some patients, particularly those recovering from traumatic brain injury.[77,79] As more attention is paid to the varying outcomes of coma, it is likely that practice norms will be influenced.

Professional Obligations and Diagnostic Discernment

It is the professional obligation of the physician caring for individuals with a disorder of consciousness to bring evolving scientific knowledge to the bedside and use it to inform the decision-making process with surrogates. It is especially critical that surrogates understand that the probability of the recovery of consciousness is dynamic and depends on considerations of etiology of injury, structural patterns of brain injury, and duration of the clinical state. Physicians should use their knowledge to orchestrate strategic discussions at key clinical milestones that have prognostic and diagnostic importance, recognizing that for the most part, these categorizations remain crude and mostly descriptive. Because of the rudimentary nature of this emerging nosology, it is inevitable that patients with variable injuries and outcomes will be included in diagnostic categories that are too broad and heterogeneous. This can make prediction difficult and undermine laudable efforts to achieve greater diagnostic refinement and precision.[177]

For these reasons, a delicate balance needs to be achieved between too quickly foreclosing any prospect of recovery and the offering of false hope. Even "favorable" outcomes, marked by survival and recovery, force difficult quality-of-life choices for those whose existence has been irrevocably altered by a disorder of consciousness and most often an alteration of the self. Translating the medical facts that are provided by clinicians into such choices is the work of surrogates.

The physician's function, assisted by members of the interdisciplinary team needed to care for these patients and the families, is *simultaneously to preserve the right to die while also affirming the right to care*.[177] This means respecting the decisions of surrogates when they believe that ongoing life-sustaining therapy would result in an existence that would have been unacceptable to the patient or inconsistent with their prior wishes. Patients should receive the appropriate amount of clinical care, diagnostic and interventional, that allows for informed decisions about treatment options, whether it be under the rubric of an informed consent or informed refusal of care.

Time-Delimited Prognostication and Evolving Brain States: Framing the Conversation

To ensure that these decisions are indeed informed, it is essential to ensure that there is proper information flow between clinical staff and surrogates when clinical findings warrant discussion or when a prognostic milestone is reached. How much information is conveyed to achieve this objective and how determinative it can be will depend upon clinical circumstances. For example, it may be justified to provide an early and definitive prognosis of permanent unconsciousness or death while a patient is comatose following an out-of-hospital cardiac arrest and if there are clear negative prognostic predictors including loss of pupillary function and corneal reflexes and bilateral absence of somatosensory-evoked responses.

In contrast, it would be inappropriate, and premature, to offer a conclusive prognosis in the comatose traumatic brain injury patient who demonstrates brainstem function and appears to be moving quickly into VS. The rate of recovery of such patients may warrant a cautiously optimistic approach[70] delineated by a *prognostic time trial* in which the clinician gives a *time-delimited prognosis*. Time-delimited prognoses are contingent upon the patient's continued evolution by certain temporal milestones.

To prepare for and organize such discussions with surrogates, we focus on major clinical and temporal milestones, which are important occasions for speaking with surrogates about the patient's current status and goals of care.

Brain death involves the most straightforward decision making. In brain death, there are no clinical goals of care as the patient cannot benefit from further therapeutic efforts and the focus for the practitioner should be to communicate these facts and address specific religious or moral concerns in individual cases. Although widely accepted in professional circles, the concept of brain death is not well understood among lay people when consent for organ donation is sought.[178] A more challenging issue is that some segments of our society reject this definition of death, most notably members of some orthodox religious groups and others with cultural roots in Asia, most notably Japan, which has only recently legalized brain death determinations.[179,180] Two states, New Jersey and New York, have accommodation clauses to accommodate religious and moral objections to determination of death by brain death testing, with New Jersey exempting this standard when it would violate religious beliefs. Working with surrogates who reject brain death standards requires cultural sensitivity and the use of cultural intermediaries to enhance communication.[181]

When speaking with surrogate decision makers for a *comatose* patient, it is important to be as specific about potential outcomes given the nature and etiology of the causative event or process while leaving open the indeterminacy of potential recovery based on time-limited observations of brain state. Because the exact fate of an individual patient for recovery or permanent unconsciousness is often indeterminate, the evolution of brain states from coma to vegetative and minimally conscious states to recovery without independence to full recovery needs to be stressed. The time evolution of states is often not appreciated by surrogates who may be unduly pessimistic or optimistic. At this juncture, it may be prudent to caution surrogates to avoid making a potentially premature decision and waiting until prognostication can be informed by *how* and *when* the patient evolves from coma.

Progression from coma to the *vegetative state* does not herald additional improvement and recovery. This is a natural state of progression in nearly all comatose patients, and movement into VS is an important clinical milestone that requires explanation. Surrogates need to appreciate that the behaviors that are seen in VS, such as sleep-wake cycles, blinking, roving eye movements, or the startle reflex, are not purposeful and do not indicate consciousness or awareness of self, others, or the environment.[182] This is a hard concept for lay people to understand. It can be explained and emphasized that these are automatic behaviors, much like breathing and the maintenance of a heartbeat, controlled by brainstem activity. Making these distinctions is important when the patient first enters VS, lest these behaviors be understood as evidence of awareness or consciousness.

Discussion should emphasize that although VS, which is as yet unmodified, may become labeled as *persistent* once it has persisted for 1 month, it is not predicted to be *permanent* until 3 months following *anoxic* injury, or 12 months when the etiology is *traumatic brain injury.*[183] In the competently assessed patient, it is clinically and ethically appropriate to assert that patients become permanently vegetative when they pass through these time intervals.[66] Although the 1994 Multisociety Task Force opined that "the persistent VS is a diagnosis and that the permanent VS is a prognosis,"[64,65] because of exceedingly rare outlier cases of late recovery from PVS, it is reasonable to maintain the permanent VS as a viable diagnostic category if an appropriate assessment has been made to be sure that the patient is not in the *minimally conscious state.*

The *minimally conscious state* presents perhaps the greatest current challenge for communication of prognosis. Although MCS is a recognized plateau from which patients may regain consistent evidence of consciousness; an awareness of self, others, and their environment; and, most critically, the ability to engage in functional communication, the wide clinical spectrum of MCS[184] includes some patients who will permanently remain unable to communicate yet retain some aspects of awareness. Because of this complexity, ethical norms for addressing patients in MCS are only now evolving and likely to change as diagnostic precision improves and therapeutic avenues open for some subcategories of patients. The recovery of functional communication appears to represent the principal goal of many but not all surrogates[70,185] involved in the care of MCS patients (additional endpoints include self-feeding, pain control, and emotional reactivity, among others). Surrogates may appropriately express the concern that waiting for further recovery from MCS may limit later opportunities to withdraw care so as not to abridge the patient's prospective wishes not to remain in VS or MCS if the condition were to be permanent.[186] Addressing these challenges will require further engagement of surrogates, physicians, and policy makers to consider palliative goals of care for the severely brain-injured patient.[187]

Emergence from MCS is a major milestone for several key reasons. First, when patients arrive at this functional level, they are able consistently to engage others. This will make the question of whether or not the patient is conscious indisputable and not open to charges of familial emotionality or denial. Second, at this more recovered state of consciousness, patients more fully recapture personhood lost as the result of their injury. As the philosopher William Winslade has observed in an early exploration of ethical issues following traumatic brain injury, "Being persons requires having a personality, being aware of ourselves and our surroundings, and possessing human capacities, such as memory, emotions,

and the ability to communicate and interact with other people."[187a] An additional point about emergence from MCS is that the potential for recovery is open ended and unpredictable. Functional capability beyond mere emergence is an area of active research with emerging evidence that the level of early impaired self-awareness may be considered as a marker for predicting complex functional activities later in the course of recovery from traumatic brain injury.[188] Thus, there is a need for ongoing assessment of capabilities and continuing physical and occupational therapy for patients who have managed to recover to this state.

A final note on *diagnostics* is in order. Families may want confirmatory studies to convince them of the solidity of the clinical diagnosis, trusting the "objectivity" of a scan over the analysis of the clinician. Expectations are raised by the advent of "neuroethics" articles in the popular culture asserting the potential of neuroimaging technologies to read minds and refine marketing techniques.[189] Because of these trends, surrogates may invest imaging technologies with more diagnostic ability than they currently possess and seek clearcut answers through this visual medium. It is important to be clear that the diagnosis and assessment of patients with disorders of consciousness *is a clinical task informed by a competent history and neurologic examination.* Although desperate families may request them, as of this writing, neuroimaging studies are only applied in research settings and at best can be ancillary to clinical evaluation. They must be interpreted in light of the history and physical examination. It is important to be transparent when discussing the capabilities of current technology to assess brain states; indicate that this is an active area of research and caution that many of the *experimental* protocols portrayed in the media are being utilized in patients who have already been diagnostically assessed.[190]

Family Dynamics and Philosophic Considerations

Beyond questions about the process of making decisions and the professional obligation to exchange information with surrogates, it is also important to appreciate that probabilities about survival and functional status do not translate easily into choices about human values. Sharing prognostic probabilities is not, in itself, sufficient to improve the deliberative process or to effect outcome decisions.

Given the complexity of the decision-making process, this is not wholly unexpected. The quality of how information was conveyed is difficult to assess and may be as critical as what has been conveyed. Families may be distrustful of clinicians and systems of care that are not designed for longitudinal chronic care.[177] They may have been the recipients of misinformation about the patient's brain state and be wary of family meetings that they worry might try to engineer a decision to withhold or withdraw care.

These would be formidable challenges even if there were continuity of care and ongoing doctor-patient/family relationships. In the setting of shifting venues of care from the acute hospital setting to rehabilitation and long-term care facilities, the challenge of building trust is formidable. To help build such relationships, it is critical to be empathic and supportive and try to imagine what has eloquently been described as "the loneliness of the long-term caregiver"[191] faced with social isolation and family members whose injury has altered them and their relationships with those who hold them dear. These longitudinal stresses and the dependency of loved ones, coupled with the prognostic uncertainties, require compassion when working with families touched by a disorder of consciousness.

Surrogates will articulate a broad range of preferences depending on the patient's values and their own sense of what constitutes proportionate care, from the rejection of brain death to the decision to remove artificial nutrition and hydration in a patient who is in a minimally conscious state. In most cases, however, most surrogates will struggle with the more nuanced question of the *degree* of loss of self that would make a life worth living.

This is a highly personal question. Families may benefit by your asking them to consider the ability to relate to others in the context of a broader consideration about the goals of care. This level is not reached until the patient has recovered to the upper end of MCS or emerged from that state. Although all may not agree with the centrality of functional communication, this may be a helpful goal of care when speaking with family members. Appreciating the cen-

trality of functional communication will also help to identify those patients who retain this ability but need assistive devices or special techniques to relate to others.[96] One of the most egregious diagnostic errors that can be made in this area of clinical practice is to mistake a *locked-in* patient for one who is vegetative.[98] Locked-in patients retain the ability for functional communication but need to be recognized in order to mobilize emerging technologies that can correlate eye movements, or even electrical brain activity, to the choice of letters on a computer screen, and thereby help locked-in patients to communicate.[94,192]

Working toward the achievement of functional communication can also help delineate objectives and time frames against which this level of function needs to be achieved lest it simply remain an elusive hope. For example, if it is agreed that functional communication is a goal of care, it might be prudent to continue to follow a patient for a year following traumatic injury in order for a patient to have the greatest chance of moving into the minimally conscious state from which a capability of functional communication might take root. If a patient remains vegetative a year after injury, the substantially reduced chances of attaining the communicative goal would help support a decision to withdraw care.

In all of these conversations, it may be helpful to reach out to the hospital's ethics committee, which will have additional expertise to help surrogates interpret technical information, such as patient diagnosis and prognosis, in light of the patient's prior wishes, preferences, and values.

REFERENCES

1. Broderick JP, Adams HP Jr, Barsan W, et al. Guidelines for the management of spontaneous intracerebral hemorrhage: a statement for healthcare professionals from a special writing group of the Stroke Council, American Heart Association. Stroke 30, 905–915, 1999.
2. *Traumatic brain injury*: Masson F, Thicoipe M, Aye P, Mokni T, Senjean P, Schmitt V, Dessalles PH, Cazaugade M, Labadens P. Aquitaine Group for Severe Brain Injuries Study. Epidemiology of severe brain injuries: a prospective population-based study. J Trauma. 51, 481–9, 2001. *Cardiopulmonary arrest*: Booth CM, Boone RH, Tomlinson G, et al. Is this patient dead, vegetative, or severely neurologically impaired? Assessing outcome for comatose survivors of cardiac arrest. JAMA 291, 870–879, 2004.

3. Jennett B, Teasdale G, Braakman R, et al. Prognosis of patients with severe head injury. Neurosurgery 4, 283–289, 1979.

4. Levy DE, Bates D, Caronna JJ, et al. Prognosis in nontraumatic coma. Ann Intern Med 94, 293–301, 1981.

5. Jennett B, Bond M. Assessment of outcome after severe brain damage. Lancet 1, 480–484, 1975.

6. Consensus conference. Rehabilitation of persons with traumatic brain injury. NIH Consensus Development Panel on Rehabilitation of Persons With Traumatic Brain Injury. JAMA 282, 974–983, 1999.

7. Jennett B. Predictors of recovery in evaluation of patients in coma. Adv Neurol 22, 129–135, 1979.

8. Brain Trauma Foundation Management and Prognosis of Severe Traumatic Brain Injury. American Association of Neurological Surgeons, 2001.

9. Gennarelli TA, Champion HR, Copes WS, et al. Comparison of mortality, morbidity, and severity of 59,713 head injured patients with 114,447 patients with extracranial injuries. J Trauma 37, 962–968, 1994.

10. Narayan RK, Greenberg RP, Miller JD, et al. Improved confidence of outcome prediction in severe head injury. A comparative analysis of the clinical examination, multimodality evoked potentials, CT scanning, and intracranial pressure. J Neurosurg 54, 751–762, 1981.

11. Braakman R, Gelpke GJ, Habbema JD, et al. Systematic selection of prognostic features in patients with severe head injury. Neurosurgery 6, 362–370, 1980.

12. Stocchetti N, Penny KI, Dearden M, et al. Intensive care management of head-injured patients in Europe: a survey from the European brain injury consortium. Intensive Care Med 27, 400–406, 2001.

13. Choi SC, Narayan RK, Anderson RL, et al. Enhanced specificity of prognosis in severe head injury. J Neurosurg 69, 381–385, 1988.

14. Marion DW, Carlier PM. Problems with initial Glasgow Coma Scale assessment caused by prehospital treatment of patients with head injuries: results of a national survey. J Trauma 36, 89–95, 1994.

15. Teasdale G, Knill-Jones R, van der SJ. Observer variability in assessing impaired consciousness and coma. J Neurol Neurosurg Psychiatry 41, 603–610, 1978.

16. Signorini DF, Andrews PJ, Jones PA, et al. Predicting survival using simple clinical variables: a case study in traumatic brain injury. J Neurol Neurosurg Psychiatry 66, 20–25, 1999.

17. Hukkelhoven CW, Steyerberg EW, Rampen AJ, et al. Patient age and outcome following severe traumatic brain injury: an analysis of 5600 patients. J Neurosurg 99, 666–673, 2003.

18. Jennett B, Teasdale G, Galbraith S, et al. Severe head injuries in three countries. J Neurol Neurosurg Psychiatry 40, 291–298, 1977.

19. van Dongen KJ, Braakman R, Gelpke GJ. The prognostic value of computerized tomography in comatose head-injured patients. J Neurosurg 59, 951–957, 1983.

20. Fearnside MR, Cook RJ, McDougall P, et al. The Westmead Head Injury Project outcome in severe head injury. A comparative analysis of pre-hospital, clinical and CT variables. Br J Neurosurg 7, 267–279, 1993.

21. Carlsson CA, von Essen C, Lofgren J. Factors affecting the clinical course of patients with severe head injuries. 1. Influence of biological factors. 2. Significance of posttraumatic coma. J Neurosurg 29, 242–251, 1968.

22. Young GB. The EEG in coma. J Clin Neurophysiol 17, 473–485, 2000.

23. Young GB, Wang JT, Connolly JF. Prognostic determination in anoxic-ischemic and traumatic encephalopathies. J Clin Neurophysiol 21, 379–390, 2004.

24. Logi F, Fischer C, Murri L, et al. The prognostic value of evoked responses from primary somatosensory and auditory cortex in comatose patients. Clin Neurophysiol 114, 1615–1627, 2003.

25. Lew HL, Dikmen S, Slimp J, et al. Use of somatosensory-evoked potentials and cognitive event-related potentials in predicting outcomes of patients with severe traumatic brain injury. Am J Phys Med Rehabil 82, 53–61, 2003.

26. Robe PA, Dubuisson A, Bartsch S, et al. Favourable outcome of a brain trauma patient despite bilateral loss of cortical somatosensory evoked potential during thiopental sedation. J Neurol Neurosurg Psychiatry 74, 1157–1158, 2003.

27. Schwarz S, Schwab S, Aschoff A, et al. Favorable recovery from bilateral loss of somatosensory evoked potentials. Crit Care Med 27, 182–187, 1999.

28. Mazzini L, Zaccala M, Gareri F, et al. Long-latency auditory-evoked potentials in severe traumatic brain injury. Arch Phys Med Rehabil 82, 57–65, 2001.

29. Perrin F, Schnakers C, Schabus M, et al. Brain response to one's own name in vegetative state, minimally conscious state, and locked-in syndrome. Arch Neurol 63, 562–569, 2006.

30. Pelinka LE, Kroepfl A, Leixnering M, et al. GFAP versus S100B in serum after traumatic brain injury: relationship to brain damage and outcome. J Neurotrauma 21, 1553–1561, 2004.

31. Shutter L, Tong KA, Holshouser BA. Proton MRS in acute traumatic brain injury: role for glutamate/glutamine and choline for outcome prediction. J Neurotrauma 21, 1693–1705, 2004.

32. Levy DE, Caronna JJ, Singer BH, et al. Predicting outcome from hypoxic-ischemic coma. JAMA 253, 1420–1426, 1985.

33. Hamel MB, Goldman L, Teno J, et al. Identification of comatose patients at high risk for death or severe disability. SUPPORT Investigators. Understand Prognoses and Preferences for Outcomes and Risks of Treatments. JAMA 273, 1842–1848, 1995.

34. Sacco RL, VanGool R, Mohr JP, et al. Nontraumatic coma. Glasgow coma score and coma etiology as predictors of 2-week outcome. Arch Neurol 47, 1181–1184, 1990.

35. Sasser H. Association of Clinical Signs with Neurological Outcome After Cardiac Arrest [dissertation]. University of Pittsburg, 1999.

36. Zandbergen EG, de Haan RJ, Stoutenbeek CP, et al. Systematic review of early prediction of poor outcome in anoxic-ischaemic coma. Lancet 352, 1808–1812, 1998.

37. Madl C, Kramer L, Domanovits H, et al. Improved outcome prediction in unconscious cardiac arrest survivors with sensory evoked potentials compared with clinical assessment. Crit Care Med 28, 721–726, 2000.

38. Rothstein TL. The role of evoked potentials in anoxic-ischemic coma and severe brain trauma. J Clin Neurophysiol 17, 486–497, 2000.

39. Rothstein TL, Thomas EM, Sumi SM. Predicting outcome in hypoxic-ischemic coma. A prospective clinical and electrophysiologic study. Electroencephalogr Clin Neurophysiol 79, 101–107, 1991.

40. Fischer C, Luauté J, Adeleine P, et al. Predictive value of sensory and cognitive evoked potentials for awakening from coma. Neurology 63, 669–673, 2004.

41. Goh WC, Heath PD, Ellis SJ, et al. Neurological outcome prediction in a cardiorespiratory arrest survivor. Br J Anaesth 88, 719–722, 2002.

42. Wijdicks EF, Parisi JE, Sharbrough FW. Prognostic value of myoclonus status in comatose survivors of cardiac arrest. Ann Neurol 35, 239–243, 1994.

43. Werhahn KJ, Brown P, Thompson PD, et al. The clinical features and prognosis of chronic posthypoxic myoclonus. Mov Disord 12, 216–220, 1997.

44. Kaplan PW. The EEG in metabolic encephalopathy and coma. J Clin Neurophysiol 21, 307–318, 2004.

45. Golby A, McGuire D, Bayne L. Unexpected recovery from anoxic-ischemic coma. Neurology 45, 1629–1630, 1995.

46. Britton JW, Ghearing GR, Benarroch EE, et al. The ictal bradycardia syndrome: localization and lateralization. Epilepsia 47, 737–744, 2006.

47. Wijdicks EF, Rabinstein AA. Absolutely no hope? Some ambiguity of futility of care in devastating acute stroke. Crit Care Med 32, 2332–2342, 2004.

48. Pullicino PM, Alexandrov AV, Shelton JA, et al. Mass effect and death from severe acute stroke. Neurology 49, 1090–1095, 1997.

49. Voetsch B, DeWitt LD, Pessin MS, et al. Basilar artery occlusive disease in the New England Medical Center Posterior Circulation Registry. Arch Neurol 61, 496–504, 2004.

50. Rabinstein AA, Tisch SH, McClelland RL, et al. Cause is the main predictor of outcome in patients with pontine hemorrhage. Cerebrovasc Dis 17, 66–71, 2004.

51. Report of World Federation of Neurological Surgeons Committee on a Universal Subarachnoid Hemorrhage Grading Scale. J Neurosurg 68, 985–986, 1988.

52. Rosen DS, Macdonald RL. Grading of subarachnoid hemorrhage: modification of the World Federation of Neurosurgical Societies scale on the basis of data for a large series of patients. Neurosurgery 54, 566–575, 2004.

53. Schievink WI, Wijdicks EF, Piepgras DG, et al. The poor prognosis of ruptured intracranial aneurysms of the posterior circulation. J Neurosurg 82, 791–795, 1995.

54. Ritz R, Schwerdtfeger K, Strowitzki M, et al. Prognostic value of SSEP in early aneurysm surgery after SAH in poor-grade patients. Neurol Res 24, 756–764, 2002.

55. Hojer C, Haupt WF. [The prognostic value of AEP and SEP values in subarachnoid hemorrhage. An analysis of 64 patients]. Neurochirurgia (Stuttg) 36, 110–116, 1993.

56. van de Beek BD, De Gans J, Spanjaard L, et al. Clinical features and prognostic factors in adults with bacterial meningitis. N Engl J Med 351, 1849–1859, 2004.

57. Pikis A, Kavaliotis J, Tsikoulas J, et al. Long-term sequelae of pneumococcal meningitis in children. Clin Pediatr (Phila) 35, 72–78, 1996.

58. Roos KL, Tunkel AR, Scheld WM. Acute bacterial meningitis. In: Scheld WM, Whitley RJ, Marra CM, eds. Infections of the Central Nervous System, 3rd ed. Philadelphia: Lippincott Williams & Wilkins, pp 347–422, 2004.

59. Xiao F, Tseng MY, Teng LJ, et al. Brain abscess: clinical experience and analysis of prognostic factors. Surg Neurol 63, 442–449, 2005.

60. Yang SY, Zhao CS. Review of 140 patients with brain abscess. Surg Neurol 39, 290–296, 1993.

61. Wingerchuk DM. The clinical course of acute disseminated encephalomyelitis. Neurol Res 28, 341–347, 2006.

62. Pulver M, Plum F. Disorders of consciousness. In: Evans WR, Baskin DS, Yatsu FM, eds. Prognosis of Neurological Disorders, 2nd ed. New York: Oxford, pp 523–534, 2000.

63. Jennett B, Plum F. Persistent vegetative state after brain damage: a syndrome in search of a name. Lancet 1, 434–437, 1972.

64. Medical aspects of the persistent vegetative state (2). The Multi-Society Task Force on PVS. N Engl J Med 330, 1572–1579, 1994.

65. Medical aspects of the persistent vegetative state (1). The Multi-Society Task Force on PVS. N Engl J Med 330, 1499–1508, 1994.

66. Jennett B. The Vegetative State: Medical Facts, Ethical and Legal Dilemmas. Cambridge: Cambridge University Press, 2002.

67. Childs NL, Mercer WN. Brief report: late improvement in consciousness after post-traumatic vegetative state. N Engl J Med 334, 24–25, 1996.

68. Rosenberg GA, Johnson SF, Brenner RP. Recovery of cognition after prolonged vegetative state. Ann Neurol 2, 167–168, 1977.

69. Matsuda W, Matsumura A, Komatsu Y, et al. Awakenings from persistent vegetative state: report of three cases with parkinsonism and brain stem lesions on MRI. J Neurol Neurosurg Psychiatry 74, 1571–1573, 2003.

70. Whyte J, Katz D, Long D, et al. Predictors of outcome in posttraumatic disorders of consciousness and assessment of medication effects: a multicenter study. Arch Phys Med Rehabil 86, 453–462, 2005.

71. Kampfl A, Schmutzhard E, Franz G, et al. Prediction of recovery from post-traumatic vegetative state with cerebral magnetic-resonance imaging. Lancet 351, 1763–1767, 1998.

72. Laureys S, Lemaire C, Maquet P, et al. Cerebral metabolism during vegetative state and after recovery to consciousness. J Neurol Neurosurg Psychiatry 67, 121–122, 1999.

73. Uzan M, Albayram S, Dashti SG, et al. Thalamic proton magnetic resonance spectroscopy in vegetative state induced by traumatic brain injury. J Neurol Neurosurg Psychiatry 74, 33–38, 2003.

74. Hansotia PL. Persistent vegetative state. Review and report of electrodiagnostic studies in eight cases. Arch Neurol 42, 1048–1052, 1985.

75. Kotchoubey B. Event-related potential measures of consciousness: two equations with three unknowns. Prog Brain Res 150, 427–444, 2005.

76. Giacino JT, Ashwal S, Childs N, et al. The minimally conscious state—definition and diagnostic criteria. Neurology 58, 349–353, 2002.

77. Giacino JT, Kalmar K. Diagnostic and prognostic guidelines for the vegetative and minimally conscious states. Neuropsychol Rehabil 15, 166–174, 2005.

78. Strauss DJ, Ashwal S, Day SM, et al. Life expectancy of children in vegetative and minimally conscious states. Pediatr Neurol 23, 312–319, 2000.

79. Lammi MH, Smith VH, Tate RL, et al. The minimally conscious state and recovery potential: a follow-up study 2 to 5 years after traumatic brain injury. Arch Phys Med Rehabil 86, 746–754, 2005.

80. Cairns H, Oldfield RC, Pennybacker JB, et al. Akinetic mutism with an epidermoid cyst of the 3rd ventricle. Brain 84, 272–290, 1941.

81. Otto A, Zerr I, Lantsch M, et al. Akinetic mutism as a classification criterion for the diagnosis of Creutzfeldt-Jakob disease. J Neurol Neurosurg Psychiatry 64, 524–528, 1998.

82. Nemeth G, Hegedus K, Molnar L. Akinetic mutism associated with bicingular lesions: clinicopathological and functional anatomical correlates. Eur Arch Psychiatry Neurol Sci 237, 218–222, 1988.

83. Castaigne P, Buge A, Cambier J, et al. Thalamic dementia of vascular origin due to bilateral softening limited to the region of the retromamillary peduncle. Apropos of 2 anatomo-clinical cases. Rev Neurol (Paris) 89–107, 1966.

84. Segarra JM. Cerebral vascular disease and behavior. I. The syndrome of the mesencephalic artery (basilar artery bifurcation). Arch Neurol 22, 408–418, 1970.

85. Katz DI, Alexander MP, Mandell AM. Dementia following strokes in the mesencephalon and diencephalon. Arch Neurol 44, 1127–1133, 1987.

86. Fisher CM. Honored guest presentation: abulia minor vs. agitated behavior. Clin Neurosurg 31, 9–31, 1983.

87. Mega MS, Cohenour RC. Akinetic mutism: disconnection of frontal-subcortical circuits. Neuropsychiatry Neuropsychol Behav Neurol 10, 254–259, 1997.

88. Fleet WS, Valenstein E, Watson RT, et al. Dopamine agonist therapy for neglect in humans. Neurology 37, 1765–1770, 1987.

89. Stuss DT, Guberman A, Nelson R, et al. The neuropsychology of paramedian thalamic infarction. Brain Cogn 8, 348–378, 1988.

90. van Domburg PH, Ten Donkelaar HJ, Notermans SL. Akinetic mutism with bithalamic infarction. Neurophysiological correlates. J Neurol Sci 139, 58–65, 1996.

91. Burruss JW, Chacko RC. Episodically remitting akinetic mutism following subarachnoid hemorrhage. J Neuropsychiatry Clin Neurosci 11, 100–102, 1999.

92. Bernat JL. Questions remaining about the minimally conscious state. Neurology 58, 337–338, 2002.

93. Onofrj M, Thomas A, Paci C, et al. Event related potentials recorded in patients with locked-in syndrome. J Neurol Neurosurg Psychiatry 63, 759–764, 1997.

94. Leon-Carrion J, Van Eeckhout P, Dominguez-Morales MDR. Review of subject: the locked-in syndrome: a syndrome looking for a therapy. Brain Inj 16, 555–569, 2002.

95. Doble JE, Haig AJ, Anderson C, et al. Impairment, activity, participation, life satisfaction, and survival in persons with locked-in syndrome for over a decade: follow-up on a previously reported cohort. J Head Trauma Rehabil 18, 435–444, 2003.

96. Bauby J-D. The Diving Bell and the Butterfly. New York: Vintage International, 1997.

97. Ware JE, Snow KK, Kosinski M. SF-36 Health Survey Manual and Interpretation Guide. 1993.

98. Laureys S, Pellas F, Van Eeckhout P, et al. The locked-in syndrome: what is it like to be conscious but paralyzed and voiceless? Prog Brain Res 150, 495–511, 2005.

99. Laureys S, Owen AM, Schiff ND. Brain function in coma, vegetative state, and related disorders. Lancet Neurol 3, 537–546, 2004.

100. Levy DE, Sidtis JJ, Rottenberg DA, et al. Differences in cerebral blood flow and glucose utilization in vegetative versus locked-in patients. Ann Neurol 22, 673–682, 1987.

101. DeVolder AG, Goffinet AM, Bol A, et al. Brain glucose metabolism in postanoxic syndrome. Positron emission tomographic study. Arch Neurol 47, 197–204, 1990.

102. Tommasino C, Grana C, Lucignani G, et al. Regional cerebral metabolism of glucose in comatose and vegetative state patients. J Neurosurg Anesthesiol 7, 109–116, 1995.

103. Rudolf J, Ghaemi M, Ghaemi M, et al. Cerebral glucose metabolism in acute and persistent vegetative state. J Neurosurg Anesthesiol 11, 17–24, 1999.

104. Laureys S, Faymonville ME, Degueldre C, et al. Auditory processing in the vegetative state. Brain 123, 1589–1601, 2000.

105. Schiff ND, Ribary U, Moreno DR, et al. Residual cerebral activity and behavioural fragments can remain in the persistently vegetative brain. Brain 125, 1210–1234, 2002.

106. Blacklock JB, Oldfield EH, Di CG, et al. Effect of barbiturate coma on glucose utilization in normal brain versus gliomas. Positron emission tomography studies. J Neurosurg 67, 71–75, 1987.

107. Alkire MT, Miller J. General anesthesia and the neural correlates of consciousness. Prog Brain Res 150, 229–244, 2005.

108. Maquet P, Degueldre C, Delfiore G, et al. Functional neuroanatomy of human slow wave sleep. J Neurosci 17, 2807–2812, 1997.

109. Laureys S, Faymonville ME, Peigneux P, et al. Cortical processing of noxious somatosensory stimuli in the persistent vegetative state. Neuroimage 17, 732–741, 2002.

110. Plum F, Schiff N, Ribary U, et al. Coordinated expression in chronically unconscious persons. Philos Trans R Soc Lond B Biol Sci 353, 1929–1933, 1998.

111. Schiff ND, Plum F. Cortical function in the persistent vegetative state. Trends Cogn Sci 3, 43–44, 1999.

112. Castaigne P, Lhermitte F, Buge A, et al. Paramedian thalamic and midbrain infarct: clinical and neuropathological study. Ann Neurol 10, 127–148, 1981.

113. Plum, F. Coma and related global disturbances of the human conscious state. In: Jones, E and Peters, P, eds. Cerebral Cortex, Vol. 9, Plenum Press, pp 359–425, 1991.

114. Menon DK, Owen AM, Williams EJ, et al. Cortical processing in persistent vegetative state. Wolfson Brain Imaging Centre Team. Lancet 352, 1148–1149, 1998.

115. Macniven JA, Poz R, Bainbridge K, et al. Emotional adjustment following cognitive recovery from 'persistent vegetative state': psychological and personal perspectives. Brain Inj 17, 525–533, 2003.

116. Menon DK, Owen AM, Pickard JD. Response from Menon, Owen and Pickard. Trends Cogn Sci 3, 44–46, 1999.

117. Schiff N, Ribary U, Plum F, et al. Words without mind. J Cogn Neurosci 11, 650–656, 1999.

118. Zeki S. The visual association cortex. Curr Opin Neurobiol 3, 155–159, 1993.

119. Owen AM, Coleman MR, Menon DK, et al. Residual auditory function in persistent vegetative state: a combined PET and fMRI study. Neuropsychol Rehabil 15, 290–306, 2005.

120. Owen AM, Coleman MR, Boly M, et al. Detecting awareness in the vegetative state. Science 313, 1402, 2006.

121. Schiff ND, Rodriguez-Moreno D, Kamal A, et al. fMRI reveals large-scale network activation in minimally conscious patients. Neurology 64, 514–523, 2005.

122. Boly M, Faymonville ME, Peigneux P, et al. Auditory processing in severely brain injured patients: differences between the minimally conscious state and the persistent vegetative state. Arch Neurol 61, 233–238, 2004.

123. Boly M, Faymonville ME, Peigneux P, et al. Cerebral processing of auditory and noxious stimuli in severely brain injured patients: differences between VS and MCS. Neuropsychol Rehabil 15, 283–289, 2005.

124. Wedekind C, Hesselmann V, Lippert-Gruner M, et al. Trauma to the pontomesencephalic brainstem-a major clue to the prognosis of severe traumatic brain injury. Br J Neurosurg 16, 256–260, 2002.

125. Bekinschtein T, Leiguarda R, Armony J, et al. Emotion processing in the minimally conscious state. J Neurol Neurosurg Psychiatry 75, 788, 2004.

126. Rees G, Kreiman G, Koch C. Neural correlates of consciousness in humans. Nat Rev Neurosci 3, 261–270, 2002.

127. Clauss RP, van der Merwe CE, Nel HW. Arousal from a semi-comatose state on zolpidem. S Afr Med J 91, 788–789, 2001.

128. Jennett B, Adams JH, Murray LS, et al. Neuropathology in vegetative and severely disabled patients after head injury. Neurology 56, 486–490, 2001.

129. Schiff ND, Plum F. The role of arousal and "gating" systems in the neurology of impaired consciousness. J Clin Neurophysiol 17, 438–452, 2000.

130. Plum F. Coma and related global disturbances of human consciousness. In: Jones E, Peters P, eds. Cerebral Cortex, Vol. 9. New York: Plenum Press, 1991.

131. Adams JH, Graham DI, Jennett B. The structural basis of moderate disability after traumatic brain damage. J Neurol Neurosurg Psychiatry 71, 521–524, 2001.

132. Voss HU, Ulug AM, Watts R, Heier LA, McCandliss B, Kobylarz E, Giacino, J, Ballon D, Schiff ND. Possible axonal regrowth in late recovery from minimally conscious state. Journal of Clinical Investigation 116, 2005–2011, 2006.

133. Dancause N, Barbay S, Frost SB, et al. Extensive cortical rewiring after brain injury. J Neurosci 25, 10167–10179, 2005.

134. Chklovskii DB, Mel BW, Svoboda K Cortical rewiring and information storage. Nature 431, 782–788, 2004.

135. Bengtsson SL, Nagy Z, Skare S, et al. Extensive piano practicing has regionally specific effects on white matter development. Nat Neurosci 8, 1148–1150, 2005.

136. Raichle ME, MacLeod AM, Snyder AZ, et al. A default mode of brain function. Proc Natl Acad Sci U S A 98, 676–682, 2001.

137. Gusnard DA, Raichle ME, Raichle ME. Searching for a baseline: functional imaging and the resting human brain. Nat Rev Neurosci 2, 685–694, 2001.

138. Gusnard DA, Akbudak E, Shulman GL, et al. Medial prefrontal cortex and self-referential mental activity: relation to a default mode of brain function. Proc Natl Acad Sci U S A 98, 4259–4264, 2001.

139. Greicius MD, Krasnow B, Reiss AL, et al. Functional connectivity in the resting brain: a network analysis of the default mode hypothesis. Proc Natl Acad Sci U S A 100, 253–258, 2003.

140. Simpson JR Jr, Snyder AZ, Gusnard DA, et al. Emotion-induced changes in human medial prefrontal cortex: I. During cognitive task performance. Proc Natl Acad Sci U S A 99, 683–687, 2001.

141. Laureys S, Faymonville ME, Ferring M, et al. Differences in brain metabolism between patients in coma, vegetative state, minimally conscious state and locked-in syndrome. Eur J Neurol 10, 224–224, 2003.

142. Smith AJ, Blumenfeld H, Behar KL, et al. Cerebral energetics and spiking frequency: the neurophysiological basis of fMRI. Proc Natl Acad Sci U S A 99, 10765–10770, 2002.

143. Logothetis NK, Pauls J, Augath M, et al. Neurophysiological investigation of the basis of the fMRI signal. Nature 412, 150–157, 2001.

144. Schiff ND, Purpura KP. Toward a neurophysiological basis for cognitive neuromodulation. Thalamus Rel Syst 2, 55–69, 2002.

145. Groenewegen HJ, Berendse HW. The specificity of the 'nonspecific' midline and intralaminar thalamic nuclei. Trends Neurosci 17, 52–57, 1994.

146. Van der Werf YD, Witter MP, Groenewegen HJ. The intralaminar and midline nuclei of the thalamus. Anatomical and functional evidence for participation in processes of arousal and awareness. Brain Res Brain Res Rev 39, 107–140, 2002.

147. Nguyen DK, Botez MI. Diaschisis and neurobehavior. Can J Neurol Sci 25, 5–12, 1998.

148. Gold L, Lauritzen M. Neuronal deactivation explains decreased cerebellar blood flow in response to focal cerebral ischemia or suppressed neocortical function. Proc Natl Acad Sci U S A 99, 7699–7704, 2002.

149. Timofeev I, Grenier F, Steriade M. Disfacilitation and active inhibition in the neocortex during the natural sleep-wake cycle: an intracellular study. Proc Natl Acad Sci U S A 98, 1924–1929, 2001.

150. McCormick DA, Shu Y, Hasenstaub A, et al. Persistent cortical activity: mechanisms of generation and effects on neuronal excitability. Cereb Cortex 13, 1219–1231, 2003.

151. Kasanetz F, Riquelme LA, Murer MG. Disruption of the two-state membrane potential of striatal neurones during cortical desynchronisation in anaesthetised rats. J Physiol 543, 577–589, 2002.

152. Robinson PA, Rennie CJ, Rowe DL. Dynamics of large-scale brain activity in normal arousal states and epileptic seizures. Phys Rev E Stat Nonlin Soft Matter Phys 65, 041924, 2002.

153. Santhakumar V, Ratzliff AD, Jeng J, et al. Long-term hyperexcitability in the hippocampus after experimental head trauma. Ann Neurol 50, 708–717, 2001.

154. Topolnik L, Steriade M, Timofeev I. Hyperexcitability of intact neurons underlies acute development of trauma-related electrographic seizures in cats in vivo. Eur J Neurosci 18, 486–496, 2003.

155. Williams D, Parsons-Smith G. Thalamic activity in stupor. Brain 74, 377–398, 1951.

156. Cohen L, Chaaban B, Habert MO. Transient improvement of aphasia with zolpidem. N Engl J Med 350, 949–950, 2004.

157. Szelies B, Herholz K, Pawlik G, et al. Widespread functional effects of discrete thalamic infarction. Arch Neurol 48, 178–182, 1991.

158. Caselli RJ, Graff-Radford NR, Rezai K. Thalamocortical diaschisis: single-photon emission tomographic study of cortical blood flow change after focal thalamic infarction. Neuropsychiatry Neuropsychol Behav Neurol 4, 193–214, 1991.

159. Ingvar DH. Reproduction of the 3 per second spike and wave EEG pattern by subcortical electrical stimulation in cats. Acta Physiol Scand 33, 137–150, 1955.

160. Kakigi R, Shibasaki H, Katafuchi Y, et al. The syndrome of bilateral paramedian thalamic infarction associated with an oculogyric crisis. Rinsho Shinkeigaku 26, 1100–1105, 1986.

161. Wilcox JA, Nasrallah HA. Organic factors in catatonia. Br J Psychiatry 149, 782–784, 1986.

162. Kamal AR, Schiff ND. Does the form of akinetic mutism linked to mesodiencephalic injuries bridge the double dissociation of Parkinson's disease and catatonia? Behav Brain Sci 25, 586–587, 2002.

163. Berthier ML, Kulisevsky JJ, Gironell A, et al. Obsessive compulsive disorder and traumatic brain injury: behavioral, cognitive, and neuroimaging findings. Neuropsychiatry Neuropsychol Behav Neurol 14, 23–31, 2001.

164. Sachs GA, Siegler M. Guidelines for decision making when the patient is incompetent. J Crit Illness 6, 348–359, 1991.

165. Terry PB, Vettese M, Song J, et al. End-of-life decision making: when patients and surrogates disagree. J Clin Ethics 10, 286–293, 1999.

166. Brock, DW. Patient Self-Determination Act. Trumping advance directives. Hastings Center Report 21, S5-S6, 1991.

167. Annas GJ. "Culture of life" politics at the bedside— the case of Terri Schiavo. N Engl J Med 352, 1710– 1715, 2005.

168. Hayward RS, Steinberg EP, Ford DE, et al. Preventive care guidelines: 1991. Ann Intern Med 114, 758– 783, 1991.

169. Wolf S, Barondess JA, Boyle P, et al. Special Report: Sources of concern about the Patient Self-Determination Act. N Engl J Med 325, 1661–1671, 1991.

170. Fins JJ, Maltby BS, Friedman E, et al. Contracts, covenants and advance care planning: an empirical study of the moral obligations of patient and proxy. J Pain Symptom Manage 29, 55–86, 2005.

171. Fins JJ, Miller FG, Acres CA, et al. End-of-life decision-making in the hospital: current practices and future prospects. J Pain Symptom Manage 17, 6–15, 1999.

172. Bedell SE, Delbanco TL. Choices about the cardiopulmonary resuscitation in the hospital. When do physicians talk with patient? N Engl J Med 310, 1089–1093, 1984.

173. Fins JJ. Constructing an ethical stereotaxy for severe brain injury: balancing risks, benefits and access. Nature Rev Neurosci 4, 323–327, 2003.

174. Annas GJ. The "right to die" in America: Sloganeering from Quinlan and Cruzan to Quill and Kevorkian. Duquesne Law Review 34, 875–897, 1996.

175. Cantor NL. Twenty-five years after Quinlan: a review of the jurisprudence of death and dying. J Law Med Ethics 29, 182–196, 2001.

176. Cranford RE. Medical futility: transforming a clinical concept into legal and social policies. J Am Geriatr Soc 42, 894–898, 1994.

177. Fins JJ. Clinical pragmatism and the care of brain damaged patients: toward a palliative neuroethics for disorders of consciousness. Prog Brain Res 150, 565– 582, 2005.

178. Siminoff LA, Mercer MB, Arnold R. Families' understanding of brain death. Prog Transplant 13, 218– 24, 2003.

179. Kimura R. Japan's dilemma with the definition of death. Kennedy Inst Ethics J 1, 123–131, 1991.

180. Gutierrez E. Japan's House of Representatives passes brain-death bill. Lancet 349, 1304, 1997.

181. Fins JJ. Across the divide: religious objections to brain death. J Religion Health 34, 33–39, 1995.

182. Jennett B, Plum F. Persistent vegetative state after brain damage. A syndrome in search of a name. Lancet 1, 734–737, 1972.

183. Kobylarz E, Schiff ND. Functional Imaging of severely brain-injured patients—progress, challenges, and limitations. Arch Neurol 61, 1357–1360, 2004.

184. Giacino J, Whyte J. The vegetative and minimally conscious states: current knowledge and remaining questions. J Head Trauma Rehabil 20, 30–50, 2005.

185. Fins JJ. A Palliative Ethic of Care: Clinical Wisdom at Life's End. Sudbury, Mass.: Jones and Bartlett, 2006.

186. Fins JJ. Rethinking disorders of consciousness: new research and its implications. The Hastings Cancer Rep 35, 22–24, 2005.

187. Fins JJ. Affirming the right to care, preserving the right to die: disorders of consciousness and neuroethics after Schiavo. Palliat Support Care 4, 169–178, 2006.

187a. Winslade, W. Confronting Traumatic Brain Injury. New Haven, Conn.: Yale University Press, 1998.

188. Sherer M, Hart T, Nick TG, et al. Early impaired self-awareness after traumatic brain injury. Arch Phys Med Rehabil 84, 168–176, 2003.

189. Farah MJ, Wolpe PR. Monitoring and manipulating brain function, new neuroscience technologies and their ethical implications. Hastings Center Report 34, 35–45, 2004.

190. Fins JJ. The Orwellian threat to emerging neurodiagnostic technologies. Am J Bioethics 5, 56–58, 2005.

191. Levine C. The loneliness of the long-term care giver. N Engl J Med 340, 1587–1590, 1999.

192. Kennedy PR, Bakay RAE. Restoration of neural output from a paralyzed patient by a direct brain connection. Neuro Report 9, 1707–1711, 1998.

193. Schiff ND. The neurology of impaired consciousness: challenges for cognitive neuroscience. In: Gazzaniga MS ed. The Cognitive Neurosciences, 3rd ed. Boston: MIT, 2004.

194. Joliot M, Ribary U, Llinas R. Human oscillatory brain activity near 40 Hz coexists with cognitive temporal binding. Proc Natl Acad Sci USA 91, 11748–11751, 1994.

Index

Page numbers followed by "t" denote tables; those followed by "b" denote boxes; and those followed by "f" denote figures

Visual obscurations, 93
Vomiting, 53–54
von Economo von San Serff, Baron Constantin,
    10b–11b, 12

Wada test, 27, 152
Wake-sleep states, 16b–17b
Wallenberg's lateral medullary
    infarction, 59
Warfarin, 123
Water intoxication, 228–229, 253–254

Wernicke-Korsakoff syndrome, 186
Wernicke's aphasia, 27
Wernicke's encephalopathy
    causes of, 223
    description of, 11
    thiamine prophylaxis, 77, 223, 313
Whipple's disease, 265–266

Xanthochromia, 82

Yawning, 53